PRACTICAL PERIPHERAL VASCULAR INTERVENTION

SECOND EDITION

PRACTICAL PERIPHERAL VASCULAR INTERVENTION

SECOND EDITION

EDITORS

IVAN P. CASSERLY, MB, BCh, FACC
Assistant Professor
Department of Cardiology
University of Colorado Hospital
Denver, Colorado

RAVISH SACHAR, MD, FACC
Interventional Cardiology
Director, Wake Heart Cerebrovascular and Peripheral Research
Wake Heart and Vascular Associates
Raleigh, North Carolina

JAY S. YADAV, MD, FACC
Chairman, Center for Medical Innovation
Piedmont Heart Institute
Atlanta, Georgia

Wolters Kluwer | Lippincott Williams & Wilkins
Health
Philadelphia • Baltimore • New York • London
Buenos Aires • Hong Kong • Sydney • Tokyo

Acquisitions Editor: Frances DeStefano
Product Manager: Leanne McMillan
Production Manager: Bridgett Dougherty
Senior Manufacturing Manager: Benjamin Rivera
Marketing Manager: Kimberly Schonberger
Design Coordinator: Teresa Mallon
Production Service: MPS Limited, a Macmillan Company

© 2011 by LIPPINCOTT WILLIAMS & WILKINS, a WOLTERS KLUWER business

Two Commerce Square
2001 Market Street
Philadelphia, PA 19103 USA
LWW.com

Printed in China

Library of Congress Cataloging-in-Publication Data
Practical peripheral vascular intervention / editors, Ivan P. Casserly, Ravish Sachar, Jay S. Yadav. — 2nd ed.
     p. ; cm.
  Rev. ed. of: Manual of peripheral vascular intervention / editors, Ivan P. Casserly, Ravish Sachar,
  Jay S. Yadav. c2005.
  Includes bibliographical references.
  ISBN-13: 978-0-7817-9914-0
  ISBN-10: 0-7817-9914-7
  1. Peripheral vascular diseases—Surgery—Handbooks, manuals, etc. I. Casserly, Ivan P.
  II. Sachar, Ravish. III. Yadav, Jay S. IV. Manual of peripheral vascular intervention.
  [DNLM: 1. Peripheral Vascular Diseases—surgery. 2. Vascular Surgical Procedures. WG 500]
  RC694.M365 2011
  616.1'31059—dc22

                                                                              2010037276

                              10 9 8 7 6 5 4 3 2 1

CONTENTS

CONTRIBUTORS

Ahmed Abdel-Latif, MD, MSPH
Interventional Fellow
Division of Cardiovascular Medicine
Gill Heart Institute
University of Kentucky
Lexington, Kentucky

Alex Abou-Chebl, MD
Associate Professor of Neurology and
    Neurosurgery
Director of Neurointerventional Services
Director of Vascular and Interventional
    Neurology Fellowships
Department of Neurology
University of Louisville School of Medicine
Louisville, Kentucky

Gary M. Ansel, MD
Clinical Director of Peripheral Vascular
    Intervention
Mid-Ohio Cardiology and Vascular
    Consultants
Columbus, Ohio

Subhash Banerjee, MD
Chief of the Division of Cardiology and
    Codirector, Cardiac Catheterization
Laboratory at VA North Texas Healthcare
    System
Assistant Professor of Medicine
University of Texas
Southwestern Medical Center
Dallas, Texas

Pareena Bilkoo, MD

Robert Francis Bonvini, MD
Interventional Cardiologist and Angiologist
Cardiology Division
University Hospital of Geneva
Geneva, Switzerland

Ivan P. Casserly, MB, BCh, FACC
Assistant Professor
Department of Cardiology
University of Colorado Hospital
Denver, Colorado

Leslie Cho, MD
Director, Women's Cardiovascular Center
Cleveland Clinic
Cleveland, Ohio

Jayer Chung, MD
Vascular Surgery Fellow
Division of Vascular Surgery and
    Endovascular Therapy
Department of Surgery
Emory University School of Medicine
Atlanta, Georgia

Christopher J. Cooper, MD
Professor of Medicine
Chief, Cardiovascular Division
University of Toledo
Toledo, Ohio

Tony S. Das, MD
Director
Peripheral Vascular Interventions
Presbyterian Heart Institute
Dallas, Texas

**Kent Dauterman, MD, FACC,
FSCAI**
Southern Oregon Cardiology
Medford, Oregon

Fadi El-Merhi, MD
Assistant Professor
Department of Diagnostic Radiology
American University of Beirut Medical Center
Beirut, Lebanon

Brian Funaki, MD
Professor of Radiology
Section Chief, Vascular and Interventional
    Radiology
University of Chicago Medical Center
Chicago, Illinois

Jeffrey Goldstein, MD
Interventional Cardiology
Peripheral Vascular Interventions
    and Disease
Prairie Cardiovascular Consultants
Springfield, Illinois

William A. Gray, MD
Director of Endovascular Services
Center for Interventional Vascular Therapy
New York-Presbyterian Hospital / Columbia
    University Medical Center
Associate Professor of Clinical Medicine
Columbia University College of Physicians
    and Surgeons New York, New York

Rajan K. Gupta, MD
University of Colorado Denver Health
    Sciences Center
Denver, Colorado

Hitinder S. Gurm, MD
Assistant Professor
Department of Cardiovascular
    Medicine
University of Michigan
Ann Arbor, Michigan

Brian G. Hynes
Interventional Cardiology Fellow
Massachusetts General Hospital
Boston, Massachusetts

Yuji Kanaoka, MD, PhD
Assistant Professor
Department of Surgery, Division of Vascular
    Surgery
Jikei University School of Medicine
Tokyo, Japan

Kenjiro Kaneko, MD
Assistant Professor
Department of Surgery, Division of Vascular
    Surgery
Jikei University School of Medicine
Tokyo, Japan

Samir R. Kapadia, MD
Director of the Sones Cardiac Catheterization
    Laboratories
Director of the Interventional Cardiology
    Fellowship Program
Robert and Suzanne Tomsich Department of
    Cardiovascular Medicine
Cleveland Clinic
Cleveland, Ohio

Karthikeshwar Kasirajan, MD, FACS
Assistant Professor of Surgery
Department of Surgery
Emory University
Faculty
Department of Surgery
Emory University Hospital
Emory University School of Medicine
Atlanta, Georgia

Ross Kessler, MD
University of Chicago
Chicago, Illinois

Melina R. Kibbe, MD
Division of Vascular Surgery
Northwestern University
Chicago, Illinois

Andrew J. Klein, MD
Staff, Interventional Cardiology
John Cochran VAMC
Assistant Professor of Medicine
St. Louis University School of Medicine
St. Louis, Missouri

Raghu Kolluri, MD, FACC, FACP
Clinical Assistant Professor
Department of Cardiovascular Medicine
Southern Illinois School of Medicine
Director, Noninvasive Vascular Laboratory
Prairie Vascular Institute
Springfield, Illinois

Ronan J. Margey, MB, MRCPI
Interventional Cardiology Fellow
Massachusetts General Hospital
Boston, Massachusetts

Ross Milner, MD
Division of Vascular Surgery and
    Endovascular Therapy
Loyola University Medical Center
Stritch School of Medicine
Maywood, Illinois

Debabrata Mukherjee, MD, FACC
Chief, Cardiovascular Medicine
Professor of Internal Medicine
Vice Chairman, Department of Internal
    Medicine
Texas Tech University
El Paso, Texas

Takao Ohki, MD, PhD
Professor
Department of Surgery, Division of
    Vascular Surgery
Jikei University School of Medicine
Tokyo, Japan

Kenneth Ouriel, MD
New York-Presbyterian Hospital
New York, New York

Joel P. Reginelli, MD
Ohio Heart and Vascular Center
Cincinnati, Ohio

Jayme Rock-Willoughby, DO
Columbus, Ohio

Marco Roffi, MD
Director, Interventional Cardiology Unit
Cardiology Division
University Hospital of Geneva
Geneva, Switzerland

Kenneth Rosenfield, MD
Director, Cardiac and Vascular Invasive
    Service
Massachusetts General Hospital
Boston, Massachusetts

Audrey Rosinberg, MD
Vascular Surgeon
Lennox Hill Heart and Vascular Institute,
New York, New York

Ravish Sachar, MD, FACC
Interventional Cardiology
Director, Wake Heart Cerebrovascular and
    Peripheral Research
Wake Heart and Vascular Associates
Raleigh, North Carolina

Jacqueline Saw, MD, FRCPC
Vancouver General Hospital
Interventional Cardiology
Clinical Assistant Professor
University of British Columbia
Vancouver, British Columbia, Canada

Mobeen A. Sheikh, MD
Clinical Instructor
Harvard Medical School
Boston, Massachusetts
Department of Cardiovascular Medicine
The Medical Group
Beverly, Massachusetts

Mehdi H. Shishehbor, DO, MPH
Staff, Interventional Cardiology &
    Vascular Medicine
Associate Program Director, Interventional
    Cardiology
Heart & Vascular Institute
Cleveland Clinic
Cleveland, Ohio

Mitchell J. Silver, DO, FACC, FABVM
MidOhio Cardiology and Vascular
    Consultants, Inc.
Columbus, Ohio

James P. Sur, MD
Provena St. Joseph Medical
Crest Hill, Illinois

Vincent V. Truong, MD
Clinical Instructor of Stroke Services
Neurointerventional Fellow
University of Louisville School of Medicine
Louisville, Kentucky

Christopher J. White, MD, FACC
Chairman
Department of Cardiology
Director
Ochsner Heart & Vascular Institute
New Orleans, Louisiana

Mark H. Wholey, MD, MBA
Pittsburgh Vascular Institute
University of Pittsburgh Medical Center
    Shadyside
Pittsburgh, Pennsylvania

Michael Wholey, MD, MBA
Central Cardiovascular Institute of San
    Antonio
San Antonio, Texas

William C.S. Wu, MD

Jay S. Yadav, MD, FACC
Chairman, Center for Medical Innovation
Piedmont Heart Institute
Atlanta, Georgia

Khaled M. Ziada, MD
Assistant Professor
Division of Cardiovascular Medicine
University of Kentucky
Lexington, Kentucky

PREFACE

Over the past decade, the application of endovascular techniques to treat patients with peripheral artery disease, aneurysmal disease, and venous disorders has grown dramatically. Improvements in catheter, sheath, wire, balloon, and stent design, as well as the advent of distal emboli protection and other novel technologies, have collectively enabled the safe, efficacious, and durable treatment of obstructive and aneurysmal arterial disease and an array of venous disorders. These advances reflect the collective efforts of specialists from the fields of interventional cardiology, vascular surgery, and interventional radiology.

One of the major challenges in the field is the insufficient numbers of accredited fellowship positions dedicated solely to percutaneous peripheral vascular intervention. As a result, operators often finish fellowships with minimal specific training in peripheral vascular disease, and have to continue the learning process "on the job." Furthermore, for those who are already in practice, retraining in peripheral vascular intervention is often a difficult and haphazard process, consisting of didactic and "hands-on" training through short courses offered in various institutions. For those who are already trained, this rapidly evolving field mandates that physicians constantly keep abreast of newer developments.

This book seeks to address some of the above challenges. First and foremost, this is a *manual* of peripheral vascular intervention, with a firm emphasis on *how to perform* peripheral vascular interventions. For this reason, we purposefully invited authors with the greatest hands-on experience to write the chapters and provide their insights. Every effort has been made to graphically illustrate the techniques and provide real-life examples of these procedures. There is also an obligation for operators to have a sound understanding of the clinical and non-invasive evaluation of patients with peripheral vascular disease, and a working knowledge of the anatomy and biology of the vascular bed in which they intend to intervene. We have therefore provided this information in as succinct a manner as possible, for each vascular bed.

We have tried to address intervention in all of the vascular territories. Carotid angioplasty and stenting has become an alternative to surgery for patients with symptomatic and asymptomatic carotid disease. As such, we hope that the chapters on carotid intervention are especially useful. Other chapters, such as those on subclavian, aortoiliac, and infrapopliteal interventions, offer insights we hope will help even experienced operators. The section on the treatment of aneurysmal disease has been significantly expanded, as has the section on the treatment of venous disorders.

Peripheral vascular intervention is an exciting and challenging field. While this book is not meant to serve as a replacement for essential didactic and hands-on training, our hope is that both trainees and experienced operators in each of the disciplines involved in performing peripheral vascular intervention will find this a useful and practical guide.

Ivan P. Casserly, MD
Ravish Sachar, MD
Jay S. Yadav, MD

ACKNOWLEDGMENTS

First, we would like to thank all of the contributing authors who took time from their busy clinical schedules and families to write their respective chapters. We understand that this represents a significant sacrifice, but hope it was also a rewarding experience. We would like to thank the many people at Wolters Kluwer who have helped bring the Second Edition to fruition. A special thanks to Fran DeStefano for her support and to Leanne McMillan for serving as product manager and being instrumental in ensuring the successful completion of this project. Most importantly we wish to thank the many patients and families who have trusted us in their moments of greatest need. It is our hope that sharing our experience in the treatment of complex vascular disease will benefit patients around the world.

Ivan P. Casserly
Ravish Sachar
Jay S. Yadav

Training and Credentialing

CHAPTER 1

Guidelines for Training and Credentialing in Peripheral Vascular Intervention

Christopher J. White

There are compelling reasons for interventional cardiologists to undertake percutaneous treatment of head to toe noncoronary atherosclerotic vascular diseases (1). Atherosclerosis is a "systemic" disease that often involves multiple vascular beds commonly causing coronary and noncoronary vascular problems in the same patient (2–4). There is general agreement that there is a shortage of trained health-care providers necessary to meet the rapidly increasing demand for percutaneous revascularization, particularly with regard to acute stroke and intracranial intervention. Interventional cardiologists possess the technical skills necessary to perform noncoronary vascular intervention but, in general, lack a comprehensive knowledge base regarding the specialty of vascular medicine. In recognition of the need for adult cardiovascular medicine trainees to gain broader expertise in vascular medicine and vascular intervention, a Core Cardiology Training Symposium (COCATS-11) has been developed (5,6).

Noncoronary vascular disease involving the extremities, visceral and renal organs, and brain is frequently an important aspect of the management of patients with heart disease. Renovascular hypertension is the most common cause of secondary hypertension in patients with atherosclerosis. Renovascular hypertension, causing resistant hypertension, negatively impacts the medical management of angina pectoris and congestive heart failure. Peripheral vascular symptoms, such as claudication, impair the effectiveness of cardiovascular rehabilitation programs. Coronary artery atherosclerosis is the most common cause of morbidity and mortality in patients with atherosclerotic peripheral vascular disease.

FEASIBILITY OF CARDIOLOGISTS PERFORMING NONCORONARY VASCULAR INTERVENTION

As experienced coronary interventionalists, we reported our initial experience in peripheral angioplasty in 164 consecutive patients over a 20-month period (7). Prior to performing angioplasty, we observed the performance of peripheral angioplasty in several angiographic laboratories performing high-volume peripheral angioplasty, we were proctored for our initial cases by a qualified outside operator, and our initial cases were reviewed and discussed with an experienced vascular surgeon.

Lower extremity percutaneous transluminal angioplasty (PTA) was performed in 116 patients, upper extremity PTA in 30 patients, and renal artery PTA in 18 patients. Successful results were obtained in 92% (191/208) of the lesions attempted, with a successful PTA in 99% (155/157) of stenoses versus 71% (36/51) of occlusions ($p < 0.01$). In no patient did a failed attempt result

in worsening of the patient's clinical condition or the need for emergency surgery. The overall major complication rate of 4.3% (7/164) was similar to other studies published in the literature.

Our experience supported the hypothesis that experienced interventional cardiologists, working in partnership with vascular surgeons, possessed the necessary technical skills to perform peripheral vascular angioplasty in a safe and effective manner. We relied on our vascular surgery colleagues to provide guidance in patient and lesion selection, which compensated for our limited knowledge regarding vascular medicine. Our results did not demonstrate a learning curve. The percentage of patients with totally occluded vessels (25%) and the average lesion length (5.8 ± 8.0 cm) attests to the relatively difficult lesions we routinely accepted for treatment.

Achieving a success rate of 92% for all lesions and a 99% success rate for stenoses suggested that coronary angioplasty skills are transferable to the treatment of noncoronary vascular lesions quite effectively. The fact that success rates were higher for non–total occlusions and lesions of shorter length were consistent with the reported outcomes for vascular intervention in the literature.

Because the risks of diagnostic aortic arch and cerebral angiography add to the risks of revascularization of the carotid artery, the most highly skilled angiographer, regardless of primary specialty, should perform these studies. We investigated the quality and risk of diagnostic cervical–cerebral angiography in the hands of experienced interventional cardiologists (8). We reviewed a total of 189 patients with 191 diagnostic catheter procedures over a 5-year period. There was only one neurologic complication (0.52%), which compares favorably to published results. There is good evidence that the catheter skills of experienced cardiologists compare well with those of other specialists for the safety and quality of noncoronary angiography.

FELLOWSHIP TRAINING IN NONCORONARY DIAGNOSTIC ANGIOGRAPHY

Cardiology fellows currently receive invasive training in both cardiac and noncardiac angiography (9). An example of this type of experience includes ascending, descending, and abdominal aortography. Additionally, angiographic studies may include selective angiography of the aortic arch vessels, mesenteric vessels, renal arteries, and iliofemoral arteries. Another example is the routine performance of selective angiography of the subclavian, internal mammary, and gastroepiploic arteries to determine patency of coronary bypass grafts. Screening renal angiography is frequently done in patients at increased risk for renal artery stenosis with clinical indications for revascularization (10). Finally, routine imaging of the iliac and femoral arteries is commonly performed if there is difficulty advancing catheters or prior to placement of vascular closure devices.

Cardiologists performing noncardiac angiography are responsible for the accurate interpretation of the images they obtain. Physicians must accept the liability for errors or omissions in their interpretation of angiography studies, just as they do for coronary angiography. Physicians who feel insecure in their ability to interpret these films may ask for assistance or overreading of the films by a qualified physician. Peer review of angiographic studies, in a nonthreatening environment, leads to improved quality of peripheral angiographic studies and provides opportunities for less experienced angiographers to enhance their understanding of peripheral vascular anatomy, collateral circulations, and anatomic variations.

FELLOWSHIP TRAINING REQUIREMENTS FOR NONCORONARY VASCULAR INTERVENTION

The American College of Cardiology (ACC)'s COCATS document provides guidelines for training in catheter-based peripheral vascular interventions (5,6). For the cardiovascular trainee wishing to acquire competence as a peripheral vascular interventionalist, a minimum of 12 months of training is recommended (Table 1.1). This period is in addition to the required core cardiology training and a minimum of 8 months in diagnostic cardiac catheterization in an Accreditation Council for Graduate Medical Education (ACGME)–accredited fellowship program (9). The prerequisite for Level 3 training in peripheral vascular interventions includes Level 1 training in vascular medicine, and Level 1 and Level 2 training in diagnostic cardiac catheterization. Requirements for Level 3 training in peripheral vascular interventions can be fulfilled during fourth year of interventional training dedicated to peripheral

---

TABLE 1.1 Recommended Fellowship Training Requirements for Cardiovascular Physicians

- Duration of training*—12 months
- Diagnostic coronary angiograms†—300 cases (200 as the primary operator)
- Diagnostic peripheral angiograms—100 cases (50 as primary operator)
- Peripheral interventional cases‡—50 cases (25 as primary operator)

*After completing core cardiovascular training with at least 8 months of cardiac catheterization.
†Coronary catheterization procedures should be completed before beginning interventional training.
‡The case mix should be evenly distributed among the different vascular beds. Supervised cases of thrombus management for limb ischemia and venous thrombosis, utilizing percutaneous thrombolysis or thrombectomy, should be included.

---

vascular interventions or concurrently with coronary interventional training (6).

It is recommended that a cardiology fellow perform 300 coronary diagnostic procedures, including 200 with supervised primary responsibility before beginning interventional training (9). The trainee in an ACGME-accredited program should participate in a minimum of 100 diagnostic peripheral angiograms and 50 noncoronary vascular interventional cases during the interventional training period (11). The case mix should be evenly distributed among the different vascular beds. Cases of thrombus management for limb ischemia and/or venous thrombosis, utilizing percutaneous thrombolysis or catheter-based thrombectomy, should be included.

Advanced training in peripheral vascular intervention may be undertaken concurrently with fourth year of training for coronary interventions (6). Peripheral vascular interventional training should include experience on an inpatient vascular medicine consultation service, in a noninvasive vascular diagnostic laboratory, and experience in longitudinal care of outpatients with vascular disease. Comprehensive training in vascular medicine (Level 2) is not a prerequisite for noncoronary interventional training.

ALTERNATIVE TRAINING PATHWAYS FOR PVD INTERVENTION

Many physicians with specialty training and board certification in interventional cardiology are currently performing peripheral vascular (noncoronary) interventional procedures. These physicians have received either formal training in accredited programs or on-the-job training. Unfortunately, there currently exists little or no cooperation between the specialty training programs with regard to peripheral vascular interventional training.

An ongoing "turf-war" over the provision of these services between competing subspecialties in many hospitals is not in the best interest of patients. Several professional societies including the ACC, the American Heart Association, the American Society of Cardiovascular Interventionists, the Society of Cardiovascular Interventional Radiologists, the Society of Vascular Surgery, and the Society for Cardiovascular Angiography and Interventions (SCAI) have published disparate guidelines for the performance of peripheral angioplasty (12–17).

The realization that there is a need for cardiologists to provide noncoronary vascular care to patients with concomitant peripheral vascular disease has prompted revision of prior guidelines that were not "cardiology" specific (11,18). This was done in order to provide a more focused view of the role of the cardiologist, specifically the interventional cardiologist, in the management of these patients. Cardiologists with widely varying backgrounds and clinical experience are currently performing peripheral vascular intervention. Competency to perform peripheral vascular percutaneous interventions can be broken down into three categories or skill sets (Table 1.2).

Unrestricted Certification

Completion of at least 100 diagnostic peripheral angiograms, with a minimum of 50 peripheral interventional procedures, has been recommended for unrestricted certification

TABLE 1.2   Skills for Optimal Endovascular Intervention

- **Cognitive:** The fund of knowledge required is derived from the specialties of vascular medicine and angiology. It includes the knowledge of the natural history of the disease, the anatomy and physiology of the affected organ systems, interpretation of noninvasive tests, and an understanding of the indications for treatment and expected outcomes (risks and benefits) of the treatment options.

- **Procedural:** These skills involve the full range of invasive percutaneous cardiovascular techniques including gaining vascular access, performing diagnostic angiography, performing angioplasty and intervention, administering thrombolytic agents, and recognizing and managing complications of these procedures.

- **Clinical:** This category encompasses the skills necessary to manage inpatients and outpatients with noncardiac vascular diseases. It includes the ability to admit patients to the hospital and provide daily care. The ability to perform a complete history and physical examination, and to integrate the patient's history, physical examination, and noninvasive laboratory data to make accurate diagnoses is required. Finally, it requires establishing a doctor–patient relationship and continuity of care in order to provide long-term care for this chronic disease.

TABLE 1.3   Suggested Alternative Pathways for Achieving Competency in Peripheral Vascular Intervention

Unrestricted Certification

- Diagnostic angiograms—100 cases (50 as primary operator)
- Peripheral interventions—50 cases (25 as primary operator)
  - Aortoiliac, brachiocephalic arteries, and extracranial carotid arteries
  - Abdominal and visceral (renal and mesenteric) arteries
  - Infrainguinal arteries
  - Thrombolysis/thrombectomy

Restricted Certification

- Diagnostic angiograms—30 cases per specific vascular territory (15 as primary operator)
- Peripheral interventions
  - Aortoiliac and brachiocephalic—15 cases (8 as primary operator)
  - Abdominal and visceral (mesenteric and renal)—15 cases (8 as primary operator)
  - Infrainguinal—15 cases (8 as primary operator)

(Table 1.3) (11). The physician should have been the supervised primary operator for one half of the procedures. These procedures should be performed under the guidance of a credentialed noncoronary vascular interventionalist.

The case mix should be evenly distributed, so as to ensure exposure to diagnosis and intervention in a variety of different vascular beds. Experience that is heavily weighted toward treatment of one specific site (e.g., renal) to the exclusion of other vascular distributions (e.g., infrainguinal) may not provide adequate expertise or preparation for the latter. To achieve the balanced experience required for unrestricted competence, the following three broadly defined vascular territories should be evenly represented: (1) aortoiliac and brachiocephalic arteries (i.e., subclavian and axillary); (2) abdominal visceral arteries (i.e., renal and mesenteric arteries); and (3) infrainguinal arteries (i.e., femoral, popliteal, tibial, and peroneal arteries). In addition, unrestricted competence requires separate supervised cases of thrombus management for limb ischemia or venous thrombosis, utilizing catheter-based thrombolysis or thrombectomy, in a nonspecified vascular bed. Familiarity with thrombolytic agents and their use is also required. Facility with other devices and technologies (e.g., mechanical thrombectomy) available for thrombus management is also desirable (11).

Obtaining competence in the performance of procedures and interventions in the cervical (i.e., subclavian, carotid, and vertebral arteries) and intracranial cerebral vessels poses unique challenges associated with gaining vascular access to the carotid and vertebral arteries and performing interventions in these circulatory beds. There are special concerns related to the morbidity and mortality associated with this vascular territory, which allows for very narrow safety margins. For physicians performing neurovascular interventional procedures, suggested requirements for achievement of competence include mastery of the cognitive and clinical skills pertaining specifically to this vascular bed and these procedures. This includes, as with other sites, an understanding of the anatomic and pathologic characteristics unique to this vascular bed and the ability to interpret relevant angiographic images. To achieve competence, additional diagnostic cerebrovascular angiograms and interventions should be performed, with appropriate documentation, follow-up, and outcomes assessment. As with procedures in other regional vascular venues, it is anticipated that for some physicians to achieve competence, supervising faculty will recommend additional cases beyond the minimum number.

Restricted Certification

Achievement of competence to perform peripheral vascular intervention need not be an all-or-none phenomenon. Rather, levels of competence in specific procedures or regional vascular territories can be achieved, particularly for those established physicians who have already completed formal training in coronary intervention or vascular surgery. A physician might become competent to perform interventions only in some regional circulations, but not in others. This is termed restricted certification. For example, one might acquire the skills to perform percutaneous renal, iliac, and subclavian intervention, yet not have adequate background or expertise to perform infrapopliteal or carotid intervention. Competence in one area may be partly or wholly transferable to another, depending upon the degree of overlap or similarity between the vascular bed, the disease state, and the knowledge and skill sets involved. For example, the technical skills required to perform iliac artery intervention are partly transferable to subclavian artery intervention, since the size of these vessels is comparable, and the therapeutic procedures are similar. In contrast, expertise in iliac artery revascularization does not confer comparable ability to perform carotid stenting, tibioperoneal angioplasty, or catheter-based thrombolysis because of the dissimilarity of these interventions and their associated vascular territories.

Restricted certification can be achieved for each of the three major vascular territories defined previously (aortoiliac and brachiocephalic vessels, abdominal visceral arteries, and infrainguinal arteries), in which competence is sought and supervised performance of a minimum of diagnostic angiograms and interventions is required (Table 1.3). One half of the diagnostic angiograms and one half of the interventions in the specific territory must have been performed as the supervised primary operator. The cognitive and clinical skills pertaining

to the particular territory should also have been mastered. Utilizing a restricted certification approach, a practicing physician possessing the requisite catheter skills can initially achieve competence in one or more selected territories and, subsequently, can elect to progress in a stepwise fashion to gain unrestricted certification.

BOARD CERTIFICATION FOR ENDOVASCULAR THERAPY

The American Board of Vascular Medicine (ABVM) was formed with sponsorship from the ACC, the Society of Vascular Medicine (SVM), and the SCAI and held its first certifying examination for cardiovascular specialists in both vascular medicine and endovascular medicine in 2005 (19). The eligibility criteria for sitting for the endovascular examination are listed in Table 1.4. ABVM certification is intended to demonstrate that a candidate has the knowledge, skills, and commitment to provide quality patient care in vascular medicine. Formal board certification is intended to establish a consistent benchmark of expertise in the field of vascular medicine.

TABLE 1.4 ABVM Endovascular Examination: Eligibility Requirements

A. Must possess a valid, unrestricted license to practice medicine in the jurisdiction of practice.

B. Hold primary board certification (ABIM, ABOIM, ABS, ABR) or specialty board certification in Cardiology, Cardiothoracic Surgery, Interventional Radiology, Vascular Surgery, or Vascular Medicine (ABVM General Examination).

C. Meet the training requirements for peripheral intervention through either the practice pathway or fellowship training pathway as outlined below.

D. Attestation of privileges or fellowship training statement as outlined below.

E. Pay the required examination (ABVM Endovascular Examination) fee.

Certification Process to Attain Status as Diplomate of ABVM

A. Meet all of the eligibility requirements.

B. Pass the computer-based endovascular examination.

Training Requirements

A. Practice Pathway
   1. Active hospital privileges for diagnostic and interventional peripheral procedures.
   2. Performance of peripheral interventional procedures for at least 12 months before application.
   3. Performance of at least 100 diagnostic peripheral arteriograms with at least 50 as the primary operator at the attending physician level (cases performed as a trainee are not counted toward this total) in the hospital where the applicant holds privileges. All qualifying procedures must have been performed within 2 years of application.
   4. Performance of at least 50 therapeutic peripheral interventional procedures, at least 25 as the primary operator at the attending physician level (cases performed as a trainee are not counted toward this total) in the hospital where the applicant holds privileges. All qualifying procedures must have been performed within 2 years of application.
   (OR)

B. Fellowship Training Pathway
   1. Successful completion of a formal ABIM-accredited fellowship that includes training in peripheral interventional procedures.
   2. Performance of the requisite number of diagnostic (100) and therapeutic (50) peripheral interventional procedures, at least half as primary operator.
   3. Written attestation of acceptable performance of peripheral procedures by the fellowship program director.
   4. Counting of cases and procedures follow the guidelines outlined in the Clinical Competence document of the ACC (http://www.vascularboard.org/cert_reqs.cfm).

PTA, percutaneous transluminal angioplasty; ABIM, American Board of Internal Medicine; ABS, American Board of Surgery; ABR, American Board of Radiology.

MAINTAINING CLINICAL COMPETENCY

Maintaining one's skill level in catheter-based peripheral vascular (noncoronary) interventions is an ongoing and continuing process. The physician's cognitive knowledge base in peripheral vascular disease management and techniques must remain up to date. The physician must commit to ongoing education and lifelong learning through documented attendance at continuing medical education seminars in the field of vascular diseases. Technical skills should be maintained via performance of a minimum of at least 25 peripheral vascular intervention cases annually with documentation of success and complication rates. Continuing appropriate board certification in his or her specific medical specialty or subspecialty as well as appropriate recertification is necessary.

CONCLUSION

There is evidence that the technical skills necessary to perform coronary intervention are transferable to the peripheral vasculature. However, an understanding of the natural history of peripheral disease, patient and lesion selection criteria, and the knowledge of other treatment alternatives are essential elements required to perform these procedures safely and effectively. For interventional cardiologists who are inexperienced in the treatment of peripheral vascular disease, appropriate preparation and training with a team approach that includes an experienced vascular surgeon are both desirable and necessary before attempting percutaneous peripheral angioplasty.

Clearly, patients with peripheral vascular disease are being underdiagnosed and undertreated. Patient care will benefit by increasing the number of physicians who can provide this needed care with either a restricted or unrestricted certification. Criticisms that the "standards" are being lowered may be countered by the implementation of ongoing quality assurance program.

There are inherent advantages for patients when the interventionalist performing the procedure is also the clinician responsible for the pre- and postprocedure care, analogous to the vascular surgeon who cares for patients before and after surgical procedures. Judgments regarding the indications, timing, and risk-to-benefit ratio of procedures are enhanced by a long-term relationship between physician and patient. Finally, in view of the increased incidence of coronary artery disease in patients with atherosclerotic peripheral vascular disease, the participation of a cardiologist in their care is appropriate.

References

1. Isner J, Rosenfield K. Redefining the treatment of peripheral artery disease. Role of percutaneous revascularization. *Circulation*. 1993;88:1534–1557.
2. Criqui MH. Peripheral arterial disease and subsequent cardiovascular mortality. A strong and consistent association. *Circulation*. 1990;82(6):2246–2247.
3. Criqui MH, Langer RD, Fronek A, et al. Mortality over a period of 10 years in patients with peripheral arterial disease. *N Engl J Med*. 1992;326(6):381–386.
4. Hertzer NR, Beven EG, Young JR, et al. Coronary artery disease in peripheral vascular patients. A classification of 1000 coronary angiograms and results of surgical management. *Ann Surg*. 1984;199(2):223–233.
5. Beller GA, Bonow RO, Fuster V. ACC revised recommendations for training in adult cardiovascular medicine. Core Cardiology Training II (COCATS 2). (Revision of the 1995 COCATS training statement). *J Am Coll Cardiol*. 2002;39(7):1242–1246.
6. Creager MA, Cooke JP, Olin JW, et al. Task force 11: training in vascular medicine and peripheral vascular catheter-based interventions endorsed by the Society for Cardiovascular Angiography and Interventions and the Society for Vascular Medicine. *J Am Coll Cardiol*. 2008;51(3):398–404.
7. White CJ, Ramee SR, Collins TJ, et al. Initial results of peripheral vascular angioplasty performed by experienced interventional cardiologists. *Am J Cardiol*. 1992;69(14):1249–1250.
8. Fayed AM, White CJ, Ramee SR, et al. Carotid and cerebral angiography performed by cardiologists: cerebrovascular complications. *Catheter Cardiovasc Interv*. 2002;55(3):277–280.
9. Jacobs AK, Babb JD, Hirshfeld JW Jr, et al. Task force 3: training in diagnostic and interventional cardiac catheterization endorsed by the Society for Cardiovascular Angiography and Interventions. *J Am Coll Cardiol*. 2008;51(3):355–361.
10. White CJ, Jaff MR, Haskal ZJ, et al. Indications for renal arteriography at the time of coronary arteriography: a science advisory from the American Heart Association Committee on Diagnostic and Interventional Cardiac Catheterization, Council on Clinical Cardiology, and the Councils on Cardiovascular Radiology and Intervention and on Kidney in Cardiovascular Disease. *Circulation*. 2006;114(17):1892–1895.
11. Creager MA, Goldstone J, Hirshfeld JW Jr, et al. ACC/ACP/SCAI/SVMB/SVS clinical competence statement on vascular medicine and catheter-based peripheral vascular interventions: a report of the American College of Cardiology/American Heart Association/American College of Physician Task Force on Clinical Competence (ACC/ACP/SCAI/SVMB/SVS Writing Committee to develop a clinical competence statement on peripheral vascular disease). *J Am Coll Cardiol*. 2004;44(4):941–957.
12. Wexler L, Levin DC, Dorros G, et al. Training standards for physicians performing peripheral angioplasty: new developments. *Radiology*. 1991;178:19–21.
13. Guidelines for percutaneous transluminal angioplasty. Standards of Practice Committee of the Society of Cardiovascular and Interventional Radiology. *Radiology*. 1990;177:619–626.
14. Guidelines for performance of peripheral percutaneous transluminal angioplasty. The Society for Cardiac Angiography and Interventions Interventional Cardiology Committee Subcommittee on Peripheral Interventions. *Cathet Cardiovasc Diagn*. 1988;21:128–129.
15. Pentecost MJ, Criqui MH, Dorros G, et al. Guidelines for peripheral percutaneous transluminal angioplasty of the abdominal aorta and lower extremity vessels. A statement for health professionals from a special writing group of the Councils on Cardiovascular Radiology, Arteriosclerosis, Cardio-Thoracic and Vascular Surgery, Clinical Cardiology, and Epidemiology and Prevention, the American Heart Association. *Circulation*. 1994;89(1):511–531.
16. Spittell JJ, Nanda N, Creager M, et al. Recommendations for peripheral transluminal angioplasty: training and facilities. American College of Cardiology Peripheral Vascular Disease Committee. *J Am Coll Cardiol*. 1993;21:546–548.
17. Levin DC, Becker GJ, Dorros G, et al. Training standards for physicians performing peripheral angioplasty and other percutaneous peripheral vascular interventions. *J Vasc Interv Radiol*. 2003;9(pt 2):S359–S361.
18. Babb JD, Collins TJ, Cowley MJ, et al. Revised guidelines for the performance of peripheral vascular intervention. *Catheter Cardiovasc Interv*. 1999;46(1):21–23.
19. American Board of Vascular Medicine. 2009 [updated 2009; cited 2009, February 22]; Available at: http://www.vascularboard.org/index.cfm.

Noninvasive Evaluation and Management of Peripheral Artery Disease

CHAPTER 2

Hemodynamic Evaluation of Peripheral Arterial Disease

Audrey Rosinberg and Melina R. Kibbe

Lower extremity peripheral arterial disease (PAD) affects 8 million people in the United States, with a prevalence of 29% (1), and is part of a spectrum of atherosclerotic disease that includes coronary and carotid artery disease. Epidemiologic studies have objectively defined the presence of PAD by an ankle–brachial index (ABI) of less than 0.9 (2). The ABI is calculated by the ratio of Doppler-recorded systolic blood pressure in the lower and upper extremities. Normally, systolic blood pressures are 10% to 15% higher at the ankle than at the arm. However, with obstructive disease in the arteries of the lower extremities, systolic blood pressure in the leg and therefore the ABI declines.

Patients may manifest PAD differently. However, in general, 10% of patients have classic symptoms of claudication, 50% have atypical symptoms other than classic claudication, and 40% are asymptomatic (1,3). In its most severe form, PAD may present as critical limb ischemia (CLI) defined by the presence of rest pain, ulceration, or frank gangrene.

PAD is not a local disease; it is a marker of overall cardiovascular health (4). Data from the Strong Heart Study and Cardiovascular Health Strategies demonstrate that the presence of PAD confers a two- to threefold increase in the risk of total mortality and cardiovascular mortality independent of any other risk factors (5). Therefore, it is important to identify asymptomatic patients in order to implement global cardiovascular risk reduction strategies. Additionally, patients may be asymptomatic because they have limited their physical activity.

Interestingly, data from epidemiologic studies of PAD also shows that patients with an ABI > 1.4 also have increased total and cardiovascular mortality (5). An ABI > 1.4 is generally indicative of noncompressible vessels due to medial calcification often found in patients with diabetes or end-stage renal disease requiring dialysis. Although these values were thought to have little diagnostic value, epidemiologic studies indicate that an ABI > 1.4 can be used to identify patients at increased risk of death (6).

Based on the large percentage of patients who are asymptomatic or have atypical symptoms, self-reported questionnaires are clearly unreliable for screening for PAD as they are only a subjective measurement. Additionally, not all patients who complain of pain in the lower extremities with ambulation have peripheral vascular disease, as this pain may be due to other neurologic or orthopedic etiologies. Noninvasive studies performed in the vascular laboratory allow for an objective assessment of PAD.

There are a variety of options available in the vascular laboratory for the hemodynamic assessment of PAD. Each test provides unique and complementary information. The tests are noninvasive, allow the clinician to confirm the presence of PAD, and, if present, determine the location and severity of the disease.

ARTERIAL HEMODYNAMIC NONINVASIVE STUDIES

Ankle–Brachial Index

The ABI is the ratio of the systolic pressure measured in the dorsalis pedis (DP) artery or the posterior tibial (PT) artery at the ankle with the cuff inflated just above the malleolus to the systolic pressure measured in the brachial artery. It is customary to use the highest pressure between the DP and PT when calculating the ABI. Additionally, in cases where the brachial pressures are different due to subclavian stenosis, it is important to use the highest brachial artery pressure in the calculation of the ABI, since this most accurately reflects the true intra-aortic pressure. The current ACC/AHA guidelines relating the severity of PAD with the ABI measurement are shown in Table 2.1 (7).

Multilevel disease can sometimes be challenging to interpret. If one segment such as the superficial femoral artery (SFA) is completely occluded, the magnitude of the pressure change distal to the occlusion will be determined by the resistance of the outflow vessels and the adequacy of collateral flow. In general, a single segment occlusion will result in a fall of the ankle pressure by one half resulting in an ABI of 0.5. However, if more than one level is occluded, the resistance of the outflow bed is additive and the fall in ankle pressure will be greater (8).

In cases of calcified arteries that are noncompressible, the ABI is often greater than 1.4 and does not provide an indication of the severity of the disease. In these cases, it is important to measure toe pressures using plethysmography (see segmental limb pressures below), as the digital vessels are typically spared of calcification (8,9).

The ABI can be used to assess the degree of success of interventions as well as follow the patient for evidence of restenosis. An improvement in the ABI greater than 0.15 is typically considered significant. Less than that typically does not represent a significant improvement due to inter- and intraobserver variability in obtaining the ABI (10). Similarly, a decrease of greater than 0.15 indicates the possibility of restenosis or progression of disease (11). As demonstrated in Figure 2.1, if all obstructions have been completely treated, the ABI should approach or exceed 1.0. However, if sites of

TABLE 2.1 Classification of Peripheral Artery Disease Based on Ankle–Brachial Index (ABI) Measurements

ABI	Severity of Peripheral Artery Disease
>1.3	Incompressible tibial vessels—uninterpretable
1.0–1.29	Normal
0.9–0.99	Equivocal
0.4–0.89	Mild-to-moderate PAD
<0.4	Severe PAD

Based on the most recent ACC/AHA classification (7).

obstruction still exist after the intervention, the ABI increases, but not to normal levels (12).

Segmental Pressures and Toe Pressures

Segmental arterial pressures can be obtained at several levels—brachial, high thigh, low thigh, below knee, and ankle (Fig. 2.2). This is referred to as the four-cuff method and provides the greatest amount of information. The blood pressure cuff is inflated until arterial flow is stopped and the Doppler signal is no longer audible. The cuff is slowly deflated until the first appearance of a systolic wave. This pressure is recorded. It is important to remember that it is the location of the cuff that determines the level of measurement, not the probe. Some vascular laboratories have modified the four-cuff

method to a two-cuff method. They use low thigh and ankle cuffs and have eliminated the high thigh and upper calf cuffs. The Doppler waveforms, discussed in more detail below, are then used to determine the presence of aortoiliac, SFA, and popliteal disease.

Segmental pressures give the clinician information on the location as well as severity of the disease. Normally one would expect similar pressure measurements at the same level in both limbs as well as between levels in the same limb. A pressure gradient of >20mmHg between adjacent cuff measurements is regarded as indicative of significant PAD in the intervening arterial segment (13). A difference of 30 mm Hg or more between levels in one limb suggests the presence of an occlusion (8). A difference of 40 mm Hg or more between similar levels of opposite limbs also suggests the presence of an occlusion (14).

A significant drop in arterial pressure between sequential cuffs signifies the presence of disease above the level of the lower cuff (Table 2.2). For example, a drop in pressure between the arm and high thigh cuffs suggests disease in the aortoiliac and/or common femoral arteries. It is important to be aware that the high thigh systolic pressure normally exceeds the brachial systolic pressure by 20% to 30%. Thus, the normal high thigh/brachial ratio is 1.2:1.3. Stenosis and occlusion of an arterial segment proximal to the high thigh cuff is typically associated with a high thigh/brachial ratio of 0.8–1.2 and <0.8, respectively (15,16). The low thigh cuff will detect disease in the SFA. The below-knee cuff will detect disease in the popliteal artery. The ankle cuff will detect disease in the tibial and peroneal vessels. For example, Figure 2.3 demonstrates segmental pressures and waveforms from a patient with isolated left SFA disease. The femoral waveform is triphasic indicating that there is no significant stenosis in the aortoiliac segment. The popliteal waveform, however, is biphasic. There is a 45-mm Hg pressure gradient between the left brachial and the left distal thigh cuff. Additionally, there is a 55-mm Hg pressure gradient between the right and left low thigh cuffs. Combining this information, this study suggests that the patient has isolated left SFA disease.

Toe pressure measurement is an important component of the segmental pressure measurements. Pressures are obtained using a small pneumatic cuff around the first or second toe. Toe pressures are particularly important when the ABI is invalid due to calcified tibial vessels as is often the case in patients with

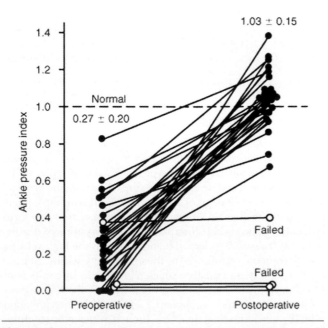

Figure 2.1 • Ankle–brachial index as measured before and after femorotibial and femoropopliteal surgical revascularization in 31 patients. Open circles indicate grafts that failed. (Reproduced with permission from Sumner DS, Strandness DE Jr. Hemodynamic studies before and after extended bypass grafts to the tibial and peroneal arteries. *Surgery.* 1979;86:442.)

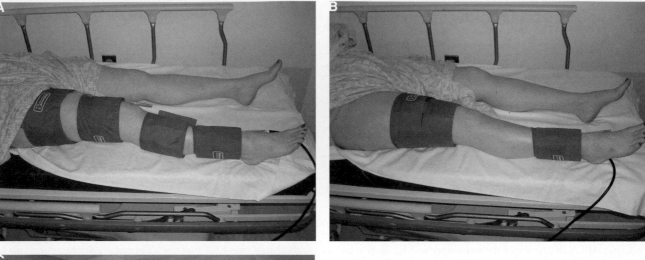

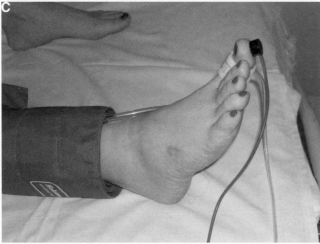

Figure 2.2 • **A:** Demonstrates the placement of the cuffs on the lower extremity in the four-cuff study in the high-thigh, low-thigh, below-knee, and ankle positions. **B:** Demonstrates the placement of the cuffs in the two-cuff study in the low thigh and ankle positions. **C:** Demonstrates photoplethysmography to obtain toe pressures.

diabetes and/or renal insufficiency, since the digital vessels are typically spared of significant calcification. Toe pressures are not different between diabetic and nondiabetic patients, and therefore are a useful indicator of the overall degree of disease. In patients with claudication, toe pressures average about 60 to 70 mm Hg. In patients with rest pain and ulceration, the toe pressures are usually less than 30 mm Hg (17). In addition, the toe pressure can give the clinician important information as to the likelihood of an ischemic ulceration healing without surgical intervention. Some authors have found a difference between toe pressures required for healing in nondiabetic versus diabetic patients. Foot lesions usually heal if toe pressures exceed 30 mm Hg in nondiabetic patients and 55 mm Hg in diabetic patients (18). Other studies, however, have not found a difference and found that greater than 90% of lesions will heal when toe pressures are greater than 30 in both diabetics and nondiabetics (9,19).

The ratio of the toe pressure to brachial pressure is referred to as the toe–brachial index (TBI). The normal TBI is 0.8 to 0.9. In patients with claudication and ischemic rest pain, the TBI is typically 0.2 to 0.5 and 0 to 0.2, respectively.

Doppler Waveforms

The Doppler waveform provides additional information to segmental pressures and ABIs, especially in cases where the vessels are not compressible. A pencil-type 5 to 8 MHz Doppler probe is generally used, and measurements are taken with the probe at an angle of 45 to 60 degrees to the artery. Both an audible interpretation as well as qualitative interpretation of the waveform is obtained. The audible interpretation consists of three distinct sounds in a normal patient. The first sound is the high velocity systolic component, followed by the smaller reverse-flow component in diastole, and finally a smaller, lower velocity component heard during late diastole. Distal to a stenosis, the flow signals are low pitched and monophasic. The audible interpretation is highly subjective and, therefore, limited. Much more useful is the qualitative analysis of the waveform.

The waveforms reflect the resistance pattern of the outflow vascular bed. The flow characteristics provide the "signature" triphasic signal. A normal triphasic signal will have three components. The first is a large forward-flow velocity peak that occurs with systole (Fig. 2.4). This is followed

TABLE 2.2 Listing of the Likely Anatomic Location of Peripheral Artery Disease Based on the Drop in Pressure between Sequential Pressure Cuffs in the Lower Extremity

Location of Pressure Drop	Likely Anatomic Location of Disease
Brachial—upper thigh	Aortoiliac, CFA
Upper thigh—lower thigh	SFA
Lower thigh—upper calf	Popliteal
Upper calf—ankle	Tibial

CFA, common femoral artery; SFA, superfical femoral artery.

by a brief period of flow reversal in early diastole, and lastly by a final period of low-frequency forward flow that is late diastole.

As atherosclerotic disease progresses, the first change seen is the loss of flow reversal resulting in a biphasic signal (Fig. 2.5). This occurs because the resistance of the outflow bed is now lower. As disease progresses further, the late diastolic forward flow is lost as well, creating a monophasic signal. As the disease progresses to total occlusion the rate of acceleration of the forward-flow wave decreases and becomes more rounded. Additionally, in monophasic waveforms, the end diastolic velocity (EDV) remains above zero (20).

The waveform proximal to a stenosis or occlusion will appear relatively normal (Fig. 2.5A and B). Distal to a stenosis

or occlusion, the waveform will appear as in Figure 2.5C–H. Thus the analysis of the waveforms at the different levels, femoral, popliteal, and pedal can localize the level of the disease. For example, in a patient with SFA disease, the femoral waveform will appear as in Figure 2.5A but the popliteal waveform will appear as in Figure 2.5E.

Since the waveform will reflect changes in resistance of the outflow vascular bed, it will be affected by both body heat as well as exercise. As body temperature increases, vasodilation will occur resulting in lower resistance. As resistance drops, the reversal of flow component disappears, resulting in a biphasic waveform. As the temperature drops, vasoconstriction will result in higher resistance, and conversely can mask the underlying disease. Thus, it is important to make sure that measurements

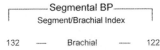

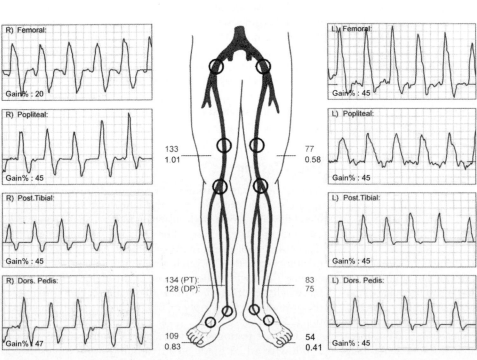

Figure 2.3 • Arterial noninvasive study demonstrating isolated left superficial femoral artery disease.

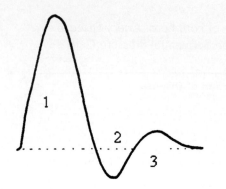

Three components

1. Large forward flow velocity peak = systole

2. Brief phase of flow reversal = early diastole

3. Low-frequency forward flow = late diastole

Figure 2.4 • Normal triphasic Doppler waveforms.

are taken in a warm room and to be sure that the patient rests for 5 to 10 minutes before obtaining measurements.

Pulse Volume Recording

Pulse volume recordings (PVRs) reflect the volume change in the limb with each cardiac cycle and are measured using a variety of plethysmographic techniques including:

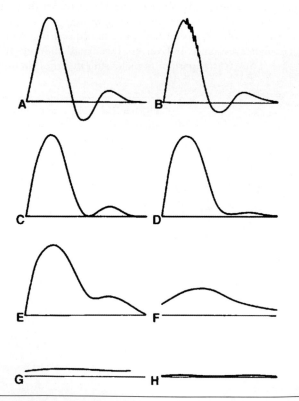

Figure 2.5 • Doppler waveforms progressing from normal **(A)** to severe peripheral arterial disease **(H)**. Note, as disease progresses, reversal of flow is lost in early diastole **(B–D)** and flattening of the waveform seen with even further progression of disease **(E–H)**. (Reproduced with permission from Johnston KW, Maruzzo BC, Kassam M, et al. Methods for obtaining, processing and quantifying Doppler blood velocity waveforms. In: Nicolaides A, Yao JST, eds. *Investigation of Vascular Disorders*. New York, NY: Churchill Livingstone; 1981:543.)

photoplethysmography, impedance plethysmography, strain gauge plethysmography, and air plethysmography. Photoplethysmography functions with an infrared light-emitting diode and measures the amount of light reflected back to the photodiode and is typically used to record PVRs from the toe(s). Air plethysmography uses pneumatic cuffs and is the most common method for acquiring PVRs from the thigh, calf, and ankle. Air plethysmography is used by some laboratories for more proximal measurements in lieu of Doppler waveforms. Impedance plethysmography measures resistance, and strain gauge plethysmography measures limb circumference. These last two modalities are not often used today.

When using air plethysmography, pneumatic cuffs are applied to the upper thigh, calf, and ankle and inflated to 65 mm Hg. Recordings are then made from each site. The normal contour consists of a steep upstroke, a sharp systolic peak, and a downslope with a sharp dicrotic notch in the middle (Fig. 2.6). The dicrotic notch represents the reverse-flow phase of diastole. As a proximal stenosis progresses, the upslope becomes less steep, the peak becomes rounded, and the dicrotic notch disappears. The amplitude decreases as the obstruction becomes more severe. PVRs are extremely accurate for identifying normal limbs and disease isolated to the below-knee arteries. However, accuracy decreases with multilevel disease to approximately 70%. When PVRs are combined with segmental limb pressures, the accuracy improves to >85% (21).

Stress Testing

Arterial noninvasive studies may miss mild disease that is only apparent with exertion. Patients who have normal arterial blood flow but have a high suspicion for PAD based on history can undergo stress testing. The basis for stress testing is that the sensitivity of pressure measurements is increased by augmenting blood flow through a stenotic segment. This can be accomplished with either exercise or through the induction of reactive hyperemia. The effect of both approaches is to reduce the resistance in the peripheral arterial bed through vasodilation (22–24).

Exercise testing is performed by having patients walk at 2 m/h with a 12% grade on a treadmill for 5 minutes. Ankle pressures are measured at baseline, immediately after exercise, then every 2 minutes for 10 minutes. A drop in the ankle

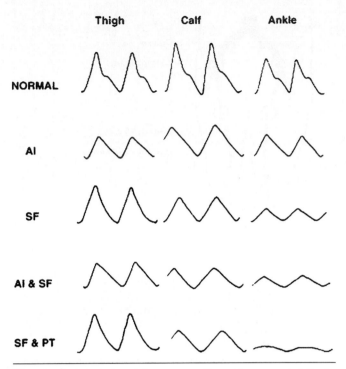

Figure 2.6 • Pulse volume recordings from normal limbs with various combinations of peripheral vascular disease. AI, aortoiliac; SF, superficial femoral; PT, popliteal-tibial. (Reprinted from Rutherford RB, Lowenstein DH, Klein MF. Combining segmental systolic pressures and plethysmography to diagnose arterial occlusive disease of the legs. *Am J Surg.* 1979;138:216, with permission from Elsevier.)

pressure of more than 20% from the baseline measurement that requires more than 3 minutes to normalize is considered abnormal. Furthermore, the magnitude of the drop in ankle pressure and the length of time required to return to baseline mirror the extent of the disease, with large pressure drops that remain low for >12 to 15 minutes being indicative of CLI (25,26). It is important to note that during exercise, brachial systolic pressures increase more relative to ankle systolic pressures. This is why it is important to use ankle pressures and not the ABI (27) during exercise testing.

Some patients may be unable to perform a treadmill test due to either cardiac or pulmonary limitations, or lower extremity symptoms. For these patients, the reactive hyperemia test is a useful alternative. This study is conducted by inflating a pneumatic cuff at the thigh to suprasystolic pressure for 5 minutes. Similar to stress testing, the ankle systolic pressure is recorded at baseline, immediately following release of the cuff, and every 2 minutes for 10 minutes. In normal patients, the ankle systolic pressure returns to baseline in less than 1 minute. In patients with significant PAD, the time to normalization of the ankle systolic pressure is prolonged to greater than 3 minutes (28). An alternative method of conducting this study is to measure the PVR in the digital vessels using plethysmography, instead of measuring the ankle pressure.

Each of these stress tests has advantages and disadvantages. Exercise testing is physiologic and reproduces the patient's

clinical symptoms. However, it is cumbersome and time consuming. Reactive hyperemia testing is less time consuming and can be used for patients who are unable to walk on a treadmill due to either cardiopulmonary limitations or physiologic limitations due to an amputation for example. However, reactive hyperemia testing is less sensitive and specific than exercise testing (29).

Potential Pitfalls of Hemodynamic Measurements

The results of arterial hemodynamic noninvasive studies must be interpreted cautiously. There are significant pitfalls that can cause erroneous interpretation of the data. When calculating the ABI, the brachial pressure must be taken in both arms. In cases where the brachial pressures are different due to subclavian stenosis, it is important to use the highest brachial pressure in the calculation of the ABI.

It is important that the high thigh cuff be placed as high as possible on the thigh. If the cuff is placed too low, a low pressure may reflect proximal SFA disease rather than aortoiliac and/or common femoral artery disease. Using an appropriately sized cuff is also important. If the cuff is too small for the thigh or ankle, the pressure will be artificially elevated. Similarly, if the cuff is too large, the pressure will be artificially lowered. The width of an appropriate-sized cuff should be at least 50% of the diameter of the limb where the measurement is being taken.

Diabetic patients and patients on dialysis are prone to developing medial calcification of the arteries resulting in incompressible vessels and falsely elevated pressures. In these patients, segmental pressures and ABIs are invalid. Toe pressures, however, typically remain reliable and can be helpful in evaluating the severity of the disease in these patients. Waveform analysis can also be used to help determine the level of the disease.

Finally, there are technical aspects to performing the examination that can affect the results. It is important that the examination be performed in a warm environment as a cold environment can cause vasospasm that will cause erroneous results. Vasospasm will result in increased arteriolar resistance leading to decreased flow and falsely low toe pressures, and it can mask mild proximal disease. Additionally, the technician must place the probe directly over the artery; otherwise, the values obtained can be artificially low. Given the variability in technique between observers and the variability in the biologic factors, only changes in ABI > 0.15 are considered significant.

In limbs with low flow due to severe PAD and/or low cardiac ejection fractions, it may be difficult to distinguish between arterial and venous flow. Venous signals are augmented with distal limb compression, whereas arterial signals are not. Duplex ultrasound can also be helpful in situations where one is unsure whether the flow is arterial or venous.

Case Examples of Hemodynamic Measurements

The best way to understand arterial hemodynamic noninvasive tests and become facile with their interpretation and clinical relevance is to practice reading as many studies as possible in the clinical setting. Figures 2.7–2.11 are examples of noninvasive hemodynamic studies for a variety of clinical scenarios.

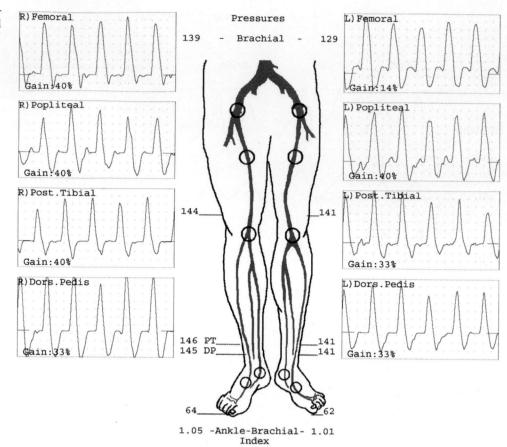

Figure 2.7 • Normal arterial noninvasive flow study.

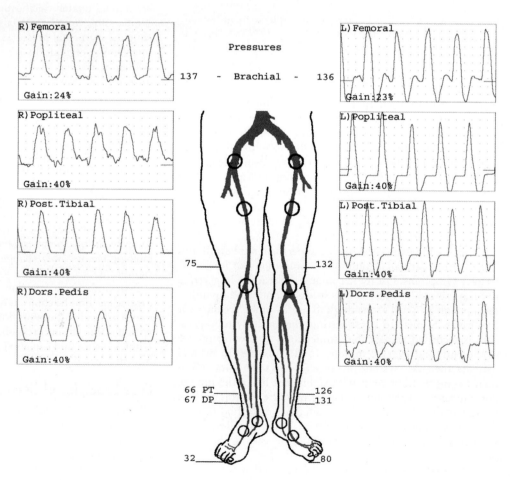

Figure 2.8 • Arterial noninvasive study demonstrating right aortoiliac disease. Note the greater than 60 mm Hg pressure gradient between the right brachial systolic pressure and the right thigh cuff pressure. There is also a 60-mm Hg pressure gradient between the right and left thigh cuffs. There is no pressure gradient between levels on the left lower extremity, indicating no significant disease of the left. Additionally, the waveforms on the right lower extremity have lost the reversal of flow in diastole and are biphasic.

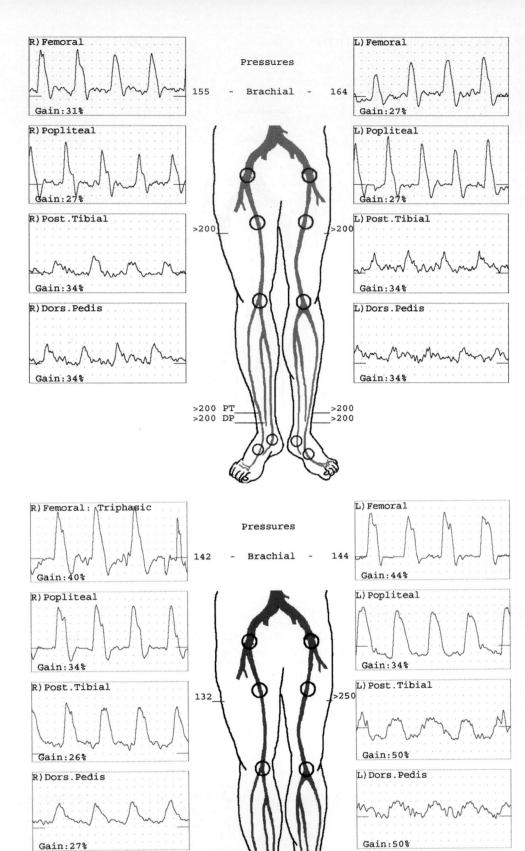

Figure 2.9 • Arterial noninvasive study demonstrating bilateral infrapopliteal disease in a patient with calcified noncompressible arteries. Note that the pressures throughout are greater than 200. The Doppler waveforms in this case are very useful. There are triphasic waveforms at the femoral and popliteal levels. At the tibial levels, the waveforms lose the reversal of flow and are flattened and monophasic. Toe pressures would provide additional useful information in this patient.

Figure 2.10 • Arterial noninvasive study demonstrating superficial femoral artery and infrapopliteal disease on the left and mild infrapopliteal disease on the right. A normal waveform is seen in the right popliteal artery, yet a biphasic waveform is seen in the left popliteal artery, indicating left superficial femoral artery disease. The tibial waveforms are diminished on the right and are associated with an ankle–brachial index (ABI) of 0.9 and a toe pressure of 36, suggesting mild infrapopliteal disease. The tibial waveforms are further diminished on the left and are associated with an ABI of 0.4 and a toe pressure of 0, suggesting severe ischemia. On the left, there is a significant drop-off in pressure to 57 mm Hg and the ABI is 0.4 compared with 0.9 on the right.

Figure 2.9 contents:

R) Femoral — Gain:31%
R) Popliteal — Gain:27%
R) Post.Tibial — Gain:34%
R) Dors.Pedis — Gain:34%

L) Femoral — Gain:27%
L) Popliteal — Gain:27%
L) Post.Tibial — Gain:34%
L) Dors.Pedis — Gain:34%

Pressures
155 – Brachial – 164
>200 — >200
>200 PT — >200
>200 DP — >200

Figure 2.10 contents:

R) Femoral: Triphasic — Gain:40%
R) Popliteal — Gain:34%
R) Post.Tibial — Gain:26%
R) Dors.Pedis — Gain:27%

L) Femoral — Gain:44%
L) Popliteal — Gain:34%
L) Post.Tibial — Gain:50%
L) Dors.Pedis — Gain:50%

Pressures
142 – Brachial – 144
132 — >250
126 PT — 57
128 DP — 43
36 — 0

0.89 -Ankle-Brachial- 0.40
Index

Figure 2.11 • Arterial noninvasive study demonstrating noncompressible calcified segmental pressures but normal waveforms throughout and preserved toe pressures. This pattern may be seen in patients with diabetes and no significant peripheral arterial disease.

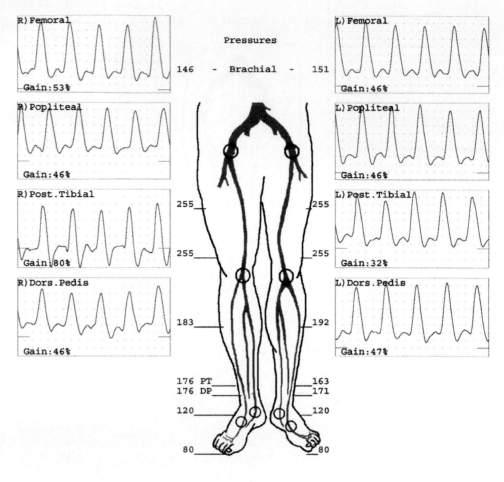

CONCLUSION

The noninvasive hemodynamic studies performed in an accredited vascular laboratory are essential to the practicing vascular surgeon and endovascular interventionalist. When used in combination, these studies can provide complementary information that can be used to diagnose and guide treatment, as well as improve patency of peripheral arterial interventions without exposing the patient to either radiation or intravenous contrast agents.

References

1. Hirsch AT, Criqui MH, Treat-Jacobson D, et al. Peripheral arterial disease detection, awareness, and treatment in primary care. *JAMA*. 2001;286:1317–1324.
2. Mcdermott M. The magnitude of the problem of peripheral arterial disease: epidemiology and clinical significance. *Cleve Clin J Med*. 2006;73:S2–S7.
3. McDermott MM, Greenland P, Liu K, et al. Leg symptoms in peripheral arterial disease: associated clinical characteristics and functional impairment. *JAMA*. 2001;286:1599–1606.
4. Heald CL, Fowkes FG, Murray GD, et al.; Ankle Brachial Index Collaboration. Risk of mortality and cardiovascular disease associated with the ankle-brachial index: systematic review. *Atherosclerosis*. 2006;189:61–69.
5. Resnick HE, Lindsay RS, Mcdermott MM, et al. Relationship of high and low ankle brachial index to all-cause and cardiovascular disease mortality. The Strong Heart Study. *Circulation*. 2004; 109:733–739.
6. O'Hare AM, Katz R, Shlipak MG, et al. Mortality and cardiovascular risk across the ankle-arm index spectrum: results from the Cardiovascular Health Study. *Circulation*. 2006;113:388–393.
7. Hirsch AT, Haskal ZJ, Hertzer NR, et al. ACC/AHA 2005 Guidelines for the management of patients with peripheral arterial disease (lower extremity, renal, mesenteric, and abdominal aortic): executive summary. *J Am Coll Cardiol*. 2006;47:1239–1312.
8. Carter SA. Clinical measurement of systolic pressures in limbs with arterial occlusive disease. *JAMA*. 1969;207:1869.
9. Ramsey DE, Manke DA, Sumner DS. Toe blood pressure: a valuable adjunct to ankle pressure measurement for assessing peripheral arterial disease. *J Cardiovasc Surg*. 1983;24:43.
10. Johnston KW, Hosang MY, Andrews DF. Reproducibility of noninvasive vascular laboratory measurements of the peripheral circulation. *J Vasc Surg*. 1987;6:147.
11. Berkowitz HD, Hobbs CL, Roberts B, et al. Value of routine vascular laboratory studies to identify vein graft stenosis. *Surgery*. 1981;90:971.
12. Sumner DS, Strandness DE Jr. Hemodynamic studies before and after extended bypass grafts to the tibial and peroneal arteries. *Surgery*. 1979;86:442.
13. Strandness DE Jr, Bell JW. Peripheral vascular disease: diagnosis and objective evaluation using a mercury strain gauge. *Ann Surg*. 1965;161(suppl 4):1.
14. Fronek A, Johansen KH, Dilley RB, et al. Noninvasive physiologic testing in the diagnosis and characterization of peripheral arterial occlusive disease. *Am J Surg*. 1973;125:205.

15. Cutjar CL, Marston A, Newcombe JF. Valu of cuff occlusion pressures in assessment of peripheral arterial disease. *BMJ*. 1973;2:392.

16. Heintz SE, Bone GE, Slaymaker EE, et al. Value of arterial pressure measurements in the proximal and distal part of the thigh in arterial occlusive disease. *Surg Gynecol Obstet*. 1978;146:337.

17. Carter SA, Lezack JD. Digital systolic pressures in the lower limb in arterial disease. *Circulation*. 1971;43:905–914.

18. Carter SA. The relationship of distal systolic pressures to healing of skin lesions in limbs with arterial occlusive disease, with special reference to diabetes mellitus. *Scand J Clin Lab Invest*. 1973;31(suppl 128):239.

19. Holstein P, Noer I, Tonnesen KH, et al. Distal blood pressure in severe arterial insufficiency: strain gauge, radioisotopes, and other methods. In: Bergan JJ, Yao JST, eds. *Gangrene and Severe Ischemia of the Lower Extremities*. New York, NY: Grune & Stratton; 1978:95–114.

20. Johnston KW, Maruzzo BC, Kassam M, et al. Methods for obtaining, processing and quantifying Doppler blood velocity waveforms. In: Nicolaides A, Yao JST, eds. *Investigation of Vascular Disorders*. New York: Churchill Livingstone; 1981:543.

21. Rutherford RB, Lowenstein DH, Klein MF. Combining segmental systolic pressures and plethysmography to diagnose arterial occlusive disease of the legs. *Am J Surg*. 1979;138:216.

22. DeWeese JA. Pedal pulses disappearing with exercise: a test for intermittent claudication. *N Engl J Med*. 1960;262:1214–1217.

23. Fronek A, Coel M, Bernstein EF, et al. The pulse-reappearance time: an index of over-all blood flow impairment in the ischemic extremity. *Surgery*. 1977;81:376.

24. Sumner DS, Strandness DE Jr. The effect of exercise on resistance to blood flow in limbs with an occluded superficial femoral artery. *J Vasc Surg*. 1970;4:229.

25. Zierler RU. Nonimaging physiological tests for assessment of lower extremity arterial occlusive disease. In: Zweibel WJ, Pellerito JS, eds. *Introduction to Vascular Ultrasonography*. Philadelphia, PA: Elsevier Saunders; 2005:275–296.

26. Zaccardi MJ, Olmsted KA. Peripheral arterial evaluation. In: Strandness DE, ed. *Duplex Scanning in Vascular Disorders*. Philadelphia, PA: Lippincott Williams & Wilkins; 2002:253–266.

27. Stahler C, Strandness DE Jr. Ankle blood pressure response to graded treadmill exercise. *Angiology*. 1967;18:237–241.

28. Hummel BW, Hummel BA, Mowbry A, et al. Reactive hyperemia vs treadmill exercise testing in arterial disease. *Arch Surg*. 1978;113:95–98.

29. Ouriel K, McDonnell AE, Metz CE, et al. A critical evaluation of stress testing in the diagnosis of peripheral vascular disease. *Surgery*. 1982;91:686.

CHAPTER 3

The Role of Vascular Ultrasonography in Peripheral Artery Disease

Ahmed Abdel-Latif and Khaled M. Ziada

Although accurate and thorough medical history taking and physical examination are crucial for diagnosing peripheral arterial disease (PAD), the limitations of clinical assessment necessitate adjunctive imaging techniques that improve the accuracy of the diagnosis and quantification of PAD. Vascular ultrasound provides a valuable tool in the assessment of various peripheral vascular beds. Despite the advances in computed tomography (CT) and magnetic resonance (MR) angiographic techniques, vascular ultrasound still represents the initial test of choice based on its noninvasive nature, accuracy, validated values, and wide availability. Beyond screening for and diagnosing PAD, imaging modalities, including ultrasound, provide essential information regarding the level and extent of the disease as well as helping plan the appropriate treatment. Moreover, noninvasive testing aids in the assessment of the success and durability of therapies. The accuracy of noninvasive tests in the diagnosis, evaluation, and follow-up monitoring of PAD has resulted in the significant reduction of the need for invasive angiography studies, with considerable savings for the health care system without compromising quality of care. The purpose of this chapter is to review the role of vascular ultrasound and its utility in the diagnosis of PAD in various vascular beds.

MODALITIES OF VASCULAR ULTRASOUND IMAGING

Ultrasound refers to sound waves with a frequency above the audible range (i.e., >20,000 cycles/sec). In clinical practice, ultrasound is generated by a piezoelectric crystal within a transducer. This ultrasound beam travels through the tissue and is reflected back to the transducer. Based on differences in the acoustic properties of the arterial wall layers and components of atherosclerotic plaque, there is heterogeneity in the reflection of the ultrasound waves, allowing the reconstruction of an image that displays the anatomic information based on different shades of gray scale (also called B-mode or brightness imaging). The resolution of the gray-scale image permits a rough evaluation of the vessel (i.e., vessel size, presence of atheroma/hematoma/aneurysm) but does not provide an accurate assessment of the severity of a stenosis within the vessel.

The ability to sample the change in frequency of the transmitted versus the received ultrasound waves (i.e., Doppler ultrasound) allows the additional assessment of blood flow velocity within the vessel. Color Doppler refers to the display technique that uses color to facilitate quick assessment of this Doppler information, allowing one to recognize the direction of flow within a vessel. By convention red and blue colors indicate blood flowing toward and away from the transducer, respectively. Turbulent flow is typically indicated by shades of green or a mosaic appearance.

Duplex ultrasound imaging combines B-mode imaging and Doppler coding of velocity shifts with pulse-wave/continuous-wave ultrasonography, and therefore, provides detailed examination of both the anatomic characteristics and the functional significance of an arterial stenosis. By superimposing the color Doppler coding on the B-mode images, the location and severity of stenosis can be identified. The combination of these modalities has significantly improved the sensitivity and specificity of ultrasound imaging in detecting hemodynamically significant stenoses against the traditional gold standard for defining stenosis severity of digital subtraction angiography (with a diameter stenosis $\geq 50\%$ considered the cutoff that defines a significant lesion).

Duplex ultrasonography has a number of practical advantages in the assessment of PAD. In addition to providing both anatomic and functional information, it is noninvasive, does not require the administration of iodinated contrast, does not expose the patient to radiation, is relatively inexpensive, is widely available (even at smaller medical centers and outpatient facilities), and is applicable in patients with claustrophobia or previously implanted devices or metal artifacts. Some limitations to this technique do exist. Since ultrasound waves cannot penetrate bone, it should not be used to image vessels within body structures (e.g., intracranial portion of carotid or vertebral artery). In addition, ultrasound penetrates gas poorly, making imaging of intra-abdominal and intra-pelvic vessels challenging, particularly in obese patients. The spatial resolution of ultrasound is also limited, making examination of smaller caliber vessels difficult (e.g., tibial vessels). Despite these limitations, Duplex ultrasound has become a valuable tool in the evaluation of patients with PAD, and in the assessment of patients following surgical and percutaneous revascularization procedures. What follows is a summary of the specific use of Duplex ultrasound in the assessment of the primary peripheral vascular territories.

THE LOWER EXTREMITY

Noninvasive evaluation of PAD of the lower extremity is traditionally achieved by multiple modalities (see Chapters 2 and 4). The Doppler and ultrasound examinations of the lower extremity are performed in the supine position. Transducers of variable frequencies are used depending on the depth of the arterial segment being examined (2 to 3 MHz for iliac arteries and 5 to 7 MHz for femoral and more distal arteries). The examination starts by identifying various arteries and arterial segments on two-dimensional (2D) or B-mode imaging. Although some degree of detail of the arterial wall and presence of plaque can be obtained, the resolution is usually not adequate to accurately define stenosis severity. Doppler signals are then obtained from these segments, with the resultant velocities and waveforms providing diagnostic information regarding flow and severity of stenosis. Color coding of the Doppler flow facilitates the examination of specific arterial segments (Fig. 3.1).

The normal Doppler peripheral arterial waveform consists of three components: rapid forward flow during systole, transient flow reversal in late systole, and a smaller forward flow phase during diastole. Hence the waveform is described as triphasic (Fig. 3.2A). The presence of a normal arterial waveform generally excludes the presence of significant arterial disease (≥50% stenosis). With mild disease, and as the artery becomes stiffer, the short late systolic flow reversal is blunted, resulting in a biphasic waveform. With more advanced disease, the flow velocity distal to the lesion is reduced and the small diastolic forward flow is blunted as well resulting in a monophasic waveform (Fig. 3.2B). In addition, the spectrum of flow velocities within the vessel is increased, resulting in "spectral broadening" or filling in of the Doppler waveform (1).

The peak systolic velocity (PSV) is measured from the Doppler waveform at the lesion site (i.e., intrastenotic) and at a normal appearing segment proximal to the lesion (i.e., prestenotic). At the lesion site, PSV increases to a degree proportional to the stenosis severity. Although the PSV at the lesion site does correlate with the severity of stenosis, the sensitivity and specificity of this variable alone are modest due to the interindividual variation in blood flow velocities. The sensitivity and specificity are improved by using the variable termed the "systolic velocity ratio" (SVR) or "peak velocity ratio" (PVR), which is the ratio of the maximum PSV at the lesion site to the maximum PSV proximal to the lesion. In most laboratories, a PVR/SVR ratio ≥ 2 is used to indicate a significant stenosis. In most clinical trials of femoropopliteal artery stenting, a PVR/SVR of ≥2.5 is used to adjudicate the presence of significant restenosis.

Therefore, a significant lesion can be identified by the morphology of the waveform, the degree of increase in PSV relative to a normal proximal segment, and the appearance of flow turbulence on color Doppler. Accordingly, a simplified approach for quantifying the severity of arterial disease has been adopted by most clinicians (2–5). Doubling of the PSV at the lesion level, loss of flow reversal, and turbulence are signs of a significant stenosis (i.e., >50% diameter stenosis). With milder stenoses (<50% diameter stenosis), the PSV is increased but to a lesser degree and the flow-reversal component of the waveform is preserved. When the arterial segment is totally occluded, no Doppler signal can be obtained and color coding demonstrates the absence of flow in the lumen

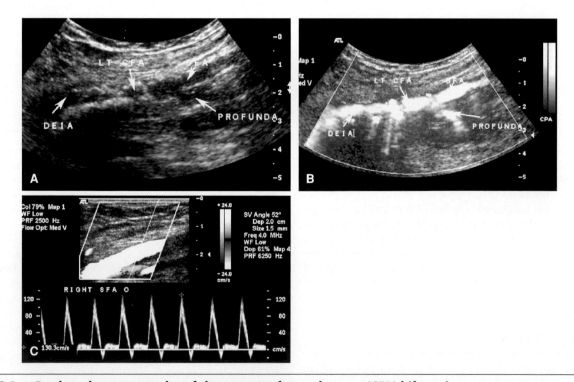

Figure 3.1 • Duplex ultrasonography of the common femoral artery (CFA) bifurcation. **A:** B-mode ultrasound image showing limited detail of the arterial lumen and wall. **B:** Color power image from the same site clearly showing the lumen of the DEIA, the CFA, and the proximal portions of the SFA and profunda femoral arteries. **C:** Routine color Doppler of the CFA bifurcation facilitating sampling of Doppler waveform from the SFA. DEIA, distal external iliac artery; SFA, superficial femoral artery.

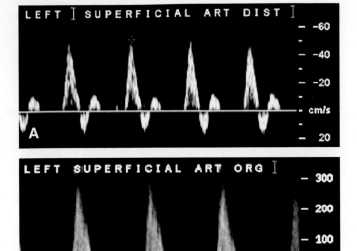

Figure 3.2 • Doppler velocity patterns in normal and diseased peripheral arteries. **A:** Normal triphasic arterial waveform demonstrating the characteristic systolic rapid forward upstroke followed by late systolic flow reversal. There is minimal diastolic blood flow as compared with low-resistance vascular beds such as the internal carotid and renal arteries. **B:** Monophasic arterial waveform with elevated peak systolic flow velocity indicating presence of significant disease. The late systolic flow reversal and early forward diastolic flow are both blunted leading to a monophasic wave.

(Fig. 3.3). Attempts to further categorize a given stenosis as <50%, 50% to 75%, and 75% to 99% have been successfully reported in the literature, although have not been widely adopted (6,7).

A meta-analysis of 16 studies showed the sensitivity and specificity of Duplex ultrasound to be 86% and 97% in aortoiliac disease and 80% and 96% in femoropopliteal disease, respectively. The sensitivity and specificity for infragenicular arterial disease were slightly lower at 83% and 84%, respectively (8).

However, it is prudent to be aware of the limitations of the technique. Lower extremity Duplex ultrasound examinations can be time-consuming, even in experienced hands (typically take 30 to 60 minutes). The frequency of incomplete studies can be significant (estimates vary from 4% to 60%) and is typically due to failure to insonate the pelvic segments, the presence of severely calcified vessel segments that cause acoustic shadowing, and the occurrence of slow flow downstream from occlusive disease (9). It is important to maintain an angle of interrogation <60 degrees during acquisition of flow velocity data to avoid obtaining spurious velocities.

THE UPPER EXTREMITY

The evaluation of the upper extremity by ultrasonography is similar to that of the lower extremity in terms of velocity cutoffs. However, because of the superficial anatomy of the arm arteries, most of the arteries distal to the clavicle can be imaged using high-frequency probes ranging from 8 to 15 MHz. Contrary to the lower extremity, atherosclerotic disease is very rare distal to the subclavian artery, except in patients with diabetes mellitus and end-stage renal disease. On the other hand, various vasculitides such as thromboangitis obliterans, scleroderma, CREST syndrome, and mixed connective tissue disease are known to have specific propensity for the small and medium-sized arteries of the upper extremity.

Subclavian artery disease is easily detected and evaluated by conventional testing and duplex scanning. Measuring the blood pressures in both arms is a useful screen, and measuring segmental pressures along the length of the arm will typically localize the diseased segment to the subclavian artery (and innominate artery on the right side). Although the origin of the left subclavian artery below the clavicle is not accessible for Doppler duplex imaging, all of the right subclavian artery and the remaining sections of the left are typically amenable. Duplex imaging of the subclavian artery provides the same information as that described with lower limb arterial imaging. The Doppler waveforms obtained from a normal subclavian artery are identical to that described earlier for lower limb arteries (i.e., triphasic). Guidelines for estimating the severity of subclavian obstructive lesions based on peak systolic velocities are similar to those used for the lower limbs. It is important to note that the systolic flow reversal phase of the Doppler signal obtained from brachial, ulnar, or radial arteries is absent in up to 50% of healthy individuals. Otherwise, qualitative changes in the waveform (e.g., spectral broadening, monophasic morphology) infer similar conclusions regarding the hemodynamic significance of obstructive disease. Palmar arch flow and digital arterial flow are best evaluated using Doppler. The contribution of the ulnar and radial arteries to palmar arch flow may be assessed using the Doppler device with sequential occlusion of the arteries.

THE CEREBROVASCULAR CIRCULATION

The majority of patients with cerebrovascular disease are asymptomatic. Physical examination is usually not reliable enough to identify most cases of occult carotid disease. Ultrasound imaging has become the most commonly used imaging modality for this indication due to its noninvasive nature, accuracy, and wide availability.

The available criteria for defining carotid disease were originally based on angiographic criteria. Among the major randomized trials reported in the 1990s that studied the role of endarterectomy in the treatment of carotid artery disease (i.e., North American Symptomatic Carotid Endarterectomy Trial (NASCET) (10), European Carotid Surgery Trial (ESCT) (11), and Endarterectomy for Asymptomatic Carotid Artery Disease Study (12)) nonuniform criteria for grading carotid artery disease were used (Fig. 3.4). As a result, a 50% and 70% stenosis based on the NASCET criteria was equivalent to a 65% and 82% stenosis, respectively, using the ECST criteria (13). Despite the differences, all provide similar prognostic information. Medicare/Medicaid and other reimbursement

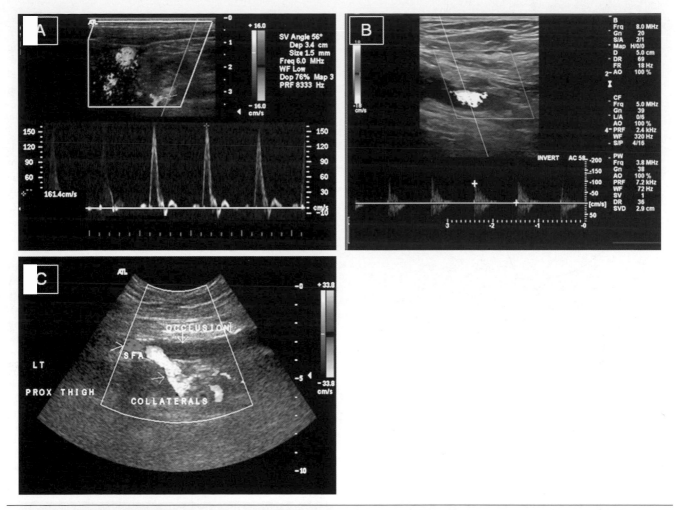

Figure 3.3 • Arterial Duplex examination (Doppler velocity and B-mode ultrasound) patterns in normal and diseased peripheral arteries.   After identifying the arterial segments to be examined, color Doppler is superimposed on the 2D image. Doppler signals are obtained from the lumen. **A:** A normal artery with laminar flow and a triphasic wave. **B:** A diseased segment with turbulence demonstrated by the mosaic appearance on the color flow. A Doppler sample distal to the lesion demonstrates reduced velocity and a monophasic wave. **C:** A totally occluded superficial femoral artery with no evidence of flow as assessed by color Doppler in the occluded segment and the collateral flow around the occluded segment of the artery.

bodies have adopted the NASCET criteria since it appears to be the most reliable and reproducible.

The Carotid Duplex Examination

The patient is placed in the supine position, turning the neck away from the side of the examination. Transducers with frequencies of 5 to 7.5 MHz are most commonly used. Initially, the common carotid artery (CCA) is identified at the base of the neck and then traced cephalad to identify the bifurcation and both internal and external carotid arteries (ICA and ECA).

After the initial scan for orientation, the CCA, carotid bulb, and ICA are then examined more closely, using B-mode or gray-scale imaging in both the longitudinal and the transverse planes. Doppler waveforms are obtained from all the arterial segments; the PSV and end-diastolic velocity (EDV) at each site are recorded. Doppler color coding may identify segments with flow turbulence, which facilitates the identification of segments with the highest velocities (14). It is important to

sweep the Doppler through the entire vessel so as not to miss a high-velocity jet.

Normal Doppler Velocity Patterns

The ICA and ECA must be identified early on in the examination process. The ICA is usually larger in size, has no branches in the neck, and courses posteriorly toward the mastoid process. Most importantly, the ICA has a low-resistance Doppler signature since it feeds a low-resistance vascular bed in the brain. The characteristic flow pattern shows high forward flow velocity during systole with continuing forward flow during diastole at a lower velocity (Fig. 3.5A). The diastolic flow is therefore above the baseline and no flow reversal is seen.

The ECA, on the other hand, supplies a high-resistance peripheral vascular bed in the neck and face. Its typical waveform has a high-velocity systolic forward flow, followed by a prominent dicrotic notch with possible late systolic flow reversal, and

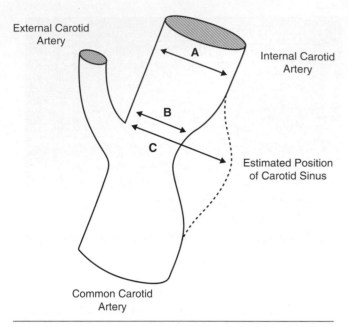

Figure 3.4 • Illustration of the methodology used to define the severity of internal carotid artery stenosis in the NASCET and ECST trials. According to the NASCET criteria, the reference diameter is measured in the internal carotid artery distal to the diseased segment. Thus, the degree of stenosis is measured as (A − B)/A. In the ESCT trial, investigators extrapolated the border of the angiogram to account for the normal dilatation at the carotid sinus and calculated the percent stenosis as (C − B)/C.

minimal low velocity forward diastolic flow (Fig. 3.5B). However, the most accurate way to discriminate the external from the internal carotid artery is to perform a temporal tap. Tapping one's finger over the superficial temporal artery (just anterior to the external auditory meatus) produces a characteristic appearance indicating that the Doppler signal is being sampled from the ECA. As the temporal artery is a branch of the ECA, velocity deflections caused by the tapping should be seen on the ECA waveform (Fig. 3.5B) (14,15).

Physiologically, approximately 80% of the CCA flow is directed to the brain; therefore, the normal Doppler waveform from the CCA has characteristics of both the ICA and the ECA flow (Fig. 3.5C). A Doppler waveform from the CCA that has the appearance of that from the ECA usually indicates the presence of an ipsilateral ICA occlusion.

Gray-Scale Imaging

The initial part of the Duplex examination of the carotid arteries is usually spent surveying the arterial segments by B-mode imaging. In clinical settings, the extent and severity of plaque are presented in descriptive or semiquantitative terms. For example, plaques may be described as extending from the CCA to the proximal third of the ICA and may be further labeled as mild, moderate, or severe. Furthermore, atherosclerosis may be circumferential or localized. As will be discussed later, it is generally possible to use the gray-scale image of the arterial wall and plaque in conjunction with color-coded flow in the lumen to have a rough estimate of the degree of diameter reduction (e.g., more or less than 50%, near-total or total occlusion) (16,17) (Fig. 3.6).

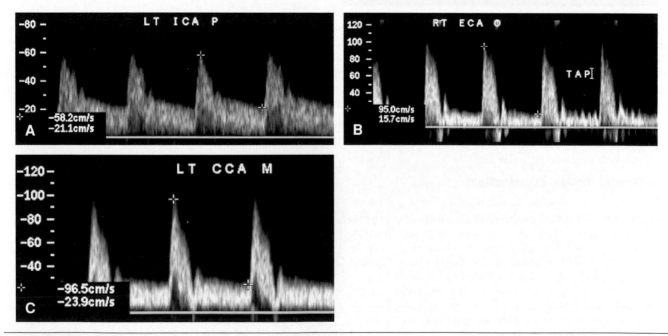

Figure 3.5 • Doppler waveforms form the carotid artery. A: Internal carotid artery flow demonstrating the characteristic low-resistance flow pattern with significant continuous diastolic flow. B: External carotid artery flow pattern demonstrating typical high-resistance vascular bed flow pattern with minimal diastolic blood flow. Note the typical effect of tapping on the superficial temporal artery on the Doppler waveform. C: Normal common carotid waveform. Common carotid artery waveform is usually a low-resistance wave since 80% of the blood flow ends in the internal carotid artery.

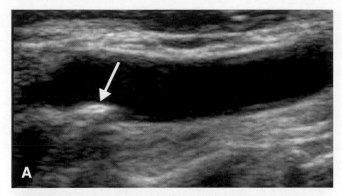

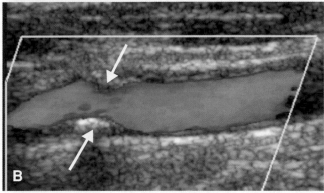

Figure 3.6 • B-mode image **(A)** and color Doppler **(B)** of the common carotid artery showing localized echogenic plaque producing mild degree of stenosis *(arrows)*.

Echogenicity of the plaque has been proposed as an indicator of plaque composition. Low echogenicity suggests a high content of lipid. Some lipid-laden plaques may be of such low echogenicity that they may not be visualized on gray-scale imaging. They are identified as a flow void on color imaging. Marked echogenicity with shadowing suggests calcification. The shadowing may be sufficiently extensive to preclude Doppler interrogation of the arterial segment under the area of calcification. Plaques predominantly composed of fibrous tissue will have an intermediate echogenicity comparable to surrounding muscular tissue but less echogenic than the arterial adventitia (16,18).

When the echogenicity of the plaque is variable, it is described as heterogenous. This is possibly caused by intraplaque hemorrhage and/or necrosis (19). Some studies have suggested that heterogenous plaques and intraplaque hemorrhage identified by gray-scale imaging are more frequently encountered in patients with clinical evidence of cerebral ischemia (20). Although surface ulceration of the plaque as detected by 2D ultrasound has been suggested as a risk factor for cerebral ischemic events (21), the data are inconsistent, and the reproducibility of this ultrasonographic finding is moderate (19,22).

Doppler Criteria for ICA Stenosis Severity

Doppler velocities provide validated and quantitative methods of grading carotid stenosis. The most common phenotypic finding is spectral broadening caused by turbulent flow at and just distal to the stenotic segment. The primary

measurement is the ICA PSV, which represents the cornerstone for grading carotid stenosis. However, the ICA EDV and the carotid index (defined as the ratio of the PSV in the ICA and the PSV in the CCA) are recommended to define the severity of carotid stenosis when technical or clinical concerns raise questions that ICA PSV may not represent the actual severity of disease (23).

The rationale for using these measurements is dependent on two pathophysiologic facts. First, the velocity of flow increases within a stenotic arterial segment, compared with the velocity of flow in a more proximal and relatively disease-free lumen. Although not linear, this relationship is proportional, such that certain ranges of flow velocities may be used to estimate the degree of diameter reduction. This applies to both the PSV and the EDV. Second, the atherosclerosis of the carotid arteries predominantly affects the carotid bifurcation, at the junction of the CCA and the ICA, and the proximal portion of the ICA. Normally, with laminar flow, there is no difference between CCA and ICA flow velocity. As the stenosis at the bifurcation increases in severity, the velocity in the ICA at the site of the stenosis increases but not that of the CCA velocity, which results in a higher ICA/CCA PSV ratio (Fig. 3.7).

Others have also examined the ICA/CCA EDV ratio, as well as the severity of spectral broadening in the ICA Doppler signal, which indicates more turbulent flow and is hence considered a sign of more severe stenosis.

Several sets of criteria have been proposed by leading vascular laboratories. The criteria most commonly followed are those proposed by Strandness (24) and Zwiebel (25). The Society of Radiologists in Ultrasound proposed a consensus set of criteria, based on the large body of evidence accumulated over the last two decades. A consensus statement by the "Society of Radiologists in Ultrasound Conference" has been adopted by the majority of vascular laboratories. The consensus statement's classification of carotid artery stenosis criteria is listed in Table 3.1. The criteria utilize both PSV and EDV cutoff values in addition to the ICA/CCA PSV ratio and take into account findings on B-mode imaging, particularly when the diagnosis of near occlusion or complete occlusion is being contemplated. It is important to exhaust all ultrasound techniques before diagnosing a total occlusion. Total occlusion is confirmed when there is no detectable patent lumen on the gray-scale image and no flow by spectral, power, and color Doppler (Fig. 3.8) (23).

The sensitivity and specificity of these criteria in diagnosing carotid stenosis vary depending on the PSV cutoffs used and can achieve 100% specificity and 96% sensitivity by adjusting the velocity according to the clinical situation (26). A meta-analysis of 41 studies found that the sensitivity and specificity of carotid duplex ultrasound for detecting a stenosis in the 70% to 99% range by angiography are 89% and 84%, respectively. The sensitivity and specificity of Doppler for detecting less severe stenoses (i.e., 50% to 69% range) are much lower (27). However, the diminished accuracy in detecting stenoses in the 50% to 69% range has no significant clinical implication in asymptomatic patients since these patients are rarely considered for revascularization.

Despite the publication of these criteria for defining lesion severity, it is critical for each laboratory to establish and validate its own criteria. The aforementioned sources of variability, both in the angiogram and in the duplex assessment,

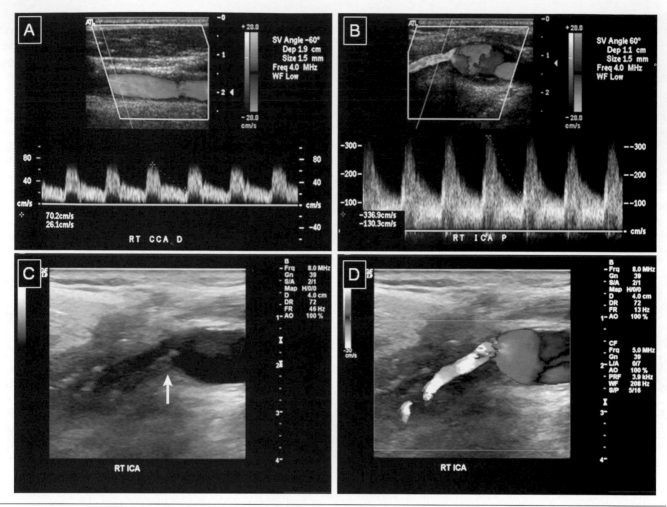

Figure 3.7 • Duplex examination of a diseased internal carotid artery. **A:** Mid common carotid artery demonstrating normal flow pattern and velocity. **B:** Proximal internal carotid artery flow demonstrating the elevated velocities consistent with proximal stenosis. The mosaic color flow reflects turbulence of flow in the stenotic segment. The peak systolic velocity is 337 cm/sec and the end diastolic velocity is 130 cm/sec consistent with >70% stenosis. The degree of stenosis is also confirmed by the ICA/CCA PSV ratio which is 4.8 consistent with >70% stenosis. **C:** B-mode image of the carotid bifurcation demonstrating complex plaque at the site of stenosis *(arrow)*. **D:** Superimposed color Doppler at the carotid bifurcation confirming the complex plaque to be the cause of the mosaic color pattern and flow disturbance.

cannot be overemphasized. The published criteria are a starting point that is fine tuned after internal quality control and correlation with CT and MR angiography, invasive angiography, and feedback following surgical endarterectomy. Therefore, physicians caring for patients with carotid disease should be familiar with the laboratory standards and criteria used to make the diagnosis. It is also imperative that angiographers and surgeons provide feedback to the vascular laboratory, in a continuous effort to improve the accuracy of reporting.

Caveats and Special Disease Subsets

The typical Doppler velocity thresholds used to define stenosis severity can lead to under- or overestimation of lesion severity in a number of conditions that ultrasound operators and interpreters need to be familiar with. Some of the more common conditions are described below.

CONTRALATERAL ICA OCCLUSION

In these cases, there is increased flow in the patent ICA and the vertebral arteries, to maintain adequate cerebral arterial perfusion. With the increased flow, the Doppler velocities in the patent ICA are elevated, giving the false impression of obstructive disease. The exact degree to which the ICA flow velocity increases in this setting is difficult to ascertain but may be dependent on the adequacy of the Circle of Willis, the contribution of vertebral flow, and the presence or absence of scar tissue in the distribution of the occluded ICA. Several investigators have modified existing Doppler cutoff values to define lesion severity within a patent ICA in the presence of a contralateral occlusion. A PSV of $\geq$140 cm/sec and EDV < 140 cm/sec were suggested as more accurate criteria to define a stenosis of 50–79%. Thresholds of PSV > 140 cm/sec and EDV > 140 cm/sec were proposed to define a stenosis between 80% and 99% (28). Other proposed criteria in

TABLE 3.1 Diagnostic Criteria for Internal Carotid Stenosis

Degree of Stenosis	Ultrasound Criteria
Normal	• PSV < 125 cm/sec • EDV < 40 cm/sec • ICA/CCA PSV ratio < 2 • No visible plaque or intimal thickening
<50% stenosis	• PSV < 125 cm/sec • EDV < 40 cm/sec • ICA/CCA PSV ratio < 2 • Visible plaque or intimal thickening
50–69% stenosis	• PSV 125–230 cm/sec • EDV 40–100 cm/sec • ICA/CCA PSV ratio 2–4 • Visible plaque
>70% stenosis	• PSV > 230 cm/sec • EDV > 100 cm/sec • ICA/CCA PSV ratio > 4 • Visible plaque
Near occlusion	• PSV > 230 cm/sec • EDV > 100 cm/sec • ICA/CCA PSV ratio > 4 • Markedly narrowed lumen on duplex ultrasound
Total occlusion	• No detectable lumen on B-mode imaging or flow on duplex ultrasound

(Adapted from Grant EG, Benson CB, Moneta GL, et al. Carotid artery stenosis: gray-scale and Doppler US diagnosis—Society of Radiologists in Ultrasound Consensus Conference. *Radiology*. 2003;229:340–346.)

this setting use a slightly higher threshold of EDV (155 cm/sec) to distinguish stenoses in the 50% to 79% from stenoses in the 80% to 99% range (29). Both of these adjusted Doppler criteria sets claim to have approximately 97% accuracy.

In order to determine how much of the increase in PSV is due to stenosis of the ICA and how much is due to compensatory flow, it may be useful to compare the velocities in the CCA. If there is a significant increase in the CCA velocities contralateral to an occluded ICA, then compensatory flow is contributing to the high velocity in the contralateral ICA. In patients with bilateral 80% to 99% stenoses who are undergoing carotid endarterectomy or stenting on one side, it is important to recheck the duplex ultrasound on the contralateral side soon after revascularization, to be certain that the stenosis is real and not due to compensatory flow (30).

FOLLOW-UP AFTER CAROTID ENDARTERECTOMY

Ultrasonography provides a sensitive and noninvasive tool for monitoring the success of carotid revascularization. Early duplex surveillance is recommended at 1 to 3 months after CEA or CAS. If the exam is normal (<50% residual stenosis), then surveillance every 1 to 2 years is adequate. If the exam is abnormal (50% to 79% residual stenosis), then surveillance every 6 months is recommended. For more severe residual stenoses (80% to 99%), confirmation of the severity followed by percutaneous or surgical revascularizations is recommended (31). However, the main advantage of surveillance carotid duplex is the early recognition and monitoring of contralateral carotid disease progression (32).

FOLLOW-UP AFTER CAROTID STENTING

The usual Doppler criteria may also create a false impression of obstructive disease following carotid stenting. In this situation, the ICA compliance is significantly reduced by the stent, and thus, the flow velocity may increase into a range that may be interpreted as a significant stenosis. Duplex examination of patients with carotid stents within days of a successful procedure (i.e., when the residual stenosis is minimal) identifies

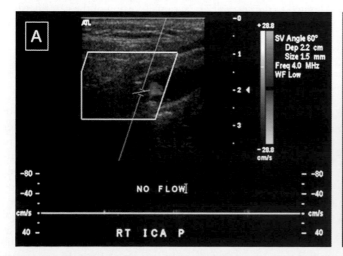
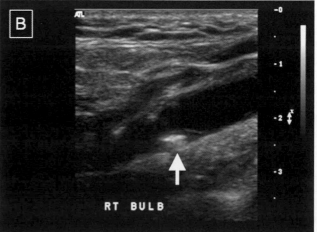

Figure 3.8 • Duplex ultrasound in a patient with occlusion of the internal carotid artery. **A:** Duplex ultrasound of an occluded right internal carotid artery. Note the absence of color Doppler flow and absence of continuous wave Doppler signals. **B:** B-mode image demonstrating the presence of complex plaque occluding the internal carotid artery lumen *(arrow)*.

a significant proportion of patients in whom the PSV is more than 125 cm/sec (31%) or the ICA/CCA PSV ratio is more than 2.0 (11%), suggesting a moderate stenosis. Recently, Lal et al. proposed new criteria to define a stenosis of at least 20%, after carotid stenting: PSV of at least 150 cm/sec and ICA/CCA PSV ratio of at least 2.16 (33). Although these preliminary data require further validation in larger data sets, it is clear that caution is warranted when interpreting Doppler velocities following carotid stenting.

COMMON CAROTID STENOSIS

Atherosclerotic obstructive disease may affect the CCA, most commonly at its origin. In these cases, and in the case of brachiocephalic stenosis, the CCA waveform may be dampened or its amplitude diminished (34). This is important, because there is no direct, gray-scale visualization of the origin of the CCA, and the changes in the waveform distal to the stenosis may represent the only clue to the diagnosis as determined by Duplex imaging. Another clue to the diagnosis is the difference between the velocity and the waveform patterns of the two CCAs. Although there may be some minor differences in the normal individual, significant differences should alert the examiner to the possibility of CCA disease. Ultrasonography should include Doppler waveforms taken as proximally as possible, using the linear transducer. If there is the suggestion that a stenosis may be present, a low-frequency transducer should be used to sample the origin of the brachiocephalic and left CCAs, directly. There are no well-defined criteria for the assessment of CCA stenoses. In cases of total ICA occlusion, when there is reduced ipsilateral flow, the CCA signal amplitude may also be diminished. If the changes are seen bilaterally, this points to a systemic phenomenon (e.g., low cardiac output or severe aortic stenosis) (17).

Vertebral Arterial Disease

Examination of the vertebral arteries usually accompanies Duplex evaluation of the carotid arteries. The vertebral arteries are located posterior to the CCA, and slightly medially. They may be visualized on gray-scale imaging from the origin to the point of entry into the skull, although the origin is technically challenging to examine. It is usually easy to obtain a Doppler signal from the vertebral artery and the normal flow velocity ranges between 20 to 40 cm/sec (Fig. 3.9A).

In the presence of significant disease, the signal is damped distal to the obstruction, and the velocity is <20 cm/sec. Although the criteria for diagnosis of vertebral lesions are not as robust as those published for carotid lesions, the accuracy of Duplex ultrasound in identifying severe lesions and total occlusions is quite high (i.e., approximately 95%). Duplex imaging, however, is not so accurate with lesions at the origin of the vertebral artery.

When the signal of vertebral flow is unusually strong and the velocity is more than 40 cm/sec, this raises the suspicion that there is increased ipsilateral flow. This may be the result of a contralateral vertebral occlusion, contralateral subclavian steal, or severe carotid disease, with the ipsilateral vertebral artery contributing significantly to collateral flow (Fig. 3.9B). In cases of subclavian steal, the direction of flow signal in the ipsilateral vertebral artery is reversed and indicates a severe stenosis in the innominate or subclavian artery proximal to the origin of the vertebral artery (35,36).

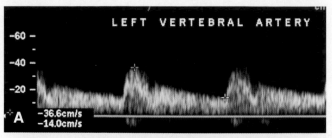
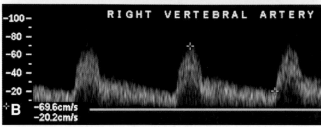

Figure 3.9 • Doppler waveforms from left **(A)** and right **(B)** vertebral arteries of the patient shown in Figure 3.8. The flow velocities in the left vertebral artery are normal. The flow velocities in the right vertebral artery are increased compared to the left because of the collateral flow from the vertebral artery to the ipsilateral carotid system.

Limitations of Carotid and Vertebral Duplex Examination

Pooled data from the literature point to significant and wide variation in the measurement properties between laboratories. These variations are clinically relevant (37). Similarly, inter- and intraobserver variability exists within technologists and interpreters alike (38). Therefore, the importance of setting individual laboratory criteria and validating them with the help of angiographers and surgeons cannot be overemphasized. Moreover, the Doppler velocities may be influenced by arterial calcifications, kinking, and tortuosity rendering the test inaccurate. The area imaged by carotid ultrasound examination is limited to the cervical extracranial portion of the carotid arteries and the intracranial portion may only be examined by transcranial Doppler (TCD).

Transcranial Doppler Examination

TCD is a technique to examine the intracranial arteries using ultrasonography. It may be performed using blind Doppler probes to detect velocity signals, but currently, it is possible to obtain the standard, spectral-Doppler signals, gray-scale images, and color-coded Doppler images, as well. Direct visualization using Duplex scanners is important, as it reduces the possibility of error in identifying specific vessels. The examination requires an acoustic window through which it is possible to isolate the intracranial vessels. The middle (MCA), anterior (ACA), and posterior cerebral arteries (PCA) are usually identified through a transtemporal window (above the zygomatic arch). The ophthalmic artery and the ICA siphon are approached via a transorbital window. The vertebral and basilar arteries are reached via a suboccipital window.

Identification of the different arteries is based on prior knowledge of their expected depth and direction of flow. For example, the normal MCA is located at a depth of 40 to 50 mm, its normal flow is toward the transducer, and its mean velocity is 30 to 80 cm/sec. The ACA is slightly deeper, and flow is directed away from the transducer in the transtemporal window. Vertebral and basilar arterial flow are both away from the transducer, with velocities ranging between 30 to 40 cm/sec. The diagnosis of an ICA stenosis depends on identifying the following: flow reversal in the ipsilateral ophthalmic artery, >50% difference between the carotid siphon velocities, >35% difference between MCA velocities, >50% difference between ACA velocities, and >35% difference between the ipsilateral MCA and PCA PSVs. These criteria have very high specificity (100%) with low sensitivity (39).

Obstructive lesions in intracranial vessels are diagnosed when there is focal turbulence and velocity increase in a specific segment of an artery, together with a drop in distal velocity. Reversal of expected direction of flow and evidence of collateral circulation development are other clues to obstructive disease.

Emerging Applications

Recently, attempts have been made to develop three-dimensional (3D) imaging of carotid arteries and carotid plaques. This has the advantage of measuring plaque volume to account for complex plaque shapes that cannot be adequately appreciated on 2D imaging. Plaque volume measurement can be used in monitoring progression or regression of disease with different therapeutic interventions (40). Interpretation of 3D ultrasound should be done with caution, as it tends to underestimate stenosis severity (41).

By averaging multiple images, compound ultrasound improves the visualization of plaque texture and surface and reduces artifacts. This improves the interobserver agreement in defining plaque echogenicity and with the advent of the more powerful computer systems, real-time compound ultrasound is now available for clinical practice (42).

THE ABDOMINAL AORTA

Similar to lower extremity arterial disease, the prevalence of small abdominal aortic aneurysms (AAA) measuring 2.9 to 4.9 cm in diameter is dependent on age and, to a lesser degree, on gender. Among men between 45 and 54 years old, the prevalence is 1.3%. This increases almost 10-fold to 12.5% among men over 75 years. In women, the prevalence is lower, ranging from 0% to 5.2% in the above age groups (2). The etiology of AAA is complex and shares its risk factors with atherosclerotic risk factors such as smoking, hypertension, coronary artery disease, and peripheral vascular disease (2). Indeed, patients with AAA have higher prevalence of systemic atherosclerosis (43,44).

Ultrasonography is a safe, accurate, and inexpensive screening test for the presence of an AAA (2). Once detected, the size of the AAA can be accurately measured and monitored over time, so that a clinical decision about timing of repair is made before it is likely to rupture. Moreover, vascular ultrasound provides important information regarding the presence of dissection or intramural thrombus, which influence the prognosis and risk of rupture of AAA (Fig. 3.10). Using a systematic approach and applying the criteria for screening programs adopted by the WHO, AAA screening is justifiable in high-risk populations (45). The US Preventive Services Task Force recently recommended a one-time screening for AAA by ultrasonography for men aged 65 to 75 years who have ever smoked (46). Similar recommendations are provided by the ACC/AHA practice guidelines with the addition of screening males > 60 years who are siblings or offspring of patients with AAA (2). The current guidelines recommend surgical or endovascular repair of infrarenal or juxtarenal AAA ≥ 5.0 to 5.5 cm in diameter and suprarenal AAA or type IV thoracoabdominal aortic aneurysms measuring 5.5 to 6.0 cm in diameter. Ultrasound monitoring is recommended every 6 to 12 months for AAA that are 4.0 to 5.4 cm in diameter and every 2 to 3 years for AAA less than 4.0 cm in diameter (2).

With sensitivity and specificity rates approaching 100% (2,46–48), ultrasound imaging is the preferred method for screening and monitoring of AAA size. CT and MRI scans are usually reserved for repair planning in patients carrying the diagnosis and needing endovascular or surgical repair. Ultrasound examinations can also be utilized for follow-up evaluation of the repaired aneurysm, using both B-mode imaging and Doppler evaluation (Fig. 3.11).

The exam is performed in the fasting state to decrease bowel gas overlap and improve imaging. The typical aortic ultrasound exam includes measuring the maximum aortic diameter in the anteroposterior, longitudinal, and transverse sections with attention to avoid oblique cuts that overestimate the diameter of the aorta. The reproducibility and inter- and intraobserver variability are excellent, making this test an excellent screening and follow-up surveillance tool. However, ultrasound is not reliable in screening or monitoring suprarenal aortic or iliac artery aneurysms and is not recommended for these indications (2).

THE RENAL ARTERIES

The overall prevalence of renal artery stenosis (RAS) in population-based studies is approximately 6% (49). The prevalence is higher among high-risk patients such as those with coronary artery disease, peripheral vascular disease, and older individuals. Although RAS is the most common treatable cause of hypertension in the adult population, it remains a significantly underrecognized condition (50). The threshold level of RAS that induces hypertension is not known and is probably different among individual patients. Ultrasound Duplex examination of the renal arteries is a helpful modality for assessing the severity and hemodynamic significance of RAS. Given its simplicity and lack of exposure to contrast or radiation, renal duplex examination is recommended as an acceptable first-line screening test for RAS (2). Duplex examination is a helpful monitoring tool following renal artery interventions and is not hampered by the effects of metal artifact (i.e., in contrast to MR angiography) (51).

Although technically challenging, renal Duplex exam provides important information when evaluating a patient with suspected RAS. Direct Doppler information from the renal artery ostium and main renal artery helps detect atherosclerotic and nonatherosclerotic (i.e., most commonly fibromuscular dysplasia) stenoses. Important indirect

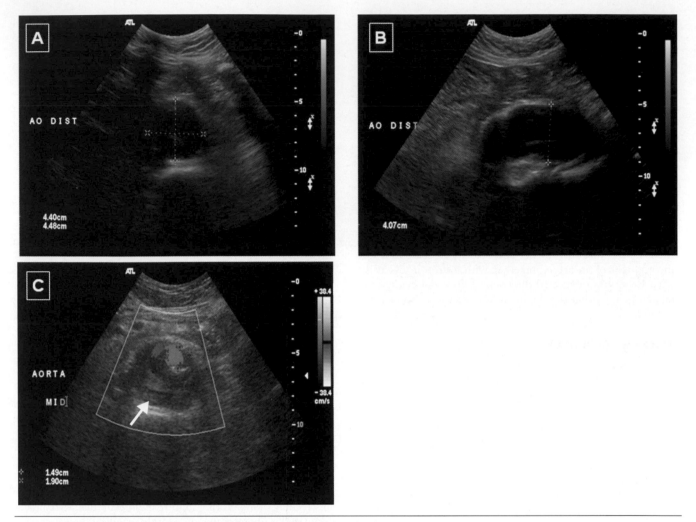

Figure 3.10 • Utility of Duplex examination of the abdominal aorta. A transverse section B-mode image of the infrarenal abdominal aorta **(A)** demonstrates an aneurysm measuring 4.5 cm in diameter. The sagittal section of the same segment **(B)** confirms the diagnosis of the aneurysm and rules out the presence of thrombus. In other aortic aneurysms **(C)**, B-mode imaging can reveal a thrombus-filled aneurysmal sac *(arrow)* and color Doppler demonstrates the flow channel.

information that helps assess the health of the parenchyma of the ipsilateral kidney is derived from assessment of the kidney size and resistive indices of the segmental arteries (see below). In addition, associated abdominal aortic pathology can be assessed.

The technical challenges encountered during imaging the renal arteries include the posterior takeoff of the renal arteries (most commonly the left renal artery), and the multiple tissue layers (abdominal wall muscles and fat) as well as bowel gas separating the ultrasound probe from the renal arteries. Therefore, imaging of the renal arteries carries a steep learning curve and is heavily operator dependent. Even with experience, renal artery studies are technically suboptimal in 5% to 12% of cases (52). Exam quality is optimized by performing the study in the morning after 12 hours of fasting. The use of color Doppler facilitates the recognition of vascular structures and helps avoid sampling of incorrect vessels. A low-frequency transducer, 2.5 to 3 MHz, is typically used to

image the deeply located renal arteries. If bowel gas is prohibitive, imaging with the patient in the lateral position may be helpful. The main and accessory renal arteries (if present) are identified with B-mode imaging, and pulsed wave and color Doppler are performed to ensure proper sampling. An alternative strategy to properly sample the renal arteries is to start by localizing them at the renal hilum and follow them back to their aortic origin. Kidney size is measured in longitudinal (i.e., superior pole to inferior pole) and transverse planes, and Doppler signals are obtained from the abdominal aorta, renal artery ostium, main renal artery, and the interlobar branches from the superior, middle, and inferior segments of each kidney (15,35).

The renal artery velocities are compared with those in the abdominal aorta at the level of the renal artery. Normally the PSV of the aorta at the level of the renal arteries is 100 ± 20 cm/sec. Similar to the internal carotid arteries, the renal artery normally has a low resistive signal since it is supplying

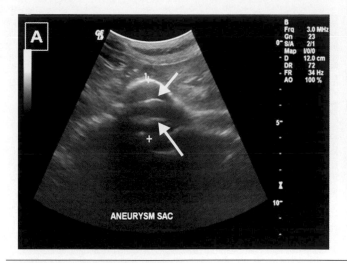
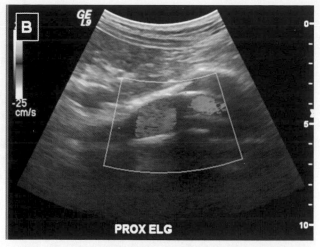

Figure 3.11 • Duplex examination of an aortic aneurysm after endoluminal graft repair. An abdominal aortic aneurysm treated with an endoluminal graft (ELG). B-mode imaging **(A)** is used to define the aneurysmal sac (between "+" cursor markers), which is excluded by the ELG (longitudinal structure traversing the center of the sac–*arrows*). The superimposed color Doppler **(B)** on the proximal ELG image demonstrates no evidence of flow into the excluded sac.

a low-resistance vascular bed (Fig. 3.12). The normal PSV in the renal arteries is 80 to 120 cm/sec and the PSV/EDV ratio is around 0.33. There should be no significant difference between the aortic and renal PSV under normal circumstances and the renal-aortic PSV ratio (RAR) is typically 1.1 ± 0.3.

Several Doppler criteria have been proposed to diagnose the presence of RAS (Table 3.2). To avoid errors caused by the large variability in normal renal artery PSV, the ratio between the PSV in the renal artery and the aorta was devised (i.e., renal aortic ratio [RAR]) (59). A RAR > 3.5 correlates with a significant stenosis (at least 60% diameter reduction). This cutoff value has a sensitivity of 84% and a specificity of 97% (53). A threshold PSV value of >180 cm/sec has also been proposed to define the presence of significant RAS, with the accuracy exceeding 90% (54). Sensitivity and specificity are improved if there is a significant reduction in the distal velocity, in addition to the proximal PSV > 180 cm/sec (57). A more commonly accepted velocity cutoff is a PSV of at least 200 cm/sec, in the presence of turbulent flow by color Doppler, which corresponds to a 60% diameter reduction with very high sensitivity and specificity (Fig. 3.13) (55). In a large prospective study to compare duplex imaging to renal DSA, the diagnosis of significant RAS (i.e., corresponding to >60% diameter stenosis by DSA) was achieved by demonstrating one or both of the following Doppler findings: a RAR ≥ 3.5 and/or a PSV ≥ 200 cm/sec (Fig. 3.13). Both sensitivity and specificity of the duplex criteria in this study were 98% (56).

Other findings that are helpful in making the diagnosis include an EDV ≥ 150 cm/sec, which corresponded to an RAS of at least 80% (56). A simple measurement of the kidney length demonstrating diminished size (i.e., less than 10 cm, or significantly smaller than the contralateral kidney) is also another clue to RAS of more than 60% or total occlusion, since such a degree of reduced arterial flow is often accompanied by loss of renal mass (60).

Overall, the sensitivity and specificity of renal artery duplex for diagnosing hemodynamically significant RAS are excellent, ranging from 84% to 98% and 62% to 99%, respectively (53,54,59,61–64). Pooled data from multiple studies showed that the PSV is more sensitive and specific than RAR (65).

The renal resistive index (RRI) is a variable derived from the Doppler signal obtained from the interlobar arteries in the renal parenchyma. It is calculated as the average of (1 + (EDV/PSV)) derived from the superior, middle, and inferior renal segments (57) (Fig. 3.14). Under normal circumstances, with a low-resistance flow pattern in the renal parenchyma, the RI is typically in the 0.5 to 0.6 range. As the flow pattern begins to assume a high-resistance pattern, reflective of parenchymal disease, the RRI increases. Although the RRI has been proposed as a tool to help determine the health of the renal parenchyma, and thus as a predictor of clinical response to renal artery revascularization, the current literature demonstrates an inconsistent relationship between RRI and clinical outcomes following renal artery revascularization. In a retrospective study, 131 patients with RAS treated with renal artery balloon angioplasty were evaluated with multiple duplex parameters including RRI. Among the 35 patients with elevated RRI (>0.8), no improvement in blood pressure control or renal function was noted as compared to those with RRI < 0.8. This was a small, retrospective study that included patients treated primarily with balloon angioplasty (57). Prospective studies did not establish a correlation between the RRI and improvement in blood pressure control or renal function following renal artery stenting (66). This is likely explained by the fact that RRI can be influenced by a number of factors including the presence of proximal RAS (falsely decrease), valvular heart disease (e.g., aortic stenosis—falsely decrease, aortic regurgitation—falsely increase), and stiff calcified aorta (falsely increase). The current guidelines do not endorse the use of RRI as a predictor of success following renal artery revascularizations (2).

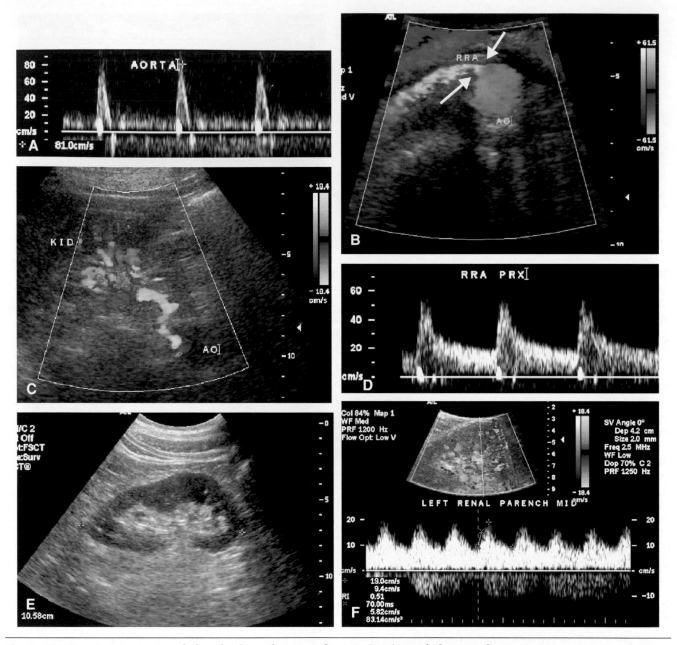

Figure 3.12 • Components of the duplex ultrasound examination of the renal arteries. **A:** Doppler waveform obtained from aorta, at the level of the renal arteries. **B:** B-mode and color Doppler allow identification of origin of the right renal artery *(arrows)*. **C:** Path of right renal artery is shown from the origin to hilum of kidney. **D:** Doppler waveform obtained from origin, proximal, mid-, and distal sections of the artery. **E:** Right kidney size measured, using B-mode image. **F:** Doppler signals obtained from segmental arteries in the upper, mid-, and lower poles of the kidney.

There are a number of limitations to Duplex imaging of the renal arteries. In addition to the technical difficulties posed by bowel gas and obesity, most studies have shown a limited sensitivity in the detection of accessory renal arteries (i.e., approximately 60%). In cases in which duplex imaging is falsely negative, the presence of RAS in an accessory artery is the most common explanation (55). Renal artery duplex imaging is very useful in follow-up monitoring after revascularization procedures (51). With the increasing use of metallic stents in renal artery revascularization procedures, MR and CT angiography often provide inadequate image quality, resulting from artifacts caused by the metal.

THE MESENTERIC ARTERIES

The gut is supplied by three main arteries that arise directly from the abdominal aorta: the celiac trunk, the superior mesenteric artery (SMA), and the inferior mesenteric artery (IMA). All of these aortic branches are susceptible to atherosclerotic

TABLE 3.2 Duplex Criteria for Diagnosis of Renal Artery Stenosis*

Reference	Criteria	Sensitivity[†]	Specificity[†]	Comments
Taylor et al. (53)	RAR > 3.5	84	97	
Hoffman et al. (54)	PSV > 180 cm/sec	95	90	
Hansen et al. (55)	PSV ≥ 200 cm/sec	93	98	Excluding kidneys with multiple vessels
	PSV ≥ 200 cm/sec	67	100	Including kidneys with multiple vessels
Olin et al. (56)	PSV ≥ 200 cm/sec and/or RAR ≥ 3.5	98	98	
	EDV ≥ 150 cm/sec			RAS ≥ 80% by DSA
Radermacher et al. (57)	PSV > 180 cm/sec and distal velocity < 25% of PSV	97	98	RAS ≥ 50% by DSA
Schwerk et al. (58)	Delta RI > 5%	100	94	Underestimates severity if bilateral RAS, RI better used for prognostication

*Renal artery stenosis (RAS) refers to stenosis ≥ 60% by angiography, unless otherwise specified.
†Using angiography as the gold standard.
RAR, renal aortic ratio; EDV, end-diastolic velocity; PSV, peak systolic velocity; DSA, digital subtraction angiography; RI, renal resistive index; RAS, renal artery stenosis.

disease, particularly at their origins (67). Acute mesenteric ischemia usually results from thrombosis or embolism to one of those arteries, which leads to a life-threatening situation in which there is rarely any time for noninvasive testing, and angiography is the preferred tool (2). In cases of chronic, progressive atherosclerosis, intestinal ischemia generally does not develop unless both the celiac artery and the SMA (and possibly the inferior mesenteric artery as well) are significantly obstructed. This is attributed to the very rich network of collaterals that prevents the development of clinically significant

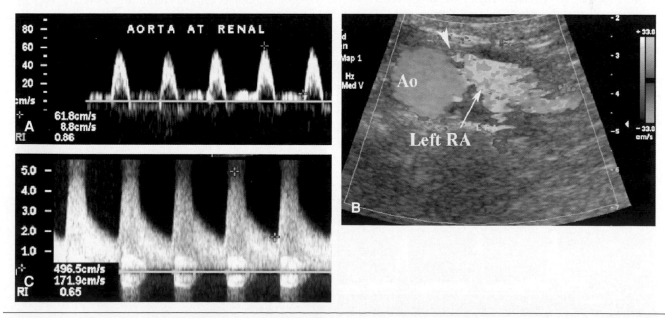

Figure 3.13 • Doppler examination from patient with severe renal artery stenosis. A: Doppler waveform obtained from abdominal aorta at the level of the aorta. B: Color Doppler image showing marked turbulent flow, at the origin of the left renal artery indicative of a severe stenosis *(arrow)*. C: Doppler waveform from the proximal left renal artery. This waveform meets all the criteria for the diagnosis of severe renal artery stenosis, specifically: PSV >200 cm/sec (496 cm/sec), EDV >150 cm/sec (171 cm/sec), and RAR >3.5 (8.1).

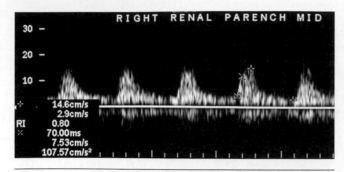

Figure 3.14 • Doppler waveform from segmental artery in mid-pole of right kidney. Compare this waveform with that in Figure 3.12F. Note that the ratio of the EDV to the PSV is much lower in this waveform, with a resistive index of 0.8, suggesting the presence of parenchymal disease in the kidney.

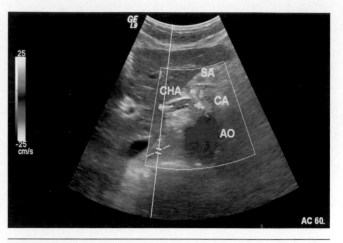

Figure 3.15 • Axial view of the proximal abdominal aorta with color Doppler flow demonstrating the origin of the celiac trunk (CA), which then bifurcates into common hepatic (CHA) and splenic (SA) arteries.

ischemia if obstructive disease is only limited to one arterial bed. Mesenteric duplex imaging can be used to accurately investigate patients presenting with unexplained chronic abdominal pain or weight loss in whom chronic intestinal ischemia is suspected (2).

Patients are required to fast for at least 6 hours prior to mesenteric artery imaging. In addition to eliminating bowel gases, this practice is critically important in the case of SMA imaging, since the Doppler velocity pattern is entirely different in the fasting and postprandial states. Technically, patients are imaged in the supine position, using a 2.0- to 3.0-MHz transducer placed in the epigastrium. B-mode and color imaging allow identification of the arteries as they arise from the abdominal aorta (Fig. 3.15), and the Doppler waveforms are obtained after ensuring that the angle of insonation is <60 degrees (Fig. 3.16) (35).

Since the majority of celiac trunk flow supplies two low-resistance beds (i.e., liver and spleen), the normal velocity

pattern in that artery is that of a low-resistance circulation (Fig. 3.16) (15,35,68). In the fasting state, SMA flow is typical of a high-resistance arterial bed. Within 1 minute of eating, and for about 6 hours afterward, the SMA arterial bed dilates significantly and turns into a low-resistance system with a low-resistance waveform (i.e., no reversal in direction of flow following systole, continuous diastolic flow, and a relatively high EDV). The Doppler velocity pattern of the IMA is normally triphasic, typical of high-resistance vascular beds (Fig. 3.16C). It is not usual for the IMA flow to change to a low-resistance pattern in the postprandial setting, since the resistance in the capillary bed of the colon is not as variable as that of the small bowel (15).

Several Doppler velocity cutoff thresholds have been used to noninvasively diagnose obstructive lesions in the mesenteric

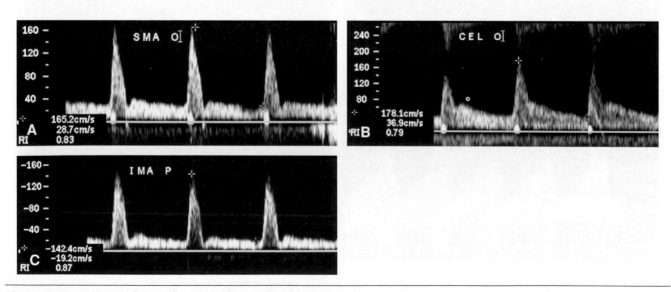

Figure 3.16 • Normal Doppler waveforms from mesenteric vessels. **A:** Superior mesenteric artery in the fasting state, with high resistance pattern. **B:** Celiac artery in the fasting state, with low-resistance pattern. **C:** Inferior mesenteric artery with high-resistance pattern.

TABLE 3.3	Diagnostic Criteria for Significant Disease in Mesenteric Arteries
Degree of Stenosis	**Ultrasound Criteria**
Celiac (>70% stenosis) (69)	• PSV ≥ 200 cm/sec • EDV ≥ 55 cm/sec
Superior mesenteric (>70% stenosis) (69–72)	• PSV > 275 cm/sec • EDV ≥ 45 cm/sec

arteries. In the case of celiac artery stenosis, the EDV is a better predictor for stenosis than the PSV (Table 3.3). An EDV ≥55 cm/sec or no detected flow has very high overall accuracy of 95%. The sensitivity and specificity of this cutoff are 95% and 100%, respectively. A PSV ≥200 cm/sec achieved an overall accuracy, sensitivity, and specificity of 93%, 93%, and 94%, respectively. The advantage of duplex scanning includes its ability to provide valuable information about the flow in branch arteries, and the reversal of blood flow in the hepatic artery carries an accuracy of 100% in diagnosing severe celiac artery stenosis or occlusion (69) (Fig. 3.17).

Most of the published parameters for mesenteric artery stenosis have been validated in the fasting state in which the SMA displays a high-resistance waveform (Table 3.3). A PSV >275 cm/sec is generally accepted as a cutoff for greater than 70% stenosis of the SMA (Fig. 3.18). The specificity increases if a higher cutoff (≥300 cm/sec) is chosen but results in lower sensitivity. In the postprandial state, the SMA displays a low-resistance waveform with high diastolic flow due to the significant dilatation in its arterial bed. In the case of significant stenosis, the increase in diastolic flow is blunted, but including postprandial duplex scanning of the SMA does not appear to allow further stratification of the stenosis, or improve the sensitivity or specificity of the test (73). An EDV ≥45 cm/sec

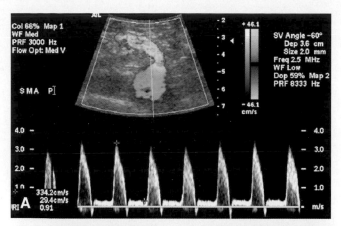

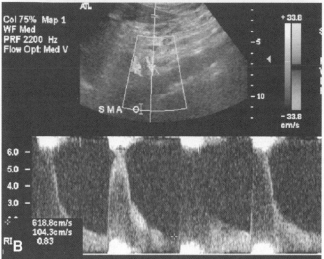

Figure 3.18 • Two examples of Doppler waveforms from patients with superior mesenteric artery stenosis. **A:** The PSV is >275 cm/sec and there is turbulence of flow in the color Doppler image. **B:** The PSV is >300 cm/sec, the EDV is >45 cm/sec, and there is turbulence of flow in the color Doppler image.

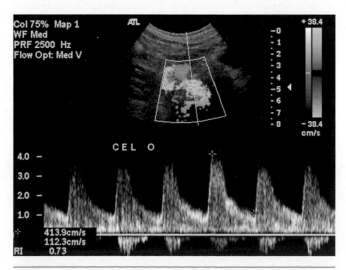

Figure 3.17 • Doppler waveform from celiac artery. The PSV is >200 cm/sec and the EDV is >55 cm/sec, indicating the presence of severe stenosis. Note the marked turbulence of flow demonstrated in the color Doppler picture above consistent with the presence of a significant stenosis.

offers the best sensitivity (90%), specificity (91%), positive predictive value (90%), and negative predictive value (91%) for diagnosing SMA stenosis ≥50% (69). Other investigators have demonstrated higher negative predictive value of duplex scanning in the setting of SMA stenosis (99%) and concluded that a negative scan virtually rules out SMA stenosis as the etiology for chronic abdominal pain (74). The overall diagnostic accuracy of mesenteric duplex scanning approaches 90% for the presence of a stenosis >70% (69–72).

The same technical considerations that applied to renal artery imaging apply to imaging the mesenteric vessels. Beyond reducing bowel gas, fasting is important in SMA imaging since the fasting and postprandial flow characteristics are entirely different. Although technically challenging, in an experienced laboratory, 98% of SMAs and 96% of celiac arteries imaged are technically adequate (69). However, vascular duplex is unable to evaluate the distal portions of the mesenteric arteries. Evaluation of the IMA is very difficult by duplex ultrasound due to its small size and short course. The IMA is an important contributor to the gut vascularity and collaterals especially in the case of SMA or celiac artery stenosis. Moreover, the mesenteric arteries commonly have anatomic variations. The proper identification of these anatomic variations is important in the diagnosis and management of mesenteric ischemia. Vascular duplex ultrasound does not provide sufficient data to diagnose or identify these variations with certainty.

References

1. Strandness DE Jr, Schultz RD, Sumner DS, et al. Ultrasonic flow detection. A useful technic in the evaluation of peripheral vascular disease. *Am J Surg.* 1967;113:311–320.
2. Hirsch AT, Haskal ZJ, Hertzer NR, et al. ACC/AHA 2005 Practice Guidelines for the management of patients with peripheral arterial disease (lower extremity, renal, mesenteric, and abdominal aortic): a collaborative report from the American Association for Vascular Surgery/Society for Vascular Surgery, Society for Cardiovascular Angiography and Interventions, Society for Vascular Medicine and Biology, Society of Interventional Radiology, and the ACC/AHA Task Force on Practice Guidelines (Writing Committee to Develop Guidelines for the Management of Patients With Peripheral Arterial Disease): endorsed by the American Association of Cardiovascular and Pulmonary Rehabilitation; National Heart, Lung, and Blood Institute; Society for Vascular Nursing; TransAtlantic Inter-Society Consensus; and Vascular Disease Foundation. *Circulation.* 2006;113:e463–e654.
3. Moneta GL, Yeager RA, Lee RW, et al. Noninvasive localization of arterial occlusive disease: a comparison of segmental Doppler pressures and arterial duplex mapping. *J Vasc Surg.* 1993;17: 578–582.
4. Pinto F, Lencioni R, Napoli V, et al. Peripheral ischemic occlusive arterial disease: comparison of color Doppler sonography and angiography. *J Ultrasound Med.* 1996;15:697–704; quiz 705–706.
5. Whelan JF, Barry MH, Moir JD. Color flow Doppler ultrasonography: comparison with peripheral arteriography for the investigation of peripheral vascular disease. *J Clin Ultrasound.* 1992;20:369–374.
6. de Smet AA, Ermers EJ, Kitslaar PJ. Duplex velocity characteristics of aortoiliac stenoses. *J Vasc Surg.* 1996;23:628–636.
7. Sacks D, Robinson ML, Marinelli DL, et al. Peripheral arterial Doppler ultrasonography: diagnostic criteria. *J Ultrasound Med.* 1992;11:95–103.
8. Koelemay MJ, den Hartog D, Prins MH, et al. Diagnosis of arterial disease of the lower extremities with duplex ultrasonography. *Br J Surg.* 1996;83:404–409.
9. Rose SC. Noninvasive vascular laboratory for evaluation of peripheral arterial occlusive disease. I. Hemodynamic principles and tools of the trade. *J Vasc Interv Radiol.* 2000;11:1257–1275.
10. North American Symptomatic Carotid Endarterectomy Trial. Methods, patient characteristics, and progress. *Stroke.* 1991;22:711–720.
11. MRC European Carotid Surgery Trial: interim results for symptomatic patients with severe (70–99%) or with mild (0–29%) carotid stenosis. European Carotid Surgery Trialists' Collaborative Group. *Lancet.* 1991;337:1235–1243.
12. Endarterectomy for asymptomatic carotid artery stenosis. Executive Committee for the Asymptomatic Carotid Atherosclerosis Study. *JAMA.* 1995;273:1421–1428.
13. Rothwell PM, Gibson RJ, Slattery J, et al. Equivalence of measurements of carotid stenosis. A comparison of three methods on 1001 angiograms. European Carotid Surgery Trialists' Collaborative Group. *Stroke.* 1994;25:2435–2439.
14. Zwiebel WJ. Normal carotid arteries and carotid exmination technique. In: Zwiebel WJ, ed. *Introduction to Vascular Ultrasonography.* 4th ed. Philadelphia, PA: WB Saunders; 2000:113–124.
15. Strandness DEJ. Noninvasive vascular laboratory and vascular imaging. In: Young JR, Olin JW, Bartholomew JR, ed. *Peripheral Vascular Diseases.* St. Louis, MO: Mosby Publishing Company; 1996:33–64.
16. Zwiebel WJ. Ultrasound assessment of carotid plaque. In: Zwiebel WJ, ed. *Introduction to Vascular Ultrasonography.* 4th ed. Philadelphia, PA: WB Saunders; 2000:125–135.
17. Zwiebel WJ. Doppler evaluation of carotid stenosis. In: Zwiebel WJ, ed. *Introduction to Vascular Ultrasonography.* 4th ed. Philadelphia, PA: WB Saunders; 2000:137–154.
18. Widder B, Paulat K, Hackspacher J, et al. Morphological characterization of carotid artery stenoses by ultrasound duplex scanning. *Ultrasound Med Biol.* 1990;16:349–354.
19. Bluth EI, Kay D, Merritt CR, et al. Sonographic characterization of carotid plaque: detection of hemorrhage. *Am J Roentgenol.* 1986;146:1061–1065.
20. Imparato AM, Riles TS, Mintzer R, et al. The importance of hemorrhage in the relationship between gross morphologic characteristics and cerebral symptoms in 376 carotid artery plaques. *Ann Surg.* 1983;197:195–203.
21. O'Donnell TF Jr, Erdoes L, Mackey WC, et al. Correlation of B-mode ultrasound imaging and arteriography with pathologic findings at carotid endarterectomy. *Arch Surg.* 1985;120: 443–449.
22. Ratliff DA, Gallagher PJ, Hames TK, et al. Characterisation of carotid artery disease: comparison of duplex scanning with histology. *Ultrasound Med Biol.* 1985;11:835–840.
23. Grant EG, Benson CB, Moneta GL, et al. Carotid artery stenosis: gray-scale and Doppler US diagnosis—Society of Radiologists in Ultrasound Consensus Conference. *Radiology.* 2003;229:340–346.
24. Strandness DEJ. Extracranial arterial disease. In: Strandness DEJ, ed. *Duplex Scanning in Vascular Disorders.* 2nd ed. New York, NY: Raven Press; 1993:113–158.
25. Zwiebel WJ. Doppler evaluation of carotid stenosis. In: Zwiebel WJ, ed. *Introduction to Vascular Ultrasonography.* 3rd ed. Philadelphia, PA: WB Saunders; 1992:123–132.
26. Suwanwela N, Can U, Furie KL, et al. Carotid Doppler ultrasound criteria for internal carotid artery stenosis based on residual lumen diameter calculated from en bloc carotid endarterectomy specimens. *Stroke.* 1996;27:1965–1969.
27. Wardlaw JM, Chappell FM, Best JJ, et al. Non-invasive imaging compared with intra-arterial angiography in the diagnosis of symptomatic carotid stenosis: a meta-analysis. *Lancet.* 2006;367:1503–1512.
28. AbuRahma AF, Richmond BK, Robinson PA, et al. Effect of contralateral severe stenosis or carotid occlusion on duplex criteria of ipsilateral stenoses: comparative study of various duplex parameters. *J Vasc Surg.* 1995;22:751–761; discussion 761–762.
29. Fujitani RM, Mills JL, Wang LM, et al. The effect of unilateral internal carotid arterial occlusion upon contralateral duplex study: criteria for accurate interpretation. *J Vasc Surg.* 1992;16:459–467; discussion 467–468.
30. Sachar R, Yadav JS, Roffi M, et al. Severe bilateral carotid stenosis: the impact of ipsilateral stenting on Doppler-defined contralateral stenosis. *J Am Coll Cardiol.* 2004;43:1358–1362.
31. Bandyk DF. Ultrasound assessment during and after peripheral interventions. In: Zwiebel W, ed. *Introduction to Vascular Ultrasonography.* 5th ed. Philadelphia, PA: WB Saunders, 2004:357–379.
32. Roth SM, Back MR, Bandyk DF, et al. A rational algorithm for duplex scan surveillance after carotid endarterectomy. *J Vasc Surg.* 1999;30:453–460.
33. Lal BK, Hobson RW 2nd, Goldstein J, et al. Carotid artery stenting: is there a need to revise ultrasound velocity criteria? *J Vasc Surg.* 2004;39:58–66.
34. Hriljac I, Gustavson S, Olin JW. Images in vascular ultrasound. Stenosis of the innominate or left common carotid artery

origin diagnosed on carotid ultrasound examination. *Vasc Med.* 2003;8:287–288.

35. Zwolak RM. Arterial duplex imaging. In: Rutherford RB, ed. *Vascular Surgery.* 5th ed. Philadelphia, PA: WB Saunders; 2000:192–214.

36. Ricci MA, Knight SJ. The role of noninvasive studies in the diagnosis and management of cerebrovascular disease. In: Rutherford RB, ed. *Vascular Surgery.* 5th ed. Philadelphia, PA: WB Saunders; 2000:1775–1789.

37. Jahromi AS, Cina CS, Liu Y, et al. Sensitivity and specificity of color duplex ultrasound measurement in the estimation of internal carotid artery stenosis: a systematic review and meta-analysis. *J Vasc Surg.* 2005;41:962–972.

38. Criswell BK, Langsfeld M, Tullis MJ, et al. Evaluating institutional variability of duplex scanning in the detection of carotid artery stenosis. *Am J Surg.* 1998;176:591–597.

39. Can U, Furie KL, Suwanwela N, et al. Transcranial Doppler ultrasound criteria for hemodynamically significant internal carotid artery stenosis based on residual lumen diameter calculated from en bloc endarterectomy specimens. *Stroke.* 1997;28:1966–1971.

40. Landry A, Spence JD, Fenster A. Measurement of carotid plaque volume by 3-dimensional ultrasound. *Stroke.* 2004;35:864–869.

41. Wessels T, Harrer JU, Stetter S, et al. Three-dimensional assessment of extracranial Doppler sonography in carotid artery stenosis compared with digital subtraction angiography. *Stroke.* 2004;35:1847–1851.

42. Kern R, Szabo K, Hennerici M, et al. Characterization of carotid artery plaques using real-time compound B-mode ultrasound. *Stroke.* 2004;35:870–875.

43. McConathy WJ, Alaupovic P, Woolcock N, et al. Lipids and apolipoprotein profiles in men with aneurysmal and stenosing aortoiliac atherosclerosis. *Eur J Vasc Surg.* 1989;3:511–514.

44. Schillinger M, Domanovits H, Ignatescu M, et al. Lipoprotein (a) in patients with aortic aneurysmal disease. *J Vasc Surg.* 2002;36:25–30.

45. Latif AA, Almahameed A, Lauer MS. Should we screen for abdominal aortic aneurysms? *Cleve Clin J Med.* 2006;73:9–10, 13, 16–17 passim.

46. U.S. Preventive Services Task Force. Screening for abdominal aortic aneurysm: recommendation statement. *Ann Intern Med.* 2005;142:198–202.

47. LaRoy LL, Cormier PJ, Matalon TA, et al. Imaging of abdominal aortic aneurysms. *Am J Roentgenol.* 1989;152:785–792.

48. Lindholt JS, Vammen S, Juul S, et al. The validity of ultrasonographic scanning as screening method for abdominal aortic aneurysm. *Eur J Vasc Endovasc Surg.* 1999;17:472–475.

49. Hansen KJ, Edwards MS, Craven TE, et al. Prevalence of renovascular disease in the elderly: a population-based study. *J Vasc Surg.* 2002;36:443–451.

50. Aristizabal D, Frohlich ED. Hypertension due to renal arterial disease. *Heart Dis Stroke.* 1992;1:227–234.

51. Olin JW. Atherosclerotic renal artery disease. *Cardiol Clin.* 2002;20:547–562, vi.

52. Pellerito J, Zweibel W. Ultrasound assessment of native renal vessels and renal allografts. In: Zweibel W, ed. *Introduction to Vascular Ultrasonography.* 5th ed. Philadelphia, PA: WB Saunders; 2004:611–636.

53. Taylor DC, Kettler MD, Moneta GL, et al. Duplex ultrasound scanning in the diagnosis of renal artery stenosis: a prospective evaluation. *J Vasc Surg.* 1988;7:363–369.

54. Hoffmann U, Edwards JM, Carter S, et al. Role of duplex scanning for the detection of atherosclerotic renal artery disease. *Kidney Int.* 1991;39:1232–1239.

55. Hansen KJ, Tribble RW, Reavis SW, et al. Renal duplex sonography: evaluation of clinical utility. *J Vasc Surg.* 1990;12:227–236.

56. Olin JW, Piedmonte MR, Young JR, et al. The utility of duplex ultrasound scanning of the renal arteries for diagnosing significant renal artery stenosis. *Ann Intern Med.* 1995;122:833–838.

57. Radermacher J, Chavan A, Bleck J, et al. Use of Doppler ultrasonography to predict the outcome of therapy for renal-artery stenosis. *N Engl J Med.* 2001;344:410–417.

58. Schwerk WB, Restrepo IK, Stellwaag M, et al. Renal artery stenosis: grading with image-directed Doppler US evaluation of renal resistive index. *Radiology.* 1994;190:785–790.

59. Kohler TR, Zierler RE, Martin RL, et al. Noninvasive diagnosis of renal artery stenosis by ultrasonic duplex scanning. *J Vasc Surg.* 1986;4:450–456.

60. Olin J, Begelman S. Renal artery disease. In: Topol E, ed. *Textbook of Cardiovascular Medicine.* 2nd ed. Philadelphia, PA: Lippincott Raven; 2002:2139–2159.

61. Carman TL, Olin JW. Diagnosis of renal artery stenosis: what is the optimal diagnostic test? *Curr Interv Cardiol Rep.* 2000;2:111–118.

62. Carman TL, Olin JW, Czum J. Noninvasive imaging of the renal arteries. *Urol Clin North Am.* 2001;28:815–826.

63. Olin JW. Role of duplex ultrasonography in screening for significant renal artery disease. *Urol Clin North Am.* 1994;21:215–226.

64. Wilcox CS. Ischemic nephropathy: noninvasive testing. *Semin Nephrol.* 1996;16:43–52.

65. Williams GJ, Macaskill P, Chan SF, et al. Comparative accuracy of renal duplex sonographic parameters in the diagnosis of renal artery stenosis: paired and unpaired analysis. *Am J Roentgenol.* 2007;188:798–811.

66. Zeller T, Muller C, Frank U, et al. Stent angioplasty of severe atherosclerotic ostial renal artery stenosis in patients with diabetes mellitus and nephrosclerosis. *Catheter Cardiovasc Interv.* 2003;58:510–515.

67. Mikkelsen WP. Intestinal angina: its surgical significance. *Am J Surg.* 1957;94:262–267; discussion 267–269.

68. Jager KA, Fortner GS, Thiele BL, et al. Noninvasive diagnosis of intestinal angina. *J Clin Ultrasound.* 1984;12:588–591.

69. Zwolak RM, Fillinger MF, Walsh DB, et al. Mesenteric and celiac duplex scanning: a validation study. *J Vasc Surg.* 1998;27:1078–1087; discussion 1088.

70. Moneta GL, Yeager RA, Dalman R, et al. Duplex ultrasound criteria for diagnosis of splanchnic artery stenosis or occlusion. *J Vasc Surg.* 1991;14:511–518; discussion 518–520.

71. Moneta GL, Lee RW, Yeager RA, et al. Mesenteric duplex scanning: a blinded prospective study. *J Vasc Surg.* 1993;17:79–84; discussion 85–86.

72. Harward TR, Smith S, Seeger JM. Detection of celiac axis and superior mesenteric artery occlusive disease with use of abdominal duplex scanning. *J Vasc Surg.* 1993;17:738–745.

73. Gentile AT, Moneta GL, Lee RW, et al. Usefulness of fasting and postprandial duplex ultrasound examinations for predicting high-grade superior mesenteric artery stenosis. *Am J Surg.* 1995;169:476–479.

74. Nicoloff AD, Williamson WK, Moneta GL, et al. Duplex ultrasonography in evaluation of splanchnic artery stenosis. *Surg Clin North Am.* 1997;77:339–355.

CHAPTER 4

CT and MR Angiography

Rajan K. Gupta, Fadi El-Merhi, and Michael Wholey

Over the past several decades, advances in medical imaging have drastically improved the ability to noninvasively evaluate the vascular tree. In particular, computed tomography angiography (CTA) and magnetic resonance angiography (MRA) have emerged as tests of choice for the anatomic assessment of a variety of vascular disorders.

Despite these advances, however, clinicians must be aware of the limitations of anatomic tests and the application of this information to their patients. When approaching vascular disease, it is critical to remember that the presence of an anatomic lesion does not always explain the patient's symptoms. Treatment of anatomic abnormalities without physiologic information and sound clinical judgment may lead to an incorrect diagnosis and inappropriate treatment of asymptomatic lesions.

Noninvasive tests to evaluate vascular disorders can be broadly divided into physiologic and anatomic tests. The noninvasive vascular lab provides a number of diagnostic tools such as the ankle brachial index, segmental limb pressures, pulse volume recordings, exercise stress testing and Doppler ultrasound (Chapters 2 and 3). These are primarily physiologic tests, although they do provide limited segmental anatomic data. Their primary role is to establish the presence of physiologically significant vascular disease, although they are also quite useful in the follow-up evaluation post-revascularization. After establishing a physiologic problem that explains the patient's symptoms, an anatomic test such as CTA or MRA can localize and characterize the disease providing an excellent road map for therapeutic intervention.

Although peripheral artery disease (PAD) is the main reason for ordering a CTA or MRA, almost 20% of arterial occlusive disease is secondary to causes other than atherosclerosis. Unlike digital subtraction angiography (DSA), volumetric tests such as CTA and MRA are able to visualize much more than the vascular lumen alone. They provide additional information about the vascular wall including the presence of soft or calcified plaque and the extent of positive remodeling. Both provide visualization of the tissues and organs surrounding the vascular segment of interest and document any pathology affecting these tissues and organs that may be indirectly causing the vascular symptoms and signs. Additionally, both modalities have been used with some success to image venous anatomy and pathology. With increasing acceptance in clinical practice, CTA and MRA are now utilized to evaluate a variety of vascular disorders (Table 4.1).

Both CTA and MRA have distinct advantages and disadvantages. The selection of which test to perform is largely based on the clinical question, patient factors, hospital factors, and physician preferences. The goal of this chapter is to provide the reader with a general overview of each test and its associated strengths and weaknesses.

COMPUTED TOMOGRAPHY ANGIOGRAPHY

CTA utilizes iodinated contrast media and ionizing radiation to obtain high-quality images of the vascular tree. Improvements in multidetector technology have revolutionized CTA in the past several decades. With 16- and 64-channel scanners, large segments of the body can be imaged with a single contrast bolus, often during a single breath-hold. Multidetector CT

TABLE 4.1 Uses of CTA/MRA

Arterial evaluation:
  Peripheral arterial disease
    Acute and chronic critical limb ischemia
    Thromboembolism
    Evaluation of previous interventions:
      Bypass grafts
      Stents/stent-grafts
  Vascular malformations
  Vasculitis
  Dissection
  Arterial entrapment syndromes
  Adventitial cystic disease
  Aneurysms
    Pretreatment planning
    Posttreatment follow-up
  Iatrogenic/traumatic injury
  Dialysis grafts and fistula

Venous evaluation:
  Stenosis/thrombosis
    Congenital or acquired (indwelling catheters) causes
    Effort thrombosis of the upper extremity
    Venous compression syndromes (SVC syndrome, May–Thurner syndrome)
    Congenital anomalies including venous malformations
    Varicose veins and incompetent valves
    Venous mapping presurgical construction of dialysis graft or fistula

angiography (MD-CTA) has been shown to have diagnostic accuracy equivalent to DSA for PAD and is an excellent tool in pretreatment planning (1–4).

A typical CTA involves a digital tomogram, an optional noncontrast acquisition, and a contrasted arterial phase acquisition, which may be empirically timed or based on bolus tracking algorithms. Bolus tracking is particularly important in patients with cardiac disease where contrast may arrive to the lower extremities slower than in the average patient. Typical injection rates are 3 to 5 cc/sec for a total volume of 70 to 120 cc of iodinated contrast. Axial images are usually reconstructed in 1- to 2-mm increments. Post-processing algorithms are used to reconstruct images in multiple planes and 3D volumes.

One of many advantages of CTA is widespread availability of multidetector CT scanners, which are often staffed and available at all times for emergent imaging (Fig. 4.1). Protocols are simple, easily reproduced, and imaging quality is often comparable across institutions. Since CT acquisition is rapid, it is substantially less prone to motion

artifact than MRA. The CT gantry is relatively large compared with an MR magnet, and CTA is better able to image those with claustrophobia or severe obesity. CTA also has higher spatial resolution and lower overall cost compared with MRA. Finally, CTA has particular utility in the evaluation of stents, stent grafts, and endoleaks (Fig. 4.2).

One of the major disadvantages of CTA is the use of iodinated contrast, which can lead to renal dysfunction,

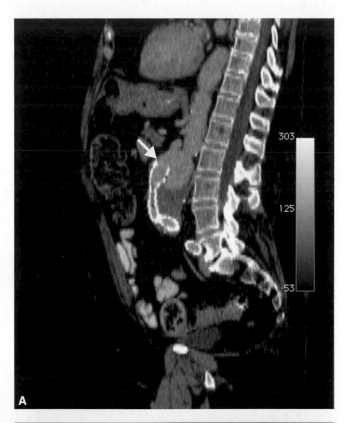

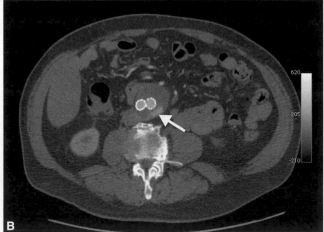

Figure 4.1 • 71-year-old patient following percutaneous intervention with pain at the access site after use of closure device. Maximum intensity projection (MIP) of a MD-CTA showing acute occlusion of the left common femoral artery *(white arrows)*. Profunda femoral artery indicated by *interrupted white arrow*. Superficial femoral artery indicated by *black arrow*.

Figure 4.2 • **A:** Sagittal reformat of CTA demonstrating distal migration of aortic stent graft with type Ia proximal endoleak. *Solid white arrow* indicates the position of the proximal margin of the stent graft. **B:** Axial CTA of aortic stent graft patient with type II endoleak in the posterior aneurysm sac from a lumbar artery *(arrow)*.

particularly in those with preexisting chronic renal insufficiency (CRI). CT imaging utilizes ionizing radiation, which contributes to an increasing dose of medical radiation to the population. CTA is prone to beam hardening or streak artifacts from calcium and bone that can limit the ability to visualize the vascular lumen. This is particularly evident in infrapopliteal calcified vascular disease where it may be impossible to determine vascular patency in heavily calcified tibial vessels. While widely quoted in the literature as a disadvantage, the ability of CTA to detect calcium can also be quite advantageous. The amount and distribution of calcium are critically important for both surgical and endovascular procedures and can greatly affect the approach to therapeutic intervention. A circumferentially calcified vessel that is widely patent may not be an appropriate target for surgical bypass, and heavy calcification may

greatly affect the success of endovascular procedures such as re-entry during subintimal recanalization, balloon angioplasty, atherectomy, or stenting (Fig. 4.3). The advantages and disadvantages of CTA are presented in Table 4.2.

MAGNETIC RESONANCE ANGIOGRAPHY

MR imaging utilizes powerful magnetic fields to measure the relaxation of protons when subject to various excitation fields. MRA has seen many improvements in the past several decades relating to high field magnets with larger fields of view, stronger and faster gradients, multichannel surface coils covering body segments of interest, parallel imaging, and moving table technology. Perhaps the greatest improvement in MRA quality and speed, however, has

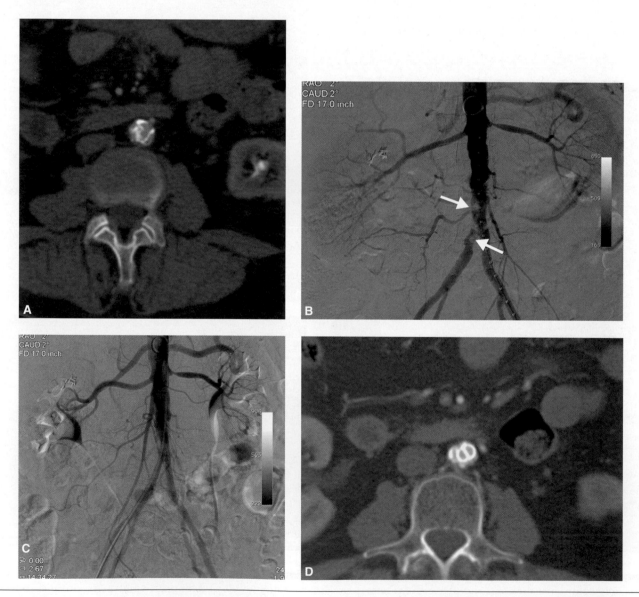

Figure 4.3 • **A:** Axial CTA in a patient with severe right greater than left claudication demonstrates severely calcified stenosis of the infra-renal abdominal aorta that extends into the right common iliac artery. **B:** Correlate angiogram demonstrating severely calcified aortoiliac disease (worst sites of calcification indicated by *arrows*). **C:** Angiogram after placement of covered balloon-expandable aortic and kissing iliac stents. **D:** Axial CTA after kissing stent placement.

TABLE 4.2 CTA—Advantages and Disadvantages

Advantages
Widespread availability and accessibility of multidetector CT scanners
Simple protocols
High spatial resolution
Rapid scanning (noncompliant patients)
Large gantry (claustrophobia, obesity)
Ability to visualize calcium
Lower cost compared with MRA

Disadvantages
Calcium limits evaluation of infrapopliteal disease
Bone/metal streak artifact
Ionizing radiation
Nephrotoxic contrast

been with the use of contrast-enhanced MRA (CE-MRA) (Fig. 4.4), which utilizes gadolinium-chelated contrast agents. CE-MRA has also been shown to have a diagnostic accuracy equivalent to conventional DSA in the evaluation of PAD and provides an excellent layout for pretreatment planning (5) (Fig. 4.5). MRA protocols are significantly more complex than CTA protocols and vary across institutions and vendors.

CE-MRA is generally superior to nonenhanced MRA as it is less prone to in-plane saturation and turbulence artifacts and requires substantially less time to image long vascular segments. CE-MRA of the lower extremities is performed using a multistation, moving-table, bolus-chase technique that is widely used and available on most magnets. Initial protocols optimized the bolus to the first abdominal aortic station. Subsequent thigh and calf stations were imaged consecutively as fast as possible, making venous contamination in the calf, and to a lesser degree in the thigh, a problem in interpretation of the arterial tree (6). Later protocols addressed venous contamination problems by using separate bolus timing injections combined with time-resolved images of the calf vessels performed prior to acquiring the CE-MRA of the more proximal arteries (7). These techniques, however, used large volumes of gadolinium contrast and increased the risks of acquiring nephrogenic systemic fibrosis (NSF) in patients with moderate to severe CRI and patients with ESRD on dialysis. NSF is further discussed later in the text in the section regarding complications.

More current protocols for CE-MRA of the lower extremities utilize a blood pressure cuff compression technique (Fig. 4.6). Blood pressure cuffs are applied to each thigh and inflated to a pressure that is sufficient to achieve venous occlusion but insufficient to cause arterial occlusion. This results in delayed venous filling allowing more time to image the thigh and calf stations before venous contamination occurs (8) (Fig. 4.7). In spite of these techniques,

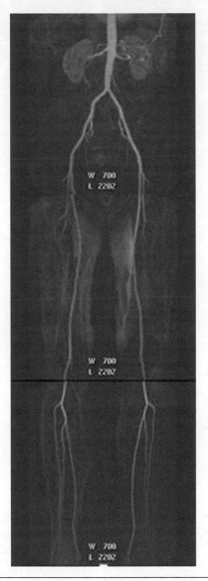

Figure 4.4 • Maximum intensity projection (MIP) reconstruction of a contrast enhanced (CE)-MRA runoff of a 46-year-old patient with atypical symptoms in the right lower extremity showing normal abdominal aorta and bilateral iliac and lower extremity arteries.

however, venous contamination can still be a problem in patients with leg hyperemia secondary to cellulitis, ulcers, or other injuries (Fig. 4.8).

A variety of noncontrast MRA techniques are available to image the vascular tree, although these are more time-consuming and subject to greater artifacts than CE-MRA. These include 2D time-of-flight (TOF) imaging (Fig. 4.9), 3D TOF, 2D phase contrast (PC), 3D PC, and balanced steady state free precession (Fig. 4.10). The most recent of the nonenhanced MRA techniques is the 3D flow-spoiled, electrocardiogram-triggered, half-Fourier fast spin echo imaging. This technique subtracts the vascular signal during diastole and systole. Imaged arteries are bright during diastole and dark during systole; so subtractions of these two images display arteries as bright. Veins are bright

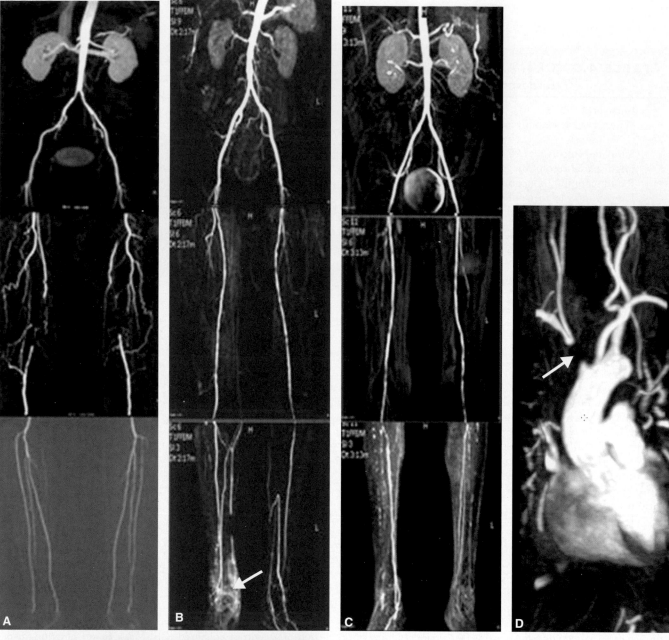

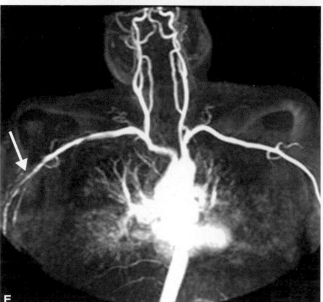

Figure 4.5 • **A:** MIP reconstruction of a CE-MRA from a 56-year-old male smoker showing bilateral chronic superficial femoral artery (SFA) occlusions. **B:** MIP reconstruction of a CE-MRA from a 59-year-old patient with bilateral lower extremity claudication and chronic nonhealing right foot ulcer showing bilateral diffuse mild SFA disease and diffuse three vessel tibial disease with hyperemia (*arrow*) secondary to a nonhealing right foot ulcer. **C:** MIP of a CE-MRA runoff from a 56-year-old patient with bilateral lower extremity claudication showing bilateral diffuse moderate SFA disease and diffuse three vessel tibial disease. **D:** MIP of a CE-MRA of the upper extremities from a 51-year-old patient showing occlusion of the innominate artery (*arrow*). **E:** MIP of a CE-MRA of the upper extremities from a 43-year-old patient showing moderate narrowing of the right subclavian artery (*arrow*).

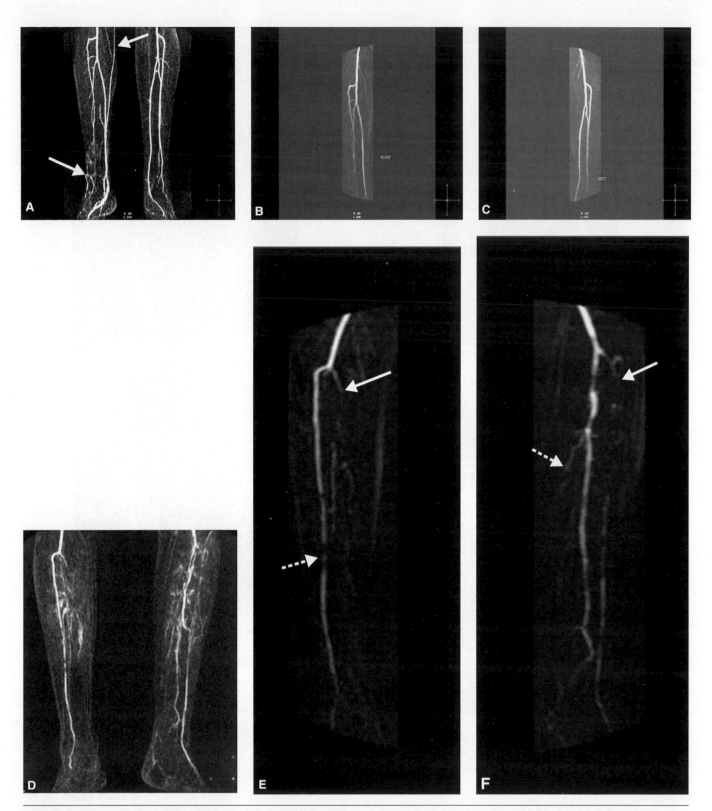

Figure 4.6 • **A:** Third station MIP image from a CE-MRA runoff without the use of thigh cuff showing venous contamination *(arrows)* involving the right calf that causes difficulty in interpretation of tibial arterial anatomy in this patient with a chronic nonhealing right foot ulcer. **B:** CE-MRA MIP of the right calf showing moderately diseased anterior tibial and mildly diseased peroneal arteries without venous contamination. **C:** CE-MRA MIP of the left calf showing normal tibial vessels. **D:** Third station MIP image from a runoff without the use of thigh cuff showing venous contamination involving both calves. **E:** CE-MRA MIP of the right calf showing occlusion of the tibioperoneal trunk *(solid arrow)* and severe disease of anterior tibial artery *(interrupted arrow)* without venous contamination. **F:** CE-MRA MIP of the left calf showing occlusion of the anterior tibial *(solid arrow)* and posterior tibial *(interrupted arrow)* arteries, and patency of the peroneal artery without venous contamination.

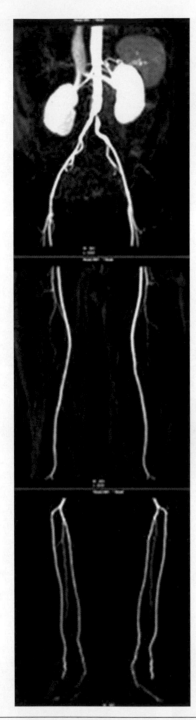

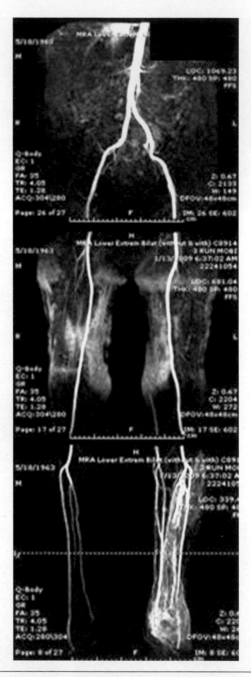

Figure 4.8 • CE-MRA MIP with venous contamination in the left calf despite the blood pressure cuff technique due to left calf cellulitis.

Figure 4.7 • CE-MRA MIP obtained with the use of blood pressure cuff compression technique where individual blood pressure cuffs were applied to each thigh and then inflated up to 60 mm Hg each. There is no evidence of venous contamination involving the calf station.

during both diastole and systole, which eliminates venous signal from subtracted images (Fig. 4.11).

Additionally, MRI flow-encoding sequences enable measurement of flow velocity (cm/sec) and flow volume (mL/sec). These techniques make use of either longitudinal

magnetization (TOF technique) or transverse magnetization (PC technique) (9). The TOF technique labels blood at one point with the vessel of interest and tracks it along a specified distance and computes the time elapsed. PC technique uses bipolar magnetic field gradients with opposite signs. This makes stationary protons accumulate a net phase of zero, whereas the moving blood will acquire a net phase shift. The phase shift is proportional to velocity. By using a modified Bernoulli equation, pressure gradients can be calculated (Fig. 4.12). Both techniques can identify the flow direction, which may be of value

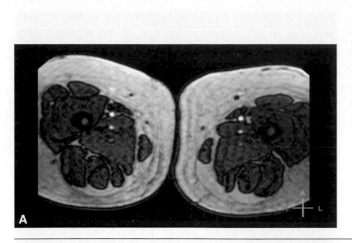

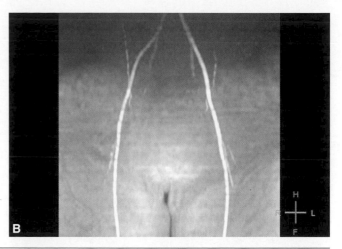

Figure 4.9 • **A:** Source image of a 2D Time Of Flight (TOF) through the pelvis and proximal thigh. **B:** MIP of 2D TOF generated from all the source images.

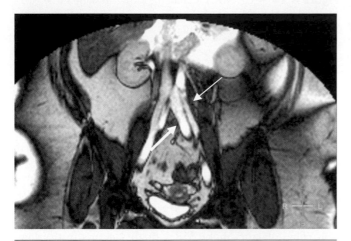

Figure 4.10 • Balanced steady state free precession coronal MR imaging showing right common iliac artery *(thin white arrow)* and right iliac vein *(thick white arrow)*.

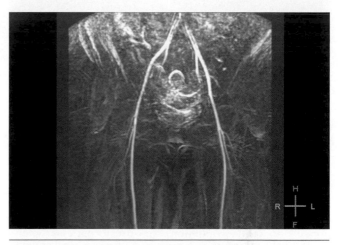

Figure 4.11 • Subtracted MIP of the 3D flow-spoiled, half-Fourier fast spin echo imaging showing normal iliac and proximal superficial femoral artery in a normal volunteer.

Figure 4.12 • Quantitative flow images of a normal volunteer obtained through the proximal superficial femoral artery. The top image represents the magnitude image and the lower image reflects the phase image. In the phase contrast image, signal intensity of each pixel is proportional to blood flow velocity with cranial flow shown as bright color and caudal flow as darker color.

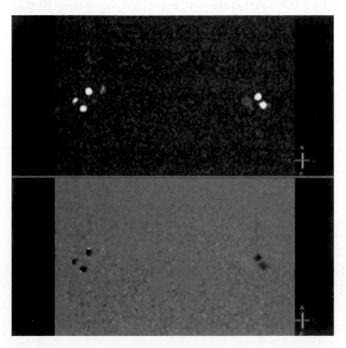

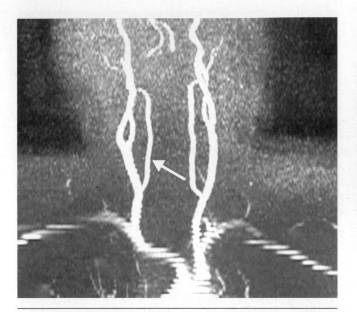

Figure 4.13 • MIP of a TOF of the cervical vessels showing antegrade flow of the right vertebral artery *(arrow)*, effectively ruling out the diagnosis of subclavian steal phenomenon.

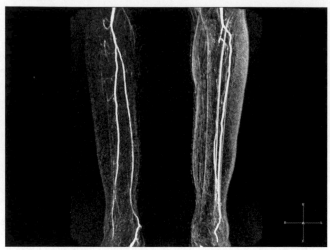

Figure 4.14 • CE-MRA MIP of the third calf station where patient jerked his left leg causing motion artifact of the left calf arteries. The right calf arteries are intact.

when evaluating disorders such as subclavian steal syndrome (Fig. 4.13).

MRA has a number of advantages (Table 4.3). No ionizing radiation is required for image acquisition. The significance of this is debatable in an older population with vascular disease and other comorbidities, although there are definite advantages for women of childbearing age and younger populations. Additionally, there is national pressure to reduce radiation exposure to patients whenever possible. Gadolinium-based contrast agents are also substantially less nephrotoxic compared with iodinated contrast agents, although the recognition of NSF has limited the use of gadolinium agents in the most vulnerable

populations where MRA was previously most utilized. MRA can also be performed without contrast, although imaging quality is sacrificed. MRA is not subject to interference from calcium, and imaging of infrapopliteal disease in patients with calcified vessels is significantly improved compared with CTA.

Disadvantages include both technical factors and patient factors (Table 4.3). MRA protocols are significantly more complex and require greater attention to detail to obtain high-quality images and prevent venous contamination. These factors make MRA quality across institutions more variable. MR magnets are generally less available than CT scanners across the country and may not be staffed at all hours for emergent tests. Patients may not be able to undergo MR imaging due to obesity and inability to fit into the magnet, claustrophobia, or MR contraindicated devices such as pacemakers. Patient cooperation is mandatory since patient movement degrades MRA images, limiting interpretation, and cannot be corrected following image acquisition (Fig. 4.14). Ferromagnetic stents, surgical clips, or orthopedic prosthetic devices may produce significant susceptibility artifact and may preclude imaging of nearby vascular structures. Signal loss in these cases is secondary to a dephasing effect, which may appear as segmental occlusions (Fig. 4.15). If evaluation of an intravascular stent is needed, CTA is a more appropriate diagnostic test.

POST-PROCESSING

Post-processing algorithms allow the display of CTA and MRA data in various ways to aid in imaging interpretation and treatment planning. Post-processing is typically performed on a dedicated workstation by technologists after image acquisition. Although valuable, these techniques are subject to the inherent limitations of the initial data set and the skill of the individual

---

TABLE 4.3	MRA—Advantages and Disadvantages

Advantages
  No ionizing radiation
  Less nephrotoxic contrast
  Ability to image without contrast
  No interference from calcium
  Dynamic imaging possible

Disadvantages
  Venous contamination
  Ferromagnetic artifacts (stents, surgical clips, orthopedic hardware)
  MRI contraindications (pacemakers)
  Smaller bore magnets (claustrophobia, obesity)
  Higher cost
  Requires a compliant patient

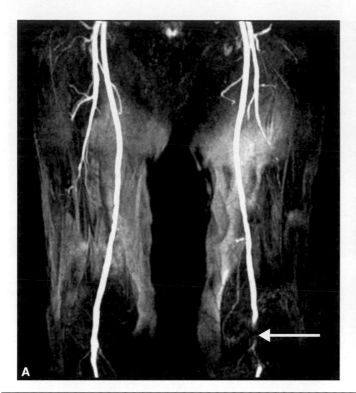

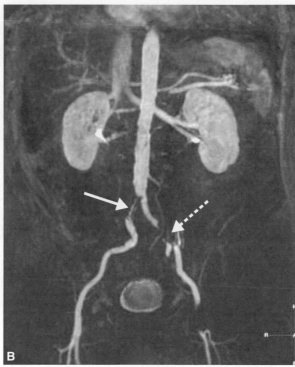

Figure 4.15 • **A:** Left knee prosthesis causing signal void in the region of the left popliteal artery *(arrow)* mimicking occlusion. **B:** CE-MRA showing signal void within the right common iliac artery *(solid arrow)* and the left external iliac artery *(interrupted arrow)* secondary to recently placed stents mimicking occlusion.

performing the reconstructions. Abnormalities noted on reconstructions should always be confirmed in the source data.

Common post-processing algorithms include multiplanar reformat (MPR), maximum intensity projection (MIP), volume rendering (VR), and intravascular projections. MPRs are images created in different 2D planes from the initially acquired data set. They are commonly created in axial, sagittal, coronal, and oblique planes. They are generally simple to perform and allow the viewer to see the source data in different projections. Coronal MPRs are often performed since they most closely resemble the viewing plane in which conventional angiographic images are displayed (Fig. 4.16). Curved MPRs can also be performed to view a curved vessel in a single plane for various purposes. These require greater time and processing. Oblique and curved MPRs are both helpful in planning of complex interventions such as stent grafts (Fig. 4.17).

MIPs are similar to reformats although they are created by displaying the highest intensity voxels on the output image in various 2D user-defined planes. The lower-intensity voxels are discarded that may result in loss of critical information. MIPs are predominantly used to increase the conspicuity of elements of the data set, such as small blood vessels and soft tissue detail (Fig. 4.18). A significant problem with MIPs is that adjacent structures may superimpose on the vessel of interest if they have a higher signal. This commonly causes an underestimation of the degree of luminal narrowing with CTA, since a calcified vessel or stent may appear as a patent vessel. This may cause overestimation of the degree of stenosis in the case of CE-MRA, since part of the vessel of interest that has a lower signal will not be displayed (Fig. 4.19).

VR creates a 3D model that can be filmed in various projections. These projections can be used to gain a rapid

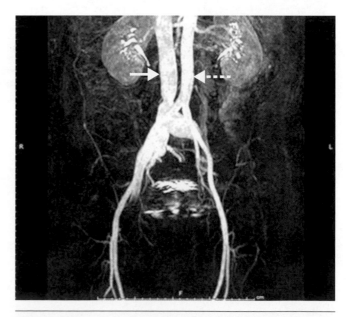

Figure 4.16 • Coronal MPR of a CE-MRA in a 59-year-old patient following right common femoral artery catheterization that experienced symptoms and signs of heart failure showing a large right common iliac artery to right common iliac vein fistula that was treated successfully with stent graft placement. Inferior vena cava indicated by *solid arrow*, and abdominal aorta indicated by *interrupted arrow*.

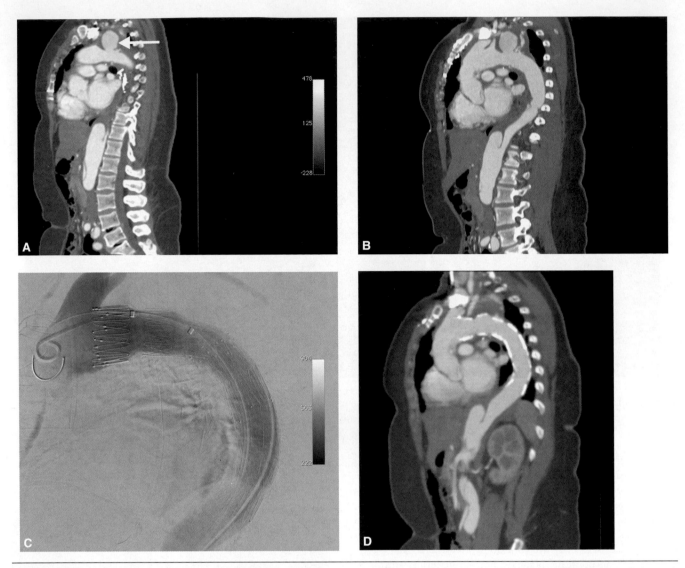

Figure 4.17 • **A:** Sagittal CT MPR of a patient with a pseudoaneurysm at the junction of a previous surgical thoracic graft *(arrow)*. **B:** Oblique CT MPR of the same patient along the axis of the aorta demonstrates the vascular anatomy better than in the sagittal view. This is helpful for treatment planning. **C:** Oblique angiogram during stent placement. The arch is bovine and the left subclavian has been covered. **D:** Oblique CT MPR after stent placement. The pseudoaneurysm is thrombosed. The left subclavian fills from a left carotid to subclavian bypass.

understanding of the overall anatomy with a single or several pictures. Volumes are often filmed around a 360-degree axis so they can be viewed as a rotating model. Data segmentation is often necessary to remove unwanted data, such as bones or organs (Figs. 4.20 and 4.21). This can be time-consuming and requires experience and attention to detail to prevent the removal of essential data. Intraluminal views of vascular structures are also possible, although they are of somewhat limited utility in vascular applications (Fig. 4.22).

COMPLICATIONS

Although both CE-MRA and MD-CTA use noninvasive techniques to image the vascular tree, both are associated with rare, potentially significant compilations. CE-MRA utilizes

gadolinium-chelated contrast agents while CTA uses iodinated contrast agents. Both are injected into a peripheral vein that put the patient at a small risk for subcutaneous contrast extravasation. All episodes of contrast agent extravasation should be examined by a physician and should not be underestimated. Although most are treated symptomatically by elevating the affected extremity and applying cold or warm compresses to the affected area, some are more serious and may require further evaluation. Large amounts of contrast extravasation may lead to skin necrosis, potentially requiring a skin graft if severe. Rarely, contrast extravasation may also lead to a compartment syndrome resulting in neurologic damage. The radiologist should evaluate the patient, determine the severity of the complication, and seek appropriate consultation from a plastic surgeon if needed.

The intravascular use of both gadolinium- and iodine-based contrast agents is associated with minor and major

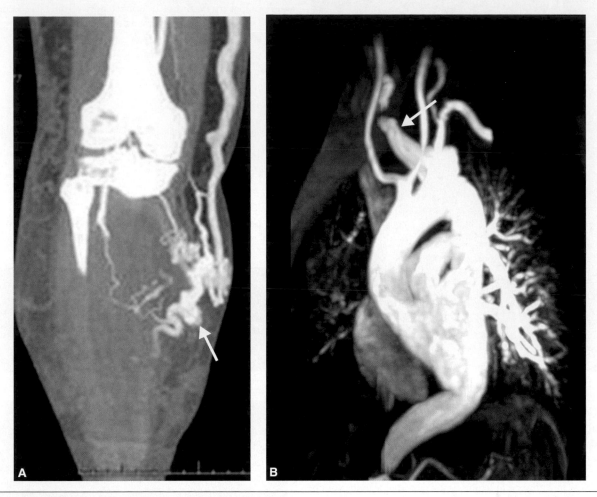

Figure 4.18 • **A:** MIP of MD-CTA runoff in a 61-year-old patient with a nonhealing wound in the stump of a below-knee amputation of the right leg showing right posterior tibial artery to right greater saphenous vein fistula *(arrow)* causing steal phenomena resulting in poor supply to the stump. **B:** MIP of a CE-MRA of an upper extremity showing an aberrant right subclavian artery *(arrow)*.

adverse drug reactions including nausea, vomiting, allergic reactions, and anaphylactic shock. Gadolinium-based agents are associated with a much lower risk of adverse reactions in comparison with the iodinated contrast agents, even in comparison to the newer, lower-risk, iso-osmolar iodinated contrast agents. Between the years 1988 and 2002, 45 million applications of IV gadolinium-chelated contrast agent were reviewed and the reported incidence of adverse events was only 0.018%. The majority (90.7%) of these reactions were minor. The remainder (i.e., 9.3%) were serious. Minor adverse events included 2.1/100,000 episodes of mucosal reactions and 3.2/100,000 episodes of urticaria. Serious events included 0.07/100,000 episodes of angioedema and 0.08/100,000 episodes of renal impairment (10).

In 1990, Katayama et al. reported adverse events associated with ionic versus nonionic iodinated contrast agents and subcategorized the adverse events in three main groups: 1) any type of reaction, which occurred in 10% of patients with ionic versus 2% with nonionic contrast; 2) severe event requiring treatment, which occurred in 0.5% of patients with ionic versus 0.1% with nonionic contrast; and 3) very severe events,

which occurred in 0.05% of patients with ionic versus 0.01% patients with nonionic contrast. The reported mortality rate was 1 in 40,000 (11).

Contrast-induced nephrotoxicity (CIN) is an additional side effect associated with the use of intravascular contrast media. CIN is defined as a rise in serum creatinine level of at least 0.25 mg/dL or a 25% rise over the baseline creatinine occurring within 3 days after intravascular contrast media administration. It is extremely rare of to have renal impairment after the use of gadolinium-chelated contrast agents in patients with a normal glomerular filtration rate (GFR) (12,13). Recently, patients developing CIN after the use of gadolinium-chelated contrast agents have been identified. Typically these patients have chronic renal insufficiency (CRI) with significant comorbidities (including diabetes mellitus and hypertension). Sam et al. concluded that underlying CRI, diabetes mellitus, and cardiovascular disease must be identified before patients receive an injection of gadolinium-chelated contrast agent and that appropriate prophylactic measures should be taken to reduce the risk of CIN. Limiting injection of gadolinium-chelated contrast agents to less than 0.4 mmol/kg is

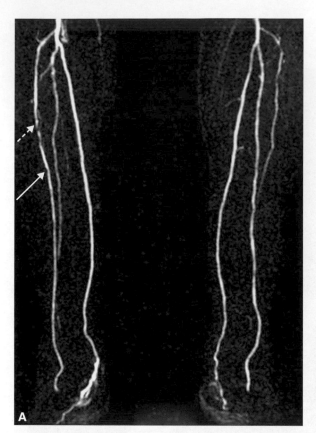

Figure 4.19 • **A:** MIP of a CE-MRA showing two consecutive focal tight stenoses *(interrupted and solid arrows)* of the proximal right anterior tibial artery. **B:** The inferior stenosis *(arrow)* has been overestimated on the MIP after reviewing the source data that were normal at that level.

Figure 4.20 • **A:** 3D volume-rendered CT image of the patient with claudication. In this image the vascular structures and bones are present. **B:** 3D volume-rendered CT image of the same patient with bones removed. Note the dense abdominal calcification above the bifurcation. Compare this to the images in Figure 4.3 of the same patient. Note how the severe stenosis is not discernable in the volume-rendered image.

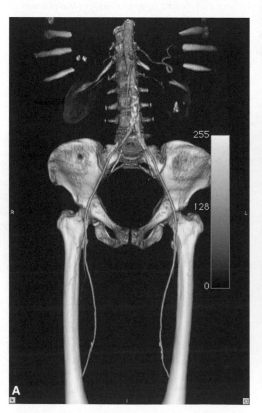

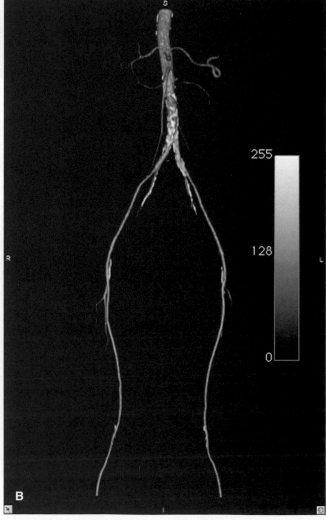

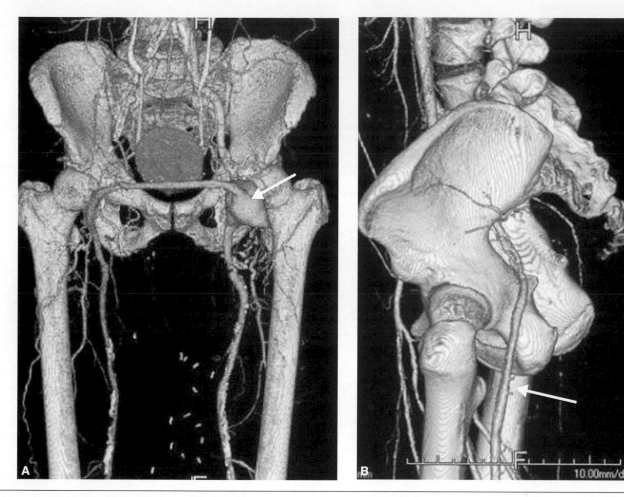

Figure 4.21 • **A:** Volume-rendered (VR) 3-D model generated from a CTA showing a mycotic pseudoaneurysm of the left arterial anastomosis of a fem-fem bypass graft *(arrow)*. The soft tissues have been segmented out. **B:** VR 3-D model generated from a CTA demonstrating a persistent sciatic artery *(arrow)*. Soft tissues have been removed.

also recommended (14,15). In contrast, even with use of the low osmolar iodinated contrast media (LOCM) that rapidly replaced the high osmolar iodinated contrast media (HOCM) in the early 1990s, the incidence of CIN in the general population following iodinated contrast exposure is 2%. Among hospitalized patients, the incidence may be as high as 11%. Additional comorbid conditions such as CRI, diabetes, and other cardiovascular disease increase the risks even further (16,17). Prophylactic IV volume expansion and use of *N*-acetylcysteine are recommended as clinically appropriate in patients with decreased creatinine clearance that are scheduled to obtain a MD-CTA with the use of iodinated contrast agents to decrease their risk of CIN. For comparison, the renal failure data reported to the Food and Drug Administration (FDA) between the years 1990 and 1994 showed an incidence of 0.122 cases per 100,000 for ionic iodinated contrast, 0.108 cases per 100,000 for nonionic iodinated contrast, and 0.02 cases per 100,000 for gadolinium-chelated contrast (18).

A risk specific to gadolinium-based contrast agents is the development of NSF. NSF is a rare disease characterized by excessive formation of connective tissue in the skin and internal organs that has been related to the use of gadolinium contrast agents in patients with moderate to severe renal insufficiency and patients with end-stage renal disease (ESRD) on dialysis. In affected patients, the skin becomes thickened, coarse and hard, sometimes leading to debilitating contractures. The disease can be progressive and in some instances fatal. The first reports began with the Dutch NSF study that was published in 2006 (19,20). The FDA promptly issued the first report three current warnings related to the health safety of gadolinium-chelated contrast agent in June 2006.

Lately, with the increasing incidence and recognition of NSF, a re-evaluation of the use of gadolinium-chelated contrast agents in CE-MRI and CE-MRA exams has been instituted on all levels. Currently, most hospitals and imaging centers that use gadolinium-chelated contrast agents in their examinations have established guidelines in concordance with the FDA recommendations and guidelines. All patients with a creatinine clearance <30 mL/min and patients on dialysis should be carefully evaluated, as they are at the highest risk. The radiologist should confirm that the study is indicated and evaluate whether alternate tests such as ultrasound,

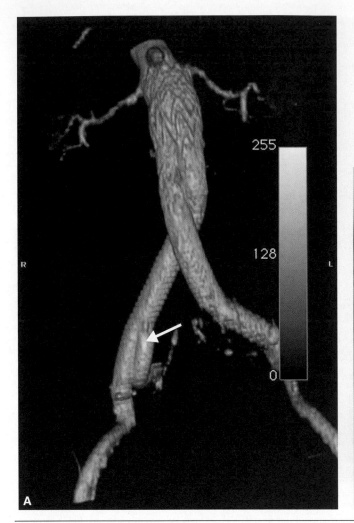
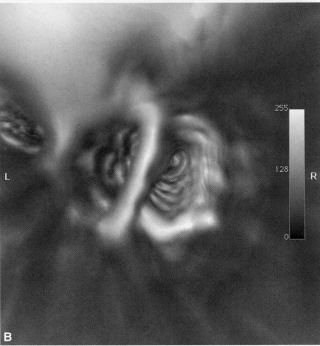

Figure 4.22 • **A:** VR CTA of bifurcated abdominal endograft. The aneurysm has been segmented out of the image to visualize the stent components. Dual covered stents have been placed into the right iliac limb to preserve flow to the right hypogastric artery *(arrow)*. **B:** Intraluminal reconstruction looking inside the main body of the graft into the bifurcated stents in the right pelvis.

noninvasive vascular laboratory evaluation, or CTA may be of lower risk. If the gadolinium-based study is still needed, however, then the patient has to be consented for the possibility of developing NSF. Although there are no published data to establish or determine the utility of dialysis to prevent NSF in ESRD patients who are on dialysis, the authors recommend performing prompt dialysis following any CE-MRI or CE-MRA exam to reduce the patient's gadolinium-chelated contrast agent body burden. Scheduling the dialysis session should be a joint effort between the ordering physician and the radiology department. In case of patients with creatinine clearance <30 mL/min who are not on dialysis yet, close follow-up is needed for any skin changes or other symptoms and signs of NSF.

CONCLUSIONS

With substantial technological advances over the past several decades, CTA and MRA have emerged as noninvasive tests of choice for the anatomic assessment of a variety of

vascular disorders. Both tests play a valuable role in the detection of peripheral vascular disease and are critical in pretreatment planning of increasingly complex and technical endovascular procedures, surgical intervention, and combined approaches to therapeutic intervention. Each test has unique advantages and disadvantages, and the test of choice is largely based on availability, hospital and patient factors, and physician preference.

References

1. Fleischmann D, Hallett RL, Rubin GD. CT angiography of peripheral arterial disease. *J Vasc Interven Radiol*. 2006;17:3–26.
2. Heijenbrok-Kal MH, Kock MC, Hunink MG. Lower extremity arterial disease: multidetector CT angiography meta-analysis. *Radiology*. 2007;245:433–439.
3. Rieker O, Düber C, Schmiedt W, et al. Prospective comparison of CT angiography of the legs with intraarterial digital subtraction angiography. *Am J Roentgenol*. 1996;166:269–276.
4. Schernthaner R, Stadler A, Lomoschitz F, et al. Multidetector CT angiography in the assessment of peripheral arterial occlusive

disease: accuracy in detecting the severity, number, and length of stenoses. *Eur Radiol*. 2008;18:665–671.

5. Langer S, Krämer N, Mommertz G, et al. Unmasking pedal arteries in patients with critical ischemia using time-resolved contrast-enhanced 3D MRA. *J Vasc Surg*. 2009;49:1196–1202.

6. Koenigkam-Santos M, Sharma P, Kalb B, et al. Lower extremities magnetic resonance angiography with blood pressure cuff compression: quantitative dynamic analysis. *J Magn Reson Imaging*. 2009;29:1450–1456.

7. Tongdee R, Narra VR, McNeal G, et al. Hybrid peripheral 3D contrast-enhanced MR angiography of calf and foot vasculature. *Am J Roentgenol*. 2006;186:1746–1753.

8. Schneider G, Prince MR, Meaney JFM, et al. *Magnetic Resonance Angiography Techniques, Indications and Practical Applications*; 2005. Available at: http://dx.doi.org/10.1007/b138651. Available to US Hopkins community.

9. Higgins CB, Roos AD. *Cardiovascular MRI and MRA*. Philadelphia, PA: Lippincott Williams & Wilkins; 2003:x, 496.

10. Knopp MV, Balzer T, Esser M, et al. Assessment of utilization and pharmacovigilance based on spontaneous adverse event reporting of gadopentetate dimeglumine as a magnetic resonance contrast agent after 45 million administrations and 15 years of clinical use. *Invest Radiol*. 2006;41:491–499.

11. Katayama H, Yamaguchi K, Kozuka T, et al. Adverse reactions to ionic and nonionic contrast media. A report from the Japanese Committee on the Safety of Contrast Media [see comment]. *Radiology*. 1990;175:621–628.

12. Niendorf HP, Alhassan A, Geens VR, et al. Safety review of gadopentetate dimeglumine. Extended clinical experience after more than five million applications. *Invest Radiol*. 1994;29(suppl 2):S179–S182.

13. Zhang HL, Ersoy H, Prince MR. Effects of gadopentetate dimeglumine and gadodiamide on serum calcium, magnesium, and creatinine measurements. *J Magn Res Imaging*. 2006;23:383–387.

14. Ledneva E, Karie S, Launay-Vacher V, et al. Renal safety of gadolinium-based contrast media in patients with chronic renal insufficiency. *Radiology*. 2009;250:618–628.

15. Sam AD II, Morasch MD, Collins J, et al. Safety of gadolinium contrast angiography in patients with chronic renal insufficiency [see comment]. *J Vasc Surg*. 2003;38:313–318.

16. Finn WF. The clinical and renal consequences of contrast-induced nephropathy. *Nephrol Dial Transplant*. 2006;21:i2–i10.

17. Mehran R, Nikolsky E. Contrast-induced nephropathy: definition, epidemiology, and patients at risk. *Kidney Int Suppl*. 2006;S11–S15.

18. Lasser EC, Lyon SG, Berry CC. Reports on contrast media reactions: analysis of data from reports to the U.S. Food and Drug Administration. *Radiology*. 1997;203:605–610.

19. Marckmann P, Skov L, Rossen K, et al. Nephrogenic systemic fibrosis: suspected causative role of gadodiamide used for contrast-enhanced magnetic resonance imaging. *J Am Soc Nephrol*. 2006;17:2359–2362.

20. Perazella MA. Nephrogenic systemic fibrosis, kidney disease, and gadolinium: is there a link? [comment]. *Clin J Am Soc Nephrol CJASN*. 2007;2:200–202.

CHAPTER 5

Medical Therapy for Peripheral Arterial Disease

Mobeen A. Sheikh

The term peripheral arterial disease (PAD) refers to noncoronary, occlusive atherosclerotic vascular disease. However, by convention most epidemiologic studies use the term PAD to refer to arterial disease of the lower extremities. It is estimated that about 10 to 11 million Americans have PAD. Unfortunately, a number of factors have contributed to the underrecognition of the true burden of PAD, including the lack of physician and patient awareness, the failure to appreciate that the majority of patients with PAD have atypical symptoms or are asymptomatic, and the underutility of safe and inexpensive noninvasive diagnostic tools such as measurement of the ankle–brachial index (ABI).

It is sometimes helpful to gain an appreciation of this in the context of other perhaps better known cardiovascular conditions such as atrial fibrillation that, by best estimates, affects 2.3 million people in the United States. A better perspective may be gleaned from a cross-sectional study of primary care practices across the United States of nearly 7000 patients that demonstrated the incidence of PAD in patients above the age of 70 years or those between the age of 50 and 69 who had a history of either smoking or diabetes to be almost one-third, yet only half of their physicians were aware of this diagnosis (1).

NATURAL HISTORY OF PAD: CONCEPT OF GLOBAL VASCULAR CARE

PAD is underdiagnosed, and as a consequence, is also undertreated. It needs to be recognized that PAD is not just a disease of the lower extremities, but in fact is a manifestation of systemic atherosclerosis and is a marker for adverse cardiovascular outcomes with a 5-year risk of cardiovascular morbidity and mortality as high as 50%. In terms of limb-related outcomes, during the same 5-year period, only a quarter of these patients will have progression in their leg symptoms and less than half of these patients will require an intervention or progress to amputation (2).

With endovascular techniques now occupying a dominant role in the management of PAD and at times assuming the role of default treatment, it is imperative to understand that in these patients their most serious problem is not their limitation in walking, but their risk of a future adverse cardiovascular event in the form of a myocardial infarction (MI), stroke, or cardiovascular-related death. Hence, the concept of "global vascular care." The first priority in formulating a treatment plan for patients with PAD should be modification of known risk factors for the progression of atherosclerosis and cardiovascular event reduction. Medical therapy is always the primary therapy for patients with PAD, including those patients who undergo an endovascular or surgical intervention. In other words it has universal application, either as a standalone or as an adjunct to more invasive forms of therapy and not as an alternative.

There are a number of features unique to patients with vascular disease, including but not limited to the fact that these patients tend to be older, have age-related issues, and also have a high prevalence of comorbid conditions. This adds to the complexity in managing patients with vascular disease.

The cornerstones of medical care in patients with PAD are

- Risk factor modification
- Pharmacologic therapy
- Exercise therapy

RISK FACTOR MODIFICATION

In the ensuing portion of this chapter, those modifiable risk factors most associated with PAD will be discussed, with an emphasis on particular nuances and variation in approach to each in light of available evidence as well as current recommendations.

Smoking Cessation

Cigarette smoking has the strongest correlation with PAD than any other cardiovascular condition. It is also directly related to progression of PAD to limb loss. In smokers, the larger inflow vessels of the lower extremity are typically involved. In patients with PAD who smoke, complete smoking cessation and long-term abstinence forms the cornerstone of therapy. It represents the most important modifiable risk factor since it can favorably alter the natural history of the disease. There are data that confirm an objective improvement in ankle pressure and treadmill walking distance when comparing those patients who stop smoking versus those who continue to smoke (3). Additionally, smoking cessation reduces the severity of limb outcomes such as critical limb ischemia and amputation (4). There is also a direct dose–response relationship between the number of cigarettes smoked and the rate of lower extremity bypass graft patency (5).

Treatment options consist of behavior-modification counseling and short-term tobacco dependency pharmacotherapy that includes sustained release bupropion hydrochloride (Wellbutrin, Zyban), nicotine supplements (gum, inhaler, transdermal patches, nasal spray), and more recently Varenicline (Chantix, Pfizer). PAD patients who smoke may also represent one of those unique patient subsets in which one should not hesitate in endorsing less conventional therapies such as hypnotherapy, acupuncture, or laser therapy.

Hyperlipidemia

The major lipid-related risk factors include elevated LDL, elevated triglyceride, and low HDL levels. Lipoprotein (a) has also been identified as an independent risk factor for PAD (6). Demonstrable evidence of the effect of lipid lowering on the progression of PAD was observed in a subgroup analysis of the 4S (Scandinavian Simvastatin Survival Study) study that showed a 38% risk reduction in the development or worsening of claudication (7). Current National Cholesterol Education Panel (NCEP) guidelines and The Adult Treatment Panel (8) (ATP) classify PAD as a "coronary artery disease equivalent" and thus shares the same aggressive targets as coronary artery disease (CAD). They recommend a target LDL-C level of <100 mg/dL, which invariably would require pharmacologic intervention. A more recently updated consensus panel has recommended lowering LDL-C levels to <70 mg/dL for high-risk patients (9), which may include patients who have undergone an endovascular intervention. The Heart Protection Study (10) brought to fore another paradigm: in patients with PAD, those who received statin therapy with simvastatin had a significantly lower rate of overall cardiovascular ischemic events, regardless of cholesterol level at baseline or the presence of manifest CAD. All current evidence points to future strategies of achieving even lower target LDL levels ("the lower the better"). Another demonstrable benefit noted in some smaller scale trials is that statins may also contribute to increasing pain-free and total walking distances as well as an improvement in overall functional status (11,12). This effect may be observed independent of the degree of lipid lowering, may manifest as soon as 3 months after sustained use, and may be consistent across different statin categories. Therefore, unless there exists a strong contraindication, all patients with PAD should be aggressively treated with a statin.

Hypertension

The goal in the management of hypertension in patients with PAD is to reduce the risk of stroke and MI. Care should be taken to avoid large decreases in blood pressure for that may cause the patient to experience a worsening of their claudication symptoms. However, it must also be pointed out that the use of beta-blockers in the management of hypertension in patients with PAD is by no means contraindicated, except perhaps in those with critical limb ischemia. This fact has been borne out in various randomized studies (13).

In patients with PAD, angiotensin-converting enzyme (ACE) inhibitors are considered the first-line antihypertensive class of choice, largely based on the outcomes of the HOPE (Heart Outcomes Prevention Evaluation) trial that demonstrated a 22% lowering in the composite endpoint of MI, stroke, and death in the PAD subgroup (14). Importantly, this was observed independent of the magnitude of blood pressure lowering and was true in patients with either symptomatic or asymptomatic forms of PAD. Similar to what has been observed in trials of statins, ACE inhibitors like ramipril have also been demonstrated to independently increase pain-free and total walking distances (15).

Another consideration is that hypertension in a patient with PAD may be secondary to renal artery stenosis, which has a higher prevalence in patients with PAD. Depending on the population studied, certain estimates would put the presence of renal artery stenosis in a PAD population to be as high as 40% in all patients referred for lower extremity angiography (16).

Diabetes

The risk of developing PAD increases in direct relationship to blood glucose impairment. Even patients with impaired glucose tolerance have an incidence of PAD nearly equal to that of those with full-blown diabetes (17). The pattern of vascular involvement typically includes the below-knee vessels including the tibial vessels, small vessels of the foot, and the microcirculation of the foot. Multilevel disease is also common.

Additionally, diabetic patients tend to progress to critical limb ischemia, the most malignant manifestation of PAD, at a greater rate than the nondiabetic population. This fact may further be complicated by sensory and/or motor neuropathy, which makes them more prone to injury and ulcer formation on the lower extremities and also contributes to delayed recognition. Diabetic patients also tend to have impaired collateral vessel formation as a compensatory mechanism that directly translates to consistently worse limb outcomes (amputation, rates of revascularization).

The role of intensive blood glucose control has been definitively proven to improve outcomes in terms of microvascular complications. However, its role in macrovascular manifestations of disease has been less clear. The Diabetes Control and Complications Trial in type I diabetic patients and the United Kingdom Prospective Diabetes Study (18) in type 2 diabetic patients, which compared conventional therapy with more aggressive therapy for blood sugar lowering, both demonstrated a trend toward the reduction of cardiovascular events such as MI, but had minimal effect on the development of PAD or complications such as death and amputation related to it. Although the macrovascular results have been underwhelming, it is still recommended to maintain tight glycemic control in diabetic patients with PAD, but also to emphasize the importance of controlling additional risk factors.

PHARMACOLOGIC THERAPY

The goals of pharmacologic therapy in claudicants are targeted toward increasing pain-free and maximal walking distances as well as improving overall functional status. Although not directed toward claudication symptoms, antiplatelet therapy is a primary consideration in all prescriptions for patients with PAD in light of the aforementioned strategy of global vascular care.

Antiplatelet Therapy

In the Physicians Health Study, low-dose aspirin demonstrated a 54% reduction in the risk of peripheral vascular surgery when compared with placebo (19), and in the antiplatelet trialists' collaboration meta-analysis, there was a 23% overall reduction in a composite of MI, stroke, and vascular death (20). When an analysis was performed on those patients enrolled in these trials on the basis of PAD only, the outcomes were similar and this was true across the dose range of 75 to 350 mg.

The search for a more efficacious antiplatelet agent with less serious adverse effects led to the CAPRIE trial (21) that compared clopidogrel, which exerts its antiplatelet effect as an antagonist to the ADP $P2Y_{12}$ receptor, with low-dose aspirin. Although this study demonstrated the superiority of clopidogrel over aspirin in terms of reducing the composite outcome of ischemic stroke, MI, or vascular death (5.3% vs. 5.8%, relative risk reduction 8.7%, $p = 0.043$, mean follow-up 1.9 years), this finding was most pronounced in the PAD population. Although not the primary intent of the CHARISMA trial, a secondary analysis of patients with a prior history of MI, stroke, or peripheral vascular disease demonstrated the superiority of dual antiplatelet therapy combining aspirin with clopidogrel over aspirin alone (7.3% vs. 8.8%, $p = 0.01$, mean follow-up 28 months) (22). Thus in patients with PAD, clopidogrel is the preferred antiplatelet agent for overall reduction of future cardiovascular events (dose 75 mg once daily), and there is also evidence to support the use of more intensive regimens combining aspirin and clopidogrel as a secondary preventive strategy.

Pentoxifylline (Trental)

Pentoxifylline is a methylxanthine derivative that has multiple hypothesized mechanisms of action including lowering plasma fibrinogen concentration, altering the deformability of red cells and white cells, and also inhibiting platelet aggregation. It is also perhaps the one medication that has been in use for the longest period of time, but at this time there is considerable evidence to suggest that it is for the most part no more effective than placebo (23).

Cilostazol (Pletal)

Cilostazol is a phosphodiesterase type 3 inhibitor approved by the FDA in 1999 for the treatment of intermittent claudication. A dose of 100 mg twice daily (or 50 mg twice for older more fragile patients) has been demonstrated in a number of randomized placebo-controlled trials to improve pain-free and maximal treadmill walking distances (24,25).

Cilostazol has a number of postulated mechanisms of action that include inhibiting platelet aggregation and the formation of arterial thrombi and smooth muscle proliferation as well as a vasodilatory action. However, there are some distinctive considerations to keep in mind while prescribing cilostazol. First, any improvement will only be noticed after 3 weeks of sustained use, but before that one may experience adverse effects in the form of headache, palpitations, diarrhea, and dizziness. Reducing the dose of cilostazol to 50 mg twice daily may help reduce these effects. This medication is also contraindicated in patients with congestive heart failure. Although not specific to cilostazol, this recommendation represents an extrapolation from earlier studies with phosphodiesterase inhibitors such as milrinone that were associated with an increased mortality due to a proarrhythmic effect in a heart failure population. Thus far, this effect has not been borne out in the safety data from clinical trials for cilostazol.

NEWER DRUGS/INVESTIGATIONAL THERAPIES

Despite significant investigation, it is perhaps disappointing to note that other than cilostazol, there are not many other medications in mainstream use that improve pain-free walking distances in patients with symptomatic PAD.

Naftidrofuryl, a 5-hydroxytryptamine receptor antagonist, is available in Europe for treating claudication. A very recently concluded meta-analysis has confirmed a clinically meaningful improvement in walking distance in patients using this medication when compared to placebo (26). Prostaglandins have been extensively studied for their role in critical limb ischemia with limited evaluation in patients with intermittent claudication. At first, the route of administration of these agents was a major issue (i.e., need for intravenous administration). With the availability of beraprost sodium, an orally active prostaglandin I2 analog, there was a lot of enthusiasm in testing its use in patients with intermittent claudication. Earlier trials had shown improvement in pain-free and maximal walking distances. However, this was not borne out in later trials despite a consistent reduction in the rate of cardiovascular events (27).

Therapeutic angiogenesis studies have yielded mixed results to date. Many angiogenic factors have been employed, including vascular endothelial growth factor, hepatocyte growth factor, fibroblast growth factor 4, and hypoxia-inducible growth factor 1. Whereas the intramuscular injection of vascular endothelial growth factor directly into the lower extremities of patients with symptomatic PAD failed to demonstrate improved walking performance or quality of life (28), the TRAFFIC study, which involved the intra-arterial administration of recombinant fibroblast growth factor 1, demonstrated moderate improvement in exercise capacity in patients after a single dose (29). Current and future studies of growth factors appear to be predominantly focused on the role of this therapy in the subset of PAD patients with critical limb ischemia who have no viable revascularization option.

Exercise

There is clear and incontrovertible evidence that an exercise program in claudicants leads to statistically significant increases in walking distance. In fact, a Cochrane database review that included 10 different trials demonstrated an increase in walking time of 150%, which exceeded that achieved with angioplasty and rivaled the outcome of surgical revascularization (30). However, with this available evidence, exercise as a prescription is underutilized and the reasons for this may be multifactorial. One important issue is that unsupervised home exercise programs have been shown not to work. Another is the issue of reimbursement. With all evidence demonstrating the benefits of an exercise program performed in a supervised environment, the Centers for Medicaid and Medicare services (CMS) does not reimburse for such programs performed purely for vascular indications. However, it must also be pointed out that there will be several patients with PAD who have contraindications to exercise from a medical standpoint. Patients with PAD tend to be older and may have severe CAD and musculoskeletal or neurologic impairments not to mention other patient-related characteristics such as patient compliance with traveling far distances and incurring personal expense.

The exercise prescription—exercise is not simply an alternative for patients with no revascularization options, but like all other forms of medical therapy has application even for those patients who undergo an invasive procedure. An effective exercise program consists of sessions that last at a minimum of 30 minutes, a minimum of three times per week for a minimum of 6 months. The objective is to walk on a treadmill until near-maximal pain is achieved. The patient then rests and attempts to walk again. This walking distance determines the baseline, and the intensity of treadmill exercise is set to the workload that initially brings on the claudication pain. As the patient is able to walk farther into the pain, increases are made either in the speed or grade of the treadmill. If the patient can already walk at 2 mph (3.2 km/h), then an increase in grade is recommended. The goal of the program is to not only increase walking distance but also walking speed. The most objective measure of improvement is walking distance, since even significant improvements in distance do not translate into increases in ankle pressures. The mechanism that leads to improvement in walking distance is poorly understood. Another bonus that cannot be overlooked is the overall beneficial effects of exercise on the entire cardiovascular system, namely decreases, in systolic blood pressure and improvement in serum cholesterol (31). A further issue to reassure patients about is that walking to the point of pain does not have any detrimental effects from what would be assumed to be ischemic injury.

SUMMARY

PAD is often undiagnosed and undertreated despite the fact that patients with PAD have a systemic vascular risk equivalent to diabetic patients and a 5-year mortality rate worse than that associated with breast cancer. Medical therapy is not an alternative to other more invasive strategies, but is applicable universally and directed toward risk factor modification with certain special considerations. Pharmacologic interventions are targeted to treating modifiable risk factors, increasing walking ability, and halting progression to more severe forms of limb ischemia. Complete cessation of all forms of tobacco, aggressive lowering of lipids, control of hypertension, optimization of glucose control in the diabetic subset, addition of antiplatelet therapy, and consideration of a supervised exercise program are optimal.

References

1. Hirsch AT, Criqui MH, Treat-Jacobson D, et al. Peripheral arterial disease detection, awareness, and treatment in primary care. *JAMA*. 2001;286:1317–1324.
2. Weitz JI, Byrne J, Clagett GP, et al. Diagnosis and treatment of chronic arterial insufficiency of the lower extremities: a critical review. *Circulation*. 1996;94:3026–3049.
3. Quick CR, Cotton LT. The measured effect of stopping smoking on intermittent claudication. *Br J Surg*. 1982;69(suppl):S24–S26.
4. Jonason T, Bergstrom R. Cessation of smoking in patients with intermittent claudication. Effects on the risk of peripheral vascular complications, myocardial infarction and mortality. *Acta Med Scand*. 1987;221:253–260.
5. Willigendael EM, Teijink JA, Bartelink ML, et al. Smoking and the patency of lower extremity bypass grafts: a meta-analysis. *J Vasc Surg*. 2005;42:67–74.
6. Valentine RJ, Grayburn PA, Vega GL, et al. Lp(a) lipoprotein is an independent, discriminating risk factor for premature peripheral atherosclerosis among white men. *Arch Intern Med*. 1994;154:801–806.
7. Pedersen TR, Kjekshus J, Pyorala K, et al. Effect of simvastatin on ischemic signs and symptoms in the Scandinavian simvastatin survival study (4S). *Am J Cardiol*. 1998;81:333–335.
8. Expert Panel on Detection, Evaluation, and Treatment of High Blood Cholesterol in Adults. Executive Summary of The Third Report of The National Cholesterol Education Program (NCEP) Expert Panel on Detection, Evaluation, and Treatment of High Blood Cholesterol in Adults (Adult Treatment Panel III). *JAMA*. 2001;285:2486–2497.
9. Grundy SM, Cleeman JI, Merz CN, et al. Implications of recent clinical trials for the National Cholesterol Education Program Adult Treatment Panel III guidelines. *Circulation*. 2004;110:227–239.
10. MRC/BHF Heart Protection Study of cholesterol lowering with simvastatin in 20,536 high-risk individuals: a randomised placebo-controlled trial. *Lancet*. 2002;360:7–22.
11. Mondillo S, Ballo P, Barbati R, et al. Effects of simvastatin on walking performance and symptoms of intermittent claudication in hypercholesterolemic patients with peripheral vascular disease. *Am J Med*. 2003;114:359–364.
12. Mohler ER, 3rd, Hiatt WR, Creager MA. Cholesterol reduction with atorvastatin improves walking distance in patients with peripheral arterial disease. *Circulation*. 2003;108:1481–1486.
13. Radack K, Deck C. Beta-adrenergic blocker therapy does not worsen intermittent claudication in subjects with peripheral arterial disease. A meta-analysis of randomized controlled trials. *Arch Intern Med*. 1991;151:1769–1776.
14. Yusuf S, Sleight P, Pogue J, et al. Effects of an angiotensin-converting-enzyme inhibitor, ramipril, on cardiovascular events in high-risk patients. The Heart Outcomes Prevention Evaluation Study Investigators. *N Engl J Med*. 2000;342:145–153.
15. Ahimastos AA, Lawler A, Reid CM, et al. Brief communication: ramipril markedly improves walking ability in patients with peripheral arterial disease: a randomized trial. *Ann Intern Med*. 2006;144:660–664.
16. Miralles M, Corominas A, Cotillas J, et al. Screening for carotid and renal artery stenoses in patients with aortoiliac disease. *Ann Vasc Surg*. 1998;12:17–22.
17. Lee AJ, MacGregor AS, Hau CM, et al. The role of haematological factors in diabetic peripheral arterial disease: the Edinburgh artery study. *Br J Haematol*. 1999;105:648–654.
18. Intensive blood-glucose control with sulphonylureas or insulin compared with conventional treatment and risk of complications in patients with type 2 diabetes (UKPDS 33). UK Prospective Diabetes Study (UKPDS) Group. *Lancet*. 1998;352:837–853.
19. Goldhaber SZ, Manson JE, Stampfer MJ, et al. Low-dose aspirin and subsequent peripheral arterial surgery in the Physicians' Health Study. *Lancet*. 1992;340:143–145.
20. Antithrombotic Trialists' Collaboration. Collaborative meta-analysis of randomised trials of antiplatelet therapy for prevention of death, myocardial infarction, and stroke in high risk patients. *BMJ*. 2002;324:71–86.
21. CAPRIE Steering Committee. A randomised, blinded, trial of clopidogrel versus aspirin in patients at risk of ischaemic events (CAPRIE). *Lancet*. 1996;348:1329–1339.
22. Bhatt DL, Flather MD, Hacke W, et al. Patients with prior myocardial infarction, stroke, or symptomatic peripheral arterial disease in the CHARISMA trial. *J Am Coll Cardiol*. 2007;49:1982–1988.
23. Ernst E. Pentoxifylline for intermittent claudication. A critical review. *Angiology*. 1994;45:339–345.
24. Dawson DL, Cutler BS, Meissner MH, et al. Cilostazol has beneficial effects in treatment of intermittent claudication: results from a multicenter, randomized, prospective, double-blind trial. *Circulation*. 1998;98:678–86.
25. Money SR, Herd JA, Isaacsohn JL, et al. Effect of cilostazol on walking distances in patients with intermittent claudication caused by peripheral vascular disease. *J Vasc Surg*. 1998;27:267–74; discussion 74–75.
26. De Backer T, Vander Stichele R, Lehert P, et al. Naftidrofuryl for intermittent claudication: meta-analysis based on individual patient data. *BMJ*. 2009;338:b603.

27. Mohler ER, 3rd, Hiatt WR, Olin JW, et al. Treatment of intermittent claudication with beraprost sodium, an orally active prostaglandin I2 analogue: a double-blinded, randomized, controlled trial. *J Am Coll Cardiol*. 2003;41:1679–1686.

28. Rajagopalan S, Mohler ER, 3rd, Lederman RJ, et al. Regional angiogenesis with vascular endothelial growth factor in peripheral arterial disease: a phase II randomized, double-blind, controlled study of adenoviral delivery of vascular endothelial growth factor 121 in patients with disabling intermittent claudication. *Circulation*. 2003;108:1933–1938.

29. Lederman RJ, Mendelsohn FO, Anderson RD, et al. Therapeutic angiogenesis with recombinant fibroblast growth factor-2 for intermittent claudication (the TRAFFIC study): a randomised trial. *Lancet*. 2002;359:2053–2058.

30. Leng GC, Fowler B, Ernst E. Exercise for intermittent claudication. *Cochrane Database Syst Rev*. 2000:CD000990.

31. Izquierdo-Porrera AM, Gardner AW, Powell CC, et al. Effects of exercise rehabilitation on cardiovascular risk factors in older patients with peripheral arterial occlusive disease. *J Vasc Surg*. 2000;31:670–677.

SECTION III

Interventional Principles and Technologies

CHAPTER 6

General Angiographic and Interventional Principles

Kent W. Dauterman and Ivan P. Casserly

Peripheral angiographic suites have evolved over the last two decades to contain a number of features that are important in performing high-quality peripheral vascular angiography and intervention. Since most operators are familiar with the basic workings of radiographic imaging systems, the purpose of this chapter will be to outline these unique features. In addition, we will provide an overview of the most commonly used equipment during peripheral diagnostic and interventional studies and describe some of the fundamental principles involved in these procedures.

RADIOGRAPHIC IMAGING

The interactive components of a radiographic imaging system are shown in Figure 6.1.

Image Intensifier

In most contemporary peripheral labs, the diameter of the image intensifier is at least 15″, providing a large field of view. This is particularly important when imaging the aorta or lower extremities. The smaller image intensifier in most cardiac catheterization laboratories (i.e., 9″) is adequate for diagnostic angiography and intervention of the carotid, vertebral, subclavian, renal, and iliac arteries.

Examination Console

During peripheral angiography, a variety of settings (i.e., kVp, mA, frames/sec) will automatically vary depending on the vascular territory of interest. These territories are usually divided as follows: cerebral, thorax, abdomen, upper extremity, and lower extremity. The tube kilovoltage will be set highest for cerebral and abdominal angiography and lowest for angiography of the extremities, with the thorax having an intermediate setting. Frame rates for peripheral angiography are generally 2 to 3 per second, but this can be adjusted for specific circumstances (e.g., increased for angiography with gadolinium contrast or decreased for venous studies in which the cineangiographic runs are long). These vascular package options can be found in the tableside or control room examination console that programs the x-ray generator.

Digital Subtraction Angiography versus Cineangiography

Cineangiography simply takes multiple x-ray pictures of the contrast-filled vessel as well as the surrounding tissue (Fig. 6.2A). For rapidly moving structures with a radiolucent background, such as the coronary arteries moving with the beating heart, this 15- to 30-frames/sec imaging modality is ideal (1).

For static vascular structures that are surrounded by radiodense structures (e.g., bone), digital subtraction angiography (DSA) is the ideal imaging modality (2). With this technique, the initial images obtained when stepping on the x-ray pedal are used to generate the baseline image from which all radio-opaque structures are subtracted. Subsequent images obtained following contrast injection will generate the subtracted images and demonstrate only the contrast-filled vascular structures (Fig. 6.2B).

This imaging modality requires that the patient does not move during image acquisition. In vascular territories where the vessels may move during respiration or swallowing (e.g., carotid, vertebral, abdomen, pelvis), the patient must also suspend these activities during image acquisition.

Trace-Subtract Fluoroscopy or "Road Mapping"

Trace-subtract fluoroscopy is the fluoroscopic equivalent of DSA. Like DSA, the initial few seconds of this mode are used to obtain a fluoroscopic image that is then subtracted (2). Once the subtracted image is seen on the screen, contrast is injected to completely fill the vessel. The pedal is then released and the subtracted image with the contrast-filled vessel remains on the screen (Fig. 6.3A). In contrast to DSA, the contrast-filled vessel will appear white as opposed to black. Subsequent activation of the fluoroscopy pedal allows visualization of catheters, wires, and interventional equipment superimposed on the saved image of the contrast-filled vessel (Fig. 6.3B). When used correctly, this technique can improve the safety of various maneuvers (e.g., advancement of wires and catheters) and help to minimize contrast usage. For optimal results, the patient must remain perfectly still between the time of contrast injection and completion of any intended maneuver.

"Road Mask" Function

A "road mask" may be generated from a DSA acquisition by selecting the single frame of the acquisition that provides optimal filling of the vascular structures of interest and activating this function, generating a vascular mask against which further interventional manipulations can be visualized (Fig. 6.4). This function provides a similar utility to the road mapping function described previously. The major difference between these two functions is that road mapping is best suited to situations where the vascular region of interest takes a prolonged time to fill with contrast, whereas the road mask function is optimal where the vascular region of interest is filled with contrast

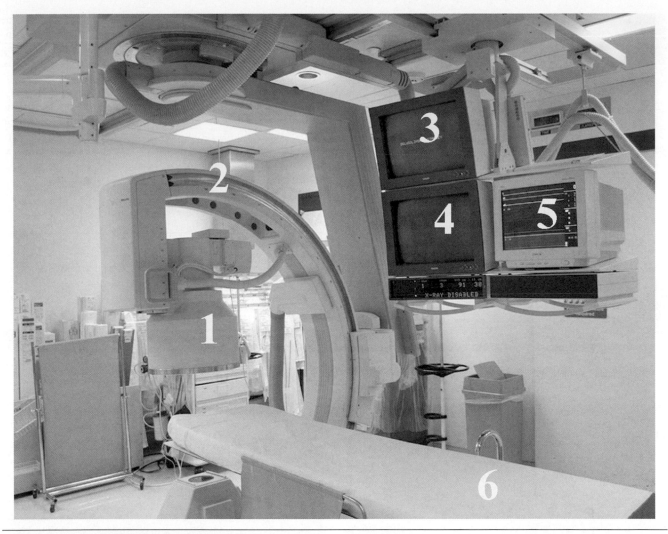

Figure 6.1 • Peripheral angiographic suite. *(1)* 15″ Image intensifier; *(2)* multiplane C-arm mounted on overhead track; *(3)* saved image monitor; *(4)* image monitor; *(5)* hemodynamic monitor; *(6)* long patient bed.

during a single frame. Both of these functions serve to minimize contrast dye loads during complicated procedures and can improve the safety of manipulations in the vascular tree.

Leg Imaging Capability

The ability to perform lower extremity angiography requires that the image intensifier be able to travel on an overhead track to the patient's feet. In addition, the table should be sufficiently long to provide working space caudal to the feet since the image intensifier is placed over the legs, thereby eliminating the usual workspace. Long wires (260 to 300 cm) are frequently used so it is important to have plenty of workspace.

There are two fundamental approaches to imaging the lower extremities: interactive mode versus stepped mode with multiple injections. When performing a "runoff" of the leg's arterial system, traditional practice has been to obtain sequential stepped static angiographic images (i.e., aortoiliac, femoral–popliteal, anterior tibial/posterior tibial/peroneal, and foot) using bolus contrast injections. This can be time-consuming and requires selective cannulation of the ipsilateral external iliac or common femoral arteries. The advantage of this method is that image

quality is usually superior, and the ability to alter the angulation of the image acquisition at different locations along the level of the lower extremity can help with vessel visualization, particularly at bifurcation points or where the vessels overly bone.

The interactive mode permits complete imaging of one or both lower extremities with a single bolus given in the ipsilateral external iliac artery or distal abdominal aorta, respectively. The first step is to engage the interactive mode in the control room and establish the beginning and end positions of the table. The bolus is then given, cineangiography is simultaneously commenced, and the bolus is chased by moving the table proximally relative to the image intensifier. The table is then automatically brought back to the starting position and a "dry" cineangiographic run is performed at the same table movement rate. The latter images are used to subtract from the initial contrast-containing images. Digital subtraction images are then obtained from the interactive run and stored. Currently, it is not possible to obtain new DSA images from the interactive run once the case has been transferred from the local storage. Problems arise if a patient has trouble holding still for the 1 to 2 minutes that it takes to complete an interactive

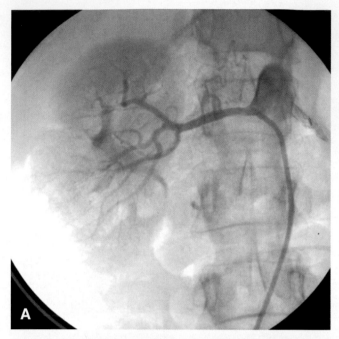

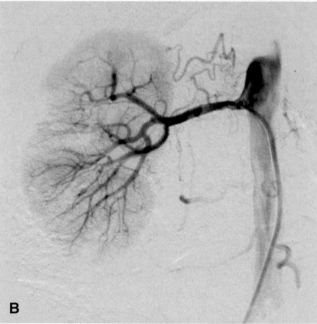

Figure 6.2 • **A:** Cineangiogram of right renal artery showing vascular and surrounding structures. **B:** Digital subtraction angiogram of right renal artery showing vascular structures with background subtracted.

run. Additionally, severe stenosis or occlusion in one extremity often results in sufficiently unequal rates of contrast runoff in both extremities that the operator needs to prioritize the leg of interest and compromise on the image quality from the contralateral leg.

Minimizing Radiation Exposure

Peripheral vascular interventions can be very long and involve significant radiation exposure for the operator, the laboratory

staff, and the patient. For the operator, maximizing the distance from the source of radiation is a fundamental principle. Wearing an appropriate "lead apron" that is checked annually for its integrity, maximizing shielding (e.g., screens, acrylic leaded shields, thyroid collars, lead glasses), collimating the image field when possible, and using low-dose pulse fluoroscopy are additional important elements in minimizing radiation exposure. Finally, consistently wearing radiation badges that monitor radiation exposure is required so that appropriate investigation of high readings can occur in an expeditious manner, and corrective actions can be instituted if required.

ARTERIAL ACCESS

One of the first steps of any endovascular procedure is determining the most appropriate site for arterial access (3,4).

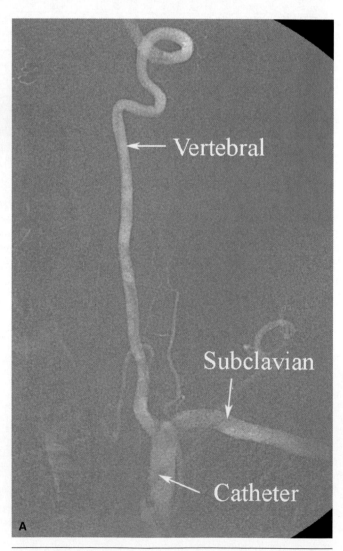

Figure 6.3 • **A:** Trace-subtract fluoroscopic image of left vertebral artery. Note that vascular structures appear white with this fluoroscopic technique.

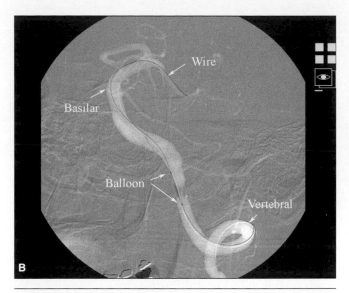

Figure 6.3 • *(continued)* **B:** Trace- subtract fluoroscopic image of intracerebral portion of the left vertebral and basilar arteries demonstrating the usefulness of this technique for wiring vessels and positioning equipment.

Common Femoral Artery

This is the most common access site used for peripheral diagnostic angiography and intervention. The common femoral artery (CFA) is centrally located and all vascular arterial systems can be reached barring occlusive and tortuous peripheral vascular disease. The advantage of this access site is the size of the CFA, which can accommodate sheath

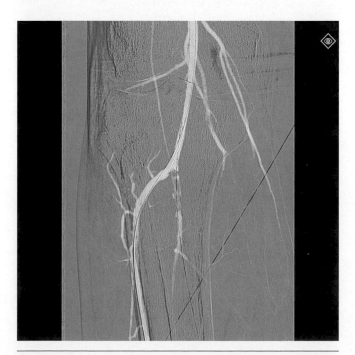

Figure 6.4 • Road mask image generated from digital subtraction angiogram of popliteal artery and proximal portion of tibial vessels.

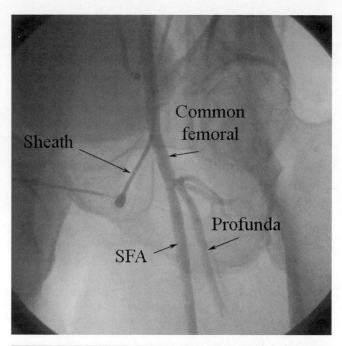

Figure 6.5 • Common femoral artery (CFA) angiogram demonstrating correct position of CFA sheath proximal to the CFA bifurcation at the level of the middle of the femoral head. SFA, superfical femoral artery.

sizes of 12 to 14 Fr. with minimal risk for ischemia. Most equipment has been developed for the femoral approach and the femoral artery approach also provides greater distance from the x-ray source and a more spacious workplace compared with the arm. On the other hand, CFA access is associated with an increased bleeding risk and delayed ambulation (5,6).

In peripheral angiography, the CFA may be accessed in a retrograde (i.e., toward the iliac artery) or antegrade (i.e., toward the foot) fashion, which impacts the access technique. In the retrograde approach, puncture of the CFA should be performed using the front-wall technique and using radiographic landmarks to maximize the chance of puncture proximal to its bifurcation (Fig. 6.5) (7,8). It is estimated the CFA bifurcation is proximal to the middle of the femoral head in 99% of patients: hence in our lab, this is the target for puncture, assuming that prior angiography or noninvasive testing has not demonstrated otherwise. In our practice, we have moved to using micropuncture access for all peripheral cases. This involves the use of 21-G needles (7 cm long) to access the artery followed by wiring of the artery with 0.018″ guidewires that have a stiff body and soft tip. The needle is exchanged for a coaxial catheter that has an inner dilator and outer sheath, with a seamless transition between these two components. The 0.018″ wire and dilator are then removed, allowing introduction of a 0.035″ wire, which allows subsequent delivery of the routine access sheath. The 0.035″ wires that we typically use for this purpose include Wholey, Versacore, Magic Torque, and SupraCore. The SupraCore wire is helpful if extra support for sheath delivery is anticipated. We would specifically warn against using J-tipped or straight wires for this purpose, since there is a high incidence of previously unrecognized iliac artery disease in patients undergoing

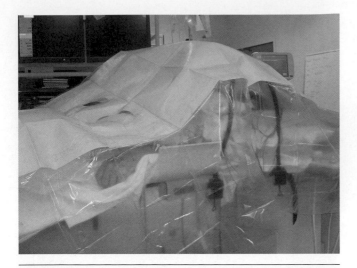

Figure 6.6 • Positioning of patient during antegrade common femoral artery access with head toward foot of table and feet toward the head of the table.

peripheral vascular procedures and dissections can easily be created by the unsuspecting operator.

Antegrade CFA access requires careful attention to detail, particularly in obese patients, where the bleeding risk is significantly increased (9). In our laboratory, the patient is draped as shown in Figure 6.6. With this arrangement, the patient's head is placed toward the foot of the table, and the patient's feet are at the head of the table. Criss-crossing flexible bars are arranged as shown to provide a "tent" effect over the patient's face and upper trunk with the goal of improving patient comfort. This arrangement has many advantages for the operator, including optimization of the length available toward the foot of the table for interventional equipment.

In order to puncture the CFA above the bifurcation, the skin puncture site of the needle is often much higher than would be anticipated by the inexperienced operator. Our practice is to use a micropuncture access set (with a 7-cm-long 21-G needle) and to perform the puncture under direct fluoroscopic guidance (Fig. 6.7). The 0.018″ wire is then advanced into the superficial femoral artery (SFA) through the micropuncture

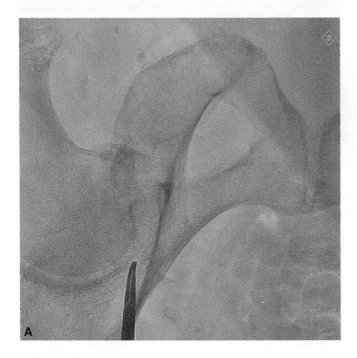

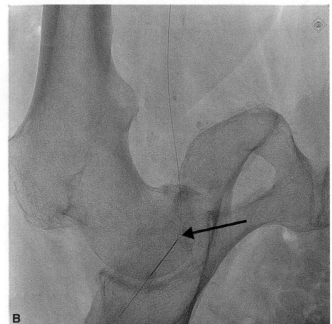

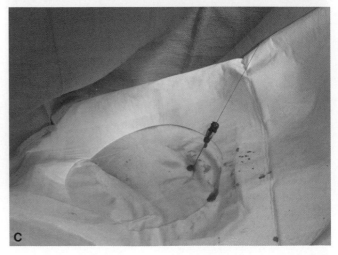

Figure 6.7 • Antegrade common femoral artery access. **A:** Fluoroscopic image demonstrating location of head of femur. **B:** Fluoroscopic image demonstrating the location of the arterial puncture at the level of the middle of the head of the femur *(arrow)*. **C:** Picture from the same patient demonstrating the location of the skin puncture by the micropuncture needle to achieve the arterial puncture shown in **B.**

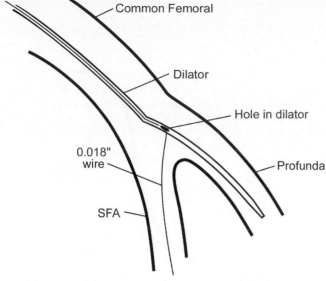

Figure 6.8 • Use of Cope–Saddekni superficial femoral artery access dilator to wire the SFA during an antegrade access of the common femoral artery.

needle. One must ensure that the 0.018″ wire is in the SFA before advancing the sheath. If there is prominent calcification in the SFA, this is straightforward. In patients with no calcium in the SFA, a useful rule of thumb is to visualize the wire coursing along the usual course of the SFA (i.e., initially medially and then laterally as it crosses the border of the femur in the typical location of Hunter's canal). The coaxial sheath is then introduced and the 0.018″ wire is exchanged for a 0.035″ wire, which is used to allow delivery of the arterial access sheath. We would strongly recommend using a stiff-bodied 0.035″ wire for the latter maneuver (e.g., SupraCore, SuperStiff Amplatz wire), as failure to deliver the sheath over the 0.035″ will require a repeat attempt at vascular access.

Body habitus strongly influences the difficulty of antegrade access. In thin individuals, access is usually straightforward. However, in obese individuals, the skin puncture site will be significantly higher than normal, and the angle at which the needle enters the CFA is significantly steeper. In some very obese patients, the 7-cm needle may not be long enough, and a 12-cm needle may be required. The steep angle of entry of the needle with the CFA in the anterior–posterior (AP) plane often makes subsequent delivery of the coaxial catheter and/or vascular access sheath (see above) very difficult. In this regard, it is very important during attempts at antegrade access that the needle be aligned with the vessel in the medial–lateral (ML) plane, as excessive angulation in both the AP and ML planes will sometimes make delivery of the sheath impossible. In patients with severe calcification of the CFA, a stiffened micropuncture coaxial sheath is often required to achieve entry to the artery and should always be available during antegrade access cases. Occasionally, the micropuncture coaxial sheath cannot be delivered over the 0.018″ wire, usually due to severe calcification that is compounded by angulation issues. In such cases, direct antegrade puncture using a conventional 18-G Cook needle, followed by introduction of a SuperStiff Amplatz wire (with 1 cm soft tip) will typically allow successful antegrade access.

The other major challenge that is sometimes encountered during antegrade access is persistent tracking of the 0.018″ guidewire into the profunda femoral branch with failure to wire the SFA. In this circumstance, special dilators (e.g., Cope–Saddekni dilator; Fig. 6.8) may help access to the SFA. Another option is to proceed with placement of the micropuncture coaxial sheath and vascular access sheath into the profunda femoral artery. After advancing a stiff-bodied 0.014″ wire (e.g., GrandSlam) into the profunda, the access sheath is withdrawn to the level of the CFA bifurcation (using small injection of contrast). A steerable 0.035″ wire (e.g., angled glidewire) supported by an angulated catheter (angled glide catheter, Bernstein) can then be used to facilitate wiring of the SFA, and subsequent delivery of the sheath.

Upper Extremity Access—Brachial and Radial

Access from the upper extremity arteries offers the advantage of early ambulation and a reduced risk of bleeding complications. The downside of these access sites is the limited sheath sizes that can be used (5 to 6 Fr. at radial, 6 to 7 Fr. at brachial), particularly in smaller female patients, and the increased risk of ischemic complications (10). Even more serious is the risk of embolization to the cerebral circulation that may occur because of instrumentation of the aortic arch or passage of equipment across the origin of the vertebral or right common carotid arteries.

Brachial artery puncture is performed with the arm and forearm extended and slightly abducted. The site of puncture should be in the area of maximal arterial pulsation but care should be taken not to stick the brachial artery significantly above the antecubital crease as it increases the risk of bleeding (Fig. 6.9). A 4-cm-long 21-G micropuncture needle is optimal for most patients. Particular attention should be paid to hemostasis following removal of brachial artery sheaths, since the location of the arteriotomy away from an easily compressible bony structure can make hemostasis difficult. Significant hematomas that cause severe patient discomfort and pseudoaneurysm formation occur following brachial access and can be minimized by applying pressure for at least 20 to 30 minutes following sheath removal.

Radial artery puncture is performed with the wrist extended (i.e., dorsiflexed) and the forearm and hand supinated. The site of puncture is generally ~1 to 2 cm proximal to the wrist crease. We use a 2.5-cm or 4-cm-long micropuncture 21-G needle for all radial artery punctures. Other operators use a peripheral IV access system (e.g., Angiocath™) to puncture the radial artery (evidenced by the back flash of blood) and advance through the posterior wall of the radial artery. The needle is then withdrawn, and the sheath is slowly withdrawn until pulsatile flow is visualized. The guidewire is then advanced into the radial artery and the radial artery sheath is placed.

Both the radial and the brachial arteries are prone to significant spasm and thrombosis in response to instrumentation. Aggressive administration of vasodilators (e.g., nitroglycerin, verapamil) and heparin (at least 3000 units) directly into the sheath is mandatory following sheath insertion to minimize these risks. During brachial artery access, operators must be aware of the potential for anomalous origin of the radial or the ulnar arteries from the axillary or high brachial artery (Fig. 6.10). In addition, the potential for wires

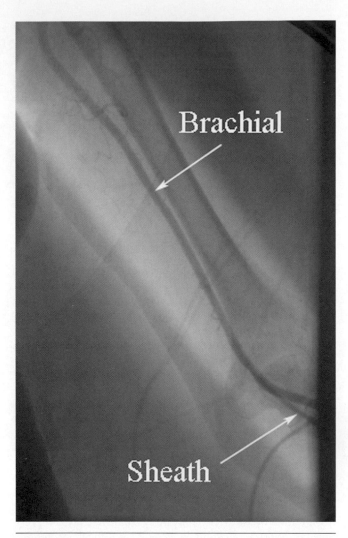

Figure 6.9 • Angiogram of left brachial artery demonstrating typical location of the brachial artery sheath during brachial artery access.

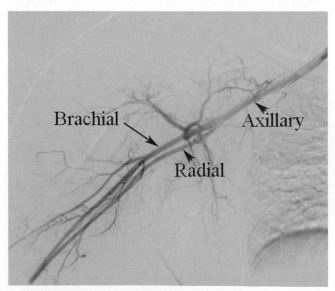

Figure 6.10 • Right axillary artery angiogram demonstrating anomalous origin of the radial artery from the axillary artery.

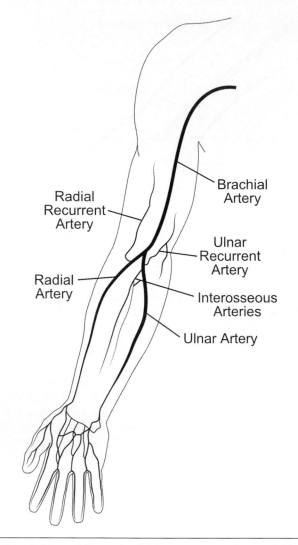

Figure 6.11 • Schematic of right upper extremity arterial supply. Note the recurrent radial branch that can be entered by wires and catheters during use of the radial artery access site and may be subject to trauma.

and catheters to track along the course of the recurrent radial branch when using radial artery access should be appreciated as this can result in trauma to this branch and hematoma formation (Fig. 6.11).

Popliteal Artery

In a small number of specific situations during lower extremity interventions, the popliteal artery may need to be accessed, usually in a retrograde fashion. The patient is placed prone on the table. Given the proximity of the popliteal vein with the popliteal artery (Fig. 6.12), ultrasound guidance (using color power Doppler function) has particular value at this access site, and if available, should be the default method used for popliteal artery access. The puncture may be performed using fluoroscopic guidance alone (assuming the popliteal artery has calcification in the wall) or using roadmap guidance following injection of contrast from another arterial site (e.g., ipsilateral CFA antegrade access or

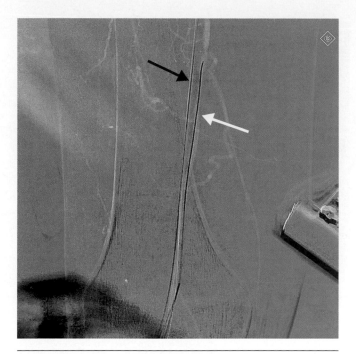

Figure 6.12 • Roadmap image demonstrating close relationship of the popliteal vein *(black arrow)* with the popliteal artery *(white arrow)*. During this case, the popliteal vein was punctured in error using roadmap guidance. Color Doppler guidance may have prevented this.

contralateral CFA access) (Fig. 6.13). A 7-cm 21-G micropuncture needle is typically used and we would avoid using sheath sizes ≥6 Fr. in this location. Careful attention to hemostasis at the arteriotomy site following sheath removal is warranted.

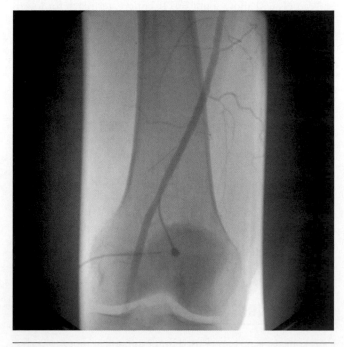

Figure 6.13 • Popliteal artery angiogram demonstrating typical location of popliteal artery sheath.

Pedal/Tibial Artery Access

Retrograde pedal (i.e., dorsalis pedis [DP]) and tibial (i.e., posterior tibial [PT]) access is performed for the treatment of complex tibial occlusive disease in patients with critical limb ischemia. The general principles for retrograde tibial/pedal access are as follows:

(a) Administer adequate sedation to ensure patient comfort and minimize patient movement during the access attempt.

(b) Use small amounts of local anesthetic to numb the puncture site at the skin. Using large amounts of local anesthetic may compress the tibial/pedal vessel that is already under low perfusion pressure due to proximal disease.

(c) Access may be guided by calcinosis in the vessel wall, roadmap guidance following injection of contrast proximally, color power Doppler guidance, and rarely following open surgical exposure.

(d) The position of the foot during access is important. For retrograde PT access, the foot should be dorsiflexed and everted. For retrograde DP access, the foot should be plantarflexed (Fig. 6.14).

(e) The authors generally use a 4-cm-long 21-G micropuncture needle and a 4-Fr. micropuncture coaxial catheter to access the DP or PT artery. The operator should concentrate on the visual guidance image (i.e., fluoroscopy, roadmap, ultrasound) and have a colleague visualize the hub of the needle for evidence of backflow, as puncture of the artery may not always be apparent to the operator by tactile feedback. Always withdraw the needle slowly if no blood return is seen, as occasionally, blood return will occur during pullback, likely due to a sidewall stick in the vessel under low perfusion pressure.

(f) The 0.018″ guidewire must be advanced with great care. If the wire does not advance beyond the tip of the needle, slowly pull back on the needle while applying gentle forward pressure on the wire.

(g) Because of the proximity of adjacent deep veins with the DP and the PT, it is common to puncture the vein during attempts at arterial access. This may not be immediately obvious in all cases, due to the low perfusion pressure in the arteries. However, wire advancement into the vein will occur without resistance (which should not occur in the artery in the presence of an occlusion), and the vein will diverge from the course of the artery at the level of the upper leg.

(h) Most operators attempt to cross the tibial occlusion using 0.014″ wires supported by 0.014″ OTW balloons using the 4-Fr. dilator sheath of the micropuncture kit. If this strategy fails, then a 4-Fr. sheath should be placed (Fig. 6.14), which will allow the use of 0.035″ wire systems supported by 4-Fr. catheters.

The choice of access site for a particular diagnostic study or interventional procedure will be outlined in the various chapters to follow. However, a number of principles are worth highlighting at this point:

(1) One must always be aware of the vascular anatomy of the patient. This can be gleaned from previous angiographic studies, as well as noninvasive studies (ultrasound, CT angiography, MR angiography). Important things to look for include known occlusions, significant stenoses,

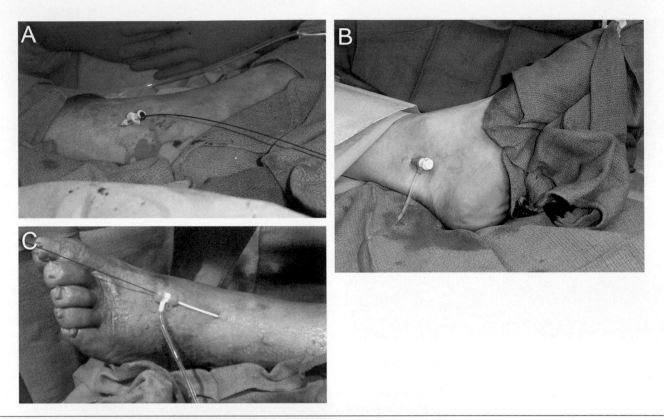

Figure 6.14 • Retrograde tibial/pedal access. **A:** Retrograde posterior tibial access with a 4-Fr. dilator in the artery. **B:** Retrograde posterior tibial access with a 4-Fr. sheath in the artery. **C:** Retrograde dorsalis pedis access with a 4-Fr. sheath in the artery.

tortuosity distal to a potential access site (e.g., subclavian artery, iliac arteries), the angulation of the aortic bifurcation (acute angulation increases the difficulty in performing crossover techniques), and the presence of known aortic arch or great vessel disease (increases the risk of cerebral embolization during upper extremity arterial access) (Fig. 6.15). In addition, it is imperative to carefully document the palpable and Dopplerable pulses present at the various potential access sites and distal to these sites prior to the procedure.

(2) The timing and nature of previous surgical revascularization procedure need to be clearly defined. For example, knowing that a patient had a femoral–femoral bypass is insufficient. Knowing the direction of flow in the graft is important since a left CFA to right CFA bypass will necessitate access on the left side (usually above the graft). The timing of any previous surgery is important as percutaneous puncture of grafts is generally avoided in the first 6 to 12 months.

(3) One must be aware of the patients' clinical history and noninvasive evaluation. For example, in lower extremity diagnostic studies, one generally obtains access from the CFA contralateral (or upper extremity access) to the extremity with the most symptoms, since this still allows for the crossover technique to be employed if an intervention is indicated.

(4) One should be aware that because of limitations of the length of interventional equipment, lower thigh, knee,

and below-knee interventions are generally not possible from the brachial access site. In addition, the left brachial access will allow about 5 to 10 cm greater reach for lower extremity intervention compared with right brachial access.

(5) The anatomy of an occlusion is often critical in determining the access approach. The points to consider are as follows:

  i. Is there enough running room between the access site and the occlusion to safely allow placement of the sheath and to provide sufficient support for wiring the lesion and delivering equipment (Fig. 6.16A).

  ii. It is important to assess from which side the occlusion should be approached. Generally, the chances of success will be greatest where there is a tapered stump without collaterals (Fig. 6.16B).

(6) When considering an intervention, one should always be aware of the sheath sizes required to deliver the equipment that one anticipates will be required to complete an intervention. For example, if the equipment requires a sheath size ≥8 Fr., femoral access will generally be required.

CHOICE OF CONTRAST AGENT

Ionic contrast is no longer used for peripheral angiography due to its high osmolality. During cerebral angiography, this type of contrast has been associated with transient blindness and

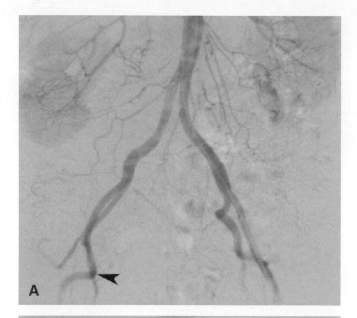

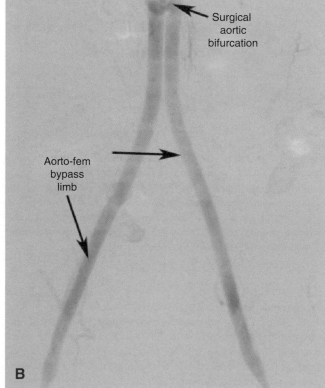

Figure 6.15 • **A:** Pelvic angiogram from a patient with right superficial femoral artery occlusion. The aortic bifurcation demonstrates an acute angle between the two common iliac arteries. The additional presence of tortuosity in the right external iliac artery (arrowhead) resulted in an antegrade common femoral artery (CFA) approach as opposed to a contralateral CFA approach. **B:** An extreme example of an acute angle at the aortic bifurcation created by a surgical aortobifemoral bypass procedure. This anatomy makes a contralateral common femoral artery approach for lower extremity intervention extremely difficult and argues in favor of a brachial artery approach or an antegrade CFA approach.

injection in the extremities is often excruciatingly painful. Its use is limited to inflation of angioplasty balloons and balloon-expandable stents during interventions. Because of the large size of the peripheral balloons and balloon-expandable stents, a mixture of 70% saline and 30% contrast is used in order to decrease the viscosity, which facilitates balloon emptying following inflation.

The best tolerated and least nephrotoxic contrast agent appears to be iodixanol (Visipaque, Amersham), which is a nonionic, isosmolar contrast agent (1). Patients rarely have any discomfort when Visipaque is injected in the peripheral circulation. However, when a catheter is placed in the mid-to-distal arm and a manual injection is performed, a 50:50 mixture of saline and contrast is given to avoid any discomfort.

For patients with chronic renal insufficiency, the optimal strategy for avoiding renal failure appears to be prehydrating and posthydrating with normal saline and minimizing the amount of contrast injected. The role of N-acetyl cysteine is questionable but is practiced by many operators (two doses of 600 mg given prior to procedure). Iodixanol should be used if possible. Gadolinium and carbon dioxide are both options for these patients but vascular imaging is often suboptimal. There is some evidence that >60 mL of gadolinium may have the same nephrotoxicity as iodinated contrast.

MANIFOLD AND HEMODYNAMIC MONITORING

A pressure/saline/contrast manifold allows continuous pressure measurement during diagnostic and interventional procedures. New automated systems (e.g., Acist CVi contrast delivery system) have also become available that have particular application in peripheral diagnostic and interventional procedures. Any dampened waveform suggests that the catheter end hole is against a vessel wall and an injection may cause vessel dissection. The system also minimizes the risk of air embolization. Continuous monitoring of the EKG, heart rate, blood pressure, and oxygen saturation often helps to detect any life-threatening issues that may arise during a procedure such as anaphylaxis, hemorrhage, pulmonary edema, or oversedation.

WIRES (0.035″, 0.018″, 0.014″)

The five primary 0.035″ wires utilized in the peripheral endovascular lab by the authors are the Wholey, Versacore, Magic Torque, SupraCore, and stiff angled glidewires (Table 6.1). The Wholey and Versacore wires are identical (different vendors) and have characteristics similar to those of the Magic Torque wire, that is, soft atraumatic coiled tip and medium supportive body. None of these wires are really steerable. The major difference between the Wholey/Versacore and Magic Torque wires is that the Wholey/Versacore wires have a white polymer covering over the wire body that tends to swell during the course of the case. This can make over-the-wire exchanges of equipment difficult. In addition, in the authors' experience, these wires appear to interact particularly badly with marker pigtail catheters—in some cases, the Wholey/Versacore wire cannot be advanced through the distal portion of the marker pigtail catheter, and on occasion, the wire has become stuck in

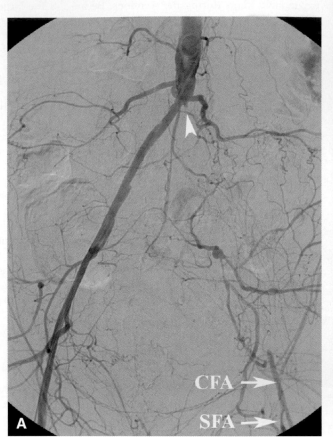
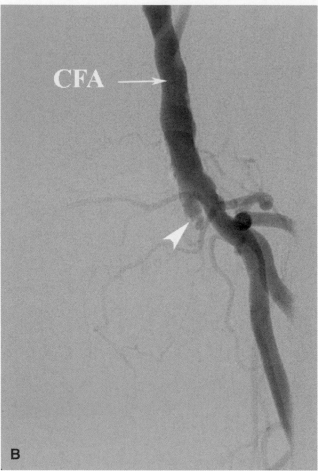

Figure 6.16 • **A:** Pelvic angiogram demonstrating a long occlusion extending from the origin of the left common iliac artery to the proximal left common femoral artery (CFA). This occlusion could be crossed using an antegrade approach with contralateral CFA access or brachial artery access. A retrograde approach would require the use of retrograde CFA access. **B:** Common femoral artery angiogram demonstrating an occlusion of the superficial femoral artery. This occlusion is favorable in that there is a clearly defined stump with no collaterals, similar to the occlusion in Figure 6.11A. Note that angulated views may be required to fully define the anatomy of the stump.

the catheter. The SupraCore wire has a soft tip and very supportive body (i.e., greater than Wholey or Magic Torque). Despite the increased support of the body of this wire, it negotiates tortuous segments very well, based on the design of the transition between the soft tip and the body. This wire has become the workhorse wire in our laboratory. The stiff angled glidewire is very steerable and trackable and provides good support. Because of its hydrophilic nature, great attention must be paid to its tip since it can dissect or perforate more easily than the other wires described. Where a steerable and trackable wire is required and support is not an issue, a floppy glidewire is safer than the stiff glidewire. The 0.035″ wires are typically used for subclavian, innominate, iliac, superficial femoral, and popliteal artery interventions.

The 0.014″ wires (Table 6.1) are suitable for carotid, vertebral, renal, and below-knee interventions. A long list of 0.014″ wires have been developed for percutaneous coronary intervention and can be safely applied in peripheral vascular intervention. It is wise to become familiar with a short list of wires that will be sufficient for the majority of procedures. This should include low, moderate, and high-support nonhydrophilic and hydrophilic wires (Table 6.1). For peripheral interventions, largely moderate or high-support wires will be used. In addition, some niche wires, such as the Synchro wire for intracerebral procedures, may be stocked. Less commonly, 0.018″ wires may be used for renal, subclavian, and popliteal interventions.

CATHETERS AND SHEATHS

Side-Hole Diagnostic Catheters

These catheters permit large volumes of contrast to be safely infused in a large artery at a rapid rate via power injection (Pig, Omniflush, Grollman, Universal Flush, Multipurpose, Straight flush). We utilize the pig catheter for ascending and arch aortography, abdominal aortography, pelvic angiography, and bilateral lower extremity runoffs (with catheter in distal abdominal aorta). When selective lower extremity angiography is performed from contralateral CFA access, we use a straight flush catheter (Fig. 6.17).

TABLE 6.1 Examples of Commonly Used Interventional Wires

Wire	Steerability	Trackability	Support	Length (cm)	Company
Wires 0.035″					
Stiff Angled Glidewire	Excellent	Excellent	Good	260	Terumo
Supracore	Poor	Good	Excellent	300	Abbott Vascular
Amplatz ExtraStiff w/ J-tip	Poor	Fair	Very Good	260	Boston Scientific
Amplatz SuperStiff (1 cm, 3 cm, 7 cm, and J-tip)	Poor	Poor	Excellent	260	Boston Scientific
Magic Torque	Fair	Good	Good	300	Boston Scientific
Wholey/Versacore	Poor	Good	Good	260	Mallinckrodt/ Abbott Vascular
Lunderquist	Poor	Poor	Excellent	260	Cook
Wires 0.018″					
Flex-T	Good	Good	Good	295	Mallinckrodt
Glidewire Gold (45 or 70 degree angle) with GT Leggiero Hydrophilic Microcatheter	Good	Excellent	Poor*	180	Terumo
Wires 0.014″					
Asahi Soft	Excellent	Good	Fair	190, 300	Abbott Vascular
Asahi Prowater	Excellent	Good	Fair	190, 300	Abbott Vascular
GrandSlam	Good	Fair	Excellent	190, 300	Abbott Vascular
Whisper (hydrophilic)	Good	Excellent	Fair	190, 300	Abbott Vascular
Shinobi (hydrophilic)	Excellent	Good	Excellent	190, 300	Cordis
Synchro Wire (hydrophilic)	Excellent	Excellent	Fair	300	Boston Scientific

*Advise exchange of Glidewire Gold for other supportive wire via microcatheter.

End-Hole Diagnostic Catheters

Selective diagnostic angiography is performed using manual injections of contrast through end-hole catheters. Good studies can usually be obtained with 4- or 5-Fr. catheters when using DSA (Table 6.2). The 4-Fr. Bernstein catheter is our workhorse catheter for imaging the carotid, vertebral, and subclavian arteries. Mesenteric and renal artery angiography is typically performed using Sos or Cobra catheters. For upper and lower extremity angiography, straight and angled glide catheters are sufficient for most procedures. The use of other catheters with more complicated shapes (e.g., Simmons, Vitek) is described in the specific chapters related to the arterial territory in which they are used (Fig. 6.18).

Guiding Catheter versus Sheath

Peripheral interventions may be performed using either a sheath or guide-based systems. Straight (e.g., Shuttle, Raabe) or shaped (e.g., Ansel, Balkan) sheaths (Table 6.3) are most commonly used. One of the major advantages of sheaths over guides is that in general, a sheath has the same internal diameter as a guiding catheter two French sizes larger (i.e., a 6-Fr. sheath has the same internal diameter as an 8-Fr. guiding catheter). However, it is generally not possible to maneuver the direction of the sheath tip, which removes some flexibility during interventional procedures. Additionally, sheaths do not offer the same degree of support as guide catheters (Figs. 6.19 and 6.20).

Sheath: Diaphragm versus Rotating Hemostatic Valve

Sheaths are designed with either a simple diaphragm or a hemostatic valve at their end. These serve as the access point for delivery of equipment. A hemostatic valve (e.g., Tuohy Borst valve) allows blood to bleed back when the valve is open, thereby reducing the risk of air and atherosclerotic debris embolization. This device should be in place when working in the aortic arch vessels and the renal and mesenteric arteries. It is less critical during lower extremity intervention. Guiding

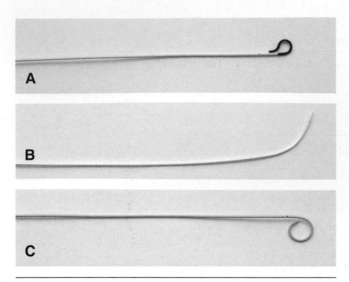

Figure 6.17 • Sample of side-hole catheters. **A:** Omni Flush. **B:** Multipurpose. **C:** Pigtail.

catheters always require a hemostatic valve be attached at their end to allow delivery of equipment.

Telescoping

Advancing large guiding catheters and sheaths into certain arteries can often be quite challenging and is often made simpler by using a "telescoping" technique (Fig. 6.21). The principle of this technique is that delivery of a sheath or guide is facilitated by building gradually increasing layers of support, using a variety of wires and catheters. This technique is most commonly practiced during delivery of carotid artery sheaths or guides or contralateral access sheaths over the aortoiliac bifurcation. For example, when one wants to deliver a sheath to the common carotid artery to allow stenting of the internal carotid artery, the following telescoping technique may be used: a diagnostic catheter is "telescoped" through the sheath. The diagnostic catheter is used to engage the CCA of interest, allowing delivery of a supportive wire to the distal CCA. The diagnostic catheter is advanced over this wire, and the sheath is then delivered over the wire/catheter combination. When using this telescoping technique, it is quite important to have a smooth transition between the guide or sheath and the telescoping catheter, particularly when advancing through tortuous and diseased vessels in order to minimize vessel trauma and embolization.

INTRAVASCULAR ULTRASOUND

Intravascular ultrasound (IVUS) is used infrequently during peripheral vascular procedures, except during percutaneous abdominal aortic aneurysm repair. IVUS can be helpful for vessel sizing, ensuring good stent apposition, and to clarify anatomic issues when angiography is indeterminate (Table 6.4). Because of the larger vessel sizes involved in peripheral vascular

TABLE 6.2 Diagnostic Catheters			
End-Hole Catheters			
Vascular Bed	**Name**	**Length (cm)**	**Comments**
Cerebral, carotid, vertebral, subclavian, and innominate	Glidecath-angled	100, 120	Great tracking ability in tortuous vessels, soft atraumatic catheter tip
	Berenstein	100	Workhorse catheter
	JR4	100,125	
	Newton (1, 2, 3, 4)	100	Similar shape as Vitek catheter
	Simmons (1, 2, 3)	100	Used for most complex aortic arch anatomies. Catheter manipulation more involved than for Vitek catheter
Renal/mesenteric	JR4	100, 125	
	Vitek	125	Default catheter for more complex aortic arch types and engagement of left common carotid artery with bovine origin
	SOS	80	Default catheter for selective renal artery angiography
	Cobra (C1, C2, C3)	65	
Upper extremity	Glidecath-angled	100, 120	
Lower extremity	IM (approach from contralateral leg)	100	Used to cross from ipsilateral iliac to contralateral iliac artery
	Multipurpose	125	Used to perform unilateral lower extremity angiography from contralateral approach with catheter in external iliac or common femoral artery

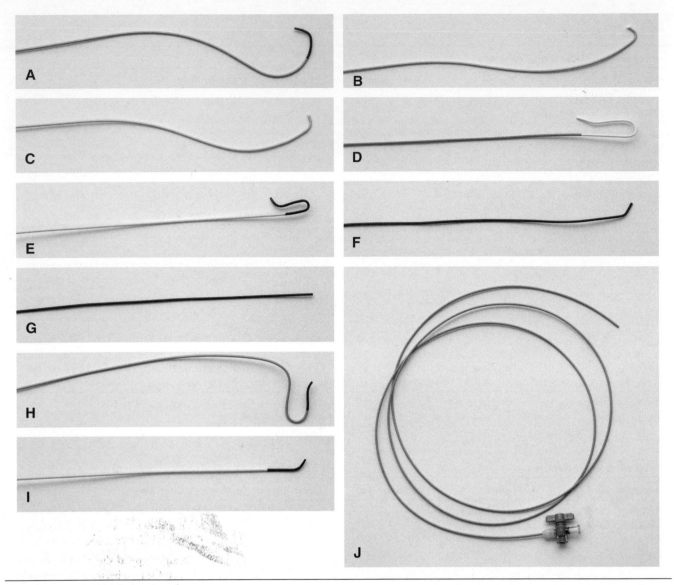

Figure 6.18 • Sample of end-hole catheters. **A:** Cobra. **B:** Multipurpose. **C:** Judkins Right. **D:** Simmons. **E:** SoS. **F:** Angled glide. **G:** Straight glide. **H:** Vitek. **I:** Berenstein. **J:** Red rubber.

procedures, peripheral IVUS catheters utilize lower-frequency transducers (typically ≤15 MHz) compared with coronary IVUS catheters (typically 30 to 40 MHz).

ADDITIONAL PEARLS

1. It is wise to establish a system for surgical backup during peripheral vascular procedures, particularly those deemed high-risk (e.g., common iliac artery or subclavian artery occlusions). Similarly, having neurovascular backup with the capability of treating intracranial complications during extracranial cerebrovascular procedures is appropriate.

2. One should be thoroughly familiar with the vascular anatomy of the vessel(s) on which you are performing a diagnostic or interventional procedure. Know which problems will arise if the artery occludes or distal embolization occurs. For example, left subclavian stenting in a patient with a patent left internal mammary artery (LIMA) graft to the left anterior descending artery could compromise the left vertebral artery, the LIMA graft, and arterial flow to the left hand.

3. Raising the table to its maximum height and minimizing the distance between the image intensifier and the patient will maximize the field of view.

4. When performing a power injection, always use a side-hole catheter to minimize the risk of vessel perforation/dissection.

5. Do not inject through end-hole catheters if you have a dampened pressure tracing.

6. For diagnostic angiography, obtain orthogonal views of suspected lesions, and identify the view that produces the least foreshortening of the lesion.

7. Always advance catheters and sheaths over a wire.

8. At the beginning of a peripheral intervention, you should be aware of the vessel diameter you are treating and the

TABLE 6.3 Guiding Catheters and Sheaths

Interventional Guiding Catheters

Vascular Bed	Name	Size (Fr.)	Length (cm)	Comments
Carotid, vertebral, subclavian, innominate	Headhunter (H1)	8, 9	90	Primary guide for engaging great vessels
	Judkins Right (JR4)	8, 9	110	
	Amplatz Left (AL1)	8, 9	110	Used in more complex great vessel and carotid interventions; see chapter 11
Renal/mesenteric	Renal Standard Curve	7, 8	55	Short tipped RES guide may also be useful
	Renal Double Curve	7, 8	55	Primary guide for renal intervention from femoral access
	Renal Multipurpose	7, 8	55	Primary guide for renal/mesenteric intervention using upper extremity access
	JR4	7, 8	110	Generally provides poor support for renal intervention
	Hockey Stick	7, 8	55	Rarely used for renal/mesenteric intervention
Iliac	Multipurpose	7, 8	110	For iliac intervention from upper extremity access.
Femoral, popliteal, below knee	Multipurpose	6, 7, 8	110	See chapters 16 and 17 for details.

Interventional Sheaths

Vascular Bed	Name	Size (Fr.)	Length (cm)	Company	Comments
Cerebrovascular/subclavian	Ansel (AN1, AN2, AN3)	6, 7	45	Cook	Curved tip. Useful for subclavian/innominate interventions from brachial/radial access
	Raabe	6, 7, 8, 9	55, 70, 80, 90	Cook	Straight tipped sheath with short distance between dilator and sheath tip
	Shuttle Sheath	6, 7, 8, 9	80, 90	Cook	Excellent tracking sheath with smooth dilator-sheath transition; sheath of choice for carotid intervention
Renal/mesenteric	Renal Standard Curve	7, 8	55	Cordis	
	Renal Double Curve	7, 8	55	Cordis	
	Renal Multipurpose	7, 8	55	Cordis	For renal/mesenteric intervention from brachial/radial access
Lower extremity	Balkan	6, 7, 8	40	Cook	Provide superior support to Pinnacle Destination sheath, but less deliverable through tortuous anatomy
	Brite Tip	6, 7, 8	35, 55, 90	Cordis	Primary sheath for ipsilateral iliac intervention
	Pinnacle Destination	5–8	45	Terumo	Primary sheath for contralateral femoral access

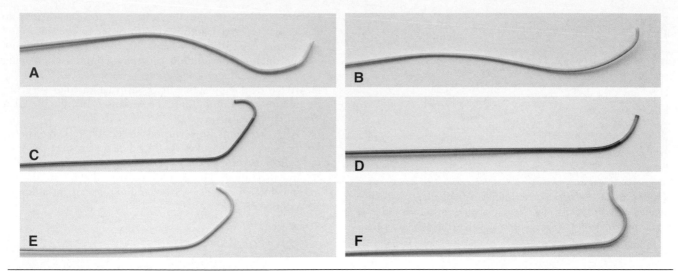

Figure 6.19 • Sample of guide catheters. **A:** Headhunter (H1). **B:** Judkins Right (JR4). **C:** Renal standard (RES). **D:** Renal multipurpose. **E:** Renal double curve (RDC). **F:** Amplatz Right (AR1).

balloon and/or stent that you are planning to use. One should then be aware of the outer diameter of these balloons/stents, since this will determine the minimum size sheath/guide catheter that will be required to deliver this equipment. An assessment of the distance of the lesion from the access site will determine the appropriate length equipment to choose. This forward planning will help

ensure that you use an appropriate access site and have the right equipment to complete a successful procedure.

9. When performing an intervention, try to have the guide catheter/sheath near the lesion (e.g., proximal SFA for mid-SFA lesion; distal common carotid for internal carotid lesion). This provides for better visualization and improved support.

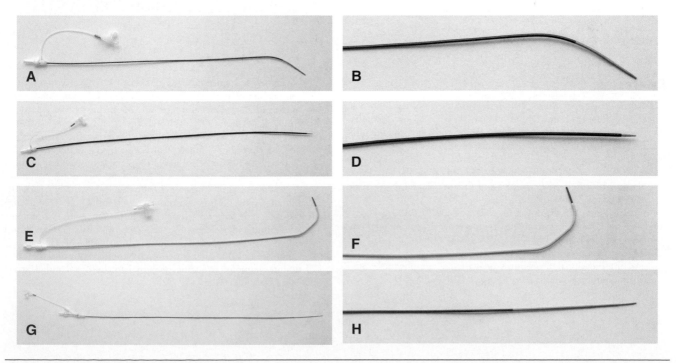

Figure 6.20 • Sample of sheaths. **A,B:** Low and high magnification view of Ansel sheath. **C,D:** Low and high magnification view of Raabe sheath. **E,F:** Low and high magnification view of renal double curve guide sheath. **G,H:** Low and high magnification view of Shuttle sheath.

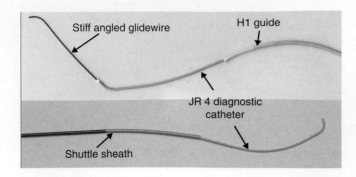

Figure 6.21 • Telescope technique. A long diagnostic catheter is advanced through the interventional guide or sheath and is used to facilitate delivery of the guide or sheath to the desired location.

10. When advancing guiding catheters and sheaths, try to have a tapered leading edge in order to prevent vessel trauma (e.g., dissection, embolization). For sheaths, use the dilator. For guiding catheters, consider telescoping with a 5-Fr. diagnostic catheter.
11. Avoid deploying stents in vessels that vascular surgeons use for anastomotic sites. These vessels include the CFA and popliteal artery.
12. After crossing an occlusion in peripheral vessels, the presence of back-flow of blood from an over-the-wire balloon or catheter does not necessarily indicate an intraluminal position. The easy movement of the wire distally into branch vessels is a better indicator of intraluminal position.

TABLE 6.4 Intravascular Ultrasound

Catheter	Console	Maximum Guidewire (OD)	Minimum Sheath Size (Fr.)	Image Depth (mm)	Transducer Frequency (MHz)	Company
Atlantis® PV Peripheral Imaging Catheter	Galaxy™ Galaxy™2	0.035″	8	24	15	Boston Scientific
Visions™ PV 018 IVUS Imaging Catheter	In Vision	0.018″	4	24	15	Volcano Therapeutics
Visions™ PV 8.2 F IVUS Imaging Catheter*	Gold™	0.038″	8	60	10	Volcano Therapeutics

*Designed specifically for assessment of abdominal aortic aneurysms.
OD, outer diameter; Fr., French.

References

1. Baim DS. Proper use of cineangiographic equipment and contrast agents. In: Baim DS, Grossman W, eds. Cardiac Catheterization, Angiography, and Intervention. 6th ed. Philadelphia, PA: Lippincott, Williams & Wilkins; 2000:15–34.
2. Wahl SI, Zinn KM. Filming and injection techniques. In: Bakal CW, Silberzweig JE, Cynamon J, et al., eds. Vascular and Interventional Radiology: Principles and Practice. 1st ed. New York, NY: Thieme Medical Publishers; 2002:17–24.
3. Patel PJ, Patel RS. Endovascular Today, May 2010:40–48.
4. Naxrins CR. Access strategies for peripheral arterial intervention. Cardiol J. 2009;16:88–97.
5. Khoury M, Batra S, Berg R, et al. Influence of arterial access sites and interventional procedures on vascular complications after cardiac catheterizations. Am J Surg. 1992;164:205–209.
6. Kiemeneij F, Laarman GJ, Odekerken D, et al. A randomized comparison of percutaneous transluminal coronary angioplasty by the radial, brachial and femoral approaches: the access study. J Am Coll Cardiol. 1997;29:1269–1275.
7. Spector KS, Lawson WE. Optimizing safe femoral access during cardiac catheterization. Catheter Cardiovasc Interv. 2001;53:209–212.
8. Garrett PD, Eckart RE, Bauch TD, et al. Fluoroscopic localization of the femoral head as a landmark for common femoral artery cannulation. Catheter Cardiovasc Interv. 2005;65:205–207.
9. Biondi-Zoccai GGL, Agostoni P, Sangiorgi G, et al. Mastering the antegrade femoral artery access in patients with symptomatic lower limb ischemia: learning curve, complications, and technical tips and tricks. Catheter Cardiovasc Interv. 2006;68:835–842.
10. Campeau L. Entry sites for coronary angiography and therapeutic interventions: from the proximal to the distal radial artery. Can J Cardiol. 2001;17:319–325.

CHAPTER 7

Balloon and Stent Technology

James P. Sur, Ivan P. Casserly, and Hitinder S. Gurm

Peripheral artery disease (PAD) has been treated percutaneously since 1964, when Charles Dotter and Melvin Judkins first described the technique of progressive serial dilatation of the arteries of the lower extremity in nine patients (1). Since that time, the techniques used to mechanically improve perfusion to the lower extremities of patients with PAD have been refined significantly, with progression from the use of dilatation catheters to balloon catheters, balloon-expandable (BE) and self-expanding (SE) stents, stent grafts and novel devices like cryotherapy balloons, medicated balloons, biodegradable stents, as well as plaque removal (atherectomy) or ablation devices.

This chapter reviews the current balloons and stents used to perform peripheral interventions and the developing balloon and stent technologies that will continue to advance the percutaneous treatment of PAD.

BALLOONS

Balloon catheters used in interventions in the periphery have similar characteristics to those designed for use in the coronary bed, except that they are available in larger diameters and lengths, and are generally less compliant. There are many balloon catheters available for use and it is important to understand the characteristics of their construction and delivery requirements (Table 7.1).

Balloon catheters used in the periphery are almost exclusively made out of plastic polymers with varying degrees of compliance (Figs. 7.1 and 7.2). The more compliant a balloon is, the less dilatation force there is at the lesion site, and the more it will stretch and expand in an area of low resistance (i.e., adjacent normal vessel). Thus, when used to treat resistant lesions that are common in the periphery, highly compliant balloons have a tendency to fail to adequately fracture the target lesion and overexpand the vessel beyond the lesion site, increasing the risk of dissection in those areas. For this reason, noncompliant balloons are usually the preferred balloon type used in the periphery because they provide a greater dilating force at the target lesion while maintaining a defined diameter in the adjacent normal vessel.

The noncompliant balloons of the periphery are usually made of polyethylene terephthalate (PET) or nylon reinforced polyurethane. This design improves the radial strength of the balloon and has a higher rate of burst pressure allowance. Some manufacturers use additional proprietary additives that serve to strengthen the balloon material and improve puncture resistance. These designs allow for a greater inflation pressure and therefore radial force with maintenance of the defined diameter.

Most peripheral balloons are deliverable through 4- to 6-Fr. sheaths (except for large caliber aortic balloons). The proximal and distal margins of the balloons are usually demarcated by markers and the balloon tips are designed to minimize the crossing profile. Most peripheral balloons are designed to be delivered over the wire. Rapid exchange balloons are most commonly utilized in the treatment of cerebrovascular, renal, or mesenteric artery disease, but some lower extremity rapid exchange balloons have recently been released (e.g., SLEEK Long, Cordis). The diameter of wire with which the balloon is compatible will depend on the vessel diameter being treated (i.e., 0.014″ and 0.018″ for smaller caliber vessels and 0.035″ for larger caliber vessels) (Table 7.1). Peripheral angioplasty balloons are usually inflated using a mixture of 70% saline and 30% contrast for ease of inflation and deflation given their longer lengths and larger diameters. These balloons also tend to have lower nominal and rated burst inflation pressures when compared to coronary balloons.

Focal Pressure Balloons — Scoring/Cutting Balloons

Routine balloon angioplasty achieves luminal gain by fracturing the plaque and creating an irregular dissection in the vessel wall. This can be particularly problematic in patients with fibrocalcific plaque where the barotrauma can be unevenly distributed. It has been argued that focal delivery of pressure can score the target lesion, creating a more controlled dissection that results in a larger luminal gain and a reduction in the incidence of flow-limiting dissections, which ultimately provides a more predictable angiographic result. In addition, these focal pressure balloons tend to achieve greater stability at the treatment site, resulting in less device slippage, and thus reduce injury in adjacent normal vessel. Much of the basic engineering data supporting the use of these devices have not been published in the peer reviewed literature and it is unclear if the plaque scoring benefits of these devices apply in calcific peripheral vessels where they are often used.

The AngioSculpt (AngioScore, Fremont, CA) and VascuTrak 2 (Bard, Tempe, AZ) balloon catheters represent the newest additions to the focal pressure balloon family. The AngioSculpt balloon catheter incorporates a laser-cut highly flexible nitinol scoring element containing three spiral struts that encircle a semicompliant balloon catheter that creates a focal concentration of dilating force along the edges of the scoring element (Fig. 7.3). The VascuTrak 2 balloon has two guidewires placed external to the semicompliant balloon to provide focal longitudinal force to score the plaque. It has been estimated that the focal stress concentration factor provided by this balloon may be 50 to 400 times that produced by a conventional balloon.

Cutting balloons (Boston Scientific, Natick, MA) have been used for nearly two decades. Initially approved for treatment of in-stent restenosis in the coronary circulation, they have

TABLE 7.1 Angioplasty Balloons Used in Peripheral Interventions

Manufacturer	Balloon Name	Diameter (mm)	Lengths (mm)	Sheath Minimum (Fr.)	Guidewire (in.)	Design	Working Length
PTA Balloons							
Abbott	Agilitrac	4–12	20, 30, 40, & 60	5–7	0.018 & 0.035	Multicompliant	80/135
Abbott	Fox PTA	3–12	20, 30, 40, 60, & 80 (5–8 mm only)	5–7	0.035	Noncompliant	80/135
Boston Scientific	Sterling	3–8 mm RX & 4–10 mm OTW	20, 30, 40, 60, 80, & 100	4–6	0.014 & 0.018	Semicompliant	40/80/135
Bard	Dorado	3–10	20, 30, 40, 60, 80, 100, 120, 150, 170, & 200	5–7	0.035	Noncompliant	40/80/120/135
Cordis	Aviator	4–7	15, 20, 30, & 40	4–6	0.014	Compliant	75/135
Cordis	SAVVY	2, 2.5, 3, 3.5, & 4–6	120, 150, & 220	4–5	0.018	Noncompliant	120/150
Cordis/J & J	SLEEK	2, 2.5, 3, 3.5, & 4	40, 80, 100, 120, 150, & 220	4	0.014	Noncompliant	150/155
Boston Scientific	UltraThin SDS	4–10	15, 20, 30, 40, 60, & 80	5–7	0.035	Noncompliant	50/75/90/135/150
ev3	NanoCross	2–4	20, 40, 80, 120, & 150	4	0.014	Noncompliant	90/150
ev3	EverCross	3–12	20, 30, 40, 60, 80, 100, 120, 150, & 200	5–7	0.035	Noncompliant	80/135
Cordis	PowerFlex P3	4–10 & 12	10, 15, 20, 40, 60, 80, & 100	5–8	0.035	Noncompliant	40/65/80/110/135
Boston Scientific	XXL	12, 14, 16, & 18	20 & 40	7–8	0.035	Noncompliant	120
Boston Scientific	PowerFlex Extreme	4–10	40, 80, & 120	5–6	0.035	Noncompliant	40/80/120
Cordis	Opta PRO	3–10 & 12	10, 15, 20, 40, 60, 80, & 100	5–8	0.035	Compliant	80/110/135
Cryotherapy							
Boston Scientific	PolarCath	2.0, 2.5, 3, 3.5, & 4–6	20, 40, 60, & 100	5–6	0.014		135/150
	PolarCath	4–8	20, 40, 60, 80, & 100	6–8	0.035		80/120

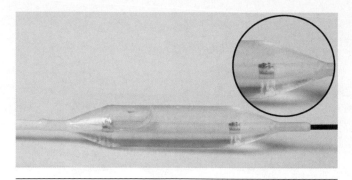

Figure 7.1 • An example of a noncompliant peripheral angioplasty balloon with polyethylene terephthalate construct with proximal and distal radiopaque markers and tapered ends.

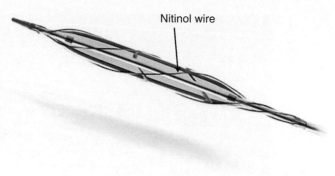

Nitinol wire

Figure 7.3 • AngioSculpt balloon—one of the three nitinol wires on surface of balloon is labeled.

increasingly found application in peripheral intervention (2). Depending on the diameter of the cutting balloon, there are three (i.e., for 1.5- to 4-mm diameter balloons) or four (i.e., for 5- to 8-mm diameter balloons) atherotomes (microsurgical blades) that are fixed longitudinally on the surface of a noncompliant balloon (Fig. 7.4). The microtomes are covered by the balloon in the wrapped defaulted state and are exposed to the vessel wall on inflation, extending 0.127 mm above the height of the balloon. Based on the assumption that the microtomes induce a longitudinal incision with less wall tension than the diffuse circumferential stress provided by conventional percutaneous transluminal angioplasty (PTA) balloons, trauma may be reduced. The current generation of cutting balloons has flexion points at 5-mm intervals along the atherotome, permitting lateral flexibility and better trackability. While the cutting balloon is routinely used in the peripheral vasculature, it is currently FDA approved for the treatment of obstructive lesions of synthetic or native arteriovenous dialysis fistulae.

Cryotherapy Balloons

There is currently one commercially available balloon device that uses compressed nitrous oxide at −10°C to deliver cryotherapy to the peripheral arteries (Fig. 7.5). This device delivers both the mechanical treatment of balloon angioplasty and the purported biologic therapy of freezing to effect treatment of the vessel. Freezing of the tissue is believed to alter the plaque's inflammatory response to angioplasty, reduce elastic recoil, and reduce smooth muscle cell proliferation by inducing apoptosis. The PolarCath Peripheral Dilatation System (Boston

Scientific) is indicated to dilate stenoses in the peripheral vasculature, including the iliac, femoropopliteal, infrapopliteal, and renal arteries. This device is also indicated for use in the treatment of restenosed areas within expanded polytetrafluoroethylene (ePTFE) graft.

The PolarCath is available in 0.014″ and 0.035″ compatible systems. The 0.014″ system is available in diameters of 2 to 4 mm (in 0.5-mm increments) and 5 and 6 mm, and lengths of 20, 40, 60, and 100 mm. These are deliverable through 5- to 6-Fr. sheaths. The 0.035″ system is available in diameters of 4 to 8 mm (in 1-mm increments) and lengths of 20, 40, 60, 80, and 100 mm. These are deliverable through 6- to 8-Fr. sheaths.

A number of nonrandomized small studies using the PolarCath device have suggested a lower incidence of clinically significant dissections and a reduced need for stenting when this device is used in the femoropopliteal artery. In one study, the 12-month freedom from restenosis was >80% (3). In a separate population with femoropopliteal disease, primary patency rates by ultrasound were ~70% at 9 months (4) and clinical patency at 3 years was 75% (5). Cryotherapy, in its initial evaluation, appears to provide similar results to PTA alone but did not perform well in heavily calcified lesions, areas of in-stent restenosis, or in vein graft lesions (6). Given its additional cost ($1700 per case on average), randomized data are needed to assess if indeed this strategy has any benefit beyond that associated with conventional PTA.

STENTS

Balloon-Expandable and Self-Expandable Stents—Materials and Design

Stents are broadly classified as either BE or SE based on how deployment is effected (Tables 7.2 and 7.3) (7). In brief, BE stents are mounted in a crimpled state on a balloon that is inflated to deploy the stent against the vessel wall. In contrast, SE stents are manufactured in an expanded state and are then crimped and constrained by a covering sheath that is retracted at the target site to allow the SE stent to expand to a predefined diameter and appose the vessel wall.

The major determinant of whether a stent will behave as a SE versus a BE stent is the material composition of the stent. In general, BE stents are made from steel that is composed of chromium and nickel (L316) (8). This is a corrosion-

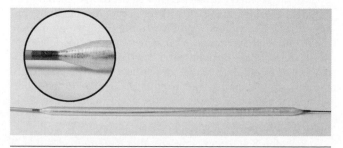

Figure 7.2 • The Dorado® balloon (Bard) has a reinforcing proprietary composite material that improves puncture resistance and permits use of higher inflation pressures.

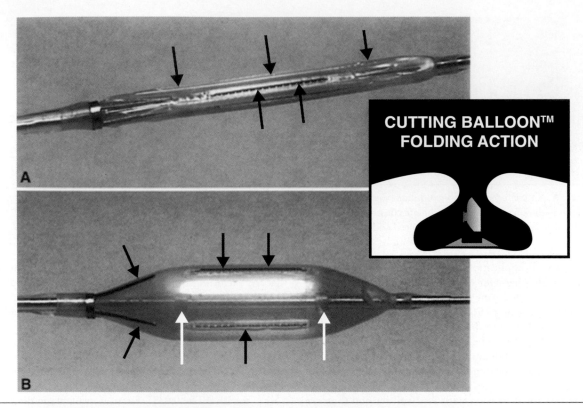

Figure 7.4 • Cutting balloon. **A:** Cutting balloon deflated. **B:** Cutting balloon inflated. Atherotomes indicated by thin black arrows. Inset—demonstrates protection of atherotomes by pockets on the balloon surface when the balloon is deflated. (With kind permission from Springer Science+Business Media: Cejna M. Cutting balloon: review on principles and background of use in peripheral arteries. *Cardiovasc Intervent Radiol.* 2005;28:400–408).

resistant material with low carbon content. Newer BE stents made of cobalt–chromium have been developed for use in the coronary and peripheral circulation. Based on the properties of cobalt–chromium, these stents have the ability to be stronger than stainless steel stents with thinner metal struts, and thus potentially can provide increased radial strength, lower crossing profiles, with enhanced flexibility and deliverability.

SE stents are typically made of nitinol, which is an alloy that consists of an ultrapure mixture of titanium (~55%) and nickel (45%). The unique properties of nitinol (i.e., shape, memory, and superelasticity) allow for SE stents to be constrained in a coaxial

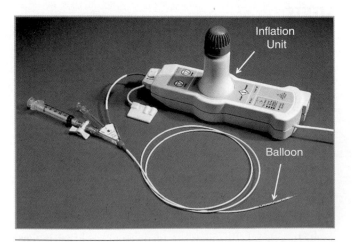

Figure 7.5 • PolarCath peripheral dilatation system.

design by an external shaft at temperatures <4°C for delivery with very low crossing profiles and for the stent to expand upon warming (>4°C) to its prespecified diameter and shape, providing lasting contact between the stent and the vessel wall.

Regardless of stent type, the majority of all stents has either a coil or slotted-tube design. A coil stent is derived from a single piece of wire. The coil design is associated with low radial strength but excellent flexibility (which enhances deliverability). This stent design has lost favor due to poor clinical performance both in the coronary and peripheral circulations (9), and such stents are currently mainly used in nonvascular applications. Slotted-tube stents are made from metal cylinders and laser is used to achieve the stent geometry desired. Initial slotted tube designs had excellent radial strength but poor flexibility (and deliverability). Over the last 15 years, significant modifications to the geometry of slotted-tube stents have occurred in an attempt to maintain the same degree of radial strength but enhance flexibility and deliverability. In the coronary circulation, the major emphasis has been on achieving these modifications in BE stents where flexibility and deliverability through tortuous and diseased small caliber vessels have been the priority. In the periphery, there has been significant interest in the modification of SE stents to improve the performance of stents in locations such as the femoropopliteal and internal carotid artery that are subject to conformational change.

The dominant stent geometry that has emerged is that of a sequential ring design (Fig. 7.6). This describes stents that are composed of a series of Z-shaped structural elements (referred to as struts), which are joined by connecting elements

TABLE 7.2 Balloon-expandable Nitinol Stents Used in Peripheral Intervention

Manufacturer	Stent Type	Diameter (mm)	Stent Length (mm)	Sheath Minimum (Fr.)	Guidewire (in.)	Design	Working Length (cm)	Radial Strength (lbs)	Stent Markers
Boston Scientific	Express Biliary	5–10	17, 25, 27, 37, & 57	6–7	0.035	Stainless steel	75/135	4.81	No
Medtronic	Bridge Assurant	6–10	20, 30, 40, & 60	6–7	0.035	Stainless steel	80/130	2.11	No
Cordis	Palmaz Genesis	5–10	19, 29, 39, 59, & 79	6–7	0.014	Stainless steel	80/135	2.58	No
Abbott	Omni Link	5–10	12, 16, 18, 28, 38, & 58	6–8	0.035	Stainless steel	80/135	1.20	No
ev3	Visi-Pro	5–10	12, 17, 27, 37, & 57	6–7	0.035	Stainless steel	80/135	4.28	Yes

(variable referred to as bridges, hinges, or nodes). Sequential ring design stents may be broadly divided into two broad categories—closed cell and open cell. In closed cell stents, all of the inflection points of the structural elements are connected by bridging elements. The original coronary stents had a closed cell design (i.e., Palmaz), which provided optimal mechanical scaffolding but resulted in poor flexibility.

Most current generation coronary and peripheral BE and SE stents have an open cell design, where some or all of the internal inflection points of the structural elements are not connected by bridging elements (10). The periodic connection between adjacent elements may occur in one of four patterns—peak-to-peak (e.g., Sentinol, Boston Scientific, or Luminexx, Bard [Fig. 7.7]), peak-to-valley (e.g., Absolute, Abbott Vascular [Fig. 7.8], or Zilver, Cook [Fig. 6B]), mid-strut to mid-strut, or a hybrid combination of these. These connections may be direct (Absolute, Abbott Vascular) or via off-set bridges (SMART, Cordis). These connectivity features are thought to contribute to what creates the radial and axial strength, the flexibility, and the likelihood of fracture of each individual stent. For example, peak-to-peak connections provide superior radial strength, whereas peak-to-valley connections provide superior scaffolding characteristics.

Other features of the SE stent design that impact performance includes the presence of flaring, and the presence and type of radiopaque markers at the stent ends. Flaring at the stent end is felt to improve the accuracy of stent placement and to reduce the risk of stent migration. Some manufacturers have looped the free strut tips to reduce tissue injury whereas others have placed radiopaque markers at the tips for better radiographic identification. One study acknowledged the improved accuracy of radiographic identification of stents with these tantalum radiopaque markers, but it raised some concern over the potential for corrosion at the junction between the body of the stent and the markers (11). Markers that are clipped on (e.g., SMART, Cordis) proved to have a more homogenous response to this testing. Regardless, this junction of the corpus of the stent to the markers raised the concern for the potential, whether by stent fracture or a mechanism associated with corrosion, for a continued stimulus for inflammation and neointimal hyper-

plasia and therefore restenosis. This would require dedicated research to further delineate the validity of this concern.

Balloon-Expandable and Self-Expanding Stents—Clinical Application

BE stents have been used in peripheral vascular interventions since 1987, when the Palmaz–Schatz stent was first tested in human iliac arteries (12). Because of their rigidity, BE stents are typically employed in peripheral intervention for the treatment of disease in relatively static arteries, such as the iliac vessels, where torsion and flexion forces are low and there is minimal risk of stent deformation or fracture (Table 7.2) (13). In contrast, these stents perform poorly at sites subject to significant deformation (e.g., superficial femoral artery [SFA], internal carotid artery), and their use at these locations has been supplanted by nitinol SE stents. There is some role for the use of BE stents below the knee, especially with improvements in the drug-eluting stent era, but their widespread use in this location is still investigational. The superior radial strength provided by the BE stainless steel design, relative to the nitinol SE stent design, allows for excellent luminal expansion, especially in larger diameter calcified vessels. Another advantage of BE stents is the ability to achieve precise placement of the stent. This is particularly important in the treatment of ostial disease (e.g., ostium or renal, visceral, and subclavian arteries, and aortoiliac bifurcation). With current antiplatelet regimens including aspirin and clopidogrel, the incidence of stent thrombosis with these stents in the periphery is very low.

SE stents are used in peripheral intervention at sites that are subject to significant deformation (e.g., external iliac artery, SFA, popliteal artery, and internal carotid artery) (Table 7) (13). There is a significant variation in the radial strength and flexibility of various SE stents, which may influence stent choice at certain locations and in certain disease anatomies. For example, a stent with high radial strength (e.g., SMART, Cordis) would be favored for the treatment of a heavily calcified iliac lesion, whereas a highly flexible stent with less radial strength would be favored in treating a noncalcified lesion in the highly mobile distal SFA and popliteal artery (e.g., Life-Stent, Bard [Fig. 7.9]).

TABLE 7.3 Self-Expandable Stents Used in Peripheral Intervention

Manufacturer	Stent Type	Diameter (mm)	Stent Length (mm)	Sheath Min (Fr.)	Guidewire (in.)
Abbott/Guidant	Absolute	5–10	20, 30, 40, 60, 80, & 100	6	0.035
Bard	LifeStent	6–10	20, 30, 40, 60, 80, 90, 100, 120, 150, & 170	6	0.035
Boston Scientific	Sentinol	5–10	20, 40, 60, & 80	6	0.035
Cook	Zilver 518	4–10	20, 30, 40, 60, & 80	5	0.018
Cook	Zilver 635	4–10, 12, & 14	20, 30, 40, 60, & 80	6	0.035
Cordis	S.M.A.R.T. Control	5–10	20, 30, 40, 60, 80 100, & 120	6	0.035
ev3	Protégé EverFlex	6, 7, & 8 (BIGGS) 9, 10, 12, & 14	20, 30, 40, 60, 80, 100, 120, & 150	6	0.035
Bard	Luminexx	4–10, 12, & 14	20, 30, 40, 60, 80, 100, & 120	6	0.035
Abbott	Xceed	510	20, 30, 40, 60, 80, 100, & 120	6	0.035
Boston Scientific	WallFlex	8 & 10	40, 60, 80, & 100	8	0.035
Boston Scientific	Wallstent	5–24	20, 40, 45, 55, 60, & 80	6	0.035

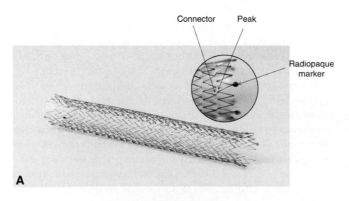

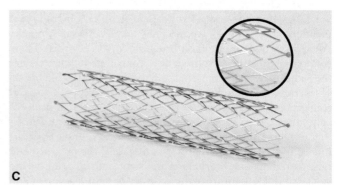

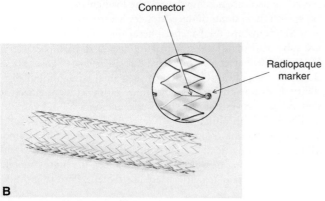

Figure 7.6 • Examples of three stents based on a symmetrical sequential ring design. **A:** SMART Control stent (Cordis) with peak-to-peak off angled connections and radiopaque markers at its flared ends. **B:** Zilver stent (Cook) with symmetric in-line stent rings connected in a peak-to-valley pattern with radiopaque markers at its unflared ends. **C:** Everflex stent (ev3) with peak-to-peak direct connections in a spiral connectivity pattern and radiopaque markers at its unflared ends.

Design	Working Length (cm)	Handle Design	Flared Ends	Connection Method	Connection Type	Pattern of Connections	Radiopaque Markers
Corrugated ring	80/135	Safety lock with thumb-wheel roller	No	Peak-to-valley	Direct	Symmetric in-line	Yes
Helical ring open cell	80/130	One-handed dial roller	Yes	Peak-to-peak	Off-set angled	Spiral	Not on long
Ring open cell	75/135	Touhy-Borst Y manifold, pin pull	No	Peak-to-peak	Direct	Symmetric in-line	No
Ring open cell	125	Pin pull with grips	No	Peak-to-valley	Direct	Symmetric in-line	Yes
Ring open cell	80/125	Pin pull with grips	No	Peak-to-valley	Direct	Symmetric in-line	Yes
Ring open cell	80/120	One-handed dial roller	Yes	Peak-to-peak	Off-set angled	Symmetric in-line	Yes
Ring open cell	80/120	Pin pull with grips	No	Peak-to-peak	Direct	Symmetric in-line	Yes
Ring open cell	80/135	One-handed thumb trigger	Yes	Peak-to-peak	Direct	Symmetric in-line	Yes
Ring open cell	80/120	One-handed dial	No	Peak-to-peak	Off-set crown	Symmetric in-line	No
Closed cell	75/135	Pull pin with retrievability	Yes	Woven	Woven	Woven, in-line overlap	No
Closed cell	75/135	Pull pin with retrievability	Yes	Woven	Woven	Woven, in-line overlap	No

Stent fracture rate is a phenomenon that has received much attention in relation to SE stents. Because these stents have been placed at sites subject to significant physical forces, stent fracture has been used as a surrogate for metal fatigue and stent failure in these locations. Although some studies have demonstrated an increased rate of restenosis associated with stent fracture (59% with fracture vs. 16% without fracture in the SFA location) (14), a causal link has not been established. There is a significant variation in-stent fracture rates across the range of available SE stents (Table 7.4) (15) that is not matched by corresponding variation in restenosis rates. However, it would appear to be a uniform goal of stent manufacturers to develop SE stents with stent fracture rates that approach zero across a range of lesion types and

stent usage (e.g., single vs. multiple overlapping stents). Regulatory agencies have also placed significant emphasis on achieving this goal, although it remains to be proved that zero rates of stent fracture will translate into improved patency rates.

When using SE stents in clinical practice, stent diameters should be chosen to be at least 1 mm larger than the reference vessel diameter to ensure stability of the stent. This persistent pressure against the vessel wall allows adequate vessel wall apposition but may lead to some reduction in its longitudinal length. In general, the stent length should be chosen to provide generous coverage of the lesion (e.g., 40-mm length stent for 25-mm length lesion). This is based on the fact that SE stents cannot be placed as accurately as BE stents. Significant foreshortening that varies from one SE stent to the other can occur. When placing overlapping SE stents, one should allow for this reduction in longitudinal length by ensuring at least 5 mm of stent overlap.

STENT GRAFTS—SELF-EXPANDABLE

There are three main SE stent grafts used in percutaneous peripheral intervention: Viabahn (Gore), Wallgraft (Boston Scientific), and Fluency (Bard).

The Viabahn Endoprosthesis (which replaced the Hemobahn device) consists of a durable reinforced ePTFE liner

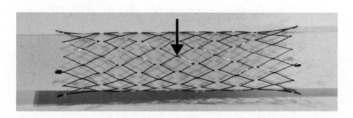

Figure 7.7 • Luminexx stent (Bard). Note presence of peak-to-peak connections between its sequential rings (*arrow*). This stent also displays an example of flared ends with radiopaque markers.

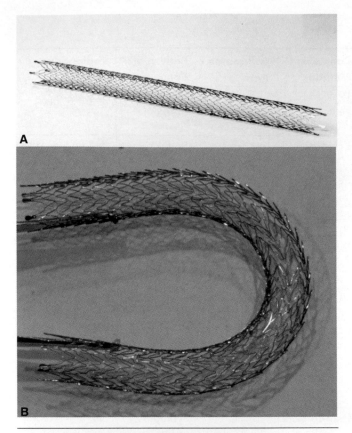

Figure 7.8 • Absolute stent (Abbott Vascular). This stent has a corrugated ring design (series of corrugated rings connected by longitudinal bridges). This stent incorporates peak-to-valley connections in a symmetric pattern **(A)**. When the stent is flexed, this stent design may have a tendency for strunt protrusion **(B)**.

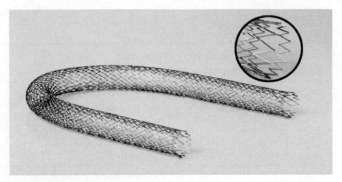

Figure 7.9 • Lifestent (Bard). This stent has a helical ring design as well as a spiral connectivity pattern that is believed to provide greater flexibility and tolerance of torsion forces. This stent is currently approved for use in the superficial femoral and above-knee popliteal arteries.

(HIT). In animal models, the heparin activity of the graft is maintained until at least 12 weeks following implantation. The technology used to provide this bioactive heparin surface is identical to that used on Gore's Propaten vascular graft that has been available in Europe since 2002. The second modification involves the proximal edge of the stent graft. Previously, this edge was a straight cut. As a result, crimping and poor apposition of the excess fabric at the proximal edge, particularly where the stent was oversized significantly, was felt to adversely affect flow dynamics and contribute to edge stenosis at this site. In the current generation, the proximal edge is now laser cut with a contoured edge and no excess of fabric at this margin. The ongoing VIPER trial (prospective nonrandomized single-arm study) is testing the clinical impact of these modifications.

The sheath sizes required to deliver Viabahn stent grafts vary from 7 to 12 Fr. depending on the graft diameter. All are delivered over a 0.035″ wire. It is important that this wire has a stiff body (e.g., SupraCore, Abbott Vascular) to ensure that the stent graft does not crimple during deployment. These stent grafts should not be used to treat noncompliant lesions, as inadequate expansion of the ePTFE liner will predispose to thrombosis. Deployment of the Viabahn stent graft is straightforward: following placement at the appropriate location, a rip cord is pulled that deploys the stent from the tip to the hub. Of note, the cord needs to be removed a significant distance before the endoprosthesis starts to deploy. Once deployment begins, one cannot move the device and it is not retractable. The Viabahn requires balloon postdilatation, usually with a balloon diameter that matches the diameter of the device delivered, to "iron out" the ePTFE. This balloon should not extend outside the device

attached to a nitinol exoskeleton (Fig. 7.10). It is available in diameters ranging from 5 to 11 mm (in 1-mm increments) and 13 mm, and in lengths of 2.5, 5, 10, and 15 cm. It is the only covered SE stent with an indication for use in the SFA and also has an indication for use in the iliac arteries. As with the other covered SE stents, the Viabahn has also been used in most large arterial beds including the subclavian, and carotid arteries for a variety of indications (e.g., aneurysms, pseudoaneurysms, and perforation).

There have been two recent modifications to this stent graft that are noteworthy (16,17). The ePTFE liner now has covalently bound bioactive heparin to prevent the development of clots on its inner surface and therefore should not be used in patients with a history of heparin-induced thrombocytopenia

TABLE 7.4 Rate of Stent Fracture in Human SFA from Two Studies Evaluating Five Commonly Used SE Nitinol Stents (15)

Stent type	1	2	3	4	5
N	24	96	45	145	116
Fracture rate (%)	29.2	27.5	53.3	2	19

SFA, superficial femoral artery; SE, self-expanding.

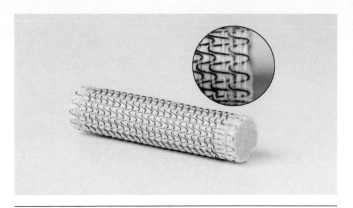

Figure 7.10 • The Viabahn Endoprosthesis consists of a self-expanding nitinol exoskeleton lined with an ePTFE graft material that is covalently bonded to heparin.

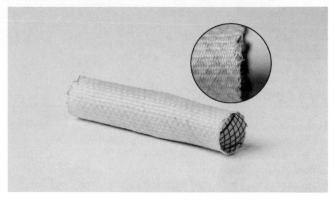

Figure 7.12 • Wallgraft (Boston Scientific). This stent graft is comprised of an endoskeleton Wallstent covered by a layer of low porosity PET graft.

edges when inflated. Because the Viabahn stent does not have markers at its ends, postdilatation without injuring the adjacent nonstented segments requires some care (i.e., using magnified views and angulations that maximize visualization of the stent margin). Aspirin and clopidogrel should be administered for a minimum of 3 months following the placement of a Viabahn device. In anatomic or clinical situations where the risk of thrombosis is deemed to be high, prolonged administration of dual antiplatelet therapy or oral anticoagulation may be used.

The Wallgraft endoprosthesis is composed of low porosity Dacron (PET) that is bonded to the outside a conventional Wallstent (Fig. 7.11) with a thin layer of Corethane (Fig. 7.12). It is available in diameters ranging from 6 to 10 mm (in 1-mm increments) and 12 and 14 mm, and lengths of 20, 30, 50, and 70 mm. The working length of the stent graft is 90 cm. The sheath size for delivery varies from 9 to 12 Fr. depending on the graft diameter. All are delivered over 0.035″ wires. Deployment is achieved by withdrawing a protective sheath using the Unistep Plus Delivery System.

Current indications for use include the treatment of occlusive iliac disease. Clinical use has extended to the treatment of aneurysms and pseudoaneurysms in appropriately sized arteries, and perforations in similar locations. This device maintains a good degree of flexibility, making it useful in arteries that are tortuous and are subject to conformational change. One of the major limitations of this stent graft (similar to its Elgiloy stent

endoskeleton) is significant foreshortening of the graft during deployment, which may lead to geographical miss. Possible foreshortening following initial successful deployment of Wallgrafts has also been reported (18). The potential impact on thrombosis risk of having an inner metal stent surface that rarely will undergo endothelialization due to its PET covering has not been born out in the literature. Common adverse effects seen with placement of this device include local pain and fever associated with the inflammatory response to the graft material.

The Fluency Plus stent graft is composed of a nitinol stent skeleton encapsulated with two ultrathin layers of ePTFE along its length except for 2 mm at either end where the stent is flared and has radiopaque tantalum markers (Fig. 7.13). It is available in diameters ranging from 5 to 12 mm (in 1-mm increments) and 13.5 mm. Available lengths include 30, 40, 60, 80, 100, and 120 mm. The delivery system comes in lengths of 80 and 117 cm. All Fluency stents are delivered over 0.035″ wires, and the deployment mechanism is similar to the Wallgraft in that a covering sheath is withdrawn to deploy the stent. This stent is not approved for vascular use but has found application in the treatment of aneurysms,

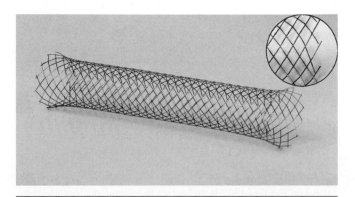

Figure 7.11 • Wallstent (Boston Scientific). This stent has a unique woven closed cell design that allows for retrieval and repositioning of the stent.

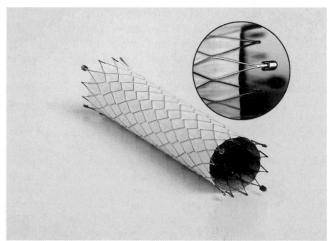

Figure 7.13 • Fluency self-expanding endograft (Bard). This stent graft is composed of a nitinol exoskeleton with a double layer of ePTFE. This lining ends 2 mm proximal to the tantalum markers.

pseudoaneurysms, and perforations in appropriately sized vessels. The advantage of this stent includes its visibility due to the radiopaque markers at the stent margins and the lack of foreshortening when compared with the Wallgraft.

STENT GRAFTS—BALLOON-EXPANDABLE

In the United States, there are two BE covered stents available for use in the peripheral circulation: the iCast (Atrium Medical Corporation) and the GraftMaster Jostent (Abbott Vascular). The iCast stent graft is composed of ultrathin 316L stainless steel stent struts that are encapsulated with a PTFE covering, resulting in the exclusion of any metal from the luminal surface of the stent. The stent graft is balloon premounted, and is available in diameters of 5 to 10 mm (in 1-mm increments) and lengths of 16, 22, 38, and 59 mm. All of these stents can be postdilatated to a diameter that is 1 to 2 mm larger than the stated diameter. However, one should be aware that postdilatation beyond the stated stent diameter will result in shortening of the stent, which should be accounted for in the initial choice of stent length. All are delivered over 0.035″ wires and can be delivered through 6/7-Fr. sheaths depending on the stent graft diameter. This makes this stent graft the lowest profile of the available stent grafts. However, due to its rigidity, it should not be deployed in locations that are subject to significant conformational change. As a result, in the periphery, the main locations in which it has been used include the distal abdominal aorta, aortoiliac bifurcation, the common iliac artery, and rarely the renal artery. The clinical indications for use have moved beyond the treatment of perforations and aneurysms to include the treatment of complex aortoiliac occlusive disease (e.g., occlusions, anatomic situations where the risk of perforation or atheroembolism is deemed to be high) and the treatment of recurrent in-stent restenosis. Although low in profile, the deliverability of this stent graft can be challenging through tortuous anatomy due to its rigidity. When delivering the iCast across the aortoiliac bifurcation, great care needs to be exercised to ensure that there is adequate wire and sheath support, particularly when treating an iliac perforation, where loss of crossover access due to prolapse of the sheath into the aorta can prove catastrophic. For this reason, when feasible, delivery of this stent graft using ipsilateral retrograde access is preferred.

The GraftMaster Jostent is composed of two 316L stainless steel stents that sandwich a central layer of PTFE (Fig. 7.14). Unfortunately, this stent is currently only approved for use in the United States for the treatment of coronary perforations (as a humanitarian device). Beyond this indication, use of the device requires an investigational device exemption that restricts its use considerably. It is available in diameters of 3 to 5 mm (in 0.5-mm increments) and in lengths of 9, 12, 16, 19, and 26 mm, and is delivered over 0.014″ guidewires through 5-Fr. sheaths. The GraftMaster Jostent is considerably more rigid than current generations of coronary bare-metal and drug-eluting noncovered stents. In the periphery, its use is largely restricted to the treatment of perforations, aneurysms, pseudoaneurysms, and fistulae in appropriately sized vessels. When used in the coronary artery, most clinicians prescribe dual antiplatelet therapy (aspirin and clopidgrel) for a prolonged period (~12 months) due to the perception of an increased risk of stent thrombosis with this stent. Restenosis rates with this stent are also felt to be high. These facts should be borne in mind when this stent graft is used in the periphery.

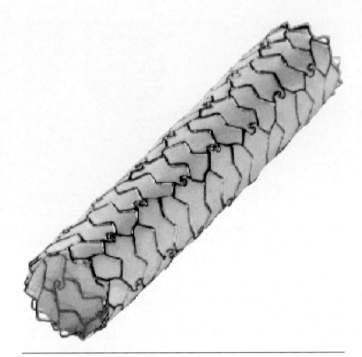

Figure 7.14 • Jostent. This stent graft is composed of two 316L stainless steel stents that sandwich a central layer of PTFE.

EMERGING DEVICES

Drug-Eluting Balloons

Given the poor long-term durability achieved with revascularization using both plain balloon angioplasty and nitinol SE stents in the femoropopliteal and infrapopliteal segments, significant interest in drug-eluting balloon technology as a strategy to achieve more durable clinical outcomes in these locations has emerged. While a complete discussion of drug-eluting balloon technology in the periphery is beyond the scope of this chapter (19–21), some salient points will be made.

Paclitaxel has emerged as the drug of choice for use in drug-eluting balloons. This is based on the strongly lipophilic nature of this drug, and the demonstration that paclitaxel is rapidly transferred to the vascular wall during transient balloon inflation (i.e., ~60 seconds) and can have a sustained antiproliferative effect on smooth muscle cells for up to 14 days with a resultant impact on restenosis. A variety of drug-eluting balloon systems have been developed by a variety of manufacturers. These systems vary in the technology used to apply the paclitaxel to the rough abluminal surface of the balloon and to control the release of the drug during balloon inflation. Currently, there is only one commercially available drug-eluting balloon in Europe (In.Pact Ampherion [Invatec Corporation]). This is a 0.014″ over the wire balloon that is available in diameters of 2 to 4 mm and balloon lengths of 40 to 120 mm, and therefore would be applicable for use in the infrapopliteal rather than the femoropopliteal location.

To date, two significant trials of drug-eluting balloon technology in the treatment of PAD have been completed: THUNDER and FemPac (22,23). In both of these studies, the active arm used a commercially available balloon that was coated with paclitaxel at a dose of 3 μg/mm². The paclitaxel was embedded in hydrophilic iopromide (a radiographic contrast agent) to increase the solubility and transfer of the paclitaxel to the vessel wall. Both studies were conducted in Europe and enrolled relatively small sample sizes ($n =154$ and $n = 87$, respectively). Although both examined two populations with femoropopliteal disease, the populations were heterogenous in that patients with claudication and critical limb ischemia (CLI) were included, and a variety of lesion types such as de novo disease, restenotic lesions, and in-stent restenosis were eligible for enrollment. Complete blinding was not possible because the drug-eluting balloon was distinguishable from the regular angioplasty balloon. Finally, follow-up was assessed at only 6 months, was incomplete, and the primary endpoint chosen was angiographic assessment of late lumen loss rather than hard clinical endpoint(s). Despite these limitations in trial design, both studies demonstrated a significant reduction in late lumen loss and target lesion revascularization rates in the active compared to the control arm(s) (Table 7.5). Interestingly, analysis of the drug-eluting balloons postintervention demonstrated that >90% of the paclitaxel dose was removed from the balloon surface following balloon inflation. Preclinical animal studies suggest that 70% to 80% of the drug may be lost in the blood stream, and that 10% to 15% of the paclitaxel drug is transferred to the lumen wall during balloon inflation using the drug-eluting balloon system used in these studies.

In conclusion, there is clearly a signal of biologic activity supporting the use of drug-eluting balloons in the treatment of infrainguinal disease. Future studies will require enrollment of much larger and homogenous populations and use of hard clinical endpoints at follow-up durations that are clinically meaningful (i.e., 1 to 5 years). Although drug-eluting balloon technology holds great promise, the major limitation of balloon angioplasty will remain—the inability to provide a mechanical scaffold that treats flow-limiting dissections which can lead to abrupt vessel closure and thereby provide a predictable acute angiographic result. Although this may be less of an issue in the periphery compared with the coronary circulation, the role of adjunctive technologies such as atherectomy and stenting will need to be defined in the context of an effective drug-eluting balloon angioplasty technology.

Bioabsorbable Stents

The rationale of using bioabsorbable stents for endovascular intervention is that they can provide the short-term mechanical scaffolding required at the time of intervention to treat flow limiting dissections, prevent abrupt vessel closure, and eliminate elastic recoil of the vessel, and then slowly resorb over time so that the longer-term limitations of having a stent in the vessel are eliminated (24,25). These limitations include the development of in-stent restenosis and late stent thrombosis. In the periphery, late stent thrombosis would appear to be a rare event, at least compared to the coronary circulation. However, in-stent restenosis in certain vessel segments that are subject to significant physical forces (e.g., femoropopliteal and infrapopliteal) is a major problem, and may result from the interaction of the presence of stent struts in the vessel with these forces. As a result, the use of bioabsorbable stents in these locations represents a very attractive potential therapeutic strategy. In addition, the ability to use bioabsorbable stents in locations where conventional stents are contraindicated (i.e., across joint spaces—common femoral artery and popliteal artery) would open up additional anatomic subsets of disease that could be treated using endovascular techniques.

The first fully biodegradable stent was made of knitted poly-L-lactic acid (PLLA) by Stack and colleagues (26), which then led Igaki and Tamai to create a zigzag helical coil configured stent made of PLLA monofilaments. Additional biodegradable polymers (e.g., polyglycolic acid, poly(D,L-lactide/glycolide) copolymer, polycaprolactone) with varying material properties have subsequently been developed for use in biodegradable polymer stents. In addition, biodegradable metallic alloys (e.g., magnesium and iron) have been used to create bioabsorbable metallic stents.

The manufacture of a safe and effective bioabsorbable stent poses significant challenges. Polymer-based bioabsorbable stents have less radial strength compared to metallic stents, resulting in early recoil following implantation. As a result, these stents are required to have thick struts, which adversely impact their profile and deliverability. These stents are radiolucent, which requires the placement of markers at either end to guide stent

TABLE 7.5 Significant Reduction in LLL and Incidence of TLR with the Use of Paclitaxel-Coated Balloons When Compared to Angioplasty (PTA) Alone from Two Randomized Controlled Trials

Trial Endpoint	Control—PTA Only	Paclitaxel Contrast	Paclitaxel-Coated Balloon	P Value
Thunder trial				
LLL 6 mo	1.7 ± 1.8 mm	2.2 ± 1.6 mm	0.4 ± 1.2 mm	<0.001
TLR 6 mo	37%	29%	4%	<0.001
TLR 24 mo	52%	40%	15%	<0.001
FemPac trial				
LLL 6 mo	1.0 ± 1.1 mm	N/A	0.5 ± 1.1 mm	0.031
TLR 6 mo	33%	N/A	7%	0.002
TLR 24 mo	50%	N/A	13%	0.001

LLL, late lumen loss; TLR, target lesion revascularization; PTA, percutaneous transluminal angioplasty.

placement. Finally, the polymers may be associated with local inflammation that can lead to restenosis. Biamino et al. reported an angiographic restenosis rate (defined as presence of >50%) of 30% in the SFA in 45 patients treated with the Igaki–Tamai stent (lesion length <7cm) (27). Unfortunately, these data have not been published and it would appear that there is a lack of further study of polymer-based absorbable stents in the periphery. Indeed, there appears to be consensus among experts in the field that polymer stents are unlikely to be a viable technology for endovascular therapy, at least in their current iteration (28).

Much of the current investigation of bioabsorbable stents has centered on absorbable metal stents (AMSs) using magnesium alloys. These metallic stents have good radial force that compare favorably to regular stainless steel stents and hence provide similar mechanical scaffolding properties. The low strut profile of these stents offers a significant advantage over polymer-based stents and makes these stents attractive for endovascular application. Since magnesium is an important micronutrient, it has been assumed that side effects from degradation products of the magnesium should be unlikely and this appears to be borne out in preclinical and clinical studies.

In terms of the peripheral application of AMS, only limited investigational work has been performed to date. A small study of 20 patients with CLI in which the Biotronik AMS was implanted in the proximal two thirds of one or more infrapopliteal vessels has been reported (29). This AMS is a tubular, slotted, BE bare-metal stent sculpted by laser from a single tube of alloy containing over 90% magnesium and rare earth elements that is completely biodegradable in humans. In the study, it was available in a 3-mm diameter and 15-mm length. At 3-month follow-up, primary clinical patency was 89.5%, and the limb salvage rate was 100%. However, a subsequent randomized comparison of this magnesium alloy AMS versus angioplasty in 117 patients with CLI failed to show a significant benefit of the AMS, with a 6-month angiographic patency rate of only 32% in the AMS arm versus 58% in the angioplasty arm (30). These results have been sobering but have not dampened the enthusiasm of proponents of this technology. Clearly, further iteration of the technology is required in terms of optimization of the magnesium alloy and design of the stent. SE AMS will be required for any application in the femoropopliteal artery, and it appears likely that the elution of antiproliferative agents by these stents will be required to achieve low rates of restenosis (31).

Drug-Eluting Stents

Given the high rates of restenosis associated with bare-metal SE stenting of the femoropopliteal artery, it is not surprising that this was the first peripheral artery in which drug-eluting stent technology was tested. Unfortunately, the results thus far have been disappointing.

The SIROCCO I trial was a randomized controlled trial that compared a sirolimus-eluting SMART SE nitinol stent with the bare-metal SMART stent in the SFA in a small sample size of 36 patients (32). Sirolimus was combined with a copolymer in a 30 to 70 drug:copolymer weight ratio on the surface of the drug-eluting stent and the amount of drug per vessel area was 90 µg/cm², which was equivalent to that used in the coronary application. However, the rate of drug-elution was significantly greater than that for the coronary drug-eluting stent platforms. This preliminary study demonstrated the feasibility and safety of the technology, and showed a trend toward benefit in reducing restenosis at 6 months. The SIROCCO II trial enrolled a further 57 patients using the same drug-eluting

stent, but with a slower elution (although still significantly greater than that for the coronary drug-eluting stent platforms). However, a benefit of the sirolimus-eluting stent in reducing restenosis at 6 months could not be demonstrated, due in large part to the very low rate of restenosis in the bare-metal arm. In a combined analysis of both phases of the SIROCCO trials, restenosis rates at 24 months were not significantly different between the bare-metal and sirolimus-eluting SMART stents (21.1% vs. 22.9%) (33).

More recently, the STRIDES trial was a multicenter European single-arm study that examined the performance of an everolimus-eluting Dynalink SE stent compared to historical controls in 104 patients with de novo or restenotic disease of the femoropopliteal artery. Although not yet published, it has been reported that improved patency rates observed at 6 months with the everolimus-eluting Dynalink stent were not maintained at 12 months. These data are certainly reminiscent of the SIROCCO studies, and reinforce the magnitude of the challenge of finding an effective drug-eluting stent for the femoropopliteal artery. Based on these data, Abbott Vascular has apparently suspended further investigation of this technology.

Perhaps the last hope for drug-eluting stent technology in the femoropopliteal artery lies with the Zilver PTX stent. This is a nitinol Zilver stent (Cook, Inc.) that has a polymer-free paclitaxel coating (34). This stent has been tested in a single-arm registry (n = 800) and a randomized comparison with plain balloon angioplasty (n = 480). Although preliminary data from the registry have been presented with encouraging results, data from the randomized study is anxiously awaited and will be critical to proving the efficacy of the drug-eluting stent platform.

The other major location in which drug-eluting stenting technology has been tested in the periphery is the infrapopliteal segment (35). Given the similarity between the diameter of infrapopliteal and coronary arteries, it is not surprising that initial testing was performed using coronary drug-eluting stents. In general, the patient populations treated have had CLI. In a large meta-analysis of observational studies to date comprising 640 patients who used coronary-type BE drug-eluting and bare-metal stents to treat infrapopliteal disease in patients with CLI, limb salvage rates of 94% and primary patency rates of 80% have been reported (36). A subset analysis showed that siroliumus-eluting stents were superior to bare-metal stents in preventing restenosis and improving primary patency. A further subset analysis suggested improved primary patency and lower rates of repeat revascularization with sirolimus-eluting (Cypher, Cordis) over paclitaxel-eluting (i.e., Taxus, Boston Scientific) stents. Rigorous prospective randomized controlled trials are needed to establish the validity of these observational data (37). In addition, these trials are required to establish the safety of the use of drug-eluting stents in heavily diseased infrapopliteal vessels in patients with CLI in whom the distal run-off is often poor. Based on the experience in the coronary circulation, these anatomies would be assumed to be associated with an increased risk of stent thrombosis. Surprisingly, this has not been suggested by observational data so far. The optimal duration of dual antiplatelet therapy following placement of drug-eluting coronary stents in this location remains unknown and is largely decided at the discretion of the operator. Based on the experience in the coronary circulation, a minimum duration of 12 months is recommended.

One of the major limitations of using coronary-type drug-eluting stents in the infrapopliteal segment is the limited stent lengths available, with the longest stent length being 38 mm. In a segment where disease is often very diffuse, longer lengths are often required. Also, there are locations in the infrapopliteal segment where BE stents may be too rigid (e.g., proximal segment of the anterior tibial artery). In the future, it is hoped that longer drug-eluting SE stents may become available for use in this location.

Outside of the femoropopliteal artery and infrapopliteal segment, there is very little investigation in the use of drug-eluting stents in the periphery. The two areas in which there is a real clinical need are for the treatment of in-stent restenosis in the renal and internal carotid arteries. With the precipitous decline in availability of intravascular brachytherapy, there are no good reliable and effective therapies available for such patients.

ACKNOWLEDGMENT

We would like to acknowledge Mr. Eugen Muntean for providing excellent photography of the balloons and stents for this chapter.

References

1. Dotter CT, Judkins MP. Transluminal treatment of arteriosclerotic obstruction: description of a new technic and a preliminary report of its application. *Circulation.* 1964;30:654–670.
2. Cejna M. Cutting balloon: review on principles and background of use in peripheral arteries. *Cardiovasc Intervent Radiol.* 2005;28: 400–408.
3. Samson RH, Showalter DP, Lepore MR, et al. CryoPlasty therapy of the superficial femoral and popliteal arteries: a single center experience. *Vasc Endovascular Surg.* 2006;40:446–450.
4. Laird J, Jaff MR, Biamino G, et al. Cryoplasty for the treatment of femoropopliteal arterial disease: results of a prospective, multicenter registry. *J Vasc Interv Radiol.* 2005;16:1067–1073.
5. DeRubertis BG, Faries PL, McKinsey JF, et al. Shifting paradigms in the treatment of lower extremity vascular disease: a report of 1000 percutaneous interventions. *Ann Surg.* 2007;246:415–422; discussion 422.
6. Samson RH, Showalter DP, Lepore M, et al. CryoPlasty therapy of the superficial femoral and popliteal arteries: a reappraisal after 44 months' experience. *J Vasc Surg.* 2008;48:634–637.
7. Duerig TW, Wholey M. A comparison of balloon- and self-expanding stents. *Min Invas Ther & Allied Technol.* 2002;11: 173–178.
8. Grewe PH, Müller KM, Deneke T, et al. Stents: material, surface texture and design, in theory and practice. *Min Invas Ther & Allied Technol.* 2002;11:157–163.
9. Palmaz JC. Influence of stent design on clinical outcome. *Min. Invas Ther & Allied Technol.* 2002;11:179–183.
10. Stoeckel D, Bonsignore C, Duda S. A survey of stent designs. *Min Invas Ther & Allied Technol.* 2002;11:137–147.
11. Wiskirchen J, Venugopalan R, Holton AD, et al. Radiopaque markers in endovascular stents–benefit and potential hazards. *RöFo.* 2003;175:484–488.
12. Palmaz JC, Richter GM, Nöldge G, et al. [Intraluminal Palmaz stent implantation. The first clinical case report on a balloon-expanded vascular prosthesis]. *Der Radiologe.* 1987;27:560–563.
13. Duda SH, Wiesinger B, Koenig C, et al. A clinical survey of vascular stents. *Min. Invas. Ther. & Allied Technol.* 2002;11:193–201.
14. Scheinert D, Scheinert S, Sax J, et al. Prevalence and clinical impact of stent fractures after femoropopliteal stenting. *J Am Coll Cardiol.* 2005;45:312–315.
15. Karnabatidis D, Katsanos K, Spiliopoulos S, et al. Incidence, anatomical location, and clinical significance of compressions and fractures in infrapopliteal balloon-expandable metal stents. *J Endovasc Ther.* 2009;16:15–22.
16. Saxon RR. The Viper Trial. *Endovascular Today*, March 2010, pp. 66–67.
17. Ansel GM, Lumsden AB. Evolving modalities for femoropopliteal interventions. *J Endovasc Ther.* 2009;16(suppl II):II82–II97.
18. Whittaker DR, McCullough JP, Wyers MC, et al. Shifting Wallgraft position: case reports and review of the forces affecting Wallgraft positioning. *J Vasc Surg.* 2006;43:383–387.
19. Waksman R, Pakala R. Drug-eluting balloon: the comeback kid? *Circ Cardiovasc Interv.* 2009;2:352–358.
20. Diehm NA, Hoppe H, Do DD. Drug eluting balloons. *Tech Vasc Interv Radiol.* 2010;13:59–63.
21. Henry TD, Schwartz RS, Hirsch AT. "POBA Plus": will the balloon regain its luster? *Circulation.* 2008;118:1309–1311.
22. Werk M, Langner S, Reinkensmeier B, et al. Inhibition of restenosis in femoropopliteal arteries: paclitaxel-coated versus uncoated balloon: femoral paclitaxel randomized pilot trial. *Circulation.* 2008;118:1358–1365.
23. Tepe G, Zeller T, Albrecht T, et al. Local delivery of paclitaxel to inhibit restenosis during angioplasty of the leg. *N Engl J Med.* 2008;358:689–699.
24. Geraghty PJ. Bioabsorbable stenting for peripheral arterial occlusive disease. *Perspect Vasc Surg Endovasc Ther.* 2006;18:295–298.
25. Waksman R. Promise and challenges of bioabsorbable stents. *Cathet Cardiovasc Interv.* 2007;70:407–414.
26. Stack RS, Califf RM, Phillips HR, et al. Interventional cardiac catheterization at Duke Medical Center. *Am J Cardiol.* 1988;62:3F–24F.
27. Biamino G, Schmidt A, Scheinert. Treatment of SFA lesions with PLLA biodegradable stents, results of the PERSEUS Study, *J Endovasc Ther.* 2005;12:I-1–I-50.
28. Peeters P, Keirse K, Verbist J, et al. Are bio-absorbable stents the future of SFA treatment? *J Cardiovasc Surg* (Torino). 2010;51: 121–124.
29. Peeters P, Bosiers M, Verbist J, et al. Preliminary results after application of absorbable metal stents in patients with critical limb ischemia. *J Endovasc Ther.* 2005;12:1–5.
30. Bosiers M, Peeters P, D'Archambeau O. AMS INSIGHT—absorbable metal stent implantation for treatment of below-the-knee critical limb ischemia: 6-month analysis. *Cardiovasc Interv Radiol.* 2009;32:424–435.
31. Brown DA, Lee EW, Loh CT, et al. A new wave in treatment of vascular occlusive disease: biodegradable stents–clinical experience and scientific principles. *J Vasc Interv Radiol.* 2009;20:315–324.
32. Duda SH, Bosiers M, Lammer J, et al. Sirolimus-eluting versus bare nitinol stent for obstructive superficial femoral artery disease: the SIROCCO II trial. *J Vasc Interv Radiol.* 2005;16:331–338.
33. Duda SH, Bosiers M, Lammer J, et al. Drug-eluting and bare nitinol stents for the treatment of atherosclerotic lesions in the superficial femoral artery: long-term results from the SIROCCO trial. *J Endovasc Ther.* 2006;13:701–710.
34. Dake MD, Ansel GM, Ragheb AO. Evaluating the Zilver PTX Stent. *Endovascular Today.* March 2010, pp. 52–57.
35. Bosiers M, Cagiannos C, Deloose K, et al. Drug-eluting stents in the management of peripheral arterial disease. *Vasc Health Risk Manag.* 2008;4:553–559.
36. Biondi-Zoccai GG, Sangiorgi G, Lotrionte M, et al. Infragenicular stent implantation for below-the-knee atherosclerotic disease: clinical evidence from an international collaborative meta-analysis on 640 patients. *J Endovasc Ther.* 2009;16:251–260.
37. Martens JM, Knippenberg B, Vos JA, et al. Update on PADI trial: percutaneous transluminal angioplasty and drug-eluting stents for infrapopliteal lesions in critical limb ischemia. *J Vasc Surg.* 2009;50:687–689.

CHAPTER 8

Debulking Technologies: Atherectomy and Laser

Andrew J. Klein, Mehdi H. Shishehbor, and Ivan P. Casserly

The first percutaneous vascular intervention was performed in the superficial femoral artery (SFA) by Charles Dotter in 1964 using a series of relatively crude dilatation devices. Despite the long-term success of this first intervention (the SFA remained open until the patient's death from heart failure 3 years later) and numerous technological advances, endovascular revascularization of the infrainguinal vessels has been plagued by suboptimal long-term patency rates (1–4). Unfortunately, stenting in this location has not yielded the favorable results obtained in the iliac arteries or in the coronary circulation. A number of reasons for this failure have been proposed. First, peripheral artery disease (PAD) of the infrainguinal vessels tends to be diffuse, is often associated with severe calcification, and has a high propensity for progression to occlusive disease (5). Second, peripheral vessels are subject to a series of complex biophysical forces (6) that are dramatic and appear to impact the success of endovascular stenting and other revascularization strategies. Third, current stent platforms are not designed to withstand these complex forces resulting in stent fracture, which is thought to be associated with in-stent restenosis (7). Therefore, many operators continue to use angioplasty alone as the primary strategy for infrainguinal revascularization, a technique that is associated with high restenosis rates, particularly in the treatment of long lesions. These are the factors that have led to interest in debulking techniques for the treatment of infrainguinal disease (8).

In clinical practice, debulking techniques may be broadly divided into two types: excisional atherectomy (i.e., physical removal of plaque) or atheroablation (i.e., disintegration or fragmentation of the plaque without its physical removal). These techniques may be used in conjunction with angioplasty and/or stenting, or as a stand-alone strategy (8). This chapter will review the four currently available atherectomy/atheroablative devices that are approved for use in the peripheral arteries.

DEBULKING TECHNIQUES—CLINICAL INDICATIONS

In clinical practice, debulking techniques in the infrainguinal vessels are used to allow for the effective acute treatment of certain anatomic disease subsets that otherwise would be difficult or impossible to treat. As a method that can minimize plaque shifting, its application is well suited in ostial SFA disease to decrease the risk of plaque shift into the profunda femoral artery. Heavily calcified plaque is another important subset, where routine angioplasty and/or stenting is often associated

with a suboptimal acute result. Debulking techniques typically allow a successful acute result without the need for stenting. Hence, their use at locations where stent use should be avoided, such as where joints are located (i.e., common femoral [CFA] and popliteal artery), is desirable. Finally, given that long overlapping stents appears to be a significant risk for the development of stent fractures and/or in-stent restenosis, the ability of debulking therapies to obviate stenting is of particular interest in patients with severe diffuse disease of the SFA/popliteal artery.

EXCISIONAL ATHERECTOMY

Directional Atherectomy-Silverhawk Atherectomy Catheter

In June 2003, the FDA gave 510(k) approval to the Silverhawk Plaque Excision System (Fig. 8.1) (ev3, Plymouth, MN) for the treatment of PAD (9). This device uses a carbide cutter at a variable height (depending on catheter type) that rotates at a speed of 8000 rpm and engages the plaque via a hinge system, in contrast to earlier devices that used balloon apposition. There are currently 12 available models of the Silverhawk family of atherectomy catheters that allow for the treatment of diseased vessels ranging from 1.5 to 7.0 mm in diameter (Table 8.1) and for the treatment of lesions of various lengths (i.e., **S**tandard nose-cone length for shorter lesions and e**X**tended nose-cone length for longer lesions). The nomenclature of these catheters can be confusing but can be explained as follows. The first letter refers to the vessel size in which the catheter is used (i.e., L, large; M, medium; S, small; E, extra small). The second letter refers to the length of the nose cone (S, standard length; X, extended length). The third letter generally refers to the variations in the design of the nose cone (F, standard nose-cone design; M, presence of MEC technology in which laser-drilled micro vent holes in the nosecone maximize tissue storage in the nose cone; C, special modification of the cutter and nose cone to allow for treatment of calcified lesions).

The device consists of a monorail low-profile catheter (advanced over any 0.014″ wire, preferably an extra-support wire) and a palm-sized drive unit with an on/off switch that activates and deactivates the cutter, respectively, and an additional switch to raise the carbide cutter from the nosecone such that atherectomy can be performed. (Fig. 8.1). Atheroma is cut and collected in a hinged nose cone that is located distal to the cutter. The number and length of cuts is determined by the operator and the device can be rotated to allow circumferential cutting of the plaque.

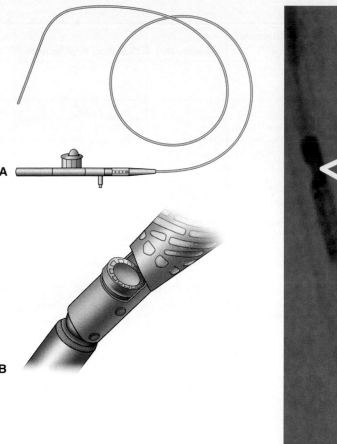

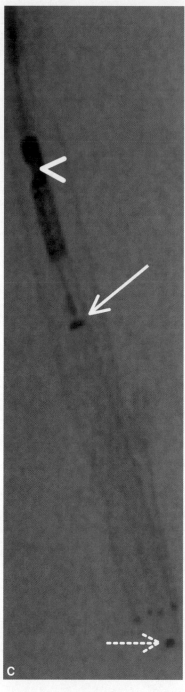

Figure 8.1 • Silverhawk Plaque Excision System. **A:** The TurboHawk atherectomy catheter that uses a carbide cutting blade specifically designed for treating calcium. **B:** Magnified view of the carbide cutting blade *(arrowhead)*. **C:** Angiographic image of the TurboHawk atherectomy device with its cutting blade *(arrowhead)* and the plunger *(arrow)* used to pack the atheroma into the nose cone of the device. The tip of the nosecone is indicated by *interrupted white arrow.*

PRACTICAL USE

The recommended sheath size for each of the Silverhawk catheters is summarized in Table 8.1 (i.e., 6 to 8 Fr.). Although an 8 Fr. sheath is recommended for the larger catheters (i.e., LS and LX), the authors have generally used 7 Fr. sheaths to deliver these catheters. As a general rule, the large catheter group (i.e., LS-C, LX-C, LS-M, and LX-M) is used in the CFA, SFA, and larger caliber popliteal arteries. The medium catheter (MS-M, MS-F) is used in the popliteal artery and the small catheter group (SS+, SX, and SXL) is suitable for use in the proximal segment of good caliber tibial vessels. The extra-small catheters

(ES+, EXL, and DS) are suitable for use in the mid and distal tibial vessels. Once the lesion has been crossed, a 0.014″ wire (preferably an extra-support wire, e.g., Grand Slam, Abbott Vascular, Santa Clara, CA) is required to allow for subsequent delivery of the catheter. Excisional atherectomy inherently has a risk of distal embolization, and therefore a careful assessment of the runoff should be made at baseline. In cases in which the use of an embolic protection device is thought necessary, the authors use a Spider FX® (eV3, Plymouth, MN) or Emboshield (Abbott Vascular, Santa Clara, CA) filter. The filter should be at least 1 mm larger than the distal vessel in which it is placed. The Spider FX filter permits crossing of the lesion with any 0.014″ wire

TABLE 8.1 Silverhawk Catheters

Catheter	Vessel Diameter (mm)	Sheath (Fr)	Crossing Profile (mm)	Tip Length (cm)
Turbo-Hawk LS-C (Super) *Large Vessel Calcium tip*	3.5–7.0	8	2.7	6
Turbo-Hawk LX-C (Super) *Large Vessel Extended Calcium tip*	3.5–7.0	8	2.7	9
Turbo-Hawk LS-C (Smooth) *Large Vessel Standard tip*	3.5–7.0	7/8	2.7	6
Turbo-Hawk LX-M (Smooth) *Large Vessel Xtended tip*	3.5–7.0	7/8	2.7	9
LS-M *Large Vessel Standard Tip with MEC™*	4.5–7.0	7/8	2.7	6
LS-F *Large Vessel Standard Flush Tip*	4.5–7.0	7/8	2.7	6
LX-M *Large Vessel Xtended Tip*	4.5–7.0	7/8	2.7	9
MS-M *Medium vessel Standard Tip with MEC™*	3.5–5.0	7/8	2.7	6
MS-F *Medium vessel Standard Flush Tip*	3.5–5.0	7/8	2.7	6
SXL *Small Vessel Xtra Long Tip*	3.0–3.5	7	2.4	7.2
SX *Small Vessel Xtended Tip*	3.0–3.5	7	2.4	4.2
SS+ *Small Vessel Standard Tip*	3.0–3.5	7	2.3	2.6
EXL *Extra Small Vessel Xtra Long Tip*	2.0–3.0	6	2.0	6
ES+ *Extra Small Vessel Standard Tip*	2.0–3.0	6	1.9	2.2
DS *Distal Vessel Standard Tip*	1.5–2.0	6	1.9	2.6

followed by exchange for the Spider filter and wire combination. The latter wire provides reasonable support for subsequent catheter delivery. Of note, if a 0.035″ wire is used to cross the lesion, a 4 Fr. glide catheter or 0.035″ Quickcross catheter can be used to exchange the 0.035″ wire for the Spider FX filter, a technique which can shorten the procedural time. When choosing the location of the landing zone of the filter of choice, it is important to be cognizant of the length of the nosecone of the Silverhawk catheter being used. It is necessary for the filter to be placed at least 1 to 2 cm plus the length of the nose cone inferior to the distal margin of the lesion being treated. For example, for

mid and distal popliteal lesions, the filter will need to be placed in a tibial vessel.

Prior to introduction into the body, the device should be flushed with heparinized saline and the drive unit should be attached to the catheter and activated to ensure proper functioning of the cutter. The catheter is then advanced such that the cutter is located approximately 1 cm superior to the proximal margin of the lesion. In this location, the tip and body of the nose cone will be situated across the proximal portion of the target lesion. Rarely, low-pressure angioplasty (using 2.0 to 3.0 mm balloon) may be required prior to atherectomy to permit device advancement, particularly when treating long occlusions or heavily calcified lesions. The authors use the roadmap function in combination with radio-opaque marker tape (e.g., LeMaitre® tape, LeMaitre, Burlington, MA) to help delineate the target area for treatment. The directionality of the cutter is adjusted as desired by rotating the back end of the catheter. When using a 2D angiographic image, one can only reliably assess whether the cutter is broadly directed medially, laterally, anteriorly, or posteriorly. The cutter is then activated and advanced in a smooth manner and at a constant speed (1 to 2 mm/sec) across the lesion. The slower the speed of catheter advancement, the deeper the cut, and vice versa. In general, the authors stop after no more than 5 cm of lesion treatment to pack the nosecone of the device. This likely reduces the risk of distal embolization of plaque elements. Following a single cut in a given direction, the deactivated device is brought back to the starting point. The device should never be pulled back while activated. The direction of the cutter can then be changed and the process repeated. Following a series of cuts, the nosecone will become full of plaque. In the larger caliber devices, this can be assessed on x-ray by noting the position of the radio-opaque marker on the plunger in the nosecone (Fig. 8.1C). The closer this marker is to the cutter, the more full the nosecone. The device is removed and the plaque removed from the nosecone using a variety of techniques, depending on the catheter type. The device is then reinserted and additional cuts can be made as desired.

CLINICAL DATA

The **T**reating Peripher**A**ls with Silverhawk: **O**utcomes Collectio**N** (TALON) is the largest prospective registry of Silverhawk use involving 601 patients from 19 different U.S. centers (10,11). All data was entered voluntarily, and outcomes were operator-reported without independent core-laboratory adjudication. Treatment was confined to the infrainguinal region (i.e., above- and below-knee). The dominant indication for treatment was claudication, with approximately one third of patients having critical limb ischemia (CLI). Short and mid-term outcomes of this registry have been reported. Acute procedural success was achieved in nearly 98% of cases. Target lesion revascularization (TLR) occurred in 10% and 20% of patients at 6- and 12-month follow-up, respectively.

In a separate analysis from this same registry including only patients with CLI, procedural success was achieved in 99% of cases (12). The primary endpoint of death, myocardial infarction, unplanned amputation, or repeat target vessel revascularization (TVR) occurred in 1% of the 69 patients at 30 days and 23% at 6 months. Notably there were no unplanned amputations in this high-risk group and amputation was avoided in 92% of limbs at 30 days and 82% of limbs at 6 months.

PROS

Given the directionality of this device and the operator-controlled cuts, this device functions well in the treatment of eccentric disease (Fig. 8.2) and in locations where plaque shift may be poorly tolerated (i.e., SFA ostium). Because of the luminal gain that can be achieved with the larger catheters, it is also particularly useful in the treatment of CFA disease. In terms of treating heavily calcified disease, the authors experience is that the TurboHawk catheters are very effective (Fig. 8.3) and achieve results superior to that achieved using

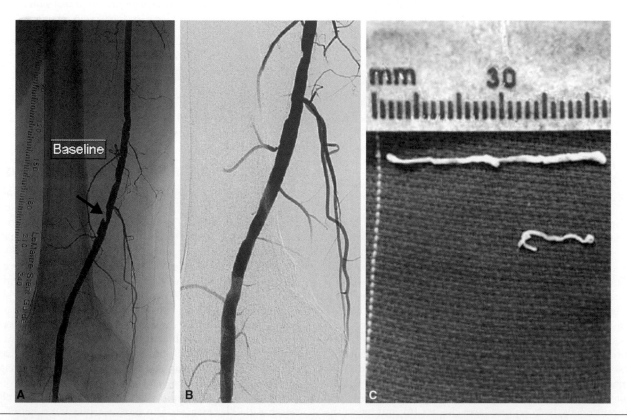

Figure 8.2 • **A:** Focal eccentric lesion of the superficial femoral artery at Hunter's Canal *(arrow)*. **B:** Excellent angiographic result post atherectomy alone using a TurboHawk® catheter. **C:** Atheromatous debris collected from the TurboHawk device.

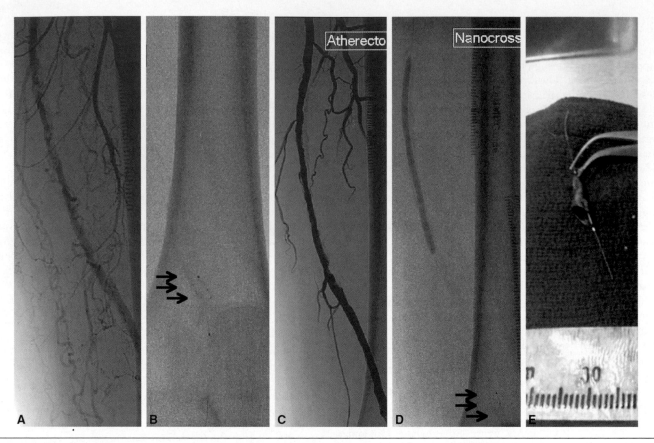

Figure 8.3 • **A:** Severe calcific disease of the distal portion of the superficial femoral artery. **B:** After the disease was crossed using a 0.014″ wire, a Spider FX filter (*black arrows*) was deployed distal to the lesion. **C:** Angiogram showing significant luminal gain post TurboHawk atherectomy. **D:** Given the extensive disease, a 4.0-mm angioplasty balloon was inflated at 3 atm for 5 min following atherectomy with little change in angiographic appearance (not shown). **E:** Image of the significant calcified atheromatous debris captured by the filter in this case. Runoff angiography disclosed no evidence of distal embolization.

either Laser or the Pathway Jetstream catheter and rival those achieved with the Cardiovascular Systems Inc. (CSI) diamondback catheter. No console is required for this catheter, which eliminates the initial funding issues associated with other debulking technologies.

CONS

The spectrum of catheters required to treat the range of vessel diameters and lesion types is problematic, as these catheters are typically purchased and laboratory costs are significant (~$3000 to $3500/catheter). This device requires removal from the body in order to clean the nosecone of atherectomized material; therefore, the treatment of long segments of disease is associated with prolonged procedural times and the risk of trauma to the catheters. This trauma can be associated with catheter failure and the need to use a new catheter, which adds significantly to the cost of the procedure. The directionality of the cutter probably does increase the risk of trauma to the media with this device. Acute perforations and arterio-venous fistula formation, and late pseudoaneurysm formation and perforation have been reported (see chapter 16), and reflect the real potential for trauma to the media using this device. These potential complications suggest that use of this device in the

subintimal space should be carried out with caution. As with other atherectomy devices, distal embolization has also been reported (10,13).

Jetstream Peripheral Vascular Atherectomy System

First approved by the FDA in 2008, the Jetstream Peripheral Vascular Atherectomy System® (Pathway Medical Technologies, Kirkland, WA) (Fig. 8.4) is unique in that it currently is approved for atherectomy in infrainguinal vessels and for thrombectomy of upper and lower extremity vessels.

The atherectomy function of the catheter is achieved by the presence of five stainless steel blades at the catheter tip that rotate at a speed of 70,000 revolutions per second. These blades are unique in that they are expandable (i.e., they assume a tangential position (blades down) when the catheter rotates in a clockwise direction with a nominal diameter of 2.1 mm and assume a radial position (blades up) when the catheter rotates in a counterclockwise direction with a maximum diameter of 3.0 mm). The blades are specifically designed to achieve differential cutting of plaque elements from the normal elastic vessel wall. The catheter also has an aspiration function that is achieved by separate pumps located in a console mounted on an IV pole, which infuse saline through the catheter and

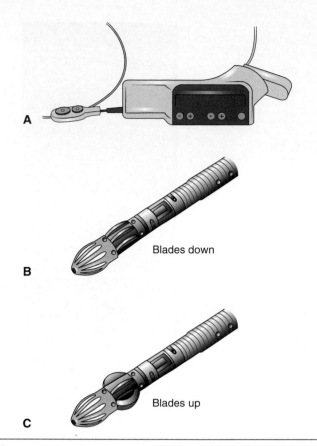

Figure 8.4 • Jetstream Peripheral Vascular Atherectomy System. **A:** The Jetstream atherectomy system showing the handheld control. **B:** The catheter tip in the blades down position. **C:** The catheter tip in the blades up position.

TABLE 8.2 Jetstream G3 and G3 SF Wire and Sheath Compatibility
Compatible Guidewires
Guidant Extra S'port 0.014″ 300 cm
ASAHI Miraclebros 3 300cm (Abbott Vascular)
ASAHI Miraclebros 6 300cm (Abbott Vascular)
Hi-Torque Spartacore 14 300cm (Abbott Vascular)
ASAHI Grand Slam Coronary Guide Wire 300 cm (Abbott Vascular)
Recommended Sheaths
7 or 8 Fr. Cook-Flexor Balkin Check-Flo (Contralateral) 40 cm
7 or 8 Fr. Cook-Flexor Check Flow Raabe 55 cm
7 Fr. Terumo-Pinnacle Destination 45 cm
7 Fr. Terumo-Pinnacle (Ipsilateral) 10 cm
7 Fr. St. Jude Medical-Maximum (Ipsilateral) 12 cm
8 Fr. Cordis Avanti (Ipsilateral) 11 cm
8 Fr. Cordis Avanti (Ipsilateral) 23 cm
8 Fr. Super Arrow-Flex 45 cm

aspirate debris from the catheter tip. One of the major modifications between the first and second (G2) generations of this device was in the location of the aspiration ports. By moving these ports from the distal tip of the catheter to just proximal to the blades resulted in improved aspiration and resolution of the issue of "vessel suckdown" in which advancement of the activated catheter appeared to be hampered by excessive suction of the vessel wall by the catheter tip. The dual function of this catheter in performing both atherectomy and aspiration explains its approval for the treatment of both atheroma and thrombus.

PRACTICAL USE

There are currently two Jetstream catheters available. The G3 catheter, which is intended for use in the CFA, SFA and popliteal vessels, can be used in the "blades down" position (Fig. 8.4B) in vessels as small as 3.0 mm and in the "blades up" position (Fig. 8.4C) in vessels with a reference vessel diameter of 4 mm. The recently released G3 SF catheter was designed for use in the below-knee vessels, with a reference vessel diameter of 2.0 to 3.0 mm. Both catheters are delivered using an 0.014″ wire in an over-the-wire (OTW) system, and require 7 Fr. sheath for delivery (Table 8.2). A dedicated 0.014″ wire (Pathway Jetwire™) was recently released by the manufacturer of the Pathway atherectomy system. Where this wire

is not available, specific wires that are compatible with the catheter are recommended by the manufacturer (Table 8.2). From this latter list of wires, in the authors' experience, the Viper family of wires (CSI, St Paul, MN) interact best with this catheter. Of note, the use of this device in the subintimal space is not recommended by the manufacturer, but has been performed (Fig. 8.5). However, if a re-entry device is used to regain entry to the true lumen, the authors would not recommend the use of this device. The device has been tested with the Spider FX embolic protection device (ev3) and the Spider wire is compatible with Jetstream G3 catheter. However, other embolic protection devices such as the Emboshield Nav[6] (Abbott Vascular) have also worked well with this device.

After crossing the lesion, the catheter is prepared outside the body by submersion in heparinized saline and "priming" of the device. The catheter tip receives continuous flush through an inner lumen and many operators add vasodilators to this flush to prevent vessel spasm. In the authors' practice, the flush solution contains the following: 1 L of normal saline, 2000 units of heparin, 5 mg of verapamil, and 1 mg of nitroglycerin. The device is then loaded and advanced over the 0.014″ wire to the target area. At this point, the interventional wire is locked on the back of the device, which prevents advancement of the wire distally during device activation and advancement. The catheter is then activated using a handheld control and is advanced at a rate of 1 mm/sec through the target area. The initial passage of the catheter should always be in the blades down position. The manufacturers recommend that the catheter be advanced using a "pecking" motion: this involves advancing the catheter tip a short distance followed by retraction of the tip by a slightly shorter

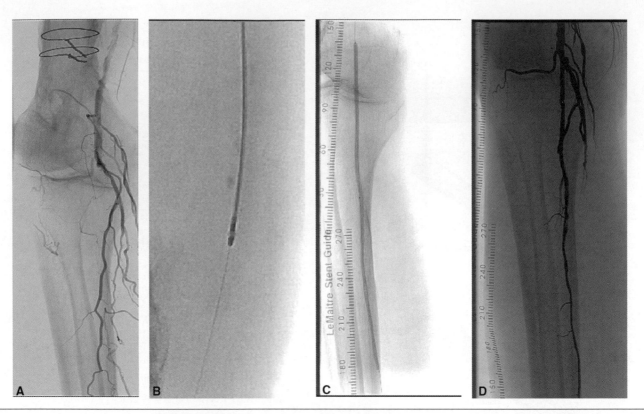

Figure 8.5 • A: Baseline angiography of a distal popliteal artery revealing an occlusion of the mid popliteal and tibioperoneal trunk. **B:** The lesion was crossed using a stiff angled glidewire and a support catheter and atherectomy was performed using a Pathway G2™ NXT catheter in the blades down position through to the peroneal artery and in the blades up position in the popliteal section of the occlusion. **C:** The entire region was then dilated with a 3.0 × 200-mm Nanocross® balloon (ev3) (as shown) and the popliteal was post dilated with a 4.0 mm balloon. **D:** Final angiogram showing an excellent result without the need for stenting with preserved single vessel runoff.

distance. This motion is particularly important when crossing a resistant portion of the lesion. It is necessary to advance the catheter slowly so as not to overcome the aspiration capability of the catheter. Following the initial pass, the device is retracted with activation of the same handheld device holding the reverse arrow that activates the aspiration function of the device alone (Fig. 8.6). The device should be withdrawn to its starting point. At this juncture, operators may wish to make another pass with the blades down or opt to activate the blades up mode.

Rarely, the device may not be able to be advanced across a lesion. In this case, predilatation with a 1.5 or 2.0 mm balloon at low pressure can be used to permit crossing of the device. Early generations of the device were hampered by a phenomenon known as "suckdown" due to excessive aspiration force of the catheter tip on the vessel wall. This appears to have been effectively addressed by design modifications to the most recent catheter tips (see above).

One of the particular quirks of this catheter is in catheter delivery and withdrawal over the aortic bifurcation. Typically, the operator will have to push a little harder to advance the catheter past this anatomic location. During withdrawal of the catheter with the reverse function activated, the catheter usually stalls just distal to the aortic bifurcation. The catheter has to be physically pulled close to the hub of the sheath. In cases where a filter is used, this maneuver should

be done carefully so as not to move the location of the filter significantly.

Following atherectomy with the Pathway Jetstream catheter, the authors routinely use prolonged low-pressure (i.e., 2 to 4 atm) angioplasty at a 1:1 balloon-to-vessel ratio (Fig. 8.7). As a matter of practical significance, if an embolic protection device is used, we recommend leaving this device in place until adjunctive angioplasty and/or stenting has been completed. In the authors' experience, it appears likely that initial atherectomy is associated with a greater degree of embolization associated with angioplasty and/or stenting than would occur with angioplasty and/or stenting stenting alone (14).

CLINICAL DATA

The pivotal study supporting the use of the Pathway Atherectomy System was performed by Zeller et al. (15). A total of 172 patients (47% diabetic) with claudication and CLI were enrolled at 9 European sites. Lesions up to 10 cm in length in the femoropopliteal and up to 3 cm in length in the infrapopliteal vessels with >70% stenosis were included. Of the 210 lesions treated, 65 (31%) were total occlusions. A significant proportion (51%) was rated to have moderate to high calcium scores. The primary outcome was freedom from major adverse events (MAE) at 30 days including clinically driven TLR, any death, TVR, myocardial infarction, and index limb amputation. The primary efficacy endpoint was a reduction in mean

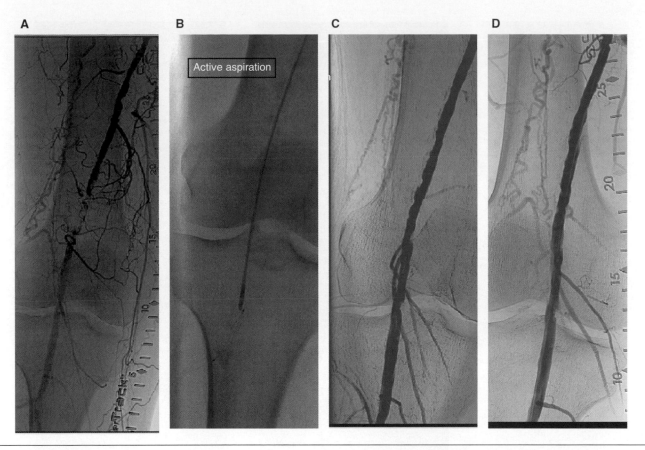

Active aspiration

Figure 8.6 • **A:** Angiography of the proximal popliteal artery revealing occlusive disease with heavy calcification. **B:** After the lesion was crossed using a 0.035″ wire and following placement of a distal embolic protection device, atherectomy was performed with the Pathway G2™ NXT atherectomy catheter in the blades down and blades up positions. Subsequent angiography revealed slow flow secondary to occlusion of the filter. The Pathway G2™ NXT atherectomy catheter was brought near to but not into the filter device and the active aspiration mode triggered. **C:** Angiographic result post atherectomy. **D:** Final result after angioplasty using 4.0 mm balloon inflated to low pressure.

percent stenosis with and without adjunctive therapy. The device was successfully used in 99% of the lesions treated with the primary MAE endpoint occurring in 1% of patients with two preplanned amputations. Clinically driven TLR occurred at 6 months in 15% and at 12 months in 26% of the cohort. Restenosis at 1 year, as assessed by Duplex ultrasound, occurred in 38.2% of lesions.

PROS

The Pathway Atherectomy System provides a unique combination of both atherectomy and aspiration; therefore, it may be associated with a lower incidence of distal embolization compared to other debulking devices. However, this has not been proven. Clinical experience with this device in the treatment of acute thrombus has been very positive. Given that the Jetstream atherectomy system is designed to perform differential cutting of plaque elements and achieves concentric (rather than eccentric) removal of plaque, the propensity for causing eccentric trauma to the media is likely to be lower than with the Silverhawk catheter system. Another advantage over the Silverhawk atherectomy catheter is that the Jetstream catheter is a front-end cutting device which reduces the likelihood of needing predilation to allow delivery of the device. The ability to use two catheters to treat a broad range of vessel diameters provides some potential cost savings.

CONS

The catheter only provides a maximal cutting diameter of 3.0 mm, which falls short of what is often required in the CFA and most SFAs. In addition, the ability to treat eccentric plaque is limited by the concentric atherectomy achieved by the catheter tip. A separate console that costs approximately $10,000 to $15,000 is required, which adds to the start-up costs of initiating this technology in most laboratories. Despite the aspiration capabilities of the catheter, distal embolization remains a concern and the authors have a low threshold for the use of embolic protection with this catheter. Advancement of the catheter must be performed slowly and prolonged procedure times are encountered in the treatment of long lesions.

ABLATIVE ATHERECTOMY

Diamondback 360° Orbital Atherectomy System

The Diamondback 360°™ Orbital Atherectomy System (CSI, St Paul, MN) (Fig. 8.8) obtained FDA approval for use in peripheral arteries in September 2007. It consists of three components: (1) a plaque ablation catheter, which consists of a flexible coil-wound drive shaft with a crown at its distal end; (2) a handle that is used to advance and retract the crown; and

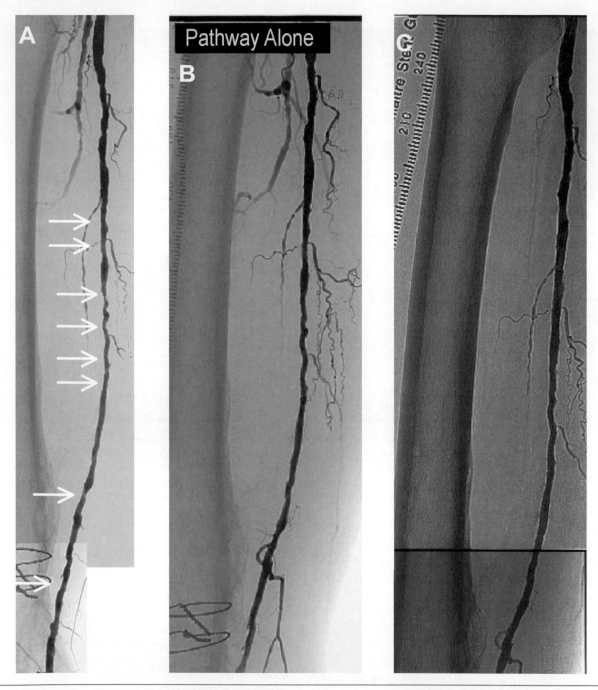

Figure 8.7 • **A:** Baseline angiography revealing a diffusely diseased superficial femoral artery with high-grade obstructive disease in the mid and distal sections (indicated by *arrows*). **B:** Repeat angiography following atherectomy using a Pathway G3 catheter in the blades down and blades up positions. **C:** Final angiography of the SFA after adjunctive low-pressure balloon angioplasty. A stent was not required.

(3) a control console, which regulates the speed of rotation of the drive shaft in the catheter and the infusion of ViperSlide™ lubricant and saline through an infusion sheath around the drive shaft, which serves to cool the crown during high-speed rotation and prevent thermal injury to the vessel wall (14). The crown is coated with diamond bits that are responsible for ablating the plaque tissue when the crown is rotated at high speed (80,000 to 200,000 revolutions per minute [rpm]). The design of the crown has undergone significant design

modification over time. Initially, the "classic" crown had a cylinder of diamond covering over the mid-segment only, whereas the newer "solid" crown has diamond bits covering the entire surface of the crown. In addition, the size of the diamond bits on the "solid crown" has been increased from 30 to 70 μm, in an attempt to improve the ablating capability of the crown. All of the crowns are specifically designed to have a nonconcentric shape. This results in the center of mass of the crown being shifted from the center of rotation during

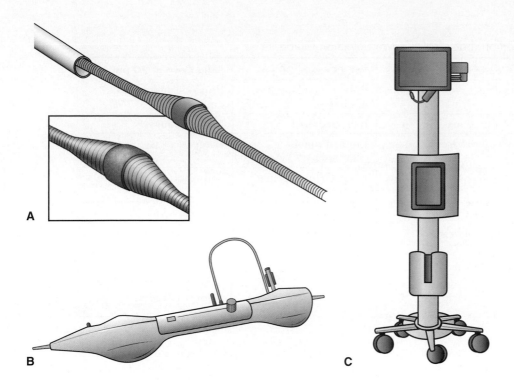

Figure 8.8 • Diamondback 360°™ Orbital Atherectomy System. **A:** Classic crown (inset with magnified image), **B:** Handle and **C:** Console.

rotation of the crown. As a result, the crown rotates in an orbit during rotation. The diameter of the orbit is determined by a number of factors: the diameter of the crown, the rotational speed (rpm) (increasing speeds associated with increasing diameter) (16), the number of passes through the lesion (increasing diameter with increasing number of passes through the lesion), and the physical properties of the lesion. This is one of the major differences between this device and the coronary Rotablator® rotational atherectomy system (Boston Scientific, Natick, MA) that rotates around the center of rotation of the burr and therefore can ablate a lumen diameter no greater than the diameter of the Rotablator burr.

The centrifugal force created by the Diamondback catheter during rotation is responsible for ablation of the plaque into microparticles. Theoretically, healthy elastic tissue in the vessel wall is not ablated by the burr (i.e., differential ablation or sanding of diseased tissue) (17). In preclinical testing, the mean size of these microparticles from the ablated plaque ranged from 1.7 to 3.1 μm. Since the average capillary diameter is between 7 and 9 μm, the expectation is that the particles generated by plaque ablation with the Diamondback catheter will pass through the distal capillaries and be removed by the reticuloendothelial system.

PRACTICAL USE

The Diamondback catheter is an OTW system that is advanced over dedicated 0.014″ wires (ViperWire™). Currently, there are two ViperWires™ available, one with a 0.017″ tip and the other with a 0.023″ tip. These enlarged tips are designed to provide a brake preventing distal embolization of the crown. In the authors' experience, the 0.023″ tip is softer and is preferred. In general, the target lesion is crossed with a separate wire, which is then exchanged for the ViperWire

(being cognizant of the diameter of the wire tip when choosing the appropriate catheter for wire exchange). When an embolic protection device is deemed necessary, the authors have successfully used an Emboshield Nav[6] filter with the ViperWire. The distal brake on the ViperWire serves the same function and the distal brake on the BareWire that accompanies the Emboshield Nav[6] filter. However, this is not formally recommended by the manufacturer.

Having successfully placed the ViperWire distal to the lesion, the Diamondback catheter is prepped. The catheter comes preattached to the handle. From the handle, extensions to the console for the infusion solution (see below) and the compressed gas turbine that powers the drive shaft are handed off to the support staff. The infusion solution is prepped by the addition of ViperSlide lubricant to normal saline. In most laboratories, nitroglycerin and verapamil are added to this solution to maximize distal vasodilatation that is thought to minimize the risk of slow flow due to distal embolization of microparticles. The infusion pump is activated on the console and when the infusion fluid is seen to emerge from the infusion sheath around the drive shaft, the crown is loaded onto the ViperWire which exits from the back of the handle. When the crown nears the access sheath, the drive shaft is tested outside the body by stepping on a foot pedal connected to the console. The catheter is then ready for insertion into the body.

Operators should choose a crown type and size according to the target vessel size, and the degree of vessel calcification and tortousity (Table 8.3). The device is advanced in a standard OTW fashion to a point just proximal to the target lesion. The crown is then advanced to engage the lesion. A short advance of the crown followed by a slightly shorter retraction is the recommended strategy for treating the length

TABLE 8.3 Diamondback 360 Crown Selection Guide

Crown	Classic Crown, 30 μm	Solid Crown, 30 μm	Solid Crown, 70 μm
Application	Smallest crossing profile	Proximal and distal sanding	Proximal and distal sanding
Mass effect	Reduced mass	Increased mass	Increased mass
Application	Distal disease	Limited runoff (<2 vessels)	Larger vessels
Plaque type	Any plaque morphology	Long, diffuse calcific disease	Soft plaque
Best applications	Ostial lesions Tortuous vessels Pilot holes	Larger luminal gains Leading edge sanding for creating pilot holes	Focal disease Requires two or more vessel runoff Soft plaque, changes vessel compliance prior to adjunctive therapy

of the target lesion. It is particularly important not to apply excessive forward force when the crown meets resistance. The goal is to ablate the proximal plaque before advancing distally. Otherwise, there is a risk of entrapping the crown. Also, it is important to advance and withdraw the crown at a similar speed, since ablation is occurring during both maneuvers. In extremely tight lesions, a pilot hole using a lower profile classic crown may be required to allow subsequent delivery of solid crowns that have a larger profile. Most operators begin at the lowest recommended rotational speed for the crown being used during the first pass across the lesion, move to the intermediate rotational speed during the second pass, and the highest rotational speed during the third pass (Table 8.4).

During the early experience with this device, there was a tendency to try to use this device as a stand-alone therapy. As a result, multiple passes at the highest rotational speed were performed with the goal of achieving the maximum luminal diameter. More recently, there has been a shift in most operators practice to use this device to modify the plaque to allow subsequent low-pressure angioplasty. This has resulted in a reduction in the number of passes with the crown and the use of smaller diameter crowns. In the authors' experience, this latter approach is strongly favored (Fig. 8.9). This is based on the experience that significant distal embolization can occur with this device, despite the preclinical data presented by the manufacturers. Shorter activation times and a less aggressive approach to ablation with an emphasis on plaque modification will likely minimize the risk of distal embolization.

CLINICAL DATA

The pivotal study in support of the Diamondback system was the OASIS (**O**rbital **A**therectomy **S**ystem for Treatment of Peripheral Vascular **S**tenosis) trial that studied 124 patients with 210 lesions (16). This was a prospective nonrandomized multicenter registry of orbital atherectomy for infrapopliteal disease. Patients with Rutherford class I–V who had a target vessel reference diameter of 1.4 to 4.0 mm and a target lesion stenosis >50% with a length <100 mm were

included. Chronic total occlusions (CTOs) were included if lesion length was <100 mm as assessed by collaterals and the lesion was successfully crossed with a guidewire. The majority of patients enrolled were Rutherford class I–III (68%) with the remaining 32% having rest pain or nonhealing ulcers. Heavy calcification was noted in 55% of the lesions intervened upon. Stand-alone atherectomy was performed in 58.2% of lesions while adjunctive angioplasty was performed in 39.3% of lesions. The primary safety endpoint of death, myocardial infarction, amputation, or repeat revascularization occurred in four patients (3.2%): two deaths, one myocardial infarction, one repeat revascularization. The primary efficacy endpoint (final percent diameter stenosis) was 17.7 ± 13.5%. At 6 months, MAE occurred in a total of 13 patients (10.4%): 3 deaths (2.4%), 3 planned minor amputations (2.4%), 7 TVRs (5.6%).

PROS

The dominant niche for the Diamondback Orbital Atherectomy System is clearly in the treatment of heavily calcified infrainguinal disease. In the authors' experience, it represents the gold standard for the treatment of such disease. Although initially approved for use in the infrapopliteal circulation, we have found that the device has its greatest utility in the treatment of calcified disease in the CFA and femoropopliteal segment. For those operators and labs familiar with the Rotablator atherectomy system, this device is very similar and is associated with a very short learning curve.

CONS

The major limitation of this device is that of distal embolization. When treating long lesions, particularly in patients with poor runoff, this risk is significant. As a result, the authors have a very low threshold for using a distal filter with this system, and have found significant debris within the filter during such cases. As a result, the authors have tended to limit the use of this device to the treatment of shorter heavily calcified lesions. Hemolysis has been observed following several cases

TABLE 8.4 Crown Sizing Guide

Crown	Crown Size (mm)	Lumen Diameter Achieved (mm)			Sheath (Fr.)	Crossing Profile (mm)
		80k (low)	*140k (medium)*	*200k (high)*		
Classic	1.25	1.4	1.7	2.10	6	1.8
	1.50	1.7	2.10	2.60	6	1.8
	1.75	1.9	2.40	3.00	6	1.8
	2.0	2.4	3.00	3.80	6	2.0
30 µm solid	1.5	1.70	2.50	3.20	6	1.8
	1.75	2.40	3.20	4.20	6	1.8
		80k (low)	*120k (medium)*	*160k (high)*		
	2.0	2.80	3.80	4.80	6	2.0
		60k (low)	*90k (medium)*	*120k (high)*		
	2.25	3.10	4.50	4.90	7	2.25
70 µm solid		*80k (low)*	*140k (medium)*	*200k (high)*		
	1.50	1.90	2.90	3.40	6	1.8
	1.75	2.40	3.70	4.10	6	1.8
		80k (low)	*120k (medium)*	*160k (high)*		
	2.0	3.40	4.80	5.20	6	2.0
		60k (low)	*90k (medium)*	*120k (high)*		
	2.25	3.90	5.30	5.80	7	2.25

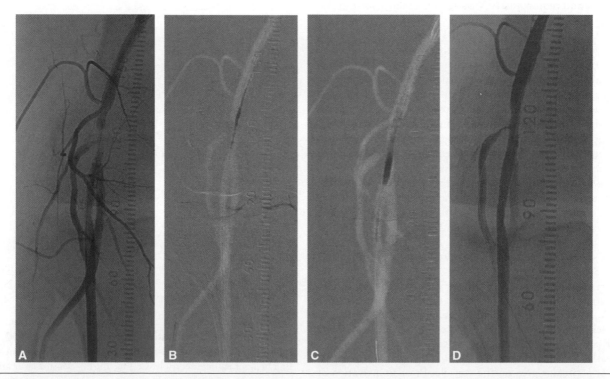

Figure 8.9 • **A:** Baseline angiography of a popliteal artery with a severe calcified focal stenosis. **B:** Image of atherectomy with Diamond-back® 1.5-mm solid crown 30 micrometer grit under roadmap function. **C:** Image of atherectomy with Diamondback 2.25-mm solid crown 70 micrometer grit under roadmap. **D:** Final angiography of the popliteal artery after adjunctive balloon angioplasty with a 4.0 mm balloon.

and patients should be warned that significant discoloration of the urine may occur following treatment. Aggressive hydration is recommended in such circumstances. The cost of the console for this system provides some inertia to initial use of this technology, and it should be accepted that most cases will require the use of more than one crown which adds to the cost of the procedure.

CVX-300 Excimer Laser System®

LASER (**L**ight **A**mplification by **S**timulated **E**mission of **R**adiation) debulking therapy was first used in an occluded SFA in 1983 (18). Since then, technological advancements have resulted in a shift to the use of primarily "cold-tipped" excimer pulse lasers which use light energy at a wavelength of 308 nm to photochemically and photomechanically debulk and ablate tissue (thrombus or plaque) without damaging the surrounding vessel wall. The photons are generated from the decay of an unstable excited dimer (i.e., xenon chloride created from a xenon/hydrogen chloride gas mixture exposed to a high voltage environment [15,000 V]) and this energy is delivered in short bursts (125 ns) that prevent photothermal (heating of surrounding tissue) ablation (19). With each pulse, 10 µm of tissue is ablated and subcellular debris (90% <10 µm in size) is washed downstream. This theoretically permits debulking without the need for embolic protection.

PRACTICAL USE

The most prevalent laser system used is the CVX-300 Excimer laser (Fig. 8.10) that interfaces with Turbo elite laser catheters (Spectranetics, Colorado Springs, CO). This system is large and bulky and requires a 220 V outlet due to the need to create the high voltage environment. In the vast majority of cases, the laser catheter is delivered over a 0.014″ wire that has crossed the target lesion. However, in contrast to all other debulking therapies, the CLiRpath laser catheters have also gained approval for use in the treatment of peripheral CTOs that are not crossable by a guidewire (19). In such circumstances, the tip of the laser catheter is delivered over a wire to the fibrous cap of the occlusion and slowly advanced ahead of the guidewire for a short distance (19). The cap may then be probed with the wire. This "step-by-step" technique can be repeated until the occlusion is successfully crossed.

The most recent generation of excimer-laser Turbo elite catheters is available with outer diameters ranging from 0.9 to 2.5 mm, and may be delivered over 0.014″ or 0.018″ guidewires. Rapid exchange or over-the-wire platforms are available. The size of the laser catheter selected is critical; the catheter diameter should not exceed 2/3 of the reference vessel diameter (Table 8.5).

Preparation of the laser catheter outside the body is relatively straightforward. The catheter is connected to the console. A Tuohy Borst adaptor is connected to the back end of the laser catheter, and tubing delivering heparinized saline under pressure is connected to the side arm of the catheter. The catheter is then calibrated by holding the catheter tip in front of a circular area on the console. Prior to activation of the catheter in the body, it is important that all of the contrast in the vessel is flushed out with normal saline. Our practice is to administer a 20 cc bolus of normal saline prior to catheter

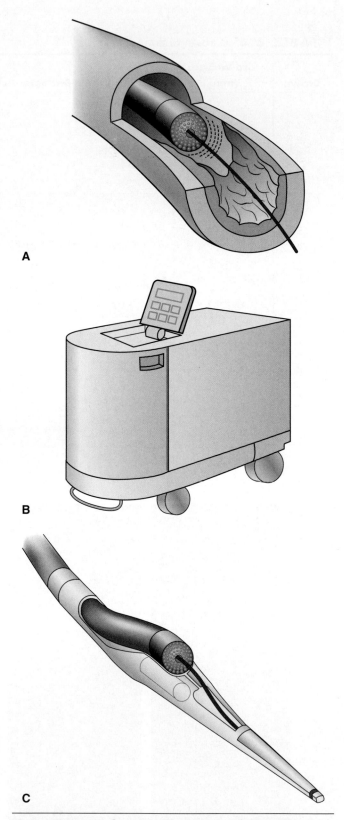

A

B

C

Figure 8.10 • Schematic illustration of CVX-300 Excimer laser system. **A:** Spectranetics Laser catheter in vessel. **B:** The laser catheter console. **C:** The Turbo-Booster laser atherectomy device to enhance luminal gain by offsetting the laser catheter.

TABLE 8.5 Laser Catheter Sizing Chart

Catheter Size (mm)	Recommended Vessel Diameter (mm)
0.9	≥1.4
1.4	≥2.1
1.7	≥2.6
2.0	≥3.0
2.3	≥3.5
2.5	≥3.8

activation to ensure complete replacement of any contrast in the vessel. This practice, together with the constant infusion of saline through the catheter during device activation, is important because transmission of laser energy to contrast and blood results in a photomechanical transformation process that can generate pressure pulses of several hundred atmospheres. This can result in acousto-mechanical vessel trauma and dissection (19). In contrast, saline is not absorbed by the 308-nm wavelength laser light (20) and studies have demonstrated that a saline "flush and bathe" reduces vessel dissection (21).

The default setting on the console is at a fluency of 45, and a frequency of 25 MHz. These settings can be increased if the laser encounters problems passing through the lesion. The maximum fluency and frequency will vary according to the catheter diameter (e.g., 0.9 mm catheter—maximum fluency 80, maximum frequency 80 MHz; 2.5 mm catheter—maximum fluency 45, maximum frequency 80 MHz). The laser catheter is advanced to a point proximal to the target lesion, typically over a supportive 0.014″ guidewire (e.g., Grand Slam). It is now recognized that slow advancement of the laser catheter (1 mm/sec) results in optimal ablation of tissue. In addition, too rapid advancement of the catheter likely increases the risk of distal embolization. In the treatment of long lesions, the slow rate of advancement results in prolonged activation times, but patience is essential to achieving the best results. Following laser atherectomy, adjunctive PTA and/or stenting may be performed at the operator's discretion, though the use of laser atherectomy has been shown to decrease the need for stenting.

A complaint against early laser catheters was the difficulty in achieving adequate luminal gain as compared with the currently available catheters. In an effort to address this shortcoming, the manufacturer created the "Turbo-Booster®" (Fig. 8.10C) which functions as a guide catheter that is used in combination with the laser catheter and offsets the laser from the guidewire axis. This permits the user to rotate the laser around the Turbo-Booster catheter permitting directionality to the photoablation. This combination permits the laser to be advanced with the catheter in a double-barrel alignment, thereby bringing the laser in contact with a different plane of the lesion, creating a larger lumen.

CLINICAL DATA

The Peripheral Excimer Laser Angioplasty (PELA) trial, a randomized prospective multicenter trial of laser versus PTA demonstrated the safety of the device in the treatment

of long SFA occlusions, with the laser group requiring less stent implantation (42% vs. 59%) (22). The LACI 2 trial (23) demonstrated the efficacy of laser debulking for limb salvage (6 month rate of 92.5%) in a CLI population. These trials are complicated by the use of older nondirectional laser catheters and thus adjunctive techniques (PTA ± stenting) were uniformly required. The most recent multicenter CLiRpath Excimer Laser to Enlarge Lumen Openings (CELLO) study, a nonrandomized open label, single group assignment study, demonstrated the safety and efficacy of the TURBO-Booster catheter in the SFA with 77% freedom from TLR at 12 months and no MAE at 30 days or 6 months (24).

PROS

Laser atherectomy is probably the least frequently used of the debulking techniques in clinical practice. In the authors' practice, it has particular utility in the treatment of long lesions with mild-to-moderate calcification where poor runoff is an issue (Fig. 8.11). This is based on our experience that distal embolization with this technique is rare. It has moderate success in treating calcified plaque, and appears useful in treating lesions with a thrombotic component. In addition, the authors find its use particularly effective for the treatment of in-stent restenosis, an application that is being evaluated in an ongoing European trial (PATENT trial).

CONS

One of the major limitations of laser atherctomy is the very high upfront cost of the laser console (list price ~$170,000). This is clearly far greater than the console price of other debulking technologies. In addition, the authors have been somewhat disappointed by the poor luminal gain achieved with this device. Although the use of the Turbo-Booster may help increase luminal gain, this catheter is not particularly user-friendly, and the precision of its use is suboptimal in that the catheter will preferentially rotate to the path of least resistance rather than ablate in the desired direction. The efficiency of this system in ablating heavily calcified plaque has also been disappointing, and in our opinion, is clearly inferior to the Diamondback system and the TurboHawk catheter.

CONCLUSION

The emerging use of debulking therapy for the treatment of infrainguinal disease over the past decade has been remarkable. It has been driven by the suboptimal long-term patency rates associated with angioplasty and stenting. These technologies have expanded the spectrum of infrainguinal disease in which a successful acute procedural result may be achieved, and have effectively decreased the proportion of cases in which stenting is required (25). However, despite the lack of any rigorous data, it appears that debulking techniques are similarly plagued by suboptimal long-term patency rates. The future viability of debulking technologies will likely be predicated on the ability to find biological therapies that can be used in conjunction with mechanical therapies that truly improve long-term patency rates. In the meantime, these technologies remain important in the treatment of specific lesion subsets, and peripheral interventionalists must tailor the use of these

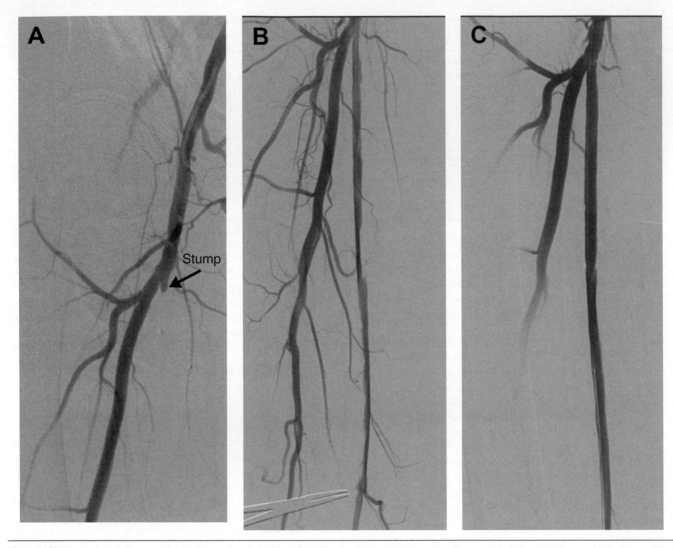

Figure 8.11 • **A:** Baseline angiography of the right superficial femoral artery (SFA) revealing a complete occlusion at the ostium with a short stump. **B:** Angiography following laser atherectomy with restoration of flow. The SFA was then post dilated with a 5.0 mm balloon at low pressure. **C:** Final SFA angiography revealing a widely patent SFA with no evidence of dissection or need for stenting.

technologies to the specific patient, and the plaque characteristics of the target lesion.

References

1. Laird JR. Limitations of percutaneous transluminal angioplasty and stenting for the treatment of disease of the superficial femoral and popliteal arteries. *J Endovasc Ther.* 2006;13(suppl 2): II30–II40.
2. Gray BH, Olin JW. Limitations of percutaneous transluminal angioplasty with stenting for femoropopliteal arterial occlusive disease. *Semin Vasc Surg.* 1997;10:8–16.
3. Dorrucci V. Treatment of superficial femoral artery occlusive disease. *J Cardiovasc Surg (Torino).* 2004;45:193–201.
4. Norgren L, Hiatt WR, Dormandy JA, et al. Inter-Society Consensus for the Management of Peripheral Arterial Disease (TASC II). *J Vasc Surg.* 2007;45(suppl S):S5–S67.
5. Klein AJ, Chen SJ, Messenger JC, et al. Quantitative assessment of the conformational change in the femoropopliteal artery with leg movement. *Catheter Cardiovasc Interv.* 2009;74:787–798.
6. Klein AJ, Casserly IP, Messenger JC, et al. In vivo 3D modeling of the femoropopliteal artery in human subjects based on x-ray angiography: methodology and validation. *Med Phys.* 2009;36:289–310.
7. Scheinert D, Scheinert S, Sax J, et al. Prevalence and clinical impact of stent fractures after femoropopliteal stenting. *J Am Coll Cardiol.* 2005;45:312–315.
8. Nguyen MC, Garcia LA. Recent advances in atherectomy and devices for treatment of infra-inguinal arterial occlusive disease. *J Cardiovasc Surg (Torino).* 2008;49:167–177.
9. Bunting TA, Garcia LA. Peripheral atherectomy: a critical review. *J Interv Cardiol.* 2007;20:417–424.
10. Zeller T, Rastan A, Sixt S, et al. Long-term results after directional atherectomy of femoro-popliteal lesions. *J Am Coll Cardiol.* 2006;48:1573–1578.
11. Ramaiah V, Gammon R, Kiesz S, et al. Midterm outcomes from the TALON Registry: treating peripherals with SilverHawk: outcomes collection. *J Endovasc Ther.* 2006;13:592–602.
12. Kandzari DE, Kiesz RS, Allie D, et al. Procedural and clinical outcomes with catheter-based plaque excision in critical limb ischemia. *J Endovasc Ther.* 2006;13:12–22.

13. Wholey M. Plaque excision in 2005 and beyond: issues of the past have yet to be resolved. *Endovasc Today.* 2005 (August):40–44.

14. Lam RC, Shah S, Faries PL, et al. Incidence and clinical significance of distal embolization during percutaneous interventions involving the superficial femoral artery. *J Vasc Surg.* 2007;46:1155–1159.

15. Zeller T, Krankenberg H, Steinkamp H, et al. One-year outcome of percutaneous rotational atherectomy with aspiration in infrainguinal peripheral arterial occlusive disease: the multicenter pathway PVD trial. *J Endovasc Ther.* 2009;16:653–662.

16. Safian RD, Niazi K, Runyon JP, et al. Orbital atherectomy for infrapopliteal disease: device concept and outcome data for the OASIS trial. *Catheter Cardiovasc Interv.* 2009;73:406–412.

17. Garcia LA, Lyden SP. Atherectomy for infrainguinal peripheral artery disease. *J Endovasc Ther.* 2009;16:II105–II115.

18. Choy DS. History of lasers in medicine. *Thorac Cardiovasc Surg.* 1988;36(suppl 2):114–117.

19. Tan JW, Yeo KK, Laird JR. Excimer laser assisted angioplasty for complex infrainguinal peripheral artery disease: a 2008 update. *J Cardiovasc Surg (Torino).* 2008;49:329–340.

20. Gijsbers GH, van den Broecke DG, Sprangers RL, et al. Effect of force on ablation depth for a XeCl excimer laser beam delivered by an optical fiber in contact with arterial tissue under saline. *Lasers Surg Med.* 1992;12:576–584.

21. Tcheng JE, Wells LD, Phillips HR, et al. Development of a new technique for reducing pressure pulse generation during 308-nm excimer laser coronary angioplasty. *Cathet Cardiovasc Diagn.* 1995;34:15–22.

22. Laird JR. Peripheral Excimer Laser Angioplasty (PELA) trial results. Transcatheter Cardiovascular Therapeutics Annual Meeting, Washington, DC, 2002.

23. Laird JR, Zeller T, Gray BH, et al. Limb salvage following laser-assisted angioplasty for critical limb ischemia: results of the LACI multicenter trial. *J Endovasc Ther.* 2006;13:1–11.

24. Dave RM, Patlola R, Kollmeyer K, et al. Excimer laser recanalization of femoropopliteal lesions and 1-year patency: results of the CELLO registry. *J Endovasc Ther.* 2009;16:665–675.

25. Casserly I. The role of atherectomy in the femoropopliteal artery. *Endovasc Today.* 2009;(September):3–7.

Cerebrovascular Intervention

CHAPTER 9

Carotid Artery Stenting: The Data

Jacqueline Saw and William Gray

Carotid artery stenting (CAS) was recently accepted as an alternative minimally invasive revascularization approach to carotid endarterectomy (CEA) for the treatment of high-risk patients with significant extracranial carotid artery stenosis and data in patients at normal risk for CEA is emerging. Although CEA is traditionally considered the "gold standard" therapy to prevent strokes in patients with carotid stenosis, this technique is invasive and may cause serious complications (death, stroke, myocardial infarction, cranial nerve palsy, wound infection, hemorrhage, etc). Consequently, carotid angioplasty and stenting was pursued almost three decades ago because it offered a less invasive approach that had the potential to be better tolerated with potentially fewer complications.

The idea of carotid angioplasty in humans was proposed in 1977 by Mathias (1), and subsequently performed by Kerber in 1980 (2). The early experience with carotid angioplasty was fraught with challenges and complications, attributed to lack of dedicated equipment, lack of protection from distal embolization, operator inexperience, and suboptimal patient selection. One of the earliest randomized carotid angioplasty trial (widely known as the "Stopped trial") was aborted after enrolling 17 patients, since 5 of the 7 carotid angioplasty procedures resulted in strokes, compared to none in the CEA arm (3). These results were likely due to the combination of operator inexperience, poor patient and lesion selection, and crude instrumentation. Fortunately, further developments in technique and equipment by early interventional pioneers have dramatically reduced acute procedural complications and improved the long-term durability of the therapy.

Emboli protection devices (EPD) and self-expanding stents are key innovations that contributed to the success of CAS and represent the standard for contemporary CAS procedures. As of mid-2008, there are six FDA-approved carotid stent and EPD systems: the AccuLink™ stent and AccuNet™ filter (Abbott Vascular, Santa Clara, CA), the Xact® stent and EmboShield™ filter (Abbott Vascular, Santa Clara, CA), the Precise™ stent and AngioGuard XP™ filter (Cordis Corporation, Warren, NJ), the Protégé® stent and SPIDER™ filter (ev3 Inc., Plymouth, MN), the Wallstent and Filterwire EZ™ filter (Boston Scientific, Nattick, MA), and the Exponent® stent and GuardWire™ device (Medtronic, Minneapolis, MN).

Since the advent of carotid angioplasty and stenting, numerous studies have been executed to evaluate the procedural complications and long-term efficacy, especially in comparison to CEA. We will review these studies systematically, including (1) early large single-center and multicenter CAS registries, (2) contemporary pivotal high-risk CAS registries (several of which led to the FDA premarket approval (PMA) of six current stent and EPD devices), (3) randomized CAS versus CEA studies, (4) other comparative CAS versus CEA studies, (5) postmarketing registries, and (6) ongoing CAS trials.

EARLY CAS REGISTRIES

Several early single-center observational studies have been published. However, these studies included only small patient numbers, had short clinical follow-up, utilized different equipment (legacy stents largely without EPD), and employed inconsistent definitions of complications (e.g., minor or major strokes, ipsilateral or all strokes). Larger multicenter registries were thus performed, for example, the Pro-CAS, ELOCAS, and the Global Carotid Artery Stent Registry, which in aggregate included over 18,000 patients with variable surgical risks and provided valuable procedural and outcome data on CAS (4–6).

ELOCAS

The European Long-term Carotid Artery Stenting Registry included 2172 CAS procedures from 1993 to 2004 at four high-volume European centers in Belgium, Germany, and Italy (4). This registry included a mixture of prospective and retrospective cases, with inconsistent neurologic assessment and no independent assessment of clinical events. Technical success rate was 99.7%, stenting was performed in 95.6%, and EPDs were used in 85.9% of cases. Symptomatic patients represented 41.6% of the cohort. The 30-day death and major stroke event-rate was only 1.2%, with no significant difference between symptomatic (1.4%) and asymptomatic patients (1.0%). The long-term death and major stroke rates were 4.1%, 10.1%, and 15.5% at 1, 3, and 5 years, respectively. Restenosis rates were low, 1% at 1-year, 2% at 3-year, and 3.4% at 5-year follow-up. Interestingly, in a nonprespecified subgroup analysis, predilatation was associated with lower stroke and death event-rate compared with direct stenting (2.7% vs. 4.6% at 1 year, $p = 0.002$).

The Global Carotid Artery Stent Registry

The Global Carotid Artery Stent Registry commenced in 1997 and initially involved 24 centers in Europe, North America, South America, and Asia and had similar limitations with respect to inconsistent neurologic evaluation and event adjudication. By September 2002, there were 53 participating centers and 12,392 CAS procedures had been performed involving 11,243 patients, symptomatic patients representing 53.2% of the cohort (5). Technical success rate was 98.9%, and EPDs were used in 38.5%. The 30-day incidence of TIA was 3.1%, minor stroke

2.1%, major stroke 1.2%, and procedural death 0.6%. The combined 30-day stroke plus procedural death incidence progressively improved over the course of follow-up, from 5.7% to 4.0%, presumably related to equipment advancement, EPD use, and operator experience. In subgroup analyses, the 30-day stroke and procedural death was 4.9% in symptomatic patients and 3.0% in asymptomatic patients, and was 2.2% in patients who had EPD use (4221 cases) versus 5.3% in patients without EPD use (6753 cases). Both symptomatic and asymptomatic patients benefited from EPD use. In symptomatic patients, the 30-day stroke and death rate was 2.7% with EPD use versus 6.0% without EPD use. In asymptomatic patients, the 30-day stroke and death rate was 1.8% with EPD use versus 4.0% without EPD use. However, there was a steep learning curve for EPD use; centers that had performed 20 to 50 cases had a 4.0% stroke and death rate compared with 1.6% in centers that had performed >500 cases. At follow-up, ipsilateral neurologic events were observed in 1.2%, 1.3%, and 1.7%, at 1, 2, and 3 years, respectively. Restenosis rate by carotid ultrasound was low at 2.4% at 3 years.

Pro-CAS

The German Prospective Registry of Carotid Artery Angioplasty and Stenting (Pro-CAS) included 3267 CAS procedures performed between 1999 and 2003 at 38 centers in Germany, Austria, and Switzerland (6). Independent neurologic assessments were voluntary, inconsistent and not standardized, and clinical events were site reported only and not independently adjudicated. Stents were used in 98% of cases, of which 89% were self-expanding stents. The use of EPDs varied widely between the centers, and was recorded at 64% starting from October 2000 (not recorded prior). The overall technical success rate was 98%. The incidence of major stroke, minor stroke, and death was 1.2%, 1.3%, and 0.6%, respectively, and the combined incidence of stroke and death was 2.8%. Symptomatic patients represented 56% of the cohort. The incidence of stroke and death was 3.1% for symptomatic patients, and 2.4% for asymptomatic patients. There was no clear advantage with EPD use in this registry. In their most recent 2008 update encompassing 5341 CAS procedures performed between 1999 and 2005, the in-hospital stroke and death event-rate was 3.6% (7). There

was a progressively lower prevalence of procedural stroke and death event rates from the inception of the trial (6.1% during the first year of enrolment) to the later years (3.0% from 2004 to 2005). Several factors were found to predict periprocedural events: center experience, age, prior symptoms, primary intervention (vs. restenotic intervention), angioplasty (vs. stent), predilatation, and heparin dose >5000 units.

CONTEMPORARY HIGH-RISK CAS REGISTRIES

With the development of dedicated carotid self-expanding stents and EPDs, contemporary registries were initiated by the respective sponsors to evaluate the safety and efficacy of these systems in a highly regulated and prospective fashion in multicenter Investigational Device Exemption (IDE) trials. These contemporary registries specifically targeted patients at high-risk for surgical endarterectomy, since intuitively these patients would have the greatest benefit from a less invasive approach. These studies included both symptomatic and asymptomatic patients with carotid stenosis severity ≥50% and >80%, respectively. The high-risk inclusion criteria included a combination of high-risk anatomic factors and medical comorbidities (Table 9.1). These studies had independent neurologic assessments pre- and postprocedures, and were monitored by safety committees and adjudicated by independent clinical events committees (which was demonstrated to increase the rate of endpoint events by ~50%). The primary safety endpoints evaluated typically comprised a composite of death, stroke, and myocardial infarction (MI) at 30 days. The primary efficacy endpoint usually included the 30-day death, stroke, and MI events, combined with death and stroke events from 31 days to 1-year post-CAS. Overall, the 30-day composite death, stroke, or MI event-rate from these registries involving high surgical risk patients range from 3.0% to 8.3% (with 30-day death or stroke rates varying between 2.8% and 7.6%), and the 1-year event-rates were 4.5% to 9.6% (Table 9.2). The results from these IDE trials utilizing specific stent and EPD platforms were predominantly used to obtain CE Mark and FDA approval in Europe and the United States, respectively.

TABLE 9.1 Typical High-Risk Criteria in Carotid Artery Stent Studies (at least 1 Required for Enrollment)

Anatomic Criteria	Medical Comorbidities
Lesion at C2 or higher	Age ≥ 80 years
Lesion below clavicle	Class III/IV congestive heart failure
Prior radical neck surgery or radiation	Class III/IV angina pectoris
Contralateral carotid occlusion	Left main/≥ 2-vessel coronary disease
Prior ipsilateral CEA	Need for urgent (<30 days) heart surgery
Contralateral laryngeal nerve palsy	LV ejection fraction ≤ 30%
Tracheostomy	Recent myocardial infarction (>1 but <30 days)
Severe tandem lesions	Severe chronic pulmonary disease

LV, left ventricular; C2, second cervical vertebra.

TABLE 9.2 High-Risk Carotid Artery Stent (CAS) Registries

	Company Device	Stent	EPD	N	Symptomatic	30-day D+S+MI	30-day D+S	1-year Outcome*
ARCHeR pooled	Guidant/ Abbott	AccuLink	AccuNet	581	24%	8.3%	6.9%	9.6%
ARCHeR 1		AccuLink OTW	None	158	–	7.6%	6.3%	8.3%
ARCHeR 2		AccuLink OTW	AccuNet OTW	278	–	8.6%	6.8%	10.2%
ARCHeR 3		AccuLink RX	AccuNet RX	145	–	8.3%	7.6%	–
BEACH	Boston Scientific	Wallstent	FilterWire EX/EZ	747	25.3%	5.8%	2.8%	9.1%
CABERNET	Boston Scientific	EndoTex NexStent	FilterWire EX/EZ	454	24%	3.9%	3.6%	4.5%
CREATE	Ev3	Protégé	Spider OTW	419	17.4%	6.2%	5.2%	7.8%
CREATE SpiderRX	Ev3	Acculink	SpiderRX	160		5.6%	–	–
EMPIRE	GORE	Any	GORE flow reversal	245	32%	3.1%	–	–
EPIC	Lumen	Any	FiberNet	237	20%	3.0%	–	–
MAVErIC 1 + 2	Medtronic	Exponent	GuardWire	498	22%	5.2%	–	–
MAVErIC Int'l	Medtronic	Exponent	InterceptorPlus	51	–	5.9%	–	11.8%
MO.MA	–	Any	Mo.Ma	157	19.7%	5.7%	5.7%	–
PASCAL	–	Exponent	Any CE-approved	115	–	8%	–	–
PRIAMUS	–	Any	Mo.Ma	416	63.5%	4.6%	4.6%	–
SECURITY	Abbott	Xact	EmboShield	305	21%	7.5%	6.9%	8.5%

* 30-day death, stroke, and MI plus ipsilateral stroke 31 to 365 days.
D, death; S, stroke; MI, myocardial infarction; EDP, embolic protection device.

ARCHeR

The ARCHeR (AccuLink™ for Revascularization of Carotids in High-Risk patients) study consisted of three sequential, multicenter, nonrandomized prospective registries. The AccuLink™ over-the-wire (OTW) self-expanding nitinol stent was used without an EPD in ARCHeR 1, and with the AccuNet™ OTW filter EPD in ARCHeR 2 (both systems by Guidant Endovascular, now Abbott Vascular). ARCHeR 3 used the rapid-exchange versions of both stent and filter systems. Of 581 patients enrolled from 2000 to 2003 at 48 sites, 24% were symptomatic. Data from the three phases were similar, and thus the results were pooled and published in 2006 (8). The 30-day major adverse event-rate (MAE) of death/ stroke/MI was 8.3% (13.1% in symptomatic patients, 6.8% in asymptomatic patients) and stroke/death rate was 6.9% (11.6% in symptomatic patients, 5.4% in asymptomatic patients). The majority of stroke events were minor (72%),

with a major stroke rate of 1.5% (4.3% in symptomatic patients, 0.7% in asymptomatic patients). The primary efficacy endpoint (composite of 30-day MAE plus ipsilateral stroke between 31 days and 1 year) was 9.6%, which was noninferior to historical controls at 14.4%. Target lesion revascularization was 2.2% at 1 year and 2.9% at 2 years. These results led to FDA approval of the AccuLink™ stent and AccuNet™ EPD in August 2004, which was the first approved CAS device platform in the United States.

BEACH

The Boston Scientific EPI: A Carotid Stenting Trial for High-Risk Surgical Patients (BEACH) enrolled 747 high-risk patients from 47 US sites. CAS was performed with the Wallstent® and FilterWire EX/EZ systems (Boston Scientific, Nattick, MA) (9). The study included three groups: 189 roll-in patients, 480 pivotal group patients, and 78 registry patients with bilateral carotid stenoses treated by staged sequential CAS. The overall 30-day composite MAE was 5.8% (death 1.5%, stroke 4.4%, MI 1.0%), with no significant difference between the three groups. There were 25.3% symptomatic patients, and they had higher 30-day stroke rate than asymptomatic patients (7.4% vs. 3.4%, $p = 0.038$), but there was no difference in the 30-day composite MAE rates (7.9% vs. 5.0%). The 1-year endpoint of 30-day MAE plus ipsilateral stroke or neurologic death from 31 days to 1 year was 8.9% for the pivotal group, and repeat revascularization rate was 4.7% (10).

CABERNET (Unpublished Data)

The CABERNET (Carotid Artery Revascularization using the Boston Scientific EPI FilterWire EX/EZ and the Endo-Tex NexStent) trial enrolled 454 high-risk patients (24% were symptomatic) from 19 sites. The 30-day composite of death, stroke, and MI was 3.9% (death 0.5%, major stroke 1.3%, minor stroke 2.1%, MI 0.2%). The first primary endpoint of 30-day death, stroke, and MI, plus ipsilateral stroke from 31 days to 1 year was 4.5%. The second primary endpoint of all death, stroke, and MI at 1 year was 11.5%. At 3 years, the major stroke rate was 2.8%, and the ipsilateral stroke rate was 4.9%. These results were presented in the Transcatheter Cardiovascular Therapeutics (TCT) meetings in 2005 and 2007. The FDA subsequently approved the NexStent and FilterWire platform in December 2006. However, it was subsequently taken off the market, and is currently not available.

CREATE

The Carotid Revascularization With ev3 Arterial Technology Evolution (CREATE) trial enrolled 419 high-risk patients in 32 centers between April and October 2004. CAS was performed with the Protégé carotid stent and the Spider FX OTW filter EPD (ev3 Inc., Plymouth, MN) (11). Technical success was achieved in 97.4% of patients. Symptomatic patients represented 7.4% of the cohort and 24% of procedures were performed for patients with restenosis after prior CEA. The primary composite endpoint of death, stroke, and MI at 30 days occurred in 6.2% (death 1.9%, nonfatal stroke 3.3%, and MI 1%). In their multivariate analysis, the duration of filter deployment, symptomatic status, and baseline renal insufficiency were independent predictors of stroke. Patients who had their filter EPD deployed for over 20 minutes had almost double the risk of stroke and death compared to patients with filter deployment times <20 minutes (12). This was the first study to show that prolonged filter deployment time predicted higher complications with CAS, although it is not certain whether the extended filter time was causally related to complications, or simply a marker of the risk of complications. CREATE 2 studied the use of the AccuLink™ stent and the rapid-exchange version of the SPIDER filter. Of the 160 high-risk patients enrolled, the 30-day composite death, stroke, and MI event-rate was 5.6% (13). The SpiderRX device was FDA approved for CAS in February 2006 and the Protégé stent in January 2007. Following FDA approval, patients are currently being enrolled in the CREATE Post Approval study.

EMPiRE (Unpublished Data)

The EMPiRE study was a prospective, single-arm, multi-center registry that evaluated the safety and efficacy of the GORE Flow Reversal System during CAS in patients who were deemed high-risk for CEA. The study included 245 patients enrolled at 28 sites from July 2006 to July 2008, and preliminary results were reported at the TCT meeting in October 2008. The mean age of the patients was 70, of which 16% were octogenarians and 32% were symptomatic. The mean procedural time was 80 minutes (ranging from 25 to 345 minutes), with a mean flow reversal time of 15 minutes. Technical success rate with the GORE Flow Reversal System was 96.3%, with 2.4% of patients not being able to tolerate the procedure. The mortality rate was 0.8%, the death and stroke rate was 2.0%, and the MAE rate was 3.7%.

EPIC (Unpublished Data)

The EPIC study (Evaluating the Use of the FiberNet Embolic Protection System in Carotid Artery Stenting) was also recently reported at the TCT meeting in October 2008. This study enrolled 237 high-risk patients (from 26 US sites) with carotid artery stenosis who underwent carotid stenting using the FiberNet Embolic Protection System (Lumen Biomedical, Plymouth, MN) and a variety of approved carotid stents. This system provides for distal protection as well as aspiration of embolic debris. The technical success rate was 97.5%, with a FiberNet device success rate of 94.1%. The mean age of the patients was 74, 21.1% were octogenarians and 20% were symptomatic. The 1-month complication rates were low: mortality 0.4%, stroke 2.1%, MI 0.9%, with overall MAE of 3.0%.

MAVErIC (Unpublished Data)

The MAVErIC (Medtronic Self-Expanding Carotid Stent System with Distal Protection in the Treatment of Carotid Artery Stenosis) trial enrolled 99 high-risk CAS patients from 16 centers in the feasibility phase (MAVErIC 1) and 399 patients from 40 centers in the pivotal trial (MAVErIC 2) using the Exponent® self-expanding stent and GuardWire® distal balloon occlusion protection device (Medtronic, Minneapolis, MN). Within the pivotal group, 22% of patients were symptomatic and 34% had restenotic lesions after prior CEA. The 30-day death, stroke, and MI event-rate was 5.3% (death 1%, stroke 3.3%, and MI 2.0%) in the pivotal MAVErIC 2 trial presented at TCT 2004. The 1-year death, stroke, and MI event-rate from the feasibility MAVErIC 1 trial was 5.1%. The 1-year results for MAVErIC 2 have not been reported.

There is also the MAVErIC 3 study, which is intended to recruit 413 CAS patients in the United States using the Exponent® stent and a different EPD, the Interceptor Plus Carotid Filter system (also by Medtronic). In the smaller MAVErIC International Study that evaluated this CAS platform in 51 patients from 11 centers in Europe, Canada, and the Middle East (14), the 30-day MAE rate was 5.9% (death 2%, stroke 3.9%, MI 2%) and 1-year MAE rate was 11.8% (death 3.9%, stroke 5.9%, and MI 5.9%).

MO.MA (Outside the United States [OUS] data)

The MO.MA registry evaluated the use of the proximal occlusion Mo.Ma (Invatec) device among 157 patients who underwent CAS using a variety of approved carotid stents in 14 European centers from 2002 to 2003. This study did not exclusively enroll high-risk patients (75.2% were high-risk and 19.7% were symptomatic). Patients with contralateral carotid occlusion, severe external carotid artery disease, or proximal common carotid artery disease were excluded from this study.

The Mo.Ma device was successfully used in 96.8% of patients, and a filter EPD was used in the unsuccessful cases. The mean duration of flow blockage was 7.6 minutes. The 30-day death and stroke rate was 5.7% (death 0.6%, major stroke 0.6%, minor stroke 4.5%), with no MI (15). A US IDE high surgical risk registry is completing enrollment.

PASCAL (OUS, Unpublished Data)

The PASCAL (Performance and Safety of the Medtronic AVE Self-Expandable Stent in Treatment of Carotid Artery Lesions) study was a European multicenter registry of 115 high-risk patients undergoing CAS with the Medtronic Exponent® stent and any CE Mark–approved EPD. The reported 30-day death, stroke, and MI rate was 8% (13). Although the study commenced in 2001, the results remain unpublished.

PRIAMUS (OUS)

The PRIAMUS (Proximal Flow Blockage Cerebral Protection during Carotid Stenting) study evaluated the Mo.Ma (Invatec) device in 416 CAS high-risk patients from four Italian centers from 2001 to 2006 (16). The study included 63.5% symptomatic patients, and did not exclude patients with contralateral carotid artery occlusion. The 30-day death, stroke, and MI event-rate was 4.6% (death 0.5%, major stroke 0.2%, minor stroke 3.8%, and no MI).

SECURITY (Unpublished Data)

The SECURITY (Registry Study to Evaluate the Em-boShield™ Bare Wire Cerebral Protection System and Xact® Stent in Patients at High Risk for Carotid Endarterectomy) trial enrolled 305 high-risk patients from 29 US centers and 1 Australian center using the Xact® stent and EmboShield™ EPD (Abbott Vascular). Technical success was observed in 96.7%, and 21% of patients were symptomatic. The 30-day composite rate of death, stroke, and MI was 7.5% (death 1.0%, major stroke 2.6%, minor stroke 4.3%, and MI 0.7%). In comparison to historical weighted controls for CEA, the primary endpoint of 30-day MAE plus ipsilateral stroke from 31 days to 1 year was lower with CAS (8.5% vs. 14%) (17). The results were presented at TCT in 2003 and subsequently submitted to the FDA and granted approval in September 2005.

RANDOMIZED CAS VERSUS CEA STUDIES

The earliest randomized trials comparing CAS to CEA were fraught with limitations and high complication rates for CAS. These early trials utilized outmoded carotid angioplasty approaches, lacked consistent use of both stents and EPDs, and included inexperienced interventional operators. In contradistinction, surgical operators were carefully chosen and most had to have demonstrated adequate CEA procedural volume and low complication rates. As such, most of these published comparative studies were of poor scientific quality and do add to the comparison of contemporary CAS versus CEA. Most would agree that comparing procedural outcomes of interventionists and surgeons of divergent skills/experience is not a reasonable comparison of the outcomes. CAS outcomes did not, until fairly recently, demonstrate a reduction and leveling off of adverse outcomes, likely due to better operator experience and patient

selection reflecting an ongoing refinement of the field. Many of the earlier randomized outcomes, then, represent a technique, and technology, in evolution and distinctly different in that regard to a more than 50-year-old operation like endarterectomy that showed a similar early experiential development. We will briefly review the early trials followed by more recently published randomized CAS versus CEA trials.

The "Stopped" Trial (1998, OUS)

This was a single-center prospective, randomized trial from Leicester, UK that started in 1996 and was originally intended to randomize 300 symptomatic patients with carotid stenosis >70% (3). However, the trial was stopped prematurely due to an excess of complications in the angioplasty arm after 23 patients were enrolled, of which only 17 patients received their allocated revascularization. There were 5 stroke events among the 7 patients who underwent carotid angioplasty, compared with no stroke events among the 10 CEA procedures. The poor outcome in the angioplasty arm is considered a marked outlier and was attributed to inexperienced operators and suboptimal technique and equipment (no EPD use), in an era when CAS was still in its infancy. Due to the extensive limitations in this small single-center study, no appropriate conclusions could be drawn.

CAVATAS (1994 to 1997, OUS)

The Carotid and Vertebral Artery Transluminal Angioplasty Study (CAVATAS) randomized standard surgical risk patients to carotid angioplasty or CEA at 22 centers throughout Europe, Canada, and Australia from 1992 to 1997 (18). This study excluded high-risk patients and enrolled predominantly symptomatic patients (90% had neurologic symptoms within 6 months). There were 246 patients who underwent CEA and 240 had angioplasty without embolic protection (only 26% had stents, which were placed after 1994). The primary endpoint of 30-day MAE rate of death plus any stroke was 9.9% with CEA and 10% with angioplasty, and the death and disabling stroke rate was similar (6%). At 3 years, the rate of death or disabling stroke was also similar, 14.3% for angioplasty and 14.2% for CEA. This study has been criticized for a number of important limitations and practice that does not reflect current standards: formal sample size calculation was not performed, the 30-day MAE rates were unacceptably high in both arms (especially since high-risk patients were excluded), stents were used in only 26% of angioplasty cases, and no EPDs were used. In spite of the higher than expected event rate in both arms, this was the first randomized trial between surgical and nonsurgical management of extracranial bifurcation carotid disease to show that an endovascular approach might be reasonable.

The Wallstent Trial (1997 to 1999, US, Unpublished)

The Wallstent study randomized 219 symptomatic patients with standard surgical risk and carotid stenosis >60% to CEA versus CAS with the Wallstent® endoprosthesis (Boston Scientific) without EPD. The primary endpoint of ipsilateral stroke, procedure-related death, or vascular death within 1 year was 12.1% with CAS versus 3.6% for CEA (p = 0.022). The rate of any stroke plus death at 30 days was also higher with CAS

(12.1% vs. 4.5% for CEA, $p = 0.049$). It was concluded that CAS was not equivalent to CEA in symptomatic low-normal risk patients, and the study was subsequently terminated prematurely before the planned enrolment of 700 patients. However, the study only has limited applicability given that inexperienced operators performed these CAS procedures, and dedicated carotid stent equipment and EPDs were not used. The study was only published in abstract form (19).

Community (Kentucky) Trial (1998, US)

This was a single-center randomized comparison of CAS (without EPD) versus CEA in a community hospital in Kentucky. In the first group consisting of 104 symptomatic patients with carotid stenosis >70% ("Community A"), 53 were randomized to CAS with the Carotid Wallstent® (Boston Scientific) and 51 to CEA (20). The event rates were low in both arms with one death in the CEA group and one transient ischemic attack (TIA) in the CAS group. There was a trend toward earlier hospital discharge with CAS (1.8 days vs. 2.7 days). In the second group ("Community B") consisting of 85 patients with asymptomatic carotid stenosis >80% randomized to CAS or CEA (21), the event rates were extremely low with no procedure-related death or stroke in either arm. At 2 years, the vessel patency rates were similar between groups with no additional strokes. This study was small and precluded definitive conclusions, but provided a basis for future trial design.

CARESS (1999 to 2002, US)

CARESS (Carotid Revascularization Using Endarterectomy or Stenting Systems) was a multicenter, prospective, nonrandomized phase I clinical trial to compare CAS to CEA, and to provide an estimate of the 30-day death and stroke event-rate for future power calculations for a larger phase II clinical trial (22,23). Treatment selection was based on patient and physician preference, with planned enrolment ratio of 2:1 for CEA to CAS. A total of 254 patients underwent CEA and 143 patients underwent CAS using the monorail Wallstent® (Boston Scientific) and GuardWire Plus EPD (Medtronic). Of the entire cohort, 85% were high-risk and 32% were symptomatic. The overall baseline characteristics were similar between the two groups except for a greater percentage of previous carotid revascularization in the CAS group. There was no significant difference in the combined death/stroke rate at 30 days (3.6% CEA vs. 2.1% CAS) or at 1 year (13.6% CEA vs. 10.0% CAS). There was also no significant difference in the composite of death, stroke, or MI at 30 days (4.4% CEA vs. 2.1% CAS) or 1 year (14.3% CEA vs. 10.9% CAS). The secondary end points of restenosis, repeat carotid revascularization, or change in quality of life were also not statistically different.

SAPPHIRE (2000 to 2002, US)

The SAPPHIRE (Stenting and Angioplasty with Protection in Patients at High Risk for Endarterectomy) trial was the first contemporary randomized study to compare CAS with a dedicated stent system and EPD with CEA (24). This study included patients with symptomatic carotid stenosis >50% or asymptomatic stenosis >80%, who were high-risk patients for CEA as dictated by anatomic factors and medical comorbidities (Table 9.2). Patients were recruited from 29 US sites, and were reviewed by a multidisciplinary team (consisting of neurologist, vascular surgeon, and interventionalist) prior to enrolment. Patients who were deemed too high-risk for CEA were entered into a CAS registry, and patients deemed too inappropriate for CAS were entered into a CEA registry. Both surgeons and interventionalists participating in this trial had to have met the AHA guidelines for achieving periprocedural stroke and death rates of <6%. The Precise™ nitinol self-expanding stent and AngioGuard™ filter EPD (Cordis Corporation, Johnson & Johnson) were used. The primary endpoint was a composite of death, stroke, and MI at 30 days, plus death or ipsilateral stroke between 30 days and 1 year. This study was designed to show that CAS was noninferior to CEA, and was terminated early in 2002 when enrolment slowed and when an interim analysis showed that the condition of noninferiority was met.

There were 307 patients randomized (156 underwent CAS and 151 underwent CEA), and 413 patients were entered into the stent ($n = 406$) and CEA ($n = 7$) registries. In the randomized study, 29.9% of patients were symptomatic in the CAS arm, and 27.7% in the CEA arm. Technical success with AngioGuard™ deployment was achieved in 95.6% of cases. The 30-day rates of death, stroke, and MI were 4.4% for CAS and 9.9% for CEA ($p = 0.06$). The 1-year primary endpoint occurred in 12.2% of patients with CAS versus 20.1% with CEA ($p = 0.004$ for noninferiority). In the noninferiority analysis, the p value was 0.053 for intention-to-treat analysis and 0.048 for per-treatment analysis. The 1-year target vessel revascularization rate was lower with CAS (0.6% vs. 4.3%, $p = 0.04$), as was the incidence of cranial nerve palsy (0% vs. 5.3%, $p = 0.003$) compared with CEA. In the high-risk CAS registry, the 30-day MAE rate was 7.8%.

These results have established CAS as a valid alternative to CEA in high-risk patients, and led to the FDA approval of CAS for this indication. Although this study is a widely accepted landmark CAS trial, there have been several criticisms of its limitations (25,26). The exclusion of a large proportion of patients from the randomized arm deemed too high-risk for CEA (entered into the CAS registry) was felt to have been biased against the types of patients enrolled into the randomized arm. However, the SAPPHIRE investigators argued that participating surgeons in this study were actually more experienced than the average, with a median volume of 30 cases annually, and the rate of cranial nerve palsy was lower than in North American Symptomatic Carotid Endarterectomy Trial (NASCET) (5.3% vs. 7.6%). The inclusion of periprocedural MI into the composite primary endpoint has also been criticized, as this endpoint was not included in traditional CEA trials. In a separate analysis excluding the 30-day MI endpoint, the SAPPHIRE event-rate was 5.5% with CAS and 8.4% with CEA ($p = NS$). Given that MI is an important morbidity frequently associated with carotid revascularization of this high-risk atherosclerotic population, its inclusion in the primary endpoint appears appropriate. Another criticism was the inclusion of a low percentage (~28%) of symptomatic patients in the study, and the lack of a medical treatment arm to help demonstrate the utility (or lack thereof) of revascularization in this high-risk population of mostly asymptomatic individuals.

Criticisms aside, this was a well-conducted randomized controlled trial of contemporary CAS against CEA in high-risk

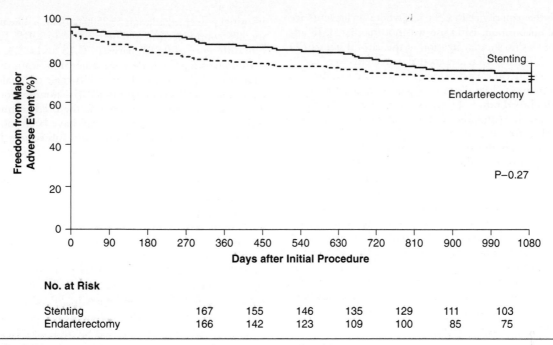

Figure 9.1 • Freedom from major adverse events at 3 years in the SAPPHIRE trial.

patients, utilizing operators with established experience and procedural outcomes, and inclusion of routine neurologic evaluations postprocedure. Long-term 3-year outcomes have been recently published, revealing no difference in the pre-specified secondary endpoint of the composite of death, stroke, or MI within 30 days, or death or ipsilateral stroke between 31 and 1080 days between the treatment groups (24.6% with CAS vs. 26.9% with CEA) and confirming long-term durability and stroke prevention efficacy of CAS equivalent to CEA (Fig. 9.1) (27). Thus, based in part on this landmark study, CAS was established as a viable alternative to CEA for high-risk patients, and arguably as the revascularization of choice in such individuals with anatomy favorable for an endovascular approach.

EVA-3S (2000 to 2005, OUS)

The Endarterectomy versus Stenting in Patients with Symptomatic Severe Carotid Stenosis (EVA-3S) study compared CAS to CEA in normal surgical risk patients with symptomatic (prior TIA or nondisabling stroke within 120 days) carotid stenosis ≥60% (28). This trial was performed at 30 centers in France and was originally designed to enroll 872 patients, with 80% power to determine if CAS was noninferior to CEA (assuming a 2% noninferiority margin, and 30 day stroke or death primary endpoint of 5.6% after CEA and 4% after CAS). Participating vascular surgeons must have performed at least 25 CEA in the preceding year, and interventionists must have performed at least 12 lifetime CAS procedures over any time span or 35 stenting procedures in the supra-aortic trunks, of which at least 5 were in the carotid artery. However, interventionalists who did not meet the credentialing requirements were still able to perform CAS and randomize patients as long as the procedures were proctored by eligible clinicians. There was no central selection process of investigator review

of eligibility, no angiographic core lab, and extremely limited funding in this trial.

The trial started in November 2000 and EPD use was initially not mandated, but became mandatory after January 2003 (29). This occurred after a preliminary analysis showed a trend toward higher 30-day death or stroke rate in 58 patients without EPD use versus 15 patients with EPD use (26.7% vs. 10.3%), with an adjusted odds ratio of 2.5 (95% CI 0.6 to 10.8).

The study was subsequently stopped prematurely in September 2005 after enrolling 527 patients, due to an excess of events in the CAS arm. The 30-day stroke or death rate was 3.9% with CEA versus 9.6% with CAS, with a relative risk of 2.5 (95% CI 1.2 to 5.1; $p = 0.01$). The 30-day risk of disabling stroke or death was 1.5% with CEA and 3.4% with CAS ($p = 0.26$). The incidence of any stroke or death at 6 months was 6.1% with CEA and 11.7% with CAS ($p = 0.02$). In the final analysis assessing EPD use, the 30-day stroke or death event-rate was 7.9% with EPD use ($n = 227$), and 25% without EPD ($n = 20$) ($p = 0.03$). Cranial nerve injury was more common after CEA (7.7% vs. 1.1%, $p < 0.001$).

The EVA-3S trial has been criticized strongly by the interventional community, predominantly due to its inclusion of interventionists with limited CAS experience. Interventionists could have done as little as five lifetime CAS procedures, or be under tutelage, to randomize and treat patients in this trial. In fact, two thirds of sites were initially under tutelage, potentially by a tutor with limited experience. This is an important limitation as there is a steep learning curve for CAS (30,31), and the results were biased in favor of CEA, which were performed by experienced surgeons. The overall stroke rate with CAS (9.2%) was much higher than contemporary CAS trials (3.6% in SAPPHIRE), where the selection of interventionists was more rigorous. As further evidence of inexperience, approximately 5% of CAS patients underwent an emergent CEA; this contrasts starkly with the experience in US trials where such events are exceedingly uncommon. EPD use was not mandated. In addition, there was no standardization of the carotid stent/EPD system (five different EPDs and six different stents were used). There is significant concern that inexperienced interventionists with obviously limited familiarity may have higher complications with this broad range of devices. In the ~10% of patients who did not receive EPD, the 30-day death or stroke rate was more than threefold that of patients who received an EPD. Another limitation with this study is that only 85% of patients were on dual antiplatelet therapy after their CAS procedure. However, the authors did comment that the primary endpoint was not significantly different between patients who received dual antiplatelet therapy and patients on monotherapy (9% vs. 11.1%), although the study was not powered to evaluate this. Finally, predilation was performed in only 17% of patients in the CAS arm, and studies have shown that lack of predilation may be an independent predictor of adverse events. The EVA-3S study remains an outlier in the "modern" era of CAS based on its excessive stroke rates in the CAS arm, as both prior and subsequent outcome data demonstrate.

SPACE (2001 to 2006, OUS)

The Stent-Supported Percutaneous Angioplasty of the Carotid Artery versus Endarterectomy (SPACE) study was published about a week after the EVA-3S study. This was also a randomized multicenter trial to assess if CAS was noninferior to CEA for the treatment of severe symptomatic carotid stenosis in low-risk patients (32). Patients were eligible if they had a neurologic event or amaurosis within 6 months with an ipsilateral carotid stenosis on ultrasound (≥70%) or angiography (≥50% by NASCET or ≥70% by ECST criteria). The primary endpoint was 30-day ipsilateral stroke or death. Vascular surgeons were required to have performed 25 consecutive successful carotid endarterectomies. Interventionalists had to show proof of 25 successful percutaneous angioplasties, although these did not need to be carotid procedures. Any CE Mark stent or EPD were allowed, and EPD use was not mandated. The noninferiority margin was set at 2.5%, with planned enrolment of 1900 patients.

The study was performed in 35 centers in Germany, Austria, and Switzerland between March 2001 and February 2006. After 1183 patients were randomized, the study was stopped prematurely due to funding problems. EPDs were used in only 27% of patients. The 30-day rate of death or ipsilateral stroke was 6.84% with CAS and 6.34% with CEA (absolute difference 0.51%, 90% CI –1.89 to 2.91%, p = 0.09). The upper 90% confidence interval of 2.91% was higher than the prespecified noninferiority threshold of 2.5%, and thus the authors incorrectly concluded that the trial failed to prove noninferiority of CAS to CEA. In fact the study was not completed as originally planned and therefore is inconclusive with regards to its hypothesis of noninferiority. At follow-up to 2 years, there was no difference in the primary endpoint plus ipsilateral strokes up to 2 years between groups (9.5% CAS vs. 8.8% CEA, HR 1.1, p = 0.62) (33).

Much like EVA-3S, the SPACE study has received a number of major criticisms. Since the study was stopped prematurely, recalculation using the actual event-rate showed that it was tremendously underpowered to test its null hypothesis, with a conditional power of only 52%. Due to the very small difference in the primary endpoint between the groups, a much larger number of patients would be required to meet

its initial power calculation (~2500 patients). The noninferiority 90% confidence interval of −1.89% to 2.91% for the absolute difference of 0.51% between CAS and CEA also crosses zero, suggesting the difference is nonsignificant or uncertain. Moreover, the authors did not specify their rationale for the assumption of a 5% event-rate and a 2.5% noninferiority margin. As the actual event-rate was 6.6%, the predetermined noninferiority margin of 2.5% used may have been too restrictive. The lack of mandated EPD use and subsequent low utilization rate of 27% was also strongly criticized. Nonrandomized registry data strongly suggest lower stroke events with EPD use (6,34), and most interventionists do believe that EPD use is crucial for contemporary CAS, especially in potentially active, recently symptomatic, plaques. Although the authors provided a comparison of event-rates between those who received EPD versus no EPD (7% in both groups), this was not a prespecified analysis and was not adjusted. This is a significant limitation as EPD use was likely reserved for patients with higher-risk characteristics, thus introducing selection bias. The technical experience of the interventionists in SPACE was also criticized, as there was no need for any prior CAS experience so long as the interventionist had proof of 25 prior percutaneous angioplasties. The average carotid stent experience of these operators was not revealed. Thus, the expertise of these interventionists in CAS is in doubt. Likewise, the infrequent use of EPD in this study may also be partially due to participation of inexperienced operators. And finally, several relevant clinical and safety endpoints were not evaluated in this study, such as periprocedural MI, cranial nerve palsy, and wound complications. This exclusion may have undermined the potential benefits of CAS in comparison to the "gold standard" of CEA.

Even despite the major limitations of the EVA-3S and SPACE trials, these results have had a significant adverse impact against CAS. However, the results from these two studies have not been deemed conclusive by the majority of the interventional community given their significant limitations, and further clarification is needed from ongoing trials of low-risk patients.

POSTMARKET SURVEILLANCE REGISTRIES

Several carotid stent and EPD platforms have been FDA approved for high-risk patients with significant carotid stenosis. However, as a condition of device approval, the FDA mandated that prospective registries be conducted to monitor device safety and efficacy outside of clinical trials. These registries are important sources of "real-world" data reflecting current clinical practice and experience. Several of these studies are ongoing, and four have been published or presented (CAPTURE, CASES-PMS, SAPPHIRE-WW, CAPTURE 2/EXACT) (Table 9.3).

CAPTURE (2005 to 2005, US)

The RX AccuLink™ stent/RX AccuNet™ EPD system (Abbott Vascular) was FDA approved in 2004 on the basis of the ARCHeR studies, and the CAPTURE (Carotid RX AccuLink™/AccuNet™ Postapproval Trial to Uncover Unanticipated or Rare Events) registry was subsequently established. This was designed to assess the safety of CAS by physicians with varying levels of experience and to identify rare or unexpected device-related complications. There were 353 interventionists

TABLE 9.3 30-Day Outcomes from Postmarketing Carotid Artery Stent Registries

	Capture N = 3500	Capture-2 N = 597	Cases N = 1493	Exact N = 1500	SAPPHIRE-WW N = 2001
Death, Stroke, and MI					
All patients	6.3%	–	5.0%	4.6%	4.4%
Symptomatic patients	12.0%	–	6.2%	–	
Asymptomatic patients	5.4%	–	4.7%	–	
Death and Any Stroke					
All patients	5.7%	5.2%	–	4.5%	4.0%
Symptomatic patients	10.6%	9.1%	–	8.6%	
Asymptomatic patients	4.9%	4.7%	–	4.0%	
Death and Disabling Stroke					
All patients	2.9%	1.3%		1.8%	
Symptomatic patients	–	1.5%	–	2.9%	
Asymptomatic patients	–	1.3%	–	1.7%	
Death	1.8%	–	1.0%	1.0%	1.1%
Stroke	4.8%	–	3.8%	3.9%	3.2%
MI	0.9%	–	0.8%	0.2%	0.7%

MI, myocardial infarction.

at 144 sites who participated and they were divided into three groups according to their level of experience. The minimum procedural experience required was 25 selective carotid angiograms, 10 peripheral procedures with self-expanding stents, and 10 with 0.014 in. systems. There was mandatory manufacturer-conducted hands-on training for all interventionalists, and less experienced physicians had to undergo a structured 2-day carotid training program with didactic and simulator-based training. Data from the first 3500 patients enrolled between October 2004 and March 2006 were published in 2007 (35). The study was intended to enroll high surgical risk patients with symptomatic (>50%) or asymptomatic (>80%) carotid stenosis. The primary endpoint was a composite of death, stroke, and MI at 30 days. Symptomatic patients represented 14% of the cohort, and 23.7% were ≥80 years of age. The primary endpoint occurred in 6.3% and was not significantly different between the three operator experience levels (5.3%, 6.0%, and 7.4% from most to least experienced, $p = 0.31$) after adjustment for baseline characteristics. The 30-day death and stroke rate was 5.7% for these high-risk patients. The primary endpoint was higher in symptomatic patients (12% vs. 5.4%). There were 10 rare events (1 stent thrombosis, 2 patients with hyperperfusion syndrome, and 7 occurrences of separation of the filter basket).

CASES-PMS (2003 to 2005, US)

Following the SAPPHIRE study, the CASES-PMS (CAS with Embolic Protection Surveillance—Post Marketing Study) was initiated in 2003 as a condition to FDA approval study for the Precise™ stent and AngioGuard™ filter EPD (Cordis Corporation, Johnson & Johnson) devices (36). There were 1493 high-risk patients (21.8% symptomatic) enrolled at 73 sites from August 2003 to October 2005. All interventionists underwent up to five training modules depending on their level of experience. Technical success with the AngioGuard™ device was 98%. The primary endpoint of death, stroke, or MI at 30 days was 5.0% (6.2% for symptomatic patients and 4.7% for asymptomatic patients), which was noninferior to the objective performance criterion of 6.3% from the stent cohort of the SAPPHIRE study. The individual endpoint of 30-day mortality was 1%, 30-day stroke was 3.8%, and 30-day MI was 0.8%. This study concluded that with a comprehensive training program, CAS could be performed in the community setting by interventionists with differing experience with safety and efficacy similar to that achieved in the SAPPHIRE study.

SAPPHIRE-WW (2006 to present, US and OUS)

The SAPPHIRE Worldwide (SAPPHIRE-WW) registry is a multicenter, prospective, observational postapproval registry to further evaluate CAS using the Precise™ stent and AngioGuard™ filter EPD involving a broader number of centers, interventional physicians, and patients ($n = 10,000$), utilizing the CASES training program. High-risk patients undergoing CAS with the above devices were enrolled from 350 US and Canadian sites since October 2006, and data from the first 2001 patients have been recently published (37). The mean age was 72, 62% were male and 27.7% were symptomatic. The 30-day death, stroke, or MI rate was 4.4%. Patients with anatomic risk had lower 30-day MAE than patients with physiologic risk (2.8% vs. 4.9%, $p = 0.03$). The multivariate predictors of 30-days MAE were symptomatic status (OR 2.30), age ≥ 80 (OR 1.92), and open-heart surgery within 6 weeks (OR 4.59).

EXACT (2005 to 2006, US)

The EXACT (EmboShield™ and Xact® Post Approval Carotid Stent Trial) was a postmarketing registry to evaluate real-world experience with the Xact® stent and EmboShield™ EPD (Abbott Vascular) following completion of the pivotal SECURITY trial. There were 1500 high-risk patients (9.9% were symptomatic) who underwent CAS at 128 sites. The 30-day results were presented at ACC 2007, but have not been published. The composite endpoint of 30-day death, stroke, and MI was 4.6%, which was lower than the 7.5% reported in the SECURITY trial (which included older patients and higher percentage of symptomatic patients—21%). Unlike CAPTURE and CASES-PMS, there was a significant difference in the 30-day death and stroke rate between the most experienced (Level 1—3.2%) and the least experienced (Level 3—8.8%) operators.

In summary, data from these postmarketing registries confirm that with appropriate training, CAS can be performed in the community setting with complication rates that are comparable, if not better, than the original pivotal SAPPHIRE randomized study and high-risk registries (Tables 9.2 and 9.3). Several other postmarketing registries are still ongoing, including the CAPTURE-2, CHOICE and PROTECT (Abbott Vascular), CREATE PAS (ev3), and CABANA (Boston Scientific) studies. If enrollment targets are achieved, these studies will recruit in aggregate 28,000 high-risk patients undergoing CAS (13).

ONGOING RANDOMIZED TRIALS OF CAS VERSUS CEA

CREST (2000 to 2008, US and Canada)

The Carotid Revascularization Endarterectomy versus Stent Trial (CREST) is currently the largest randomized trial comparing CAS to CEA. This is a North American study sponsored by the US National Institute of Neurological Disorders (NINDS)/National Institute of Health (NIH) and Abbott Vascular. The trial was initially conceived and designed in the mid-1990s and was in the planning, development, and funding stages for several years before enrolling the first patient in December 2000 (38). It required 8 years to complete enrolment of 2516 patients into the main study in July 2008. This study was designed to evaluate standard surgical risk patients, and originally intended to enroll only symptomatic patients with carotid stenosis ($\geq 50\%$ on angiography or $\geq 70\%$ by ultrasound, CT, or MRA). In 2004, the trial was expanded to include asymptomatic patients (carotid stenosis $\geq 60\%$ by angiography, or $\geq 70\%$ by ultrasound, or $\geq 80\%$ by CT/MRA) to improve enrolment and broaden the study population. The CAS devices used were the RX AccuLink™ stent and RX AccuNet™ EPD (Abbott Vascular). The primary endpoint is the composite of death, stroke, and MI at 30 days, plus ipsilateral stroke in the follow-up period to 1 year. Application has been made to the NINDS to carry follow-up in an extended fashion.

Unlike the SPACE and EVA-3S studies, all participating interventionists are required to undergo a rigorous credentialing process, with a minimum of 30 lifetime procedures (20 cases using the AccuLink™/AccuNet™ system) and have to enroll at least three patients in the lead-in phase. Interventionists were approved for the randomized phase only after careful case review by a multidisciplinary interventionist panel and if the lead-in cases were satisfactory.

Results from the first 749 patients (30.7% symptomatic) treated with CAS in the lead-in phase of CREST have been published (39). Of note, EPD was utilized in 88.1% of these CAS cases, and technical success was 99.7%. The overall 30-day stroke and death rate was 4.4%. This was significantly higher for octogenarians (12.1%) ($n = 99$) compared to patients <80 years of age (3.2%), despite adjusting for EPD use, gender, symptom status, and severity of stenosis (40). The results on octogenarians undergoing CAS remains conflicting in the literature, and further data are required for more conclusive recommendations. As a result, caution should be exercised in selecting octogenarians for CAS.

ICSS/CAVATAS-2 (200– to 200–, OUS)

The International Carotid Stenting Study (ICSS or CAVATAS-2) is a European, multicenter, randomized trial coordinated by the Institute of Neurology in London, UK. This study is planning to enroll 1500 low or standard-risk patients with symptomatic carotid stenosis >50% (by NASCET criteria) suitable for either CAS or CEA. There is no specification on the type of stent or EPD used. The primary outcome is death or disabling stroke with follow-up to 5 years. Secondary outcome measures will be any stroke, death, or MI at 30 days, treatment-related cranial nerve palsy or hematoma, restenosis $\geq 70\%$ on ultrasound, and stroke or TIA during follow-up. The study recently completed enrolment, with 1711 patients randomized at 53 centers and 16 countries.

ACT-1 (2005 to present, US)

The Asymptomatic Carotid Stenosis Stenting versus Endarterectomy Trial (ACT-1) is a North American Phase III multicenter trial of CAS versus CEA in asymptomatic patients (no symptoms related to the carotid artery within 180 days). Patients are included if they are suitable for either CAS or CEA procedures. Those over 80 years old or at high risk for CAS or CEA are excluded. The devices used in the CAS arm are the Xact stent and EmboShield EPD (Abbott Vascular), and the study is sponsored by Abbott Vascular. The study started in April 2005 and plans to randomize 1858 patients to CAS or CEA on a 3:1 basis. The study is still ongoing, and 863 patients have been enrolled to date. The primary outcome is the composite of death, stroke, or MI at 30 days, and ipsilateral stroke between 31 and 365 days.

ACST-2 (2007 to present, OUS)

The Asymptomatic Carotid Surgery Trial–2 (ACST-2) is a European randomized trial comparing CAS to CEA in asymptomatic patients with carotid stenosis. The planned enrolment is 5000 asymptomatic low-risk patients, and enrolment started in July 2007. The primary endpoint will be the 30-day composite rate of death, stroke, and MI, and long-term freedom from stroke up to 5 or more years.

TACIT

The Transatlantic Asymptomatic Carotid Intervention Trial (TACIT) is a prospective, Phase III, multicenter, randomized trial of patients with asymptomatic carotid stenosis ≥60% (on duplex ultrasound), and is the only randomized CAS trial that is inclusive of a medical treatment arm (41–44). Although there have been advances in medical therapy since ACAS and ACST, its role vis-à-vis revascularization has not been proven. Thus, this study will randomize patients to three treatment strategies: (1) contemporary medical therapy, (2) medical therapy + CEA, (3) medical therapy + CAS. The investigators plan to enroll 3700 asymptomatic patients from ~125 sites in the United States and Europe, and evaluate periprocedural death and stroke outcomes out to 5 years. Medical therapy will include contemporary antiplatelet therapy, cholesterol-lowering agents, antihypertensives, glycemic control, and smoking cessation. Of note, the severity of carotid stenosis in these asymptomatic patients only needs to be ≥60%, which is a very low threshold for performing carotid revascularization. Most centers do not perform carotid revascularization for asymptomatic patients until the stenosis severity is ≥80%, and there is concern that this low threshold may bias the results toward the medical treatment arm since event rates in this group may be limited. Recent reports have suggested that this study may be in jeopardy due to problems with funding.

CONCLUSION

In summary, there have been considerable advances in the development of CAS, encompassing improvement in equipment and design, technical operator experience, and patient selection. Each of these plays crucial roles in the evolution of carotid stenting as a valid rival to endarterectomy, with contemporary data showing impressive modern-day safety and efficacy for the treatment of carotid stenosis. Most clinicians would agree that CAS is the revascularization of choice for high surgical risk patients. Several well-designed and rigorous large randomized trials are ongoing or have recently completed enrolment of standard surgical risk patients, and these data are anticipated to address management of this substantial group of carotid stenosis patients.

References

1. Mathias K. A new catheter system for percutaneous transluminal angioplasty (PTA) of carotid artery stenoses. *Fortschr Med.* 1977;95:1007–1011.
2. Kerber CW, Cromwell LD, Loehden OL. Catheter dilatation of proximal carotid stenosis during distal bifurcation endarterectomy. *Am J Neuroradiol.* 1980;1:348–349.
3. Naylor AR, Bolia A, Abbott RJ, et al. Randomized study of carotid angioplasty and stenting versus carotid endarterectomy: a stopped trial. *J Vasc Surg.* 1998;28:326–334.
4. Theiss W, Hermanek P, Mathias K, et al. Pro-CAS: a prospective registry of carotid angioplasty and stenting. *Stroke.* 2004;35: 2134–2139.
5. Bosiers M, Peeters P, Deloose K, et al. Does carotid artery stenting work on the long run: 5-year results in high-volume centers (ELOCAS Registry). *J Cardiovasc Surg (Torino).* 2005;46: 241–247.
6. Wholey MH, Al-Mubarek N. Updated review of the global carotid artery stent registry. *Catheter Cardiovasc Interv.* 2003;60: 259–266.
7. Theiss W, Hermanek P, Mathias K, et al. Predictors of death and stroke after carotid angioplasty and stenting: a subgroup analysis of the Pro-CAS data. *Stroke.* 2008;39:2325–2330.
8. Gray WA, Hopkins LN, Yadav S, et al. Protected carotid stenting in high-surgical-risk patients: the ARCHeR results. *J Vasc Surg.* 2006;44:258–268.
9. White CJ, Iyer SS, Hopkins LN, et al. Carotid stenting with distal protection in high surgical risk patients: the BEACH trial 30 day results. *Catheter Cardiovasc Interv.* 2006;67:503–512.
10. Iyer SS, White CJ, Hopkins LN, et al. Carotid artery revascularization in high-surgical-risk patients using the Carotid WALL-STENT and FilterWire EX/EZ: 1-year outcomes in the BEACH Pivotal Group. *J Am Coll Cardiol.* 2008;51:427–434.
11. Safian RD, Bresnahan JF, Jaff MR, et al. Protected carotid stenting in high-risk patients with severe carotid artery stenosis. *J Am Coll Cardiol.* 2006;47:2384–2389.
12. Yadav JS. New insights into improving acute and long-term outcomes of carotid stenting. *J Am Coll Cardiol.* 2006;47:2397–2398.
13. Endovascular Today. CAS Clinical Trial and Registry Update. *Endovascular Today* 2007;6:76–79.
14. Hill MD, Morrish W, Soulez G, et al. Multicenter evaluation of a self-expanding carotid stent system with distal protection in the treatment of carotid stenosis. *Am J Neuroradiol.* 2006;27:759–765.
15. Reimers B, Sievert H, Schuler GC, et al. Proximal endovascular flow blockage for cerebral protection during carotid artery stenting: results from a prospective multicenter registry. *J Endovasc Ther.* 2005;12:156–165.
16. Coppi G, Moratto R, Silingardi R, et al. PRIAMUS—proximal flow blockage cerebral protection during carotid stenting: results from a multicenter Italian registry. *J Cardiovasc Surg (Torino).* 2005;46:219–227.
17. Xact® Carotid Stent System—P040038. Summary of Safety and Effectiveness data. 2005.
18. CAVATAS Investigators T. Endovascular versus surgical treatment in patients with carotid stenosis in the Carotid and Vertebral Artery Transluminal Angioplasty Study (CAVATAS): a randomised trial. *Lancet.* 2001;357:1729–1737.
19. del Zoppo GJ, Poeck K, Pessin MS, et al. Recombinant tissue plasminogen activator in acute thrombotic and embolic stroke. *Ann Neurol.* 1992;32:78–86.
20. Brooks WH, McClure RR, Jones MR, et al. Carotid angioplasty and stenting versus carotid endarterectomy: randomized trial in a community hospital. *J Am Coll Cardiol.* 2001;38:1589–1595.
21. Brooks WH, McClure RR, Jones MR, et al. Carotid angioplasty and stenting versus carotid endarterectomy for treatment of asymptomatic carotid stenosis: a randomized trial in a community hospital. *Neurosurgery.* 2004;54:318–324; discussion 324–325.
22. CARESS Steering Committee. Carotid revascularization using endarterectomy or stenting systems (CARESS): phase I clinical trial. *J Endovasc Ther.* 2003;10:1021–1030.
23. CARESS Steering Committee. Carotid Revascularization Using Endarterectomy or Stenting Systems (CARESS) phase I clinical trial: 1-year results. *J Vasc Surg.* 2005;42:213–219.
24. Yadav JS, Wholey MH, Kuntz RE, et al. Protected carotid-artery stenting versus endarterectomy in high-risk patients. *N Engl J Med.* 2004;351:1493–1501.
25. Cambria RP. Stenting for carotid-artery stenosis. *N Engl J Med.* 2004;351:1565–1567.
26. Hamdan AD, Pomposelli FB Jr., Gibbons GW, et al. Renal insufficiency and altered postoperative risk in carotid endarterectomy. *J Vasc Surg.* 1999;29:1006–1011.

27. Gurm HS, Yadav JS, Fayad P, et al. Long-term results of carotid stenting versus endarterectomy in high-risk patients. *N Engl J Med*. 2008;358:1572–1579.

28. Mas JL, Chatellier G, Beyssen B, et al. Endarterectomy versus stenting in patients with symptomatic severe carotid stenosis. *N Engl J Med*. 2006;355:1660–1671.

29. Halliday A, Mansfield A, Marro J, et al. Prevention of disabling and fatal strokes by successful carotid endarterectomy in patients without recent neurological symptoms: randomised controlled trial. *Lancet*. 2004;363:1491–1502.

30. Kopp CW, Steiner S, Nasel C, et al. Abciximab reduces monocyte tissue factor in carotid angioplasty and stenting. *Stroke*. 2003;34:2560–2567.

31. Verzini F, Cao P, De Rango P, et al. Appropriateness of learning curve for carotid artery stenting: an analysis of periprocedural complications. *J Vasc Surg*. 2006;44:1205–1211; discussion 1211–1212.

32. Ringleb PA, Allenberg J, Bruckmann H, et al. 30 day results from the SPACE trial of stent-protected angioplasty versus carotid endarterectomy in symptomatic patients: a randomised non-inferiority trial. *Lancet*. 2006;368:1239–1247.

33. Eckstein HH, Ringleb P, Allenberg JR, et al. Results of the Stent-Protected Angioplasty versus Carotid Endarterectomy (SPACE) study to treat symptomatic stenoses at 2 years: a multinational, prospective, randomised trial. *Lancet Neurol*. 2008;7:893–902.

34. Kastrup A, Groschel K, Kraph H, et al. Early outcome of carotid angioplasty and stenting with and without cerebral protection devices. A systematic review of the literature. *Stroke*. 2003;34:813–819.

35. Gray WA, Yadav JS, Verta P, et al. The CAPTURE registry: results of carotid stenting with embolic protection in the post approval setting. *Catheter Cardiovasc Interv*. 2007;69:341–348.

36. Adams GL, Mills JS, Melloni C, et al. Highlights from the 56th annual scientific sessions of the American College of Cardiology: March 25 to 27, 2007, Atlanta, Georgia. *Am Heart J*. 2007;154:247–259.

37. Katzen BT, Criado FJ, Ramee SR, et al. Carotid artery stenting with emboli protection surveillance study: thirty-day results of the CASES-PMS study. *Catheter Cardiovasc Interv*. 2007;70:316–323.

38. Massop D, Dave R, Metzger C, et al. Stenting and angioplasty with protection in patients at high-risk for endarterectomy: SAPPHIRE Worldwide Registry first 2,001 patients. *Catheter Cardiovasc Interv*. 2009;73:129–136.

39. Hobson RW II, Howard VJ, Brott TG, et al. Organizing the Carotid Revascularization Endarterectomy versus Stenting Trial (CREST): National Institutes of Health, Health Care Financing Administration, and industry funding. *Curr Control Trials Cardiovasc Med*. 2001;2:160–164.

40. Hobson RW IInd, Howard VJ, Roubin GS, et al. Carotid artery stenting is associated with increased complications in octogenarians: 30-day stroke and death rates in the CREST lead-in phase. *J Vasc Surg*. 2004;40:1106–1111.

41. ICSS—International Carotid Stenting Study. Accessed at http://www.cavatas.com/.

42. ACT I: Asymptomatic Carotid Stenosis, Stenting Versus Endarterectomy Trial. Accessed at http://www.clinicaltrials.gov/ct/show/nct00106938?term=asymptomatic+carotid+stenosis&rank=3#locn.

43. Asymptomatic Carotid Surgery Trial (ACST-2). A large, simple randomised trial to compare carotid endarterectomy versus carotid artery stenting to prevent stroke. Accessed at http://www.acst.org.uk/.

44. Transatlantic Asymptomatic Carotid Intervention Trial (TACIT) website. Accessed at http://bibamed.agcl.com/cx_2007/mon%201000%20katzen.pdf.

CHAPTER 10

Carotid Artery Stenting: Basic Techniques

Ivan P. Casserly and Jay S. Yadav

In 1905, Chiari reported that embolization of thrombotic material that formed on the surface of atherosclerotic plaque in the carotid sinus was a cause of apoplexy (i.e., sudden impairment of neurologic function, i.e., stroke). Further published work by Miller Fisher in the 1950s solidified the association between carotid artery disease and stroke and led to the development of carotid endarterectomy (CEA) as a treatment option for patients with carotid artery disease. It took nearly 50 years before large, randomized, clinical trials demonstrated that this therapy improved outcomes for symptomatic patients with moderate to severe carotid stenosis, and asymptomatic patients with severe carotid stenosis. Based on these data, CEA established itself as the gold standard for carotid revascularization.

Coincident with the development of endovascular therapies at other vascular sites, a small number of investigators began to perform angioplasty of the carotid artery in the early 1980s (1). These investigators faced a number of unique challenges. The hazard of distal embolization and resultant stroke at the time of endovascular intervention limited the ability to offer this therapy to surgically eligible patients, where cross-clamping of the carotid distally provides protection against embolization. By the early 1990s, it was clear that percutaneous carotid intervention would not become a viable therapy without addressing this limitation. A variety of embolic protection devices (EPDs) were developed that served to limit or prevent distal embolization. Unfortunately, it took nearly a decade to get FDA approval for these devices.

As in other vascular territories, the use of stents in the carotid artery gained acceptance in the mid-1990s, as operators sought to achieve a predictable angiographic result, treat procedural complications such as abrupt closure and dissection, eliminate vessel recoil, and reduce the risk of restenosis. However, conventional balloon-expandable stents in the carotid location proved suboptimal for two reasons: (1) conventional balloon-expandable stents were too rigid and resulted in kinking of the internal carotid artery (ICA) in the length between the stent and the petrous portion of the artery, particularly in tortuous vessels (Fig. 10.1) and (2) balloon-expandable stents were associated with a high incidence of loss of apposition between the stent and the vessel wall. These considerations led to the development of nitinol self-expanding stents that have performed well in the carotid location and several have received FDA approval for use in the carotid location.

In addition to the technical issues related to the procedure, percutaneous carotid intervention has had to overcome a number of political hurdles. Among providers in the surgical community, there has been an understandable reluctance to abandon the old gold standard of CEA for the treatment of carotid disease. Among endovascular specialists, there have been significant turf wars about who should be allowed to perform these procedures. The current limited coverage policy for carotid intervention, determined by the Centers for Medicare and Medicaid Services (CMS) (following FDA approval), has also hampered the dissemination of this technique.

Having met the major technical challenges of the procedure and slowly addressed the political issues, proponents of percutaneous carotid intervention have made it a reality. A major shift toward carotid stenting for patients deemed high risk for CEA has occurred and is supported by an increasing body of evidence. The evidence for carotid artery stenting (CAS) is summarized in Chapter 9. The goal of the current chapter is to provide a comprehensive description of the technique of CAS, and the periprocedural management of these patients.

ANATOMIC CONSIDERATIONS

The right common carotid artery (CCA) arises in a remarkably constant fashion from the bifurcation of the innominate artery (Fig. 10.2). It may rarely arise as a separate branch off the aortic arch, or in conjunction with the left CCA (i.e., common carotid trunk) (Fig. 10.3).

In contrast, the origin of the left CCA is variable. In approximately 75% of cases, it arises as the second great vessel off the aortic arch, in a plane posterior to the innominate artery (Fig. 10.2). In the remaining cases, the left CCA shares its origin off the aortic arch with the innominate artery (i.e., ~10% to 15%) or arises from the innominate artery (i.e., bovine origin, ~10%) (Fig. 10.4).

At the level of the upper border of the thyroid cartilage, each CCA bifurcates into an external and internal branch. During diagnostic angiography, the angle of the mandible serves as a useful landmark for the carotid bifurcation, although significant variation in the level of the carotid bifurcation is common. The external carotid artery (ECA) is easily recognized, owing to its numerous branches to the face, scalp, and thyroid. A basic understanding of the anatomy of the ECA is important, because this vessel and its branches are often instrumented with wires and catheters during carotid intervention (see below). Anterior branches arise in the following order: the superior thyroid, lingual, and facial. The occipital branch arises posteriorly, at the level of the facial artery. The ECA terminates by giving off the internal maxillary branch

Figure 10.1 • Schematic illustrating the effect of rigid stainless steel, balloon-expandable (**B**), and self-expanding nitinol stents (**C**), when used to treat stenosis (**A**) in the carotid location. Nitinol stents conform to the tortuosity in the carotid artery, minimizing any kinking distally.

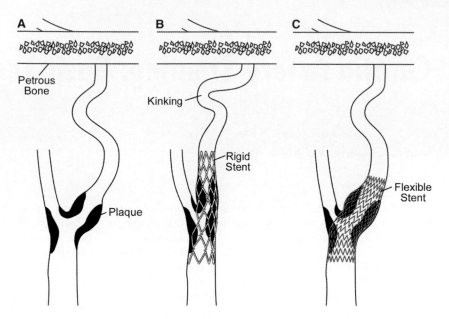

that is directed anteriorly, and the superficial temporal branch that runs toward the temporal scalp region (Fig. 10.5).

Under normal conditions, the ICA contains a bulbous dilation at its origin, referred to as the carotid sinus. The adventitia in this region contains the mechanoreceptors responsible for blood pressure regulation. In its proximal portion, the ICA lies posterior and medial to the ECA. These relationships may be appreciated in the lateral and posteroanterior (PA) projections by angiography, respectively.

By convention, the ICA is divided into four sections (Fig. 10.6) as follows:

1. The *prepetrous* or *cervical portion*. This defines the segment of vessel between the CCA bifurcation and the petrous bone and contains no arterial branches. Most carotid intervention involves treatment of atherosclerosis of the ostium and proximal portion of this segment of vessel.

2. The *petrous portion*. This refers to the L-shaped section of vessel (i.e., rotated 90°) that courses through the petrous bone.
3. The *cavernous portion*, which courses through the cavernous sinus.
4. The *supraclinoid portion*, which gives off the important ophthalmic, posterior communicating, and anterior choroidal branches and terminates in the middle and anterior cerebral arteries.

The ophthalmic artery supplies the ipsilateral retina and optic nerve and is an important route for collateral flow between the ECA and ICA (via maxillary branches) when the ICA is occluded. Similarly, the posterior communicating branch links the ICA with the posterior cerebral artery, providing an important collateral link between the anterior and posterior cerebral circulations. The area of the brain supplied by the anterior and middle cerebral arteries is termed the *carotid territory*.

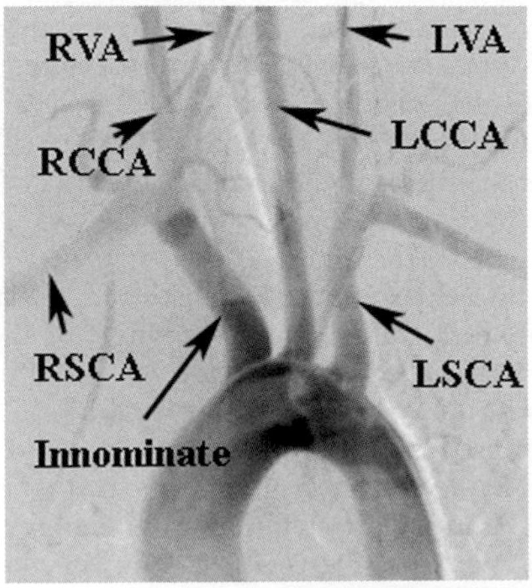

Figure 10.2 • Normal anatomy of the aortic arch and great vessels. LCCA, left common carotid artery; RCCA, right common carotid artery; LVA, left vertebral artery; RVA, right vertebral artery; LSCA, left subclavian artery; RSCA, right subclavian artery.

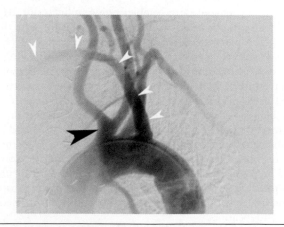

Figure 10.3 • Arch aortogram from patient with common carotid trunk *(black arrowhead)* and anomalous origin of the right subclavian artery, distal to the origin of the left subclavian artery *(white arrowheads)*.

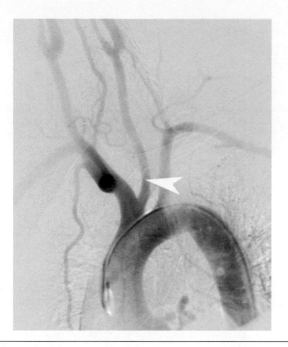

Figure 10.4 • Arch aortogram with bovine origin of the left common carotid artery off the innominate artery *(arrowhead)*.

CURRENT INDICATIONS FOR CONTEMPORARY CAROTID INTERVENTION

Currently, there are five carotid artery stent and filter systems that have been approved by the FDA for CAS for the treatment of symptomatic carotid stenosis ≥50% and asymptomatic carotid stenoses ≥80% in patients who are at high risk for CEA (Tables 10.1 and 10.2). Despite this, the CMS has continued to restrict coverage for CAS in the United States to symptomatic

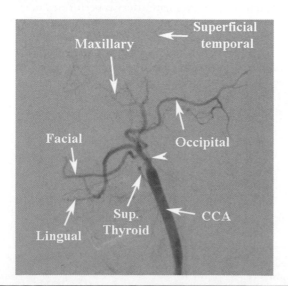

Figure 10.5 • Anatomy of the external carotid artery. Angiogram of the common carotid artery (CCA) shows occlusion of the internal carotid artery *(white arrowhead)* facilitating identification of the branches of the external carotid artery.

patients with ≥70% stenosis who are at high risk for CEA. Provided patients are participating in an investigational device exemption (IDE) trial or FDA-approved postapproval study, coverage is provided for the following subgroups of patients:

1. Symptomatic patients with 50% to 69% stenosis who are at high risk for CEA
2. Asymptomatic patients with ≥80% stenosis who are at high risk for CEA

CAS in symptomatic and asymptomatic patients at normal risk for CEA is currently not approved by the FDA. A decision based on data from the CREST and ICSS trials (and perhaps the EVA-3s and SPACE trials), and the ACT I trial is awaited. It remains unclear how CMS will respond if the FDA provides approval for CAS in these patient subsets.

Carotid Artery Stenting— Appropriate Case Selection

One of the concepts that has recently emerged in the field of carotid artery revascularization is that patients often have distinct risks for both CEA and CAS. Although these two methods of revascularization do share some common risk variables (e.g., age, cerebrovascular reserve), the risk for CEA is heavily influenced by patient comorbidity and specific anatomic factors such as prior radiation, prior endarterectomy, high anatomic location above the angle of the mandible, and low anatomic location (i.e., origin of great vessels, and proximal/mid-CCA). The risk for CAS is generally more heavily influenced by anatomic factors that are distinct from those for CEA including: aortic arch type, burden of atheroma and degree of calcification in the aortic arch, tortuosity in the CCA and ICA distal to the lesion, dense calcification of the carotid lesion, and presence of thrombus in the carotid lesion (Fig. 10.7). These latter anatomic factors influence the difficulty in delivering a guide or sheath to the distal CCA, the ability to place an embolic protection system, and the effectiveness of treating the carotid lesion. Although CEA and CAS have been viewed as competitive strategies for carotid revascularization by many in the medical community, it makes more sense to view these strategies as being complementary. It is incumbent on the treating physician to assess the specific risk for each patient for both CEA and CAS based on an analysis of clinical and anatomic variables, and the skill, experience, and clinical outcomes achieved by endovascular specialists and vascular surgeons at their institution. This approach is likely to result in optimal outcomes for patients.

DIAGNOSTIC CAROTID ANGIOGRAPHY

Prior to performing a diagnostic carotid angiogram, one should first make an assessment of the anatomy of the aortic arch. Noninvasive studies such as computed tomography (CT) or magnetic resonance angiography (MRA) that provide a 3D assessment of the arch are ideal for this purpose. In addition, CT angiography provides detail about the degree of calcification and the burden and distribution of plaque in the aortic arch. Conventional aortic arch angiography provides a 2D assessment of the arch that often underestimates the degree of

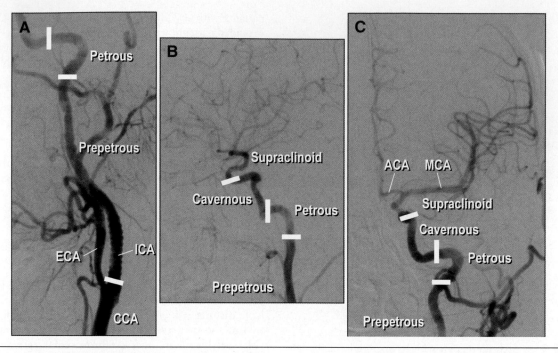

Figure 10.6 • Anatomy of the internal carotid artery (ICA). **A:** LAO oblique view showing the proximal portion of the left ICA. **B:** Lateral view of distal portion of the left ICA. **C:** Posteroanterior (PA) cranial view of the distal left ICA and its cerebral branches. ICA, internal carotid artery; ECA, external carotid artery; CCA, common carotid artery; MCA, middle cerebral artery; ACA, anterior cerebral artery.

tortuosity in the CCA and innominate artery, and the plaque burden in the aortic arch. Rotational or biplane angiography of the aortic arch, if available, is preferable.

The information that needs to be gleaned from the aortic arch assessment includes (1) the aortic arch type (Fig. 10.8), (2) the presence of any variant anatomy in the origin of the great vessels off the aortic arch, and (3) the presence of atherosclerotic disease or tortuosity in the proximal portions of the great vessels. These factors strongly influence the choice of diagnostic catheter (Fig. 10.9) and the interventional strategy selected.

For all patients with type I aortic arch anatomy and most patients with type II, our practice is to use a 4-Fr. Bernstein diagnostic catheter for carotid angiography. The exception to this rule involves patients with a bovine origin of the left CCA, where a Vitek® catheter is often required, regardless of the aortic arch type. In patients with type III aortic arches, a Vitek

catheter is usually required. Rarely, a Simmons 1 or Simmons 2 catheter is required.

Selective angiography of the left CCA and bifurcation are performed with the diagnostic catheter at the origin of the vessel, although in some cases the catheter may need to be advanced over an angled glidewire toward the midportion of the vessel. For right CCA angiography, the innominate artery is first engaged with the diagnostic catheter. Typically, a road map of the innominate artery is performed in the right anterior oblique (RAO) projection, which generally splays the origins of the right subclavian artery and right CCA. A stiff-angled glidewire is advanced into the right CCA, and the catheter is advanced over the wire to the midportion of the vessel to allow selective angiography.

In most patients, ipsilateral oblique (30° to 45°) and left lateral views of the CCA of interest are adequate to define

TABLE 10.1 Summary of FDA-Approved Carotid Artery Stents

Stent	Manufacturer	Stent Design	Cylindrical/Tapered
Precise	Cordis	Open cell	C
Acculink	Abbott Vascular	Open cell	T, C
Xact	Abbott Vascular	Closed cell	T, C
Wallstent	Boston Scientific	Closed cell	C
Protégé	ev3	Open cell	T, C

C, cylindrical; T, tapered.

TABLE 10.2   Criteria Used to Define Patients at High Risk for Carotid Endarterectomy

High-Risk Criteria
Clinical
Age >80 years
Congestive heart failure (class III/IV)
Known severe left ventricular dysfunction, LV EF <30%
Open-heart surgery needed within 6 weeks
Recent MI (>24 hours and <4 weeks)
Unstable angina (CCS class III/IV)
Severe pulmonary disease
Contralateral laryngeal nerve palsy
Anatomic
Previous CEA with recurrent stenosis
High cervical ICA lesions or CCA lesions below the clavicle
Contralateral carotid occlusion
Radiation therapy to neck
Prior radical neck surgery
Severe tandem lesions

ICA, internal carotid artery; CCA, common carotid artery; LV EF, left ventricular ejection fraction; MI, myocardial infarction; CEA, carotid endarterectomy; CCS, Canadian Cardiovascular Society

the anatomy of the carotid bifurcation. Additional views (e.g., straight anteroposterior, contralateral oblique, or adding cranial or caudal angulation to standardized views) may be required to define a lesion of interest, especially in situations where significant tortuosity distorts the normal geometric relationship between the ICA and ECA. The anatomic features that require assessment during angiography of the carotid bifurcation, and the potential influence of these features on the interventional strategy or technique employed, are summarized in Table 10.3.

Additionally, a baseline angiogram of the anterior cerebral circulation is routinely performed prior to any planned carotid intervention. This serves as a reference against which the postprocedural cerebral angiogram may be compared, thus facilitating the prompt diagnosis of distal embolization related to the procedure. Additionally, the presence of associated, significant intracranial or distal extracranial atherosclerotic artery disease, or other vascular pathology that might influence management, will be uncovered. A shallow PA cranial view (i.e., with enough cranial angulation to position the petrous bone at the base of the orbit) and left lateral views are the standard projections used by most operators. To obtain good quality cerebral angiograms, the diagnostic catheter ideally should be placed in the distal CCA. For this reason, we typically delay cerebral angiography on the side of the carotid intervention until there is placement of the sheath or guide in the distal CCA. In patients with significant renal dysfunction, intracerebral angiograms may be omitted, understanding the implications of this decision.

CAROTID INTERVENTION

Pharmacology

In the practice of the authors, all patients receive aspirin and clopidogrel for at least 3 days prior to the CAS procedure. For most patients, all antihypertensive medications are stopped on the morning of the procedure, anticipating the hypotensive response that typically occurs following stent placement in the region of the carotid bulb for the treatment of de novo atherosclerotic disease (see below). Intravenous fluids are administered for 3 to 4 hours prior to the procedure with the goal of attenuating the hypotensive response to stenting.

In the absence of contraindication, a small bolus of heparin (i.e., 2000 to 3000 units) is administered prior to arch aortography or diagnostic carotid angiography, and this is supplemented during the intervention to achieve an ACT of 275 to 300 seconds. In patients with a contraindication to heparin, CAS may be performed using the direct thrombin inhibitor, bivalirudin. However, there currently are insufficient data documenting the safety of bivalirudin for *routine* use during CAS.

Delivery of Sheath or Guide to CCA

With rare exception, carotid intervention is performed using femoral arterial access. Having achieved access, the first task is the successful delivery of a sheath or guide to the distal CCA. With currently available stent delivery systems, balloon dilation catheters, and filters, the inner diameter of an 8-Fr. guide

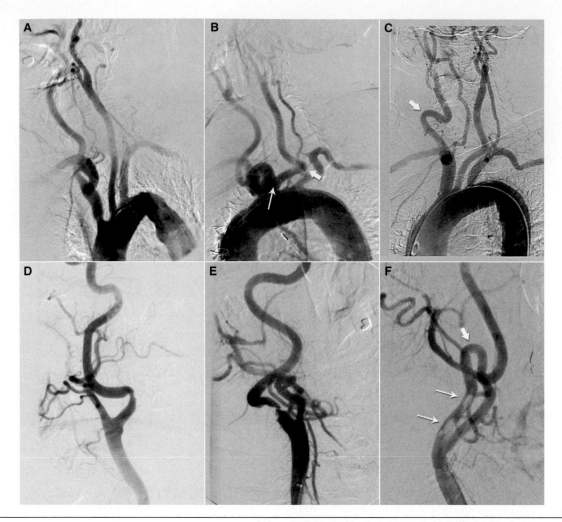

Figure 10.7 • Example of anatomic variations that increase procedural risk during carotid artery stenting. **A:** Type III aortic arch. **B:** Bovine origin of left common carotid artery *(narrow arrow)* and severe tortuosity in left common carotid artery *(thick arrow)*. **C:** Severe tortuosity in right common carotid artery *(arrow)*. **D:** Marked angulation in internal carotid artery (ICA) at site of stenosis. **E:** Tandem areas of angulation distal to ICA stenosis. **F:** Dense circumferential calcification at lesion site *(narrow arrows)* and severe tortuosity distal to ICA stenosis.

or 6-Fr. sheath is required to allow easy delivery of required devices. Although the particular choice of the use of a guide or sheath is often determined by operator bias, there are objective advantages and disadvantages to either, which are summarized in Table 10.4.

The authors have moved from the practice of using guide catheters to using sheaths for most CAS procedures. With the current array of available wires and catheters, sheaths can be successfully delivered in the vast majority of cases. The lower profile of sheaths and the smooth transition between the sheath and either its dilator or designated catheter make this a safer option for most patients. Sheaths should be favored in patients with severe peripheral vascular disease owing to the smaller arteriotomy required. They should also be considered in patients with CCA disease because of the smaller outer diameter of the 6-Fr. sheath, compared with an 8-Fr. guide.

Figure 10.8 • Illustration of aortic arch types.

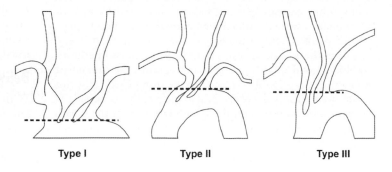

Type I   Type II   Type III

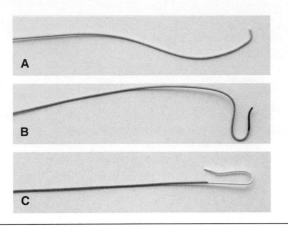

Figure 10.9 • Diagnostic catheters used during carotid artery angiography. A: JR 4. B: Vitek. C: Simmons 1.

Guides should certainly be considered in situations where added support is required (e.g., significant tortuosity distal to ICA lesion, critical ICA stenosis) and in more complex anatomies (see below).

The specific details of sheath and guide delivery to the target CCA are outlined below. Although there are innumerable ways to achieve this goal, some basic rules for sheath and guide delivery should be obeyed: (1) At no time should any wire or catheter be advanced past a significantly diseased area in the distal CCA or ICA to achieve sheath or guide delivery. (2) Manipulation of catheters and wires in the aortic arch and CCA should be kept to a minimum. (3) The strategy that involves the minimum number of maneuvers to achieve sheath/guide delivery is optimal. Learning which specific strategy will achieve

the highest likelihood of success in sheath or guide delivery for a given anatomic situation is one of the critical elements that distinguishes experienced from inexperienced operators.

STANDARD SHEATH TECHNIQUE

In our practice, the sheath that is used for CAS procedures is a 6-Fr., 90-cm-long Shuttle sheath (Cook Inc., Bloomington, IN). The method of delivery may vary considerably, but the two basic strategies used by the authors are as follows:

(1) A diagnostic catheter is used to engage the carotid artery of interest. A road map of the CCA is then performed at low magnification, in a view that allows clear visualization of the origins of the ICA and ECA (typically the ipsilateral oblique view) and the aortic arch. Under road map guidance, an angled stiff-bodied glidewire is advanced through the diagnostic catheter into the ECA or distal CCA (i.e., if the ECA is diseased or occluded, or the distal CCA has significant disease). Inclusion of the aortic arch within the field of view is important so that the behavior of the diagnostic catheter and sheath during attempts at delivery can be monitored, particularly in patients with complex arch anatomies. In this regard, one should be aware that the arch is significantly foreshortened in the RAO view. As a result, manipulations through the aortic arch using the RAO view for guidance need to be monitored with extra care. Although the lateral view often provides the best display of the origin of the ICA and ECA, this view should not be used to guide these maneuvers, as the majority of the CCA and the entire arch cannot be visualized in this view. The diagnostic catheter is then advanced into the ECA or distal CCA over the stiff-angled glidewire, which is exchanged for a more supportive wire. Formerly,

TABLE 10.3 Influence of Assessments Made during Diagnostic Carotid Angiography on Carotid Interventional Procedures

Angiographic Assessment	Impact on Interventional Procedure
Assess lesion characteristics	
Precise location of the lesion, with definition of the proximal and distal extent of lesion	Influences planned location for stent placement and stent length
	Influences strategy for delivery of guide/sheath to distal CCA
Approximate length of lesion	Stent length
Complex lesion ulceration	Predict difficulty of crossing lesion with filter device
Severity of stenosis	Predict difficulty of crossing lesion with filter device
	Predict need for predilation of lesion prior to filter delivery
Calcification	Predict ability to achieve good stent expansion
Diameter of CCA and ICA	Influences choice of stent diameter and filter diameter
Assess the entire prepetrous portion of the ICA	Influences the choice of landing zone for the filter device
Tortuosity distal to the lesion and proximal to the landing zone for filter	Favors use of guide to provide support Predict degree of difficulty in delivering filter
Patency of external carotid artery	Influences strategy for delivery of guide/sheath to distal CCA

TABLE 10.4 Advantages and Disadvantages of Guide- and Sheath-Based Approaches to Carotid Artery Stenting Procedures

	Guide	Sheath
Advantages	• Torque control of tip allows orientation of guide with respect to the ICA • Provides superior support • More resistant to kinking in tortuous vessels or type III arches	• 6-Fr. sheath adequate for carotid intervention minimizing arteriotomy size and risk of limb ischemia in patients with PAD • Smooth transition between dilator and sheath advantageous in patients with diseased CCA • Easier to deliver through CCA tortuosity
Disadvantages	• 8-Fr. guide required for carotid intervention • Transition from diagnostic catheter to guide less optimal than with sheath and dilator	• Provides less support than guide • More likely to be displaced proximally into CCA during intervention • No torque capability

ICA, internal carotid artery; CCA, common carotid artery; PAD, peripheral artery disease.

the authors had used a SuperStiff Amplatz wire (Boston Scientific) (with 7-cm soft tip) for this purpose, but more recently, the SupraCore wire (Abbott Vascular) has been used and has performed well. The diagnostic catheter and short femoral sheath are then removed and the 6-Fr. Shuttle sheath (with dilator) is delivered from the groin access site to the desired location in the CCA.

In more complex anatomies, the Shuttle sheath and its dilator may be delivered to the descending thoracic aorta at which point, the dilator is exchanged for 6.5Fr. JB 1 catheter that is advanced into the ECA or distal CCA, and the Shuttle sheath can then be advanced over the JB 1 catheter/wire combination. The 6.5Fr. JB 1 catheter has been designed specifically for use with the 6-Fr. Shuttle sheath and provides a low profile transition with the sheath.

It is important to be aware that the dilator of the Shuttle sheath extends approximately 3 cm beyond the tip of the Shuttle sheath and does not have a radiopaque marker. Fluoroscopically, its position may be inferred from the straightening effect the dilator tip has on the wire. It is recommended that the tip of the dilator should not extend beyond the distal target for the sheath. Thus, when the tip of the sheath reaches the mid-CCA, the dilator is detached from the sheath, and the sheath is advanced, independently, over the dilator for the last 3 cm of its course in the distal CCA.

(2) In the second strategy, the 90-cm Shuttle sheath is initially delivered to the descending thoracic aorta over a 0.035″ wire. The dilator of the Shuttle sheath is removed and a 125-cm long, diagnostic catheter (JR4, Vitek, JB 1) is then advanced through the Tuohy-Borst adapter at the end of the sheath and is used to selectively engage the innominate or left CCA. Where possible, the 6.5Fr. JB 1 catheter should be used because of the low profile transition with the sheath (see above). Using the methodology described above, a stiff-angled glidewire is advanced through the diagnostic catheter into the ECA or distal CCA, and the diagnostic catheter is then advanced over the glidewire to the ECA or distal CCA. At this point, the sheath may be directly advanced over the glidewire–catheter combination (particularly if a JB 1 catheter has been used). If a diagnostic catheter other than a JB 1 catheter has been used, then it is recommended that this diagnostic catheter be removed (due to the potential hazard of uplifting plaque from the potential space between the diagnostic catheter and sheath) and the dilator of the Shuttle sheath (or the 6.5Fr. JB 1 catheter) be introduced and advanced over the glidewire. If enhanced wire support is required, the glidewire can be exchanged for a more supportive wire (e.g., SupraCore, SuperStiff Amplatz).

STANDARD GUIDE TECHNIQUE

Our guide of choice is the H-1 guide (Fig. 10.10). The standard technique for delivery is as follows (Fig. 10.11): a long (i.e., 125 cm) diagnostic catheter is advanced through a Tuohy-Borst type adapter at the hub of the guide, such that its tip extends beyond the tip of the guide (Fig. 10.12). One should use

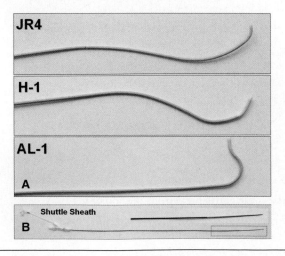

Figure 10.10 • Picture of guide catheters **(A)** and Shuttle sheath **(B)** used during carotid intervention.

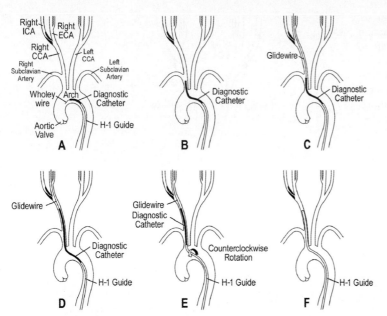

Figure 10.11 • Schematic of technique used to deliver a guide to the distal common carotid artery and internal carotid artery. See text for details. ICA, internal carotid artery; ECA, external carotid artery; CCA, common carotid artery.

the diagnostic catheter that successfully engaged the carotid of interest during the diagnostic angiogram (see above). Over a soft-tipped 0.035″ wire (e.g., Wholey, Versacore), the catheter–guide combination is delivered into the thoracic aorta. The diagnostic catheter is engaged into the ostium of the innominate or left CCA. It is important to keep the tip of the guide approximately 6 to 7 cm proximal to the tip of the catheter, to enable adequate manipulation of the catheter tip. A road map of the CCA is then performed at low magnification, in a view that allows clear visualization of the origins of the ICA and ECA and the aortic arch.

Using this road map, a stiff-angled glidewire is then advanced through the diagnostic catheter into the ECA. In situations where the ECA has severe proximal disease or is occluded, or the distal CCA has significant disease, the stiff-angled glidewire should instead be positioned in the distal CCA, proximal

to any disease. At this point, the diagnostic catheter is slowly advanced over the wire to the distal CCA or ECA (when patent and not significantly diseased). The guide is then carefully advanced, using slow counterclockwise rotation over the catheter–wire combination, to the distal CCA. Finally, the catheter–wire combination is carefully removed under fluoroscopic guidance.

Modifications to the Standard Guide Technique

Modifications to the above technique will be required in a number of situations, most notably in patients with more difficult aortic arch types (e.g., bovine origin of the left CCA), tortuosity of the innominate or CCA, and an ECA that is unavailable for use. The following section describes the most common modifications to the technique outlined above, which are divided into grades I to III in increasing order of complexity and risk.

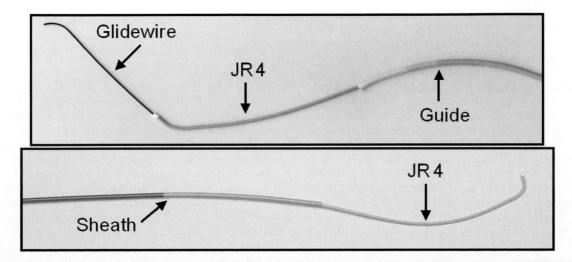

Figure 10.12 • Illustration of diagnostic catheter advanced through the guide catheter and Shuttle sheath, for the telescoping technique used to deliver the sheath or guide to the common carotid artery during carotid intervention. See text for details.

Grade I Modification In patients with type III arches or severe CCA tortuosity, the support provided by the combination of the diagnostic catheter and glidewire may be inadequate to allow delivery of the guide catheter. In this situation, with the diagnostic catheter in the ECA or distal CCA, the glidewire is exchanged for a stiff Amplatz® wire with a 7-cm soft tip, and the guide is advanced over the catheter–stiff Amplatz wire combination. Following delivery of the guide, the process of removal of the catheter–wire combination is carefully observed under fluoroscopy, and accomplished with slight backward tension on the guide, owing to the tendency of the guide to prolapse forward.

Grade II Modification In patients with the complex anatomy types outlined above, the diagnostic catheter will occasionally provide inadequate support, in itself, to allow delivery of the stiff-angled glidewire into the ECA or distal CCA. In this circumstance, one may have to engage the innominate or left CCA, directly, with the guide catheter. Great care with this maneuver is required because there is an increased risk of guide-related trauma. Although an H-1 guide may occasionally be successful, in the authors' experience, typically, an AL1 guide is required in this situation (Fig. 10.10). The terminal tip of the AL1 guide is removed using a metal wire introduced into the catheter tip, and a blow heater to mold the tip. With the AL1 or H-1 guide at the origin of the innominate or left CCA, the ECA or distal CCA is wired. If the ECA is available, it is worth spending the time to advance the wire far distally into one of the major branches of the ECA (e.g., occipital) for enhanced support. The diagnostic catheter is then advanced as far as possible. At this point, it is best to exchange the glidewire for a stiff Amplatz wire (i.e., generally, with a 7-cm soft tip) or SupraCore wire in anticipation of the extra support required to deliver the guide to the distal CCA. If an H-1 guide has been used, it may be advanced safely over the catheter–stiff wire combination. However, this maneuver should never be attempted with the AL1 guide. Owing to the shape of this guide, the risk of trauma to the CCA during such an attempt is prohibitively high. Therefore, with the catheter and stiff Amplatz wire in the ECA or distal CCA, the AL1 guide should be exchanged for an H-1 guide, which is subsequently advanced to the distal CCA.

Grade III Modification Very rarely, the anatomic considerations outlined above may make it impossible to deliver a guide catheter into the distal CCA. If that situation exists, it may be elected to abandon the procedure or to attempt to perform the procedure with the guide (i.e., typically an AL1) positioned in the origin of the CCA or innominate artery (Fig. 10.13).

Clearly, only the most experienced operators are qualified to make this judgment and attempt such procedures. If the procedure is attempted, an extra-support 0.014″ wire (e.g., Ironman®) advanced into the ECA provides the added support to facilitate delivery of equipment into the carotid bifurcation. Alternatively, if one increases the size to a 9-Fr. guide, a 0.035″ wire may be advanced into the ECA, for superior support. Great care needs to be exercised during these procedures, as any maneuver that tends to back the guide away from the ostium of the great vessel (e.g., stent delivery) will also tend to drag the filter or distal balloon occlusion device proximally, potentially across the bifurcation lesion. For this reason, one should try to use a low-magnification view during critical maneuvers, keeping the guide and EPD in view simultaneously.

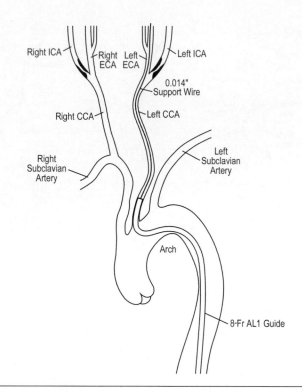

Figure 10.13 • Illustration of the modification to the standard guide technique in patients with type III arches that do not allow delivery of a guide to the common carotid artery. See text for details.

In the authors' experience, the techniques for sheath delivery outlined above will allow successful completion of approximately 90% to 95% of all CAS procedures. Although the use of the guide techniques described allows for a much greater variety of strategies toward achieving the goal of delivery to the distal CCA and is particularly useful in more complex anatomies, it should only be performed by operators with training or proctoring in these techniques.

Embolic Protection Devices

Having secured delivery of a sheath or guide to the distal CCA, the next task during carotid intervention is to place an EPD, to prevent or limit distal embolization during the angioplasty and stenting portion of the procedure. A variety of EPDs are available and are summarized in the following section.

FILTER-TYPE EPDs

Filter-type EPDs are the most popular and user-friendly of the carotid EPDs and have the largest body of data to support their use in carotid intervention (Table 10.5 and Fig. 10.14).

In design, these devices most commonly contain a polyurethane membrane with pores of fixed size—ranging from 80 to 140 μm between devices—which is supported by a nitinol frame. The Spider EPD is unique in that the filter pores are formed by a nitinol mesh. The filter is integrated with a 0.014″ guidewire with a 3- to 4-cm malleable floppy tip. With the exception of the Emboshield and Spider devices, the filter is fixed to the wire.

The technique for delivery of the filter-type EPD varies according to the design of the system. In systems such as the

TABLE 10.5   Summary of Filter-Type Embolic Protection Devices Used during Carotid Intervention

Filter	Manufacturer	Diameters	Pore Size (μm)	Filter and Guidewire Integrated	Filter Type
FilterWire® EZ	Boston Scientific, Natick, MA	3.5–5.5	110	Yes	Unsupported
Angioguard® XP Angioguard® RX	Cordis, Warren, NJ	4, 5, 6, 7, 8	100	Yes	Supported
EmboShield Nav6™	Abbott Laboratories, Abbott Park, IL	5, 7.2	140	No	Supported
Spider®	ev3, Plymouth, MN	3, 4, 5, 6, 7	70–200	Yes	Supported
Accunet® OTW	Guidant, Indianapolis, IN	4.5, 5.5,	150	Yes	Supported
Accunet® RX		6.5, 7.5			

Accunet, FilterWire EZ, and Angioguard, the filter is delivered in a collapsed form across the carotid lesion on the attached guidewire. With the Emboshield system, a unique 0.014″ wire (BareWire™) is used to cross the lesion first, and the filter is delivered in a collapsed form over this wire and deployed over the distal portion of the wire. The Spider system allows the lesion to be crossed using any 0.014″ wire, followed by a 2.9-Fr. delivery catheter, which allows delivery of the Spider filter, which is integrated with a dedicated 0.014″

wire, that allows a small range of independent motion of the wire and filter.

Predilatation of the carotid lesion prior to delivery of the filter-type EPD is required in <1% to 2% of cases. If required, a small-caliber coronary balloon (i.e., 2.0-mm diameter) that minimizes the risk of distal embolization should be used. Regardless of the filter-type EPD used, the filter should ideally be deployed in a straight and nondiseased portion of the cervical ICA (Fig. 10.15), which is typically just proximal to

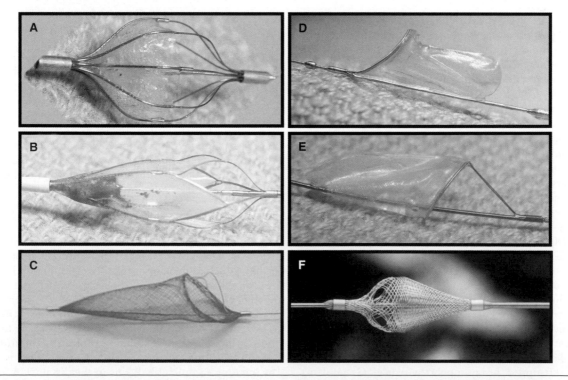

Figure 10.14 • **Examples of filter-type embolic protection devices used during carotid intervention.**   **A:** Angioguard® XP (Cordis, Warren, NJ). **B:** Accunet® (Guidant Corporation, Santa Clara, CA). **C:** Spider® (ev3, Plymouth, MN). **D:** FilterWire EX® (Boston Scientific, Natick, MA). **E:** FilterWire EZ® (Boston Scientific, Natick, MA). **F:** Interceptor® (Medtronic, Minneapolis, MN).

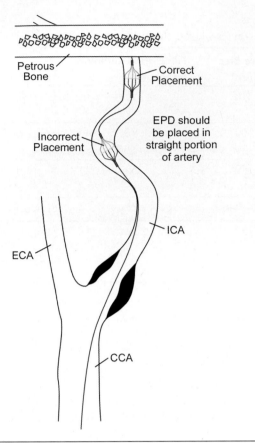

Figure 10.15 • Schematic of internal carotid artery demonstrating correct placement of filter-type embolic protection device.

the petrous portion of the vessel. The presence of tortuosity or disease in the cervical portion of the ICA may require an alternate placement, but there must be at least 3 to 4 cm of distance between the proximal margin of the filter and the distal margin of the ICA lesion to allow subsequent delivery of interventional equipment. In the authors' experience, one always tends to underestimate the distance required between the filter landing zone and the treatment site due to the dead space proximal to the filter system and at the distal end of the stent delivery system.

Delivery of the filter through tortuosity distal to the ICA lesion is sometimes impossible (Fig. 10.16). There are defined maneuvers that may be used to overcome this problem but should only be employed by experienced operators. Initially, a soft-tipped, 0.014″, low-support wire (e.g., Asahi Soft, Asahi Prowater) is advanced through the lesion and positioned in the petrous portion of the ICA. Occasionally, this wire may provide a sufficient straightening effect on the cervical ICA to allow delivery of the filter. If this fails, a coronary over-the-wire balloon is advanced over this wire to its tip, and a further attempt at filter delivery is made, using the wire-and-balloon combination to provide support and a straightening effect. If this fails, the final maneuver is to exchange the low-support wire for a soft-tipped, heavy-support wire (e.g., GrandSlam). This wire usually provides sufficient support and straightening effect, alone, without the balloon. Excessive straightening of the cervical ICA may be problematic, as it may produce severe

kinking of the vessel that both interferes with antegrade flow and makes delivery of the filter more difficult. Once the filter has been successfully delivered, it is important to remember to bring the support wire proximal to the filter, so that it does not compromise the apposition of the filter with the wall of the vessel.

The major advantage of filter-type EPDs is that they allow continued antegrade flow during carotid intervention, an important consideration for patients with compromised collateral flow to the ipsilateral carotid territory (e.g., patients with contralateral carotid disease or occlusion). Although the crossing profile of these EPDs is slightly greater than distal balloon occlusion devices, in the authors' experience, predilation of the carotid lesion to facilitate delivery of the filter is required is rare. Finally, it is important to emphasize that filter-type EPDs serve as embolic limitation devices that prevent embolization of particles greater than approximately 80 to 100 µm in diameter, while allowing particles of smaller diameter to pass through.

DISTAL OCCLUSION BALLOON EPDs

Distal occlusion balloon EPDs were the first EPD used during a carotid intervention (circa 1998). There is currently only one example of this EPD type available: the GuardWire®. In essence, this device contains a compliant balloon that is inflated and deflated through a hollow, nitinol hypotube, located in a 0.014″ angioplasty-style wire. The GuardWire is advanced in its deflated state across the carotid lesion. A marker indicating the position of the balloon is placed in the same location in the prepetrous portion of the cervical ICA, as would a filter-type device. The balloon is then inflated, producing complete cessation of antegrade flow. Following the angioplasty and stenting portions of the procedure, a monorail-export catheter is used to aspirate the column of blood proximal to the filter, thus removing any debris that may have embolized from the carotid plaque. The balloon is then deflated and the GuardWire removed. The Guard-Wire has a lower crossing profile, compared with filter-type EPDs. In theory, this type of EPD should serve as a true embolic prevention device, by removing all embolized debris regardless of particle size. In practice, the device functions more as an embolic limitation device. Its major limitation is that complete cessation of antegrade ICA flow may be poorly tolerated in patients with compromised collateral flow to the anterior cerebral circulation.

PROXIMAL OCCLUSION DEVICES

Proximal occlusion devices are the most recent group of EPDs developed for carotid intervention and appear to be gaining increasing popularity that is supported by an increasing body of data with their use (2,3). Two examples of such devices currently exist: The MO.MA® system (Invatec) and the Parodi® Anti-Embolism System (Gore) (Fig. 10.17). These devices function by generating retrograde flow in the ICA, which theoretically should protect the brain from distal embolization during the intervention. This is achieved by inflating compliant balloons in the distal CCA and ECA, which interrupts antegrade ICA and retrograde ECA flow and allows retrograde flow along the ICA from the circle of Willis.

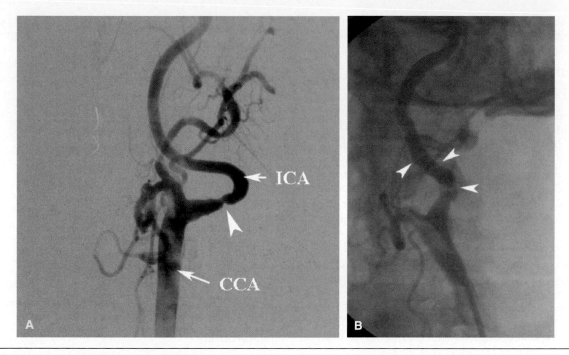

Figure 10.16 • **A:** Common carotid artery angiogram from a patient with severe tortuosity distal to a focal internal carotid artery lesion *(arrowhead)* that would not allow delivery of the filter device. **B:** Angiogram following placement of a stiff Ironman® wire in the internal carotid artery, demonstrating the straightening effect on the artery. Also note the kinking *(arrowheads)* in the artery created by the wire.

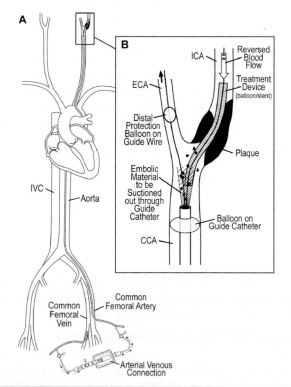

Figure 10.17 • Illustration of proximal balloon occlusion–type embolic protection device (Parodi System). Occlusion of the common carotid artery (CCA) and external carotid artery (ECA) blocks antegrade flow in the internal carotid artery (ICA) (see magnified view of carotid bifurcation in **B**). The connection between the catheter placed in the CCA and the common femoral vein creates a gradient for retrograde flow along the ICA, providing embolic protection during the procedure.

The MO.MA® system requires delivery through a 9-Fr. sheath. There are two noncompliant balloons on the distal portion of the shaft—the proximal balloon is inflated in the distal CCA (designed for reference vessel diameter of 5 to 13 mm) and the distal balloon inflates in the ECA (designed for reference vessel diameter of 3 to 6 mm). These balloons are separated by a 6-cm length, in which there is an exit port that allows access to the ICA. With inflation of both balloons, both antegrade ICA and retrograde ECA flow cessation, *passive* retrograde ICA flow is achieved. Adequate expansion of both balloons is confirmed radiographically by a change in the balloon shape from circular to cylindrical. Once cessation of flow has been achieved, the lesion is treated in the usual manner. Aspiration of 60 cc of blood through the central lumen of the catheter is then performed prior to deflation of the occlusion balloons.

The Parodi system differs from the MO.MA® system in one fundamental respect—this system allows active internal carotid flow reversal by connection of the lumen of the catheter through a blood-return system to the femoral vein. This provides a gradient for flow between the ICA and the femoral vein, ensuring continued retrograde ICA flow during balloon angioplasty and stent placement.

These devices are more cumbersome and technically challenging to use compared with filter-type EPD systems. Sheath size compatibility remains significantly larger with these systems (i.e., 9 Fr. vs. 6 Fr.), and since there is no antegrade flow during flow cessation, visualization of the lesion during stenting is suboptimal. In addition, they require an adequate collateral circulation in the circle of Willis to ensure retrograde flow along the ICA, which is not present in a small percentage of patients (~5%). However, in theory, these systems should provide more effective prevention from embolization. These devices may find particular use for patients in whom tortuosity or disease distal to the carotid bifurcation lesion prevents the use of other EPDs, and in thrombotic lesions where filter-type EPD use is contraindicated.

Angioplasty and Stenting
BALLOON PREDILATION

Following placement of the EPD, it is generally recommended that pre-dilation of the lesion be performed prior to stent placement (Fig. 10.18). The primary purpose of predilation is to ensure the subsequent delivery of the stent. In general, the greater the degree of lesion calcification and severity of stenosis, the more likely that predilation will be necessary, to allow successful stent delivery. Predilation also serves several useful secondary functions: (1) it provides a rough assessment of the length of the lesion, and diameters of the ICA and CCA, which influences the choice of stent length and diameter; (2) the hemodynamic response to predilation provides some insight into the likely hemodynamic consequences of stent deployment and postdilation, enabling the operator to take appropriate prophylactic measures (e.g., the administration of intravenous atropine or more aggressive fluid management); and finally (3) the ease with which balloon predilation achieves its nominal diameter gives some assessment of the rigidity of the plaque.

Predilation is generally performed using a 4.0-mm diameter coronary balloon (e.g., Maverick®). Balloon lengths for predilation are also conservative, with a targeted balloon:lesion length of approximately 1:1. The balloon is inflated to nominal pressure for 10 to 15 seconds.

STENT DEPLOYMENT

Following predilation, carotid bifurcation lesions are stented using a variety of self-expanding nitinol stents. These stents are available in cylindrical and tapered shapes (Fig. 10.19).

The lengths and diameters typically employed in the carotid location vary from 20 to 40 mm and from 5 to 10 mm, respectively. In addition to the lesion length and vessel diameter, the most important determinant of stent length and diameter is lesion location (Fig. 10.20).

The majority of carotid bifurcation lesions involve the ostium of the ICA, and in such situations, a longer stent that extends from the distal CCA into the ICA should be chosen. In this circumstance, assuming that a cylindrical stent is the only stent available, the stent diameter chosen should match the estimated diameter of the distal CCA. With tapered stents, which are ideally suited for this purpose, the larger diameter of the taper should match the CCA diameter, and the smaller diameter of the taper should match the ICA diameter.

For lesions that are truly confined to the ICA, a cylindrical stent confined to the ICA is entirely appropriate, and the stent diameter may match the ICA diameter. It should be stressed that self-expanding stents appose the arterial wall less well than balloon-expandable stents. For this reason, the authors generally add 1 mm to the estimated vessel diameter size, to arrive at the stent diameter to be used.

Stent placement using self-expandable stents is less precise than with balloon-expandable stents. There is often a tendency for self-expanding stents to move forward during deployment. Pulling back on the stent to the correct position, prior to deployment, will minimize this phenomenon. In addition, the initial phase of deployment should be done slowly and carefully, as one may continue to adjust the stent position up until the deployment of the first few stent cells. One should be aware that once any of the cells are deployed, the stent should not be pushed forward but typically may be pulled backwards, provided only a few cells have been deployed. When positioning the stent, one should avoid allowing the proximal margin of the stent to straddle the distal CCA, as this may complicate retrieval of filter-type EPDs by impeding delivery of the retrieval sheath (Fig. 10.21). It may also impede delivery of the export catheter when using a distal balloon occlusion EPD.

There has been some debate regarding the use of carotid stents with closed-cell versus open-cell design. In clinical practice, the open-cell design stents are easier to use and have certain anatomic advantages over closed-cell designs. In particular, in locations where there are sudden transitions between vessel segments of markedly different diameters (i.e., CCA/ICA junction, following prior endarterectomy), the open-cell stent (sized to the CCA diameter) provides better and more complete stent apposition than the closed-cell stent. In addition, open cell stents result in less kinking in vessels with tortuous anatomy.

POSTDILATION

Most operators dilate the stent following deployment, using 4.0- to 5.0-mm diameter balloons (e.g., Sterling, Aviator, Viatrec) inflated to nominal pressure for 10 to 15 seconds. There has generally been a shift toward using smaller diameter balloons for postdilation, with the goal of minimizing distal embolization, and relying on the continued outward force generated by the self-expanding nitinol stent to achieve adequate luminal expansion in the longer term. Generally, the balloon length should be shorter than the stent length to minimize the risk of dissection caused by angioplasty beyond the limits of the stent. In contrast to coronary intervention, mild residual stenosis (i.e., up to 20%) is generally tolerated during carotid stenting, owing to the low risk of restenosis.

In heavily calcified lesions that do not expand well in response to stenting, resulting in a larger residual stenosis, one needs to be wary against overaggressive postdilation of the stent. This may produce a tear in the media or adventitia of the vessel, which typically results in a contained vessel perforation. The authors advocate a conservative approach to balloon postdilation in symptomatic patients and patients with soft plaque; the reasoning is that aggressive postdilation in these situations increases the likelihood of excessive extrusion of plaque elements, which increases the risk for distal embolization. In these situations, if an adequate angiographic result is achieved with stenting alone, one may elect to avoid postdilation altogether.

Removal of EPD and Final Angiography

Following the angioplasty and stenting portion of the procedure, the filter-type EPD is collapsed and removed using a retrieval sheath. Most retrieval sheaths are available in a straight or angled shape to allow the retrieval sheath advance past the stent. Rarely, the patient may either have to turn their head, or external compression may have to applied to the carotid, in order to facilitate this maneuver. Careful angiography of the lesion site and ipsilateral anterior cerebral circulation is performed. The authors also suggest performing angiography of the ipsilateral CCA to document the absence of trauma to the CCA from delivery of the sheath or guide.

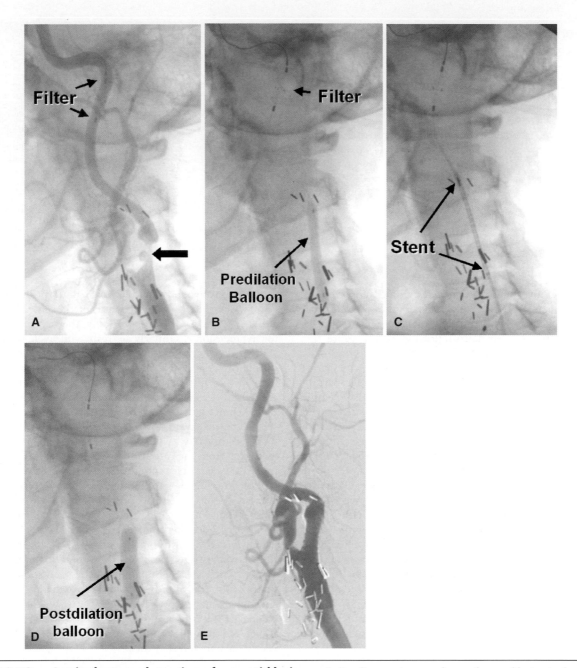

Figure 10.18 • Angioplasty and stenting of a carotid lesion. **A:** Baseline angiogram shows ulcerated lesion in the proximal internal carotid artery (ICA) and the filter placed in the prepetrous portion of the cervical ICA. **B:** The lesion is predilated with a 4.0 × 30-mm balloon. **C:** An 8.0 × 30-mm stent is placed across the lesion, extending into the common carotid artery. **D:** Postdilation with a 5.5 × 30-mm balloon. **E:** Final angiogram following removal of filter.

MANAGEMENT OF COMPLICATIONS OF CAROTID INTERVENTION

Hemodynamic Complications

HYPOTENSION AND BRADYCARDIA

Angioplasty and stenting in the region of the carotid sinus result in stretching of mechanoreceptors at this location. This generates afferent impulses in the glossopharyngeal nerve (i.e., CN IX) that activate the vasomotor center in the medulla. The efferent output from this area activates the vagus nerve (i.e., CN X) and reticulospinal tract, resulting in peripheral vasodilation and a reduction in heart rate and contractility of the heart (Fig. 10.22).

This mechanism underlies the combination of transient hypotension and bradycardia that is frequently observed (i.e., ~40% of cases) during CAS and during the postprocedural period (4–8). It also explains why hypotension and bradycardia are most commonly seen during the treatment of bifurcation lesions involving the ICA ostium, as opposed to procedures on isolated ICA lesions. The effect is seen following predilation,

Figure 10.19 • Cylindrical (**upper**) and tapered (**lower**) nitinol self-expanding carotid stents.

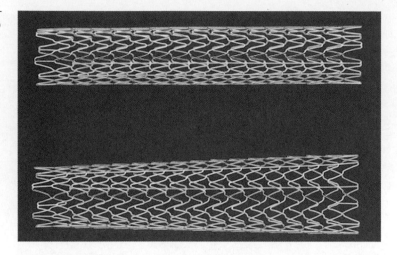

stent placement, and postdilation. Since postdilation typically produces the maximal stretch on the carotid sinus, the maximal effect is usually seen at this point in time. More modest effects may be seen up to 24 to 48 hours following the procedure.

Some operators routinely administer atropine prior to the angioplasty and stenting portion of the procedure in an effort to prevent procedure-related hypotension and bradycardia. In the authors' experience, this is unnecessary. Indeed, routine administration of atropine may increase procedure-related morbidity, since in elderly patients, atropine is associated with significant side effects, including urinary retention, confusion, and severe dry mouth. In patients with critical coronary artery disease, the tachycardia induced by atropine may precipitate coronary ischemia. It is preferable to administer prophylactic atropine only in select situations, including (1) in patients with exaggerated hypotensive or bradycardia response to predilation or stent deployment and (2) in patients with critical aortic stenosis. In the latter situation, even brief episodes of hypotension and bradycardia may be poorly tolerated and result in hemodynamic collapse. Using this approach, atropine is administered in approximately 5% of the cases seen by the authors.

Procedure-related hypotension is certainly mitigated by aggressive, preprocedural hydration. All patients commence receiving intravenous fluids 2 to 3 hours prior to the procedure, which are continued during the procedure (i.e., at ~100–200 mL/h). Intraprocedurally, the first line of therapy for hypotension is similarly aggressive intravenous hydration. If the patient becomes symptomatic, or if severe asymptomatic hypotension develops (i.e., systolic blood pressure [SBP] lower than 75 mm Hg), intravenous dopamine is commenced (i.e., at the rate of 5 μcg/kg) and titrated to achieve an SBP higher than 90 mm Hg, or to alleviate symptoms.

Hypotension in the postprocedural period should always be carefully evaluated. Typically, hypotension caused by stretch from the carotid stent will first manifest during the procedure and persist into the postprocedural period. It is important to remember to withhold all blood pressure medications and aggressively hydrate the patient with intravenous fluids. For asymptomatic patients with severe hypotension, we use oral pseudoephedrine, 60-mg tablet every 4 hours. If the patient becomes symptomatic, intravenous dopamine should be given and titrated to achieve an asymptomatic status. When administering these sympathomimetic agents, one should be aware of the risk of inducing coronary ischemia, since 50% to 60% of patients with carotid artery disease will have significant coronary artery disease. Bradycardia postintervention rarely, if ever, requires intervention, other than to modify the dose of AV-nodal antagonist agents.

HYPERTENSION

Hypertension is a frequent finding during, and following, CAS. Most commonly, it reflects a persistence of the patients' baseline condition (7). Although acute hypertension caused by CEA has been described and attributed to transient dysfunction of adventitial baroreceptors at the endarterectomy site (9), there is no report of evidence that this phenomenon occurs with carotid intervention.

The importance of periprocedural hypertension is emphasized by the strong association between hypertension and hyperperfusion to the ipsilateral cerebral hemisphere (10). This complication was first described in patients undergoing CEA. Mechanistically, it is explained as follows: (1) the presence of a critical carotid stenosis compromises cerebral blood flow; (2) compensatory dilation of the cerebral vessels occurs in an attempt to maintain the baseline flow (11); (3) chronic

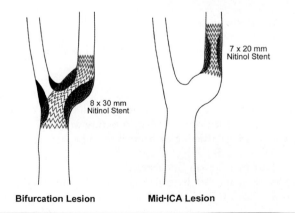

Bifurcation Lesion   **Mid-ICA Lesion**

Figure 10.20 • Schematic of internal carotid artery, demonstrating appropriate stent placement, sizing, and length, based on lesion location.

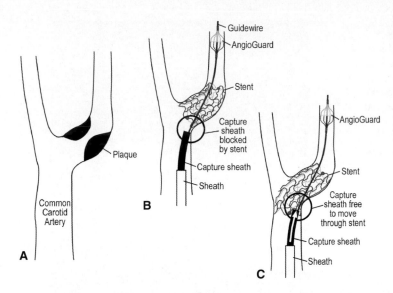

Figure 10.21 • Illustration of the problem created by placing a stent at the ostium of the internal carotid artery. A shows carotid bifurcation with typical location of plaque at ostium of the internal carotid artery. Following stent placement, the stent struts, inferiorly, may interfere with advancement of the filter retrieval sheath **(B).** By placing the proximal portion of the stent in the distal common carotid artery, this problem is overcome **(C).**

dilation of the vessels results in a loss of their normal vasomotor response (i.e., their ability to vasoconstrict and limit cerebral flow); and (4) the sudden removal of carotid stenosis by CAS restores carotid flow, and in the presence of dilation of the cerebral vessels, there is hyperperfusion to the brain.

Retrospective registry data suggest an incidence of hyperperfusion following CAS of between 1% and 5% (10). Based on the CEA experience and limited carotid intervention data, it appears that hypertension in conjunction with the treatment of a critical, ipsilateral carotid stenosis (i.e., of greater than 90%), and the presence of a contralateral stenosis (i.e., of more than 80%), or occlusion, predicts the group at highest risk for this complication (12). Clinically, patients complain of a headache that lateralizes to the side of the intervention. The headache has a throbbing quality and may be located in the facial, temporal, or retro-orbital regions. Nausea, vomiting, focal neurologic deficits, or seizures often accompany the headache.

The absence of abnormal findings on CT of the head and increased flow velocities in the ipsilateral middle cerebral artery, as assessed by transcranial Doppler, provide supportive evidence for the diagnosis of hyperperfusion (13). Prompt diagnosis and emergent management are the keys to a successful outcome from this complication. Aggressive treatment with intravenous antihypertensive medication is mandatory. Several antihypertensive agents are associated with increased cerebral

blood flow and are therefore contraindicated (e.g., glycerol trinitrate, nitroprusside, calcium channel antagonists, angiotensin-converting enzyme inhibitors). Recommended agents include β-blockers, labetalol (mixed α- and β-adrenergic antagonist), and clonidine (central α$_2$-adrenergic antagonist) that have favorable effects on cerebral blood flow and cerebral perfusion pressure in this clinical situation. Following the acute control of hypertension, aggressive reinstitution of the patient's baseline oral, antihypertensive regimen is also important. If neurologic symptoms are prominent, typically, the patient's routine postprocedural aspirin and clopidogrel therapy is held until the neurologic symptoms resolve and the blood pressure is controlled. This is because the most feared complication of the hyperperfusion syndrome is cerebral hemorrhage (10,14–17). This diagnosis carries a very high mortality rate (i.e., ~30% to 80%), and among those who survive, 20% to 40% have significant residual neurologic dysfunction (18). In the single institution registry of 450 carotid interventions, intracranial hemorrhage occurred in three of the five patients with hyperperfusion syndrome (i.e., 0.67%). Although this frequency is low, the morbidity and mortality associated with the condition underscore the importance of meticulous attention to hypertension management and the necessity for early recognition and appropriate management of hyperperfusion syndrome.

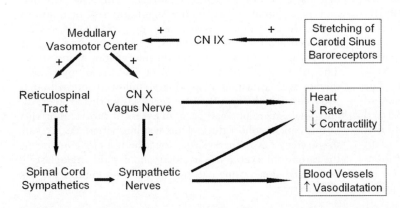

Figure 10.22 • Diagrammatic representation of the effect of activation of mechanoreceptors in the carotid sinus during carotid intervention.

Stroke

Stroke is the major feared complication of CAS. In the high-risk carotid stent registries to date, the 30-day incidence of stroke with CAS is approximately 3% (19,20), which compares favorably to the rate of 3.3% in the CEA arm of the SAPPHIRE trial (21). One may not use the stroke rates reported from the CEA trials of the 1990s for comparison, however, as the patient populations were different. It is encouraging that the majority of strokes following CAS are classified as minor (i.e., resolution within 30 days, or NIH Stroke Scale 3 or less).

Distal embolization of extruded atherosclerotic debris during angioplasty and CAS is a universal finding in carotid intervention and is clearly the dominant mechanism of procedure-related stroke. However, it is important to be aware of other potential etiologies, most notably, the manipulation of wires, catheters, and guides in the aortic arch and CCA. These manipulations are not protected by an EPD. Distal embolization of debris, at the time of these manipulations, should certainly be implicated as the likely mechanism in patients who experience strokes outside of the territory of the treated carotid artery (i.e., posterior or contralateral anterior circulation stroke) (22). This phenomenon also explains why even an EPD that functions perfectly may not be expected to reduce the risk of stroke during CAS to zero.

If a neurologic deficit occurs during the carotid procedure, cerebral angiography should be performed, as further management is largely dictated by these angiographic findings. In the presence of a normal angiogram, the clinical outcome in these patients is predictably excellent, and they should be managed conservatively. If a large artery (i.e., 2 to 2.5mm diameter, or greater) occlusion that is the result of distal embolization is identified, it is reasonable for a suitably qualified interventionalist to attempt recanalization—using a combination of mechanical (i.e., thrombectomy, angioplasty) and pharmacologic (i.e., thrombolytic, glycoprotein IIb/IIIa) therapies (Fig. 10.23).

Unfortunately, there are no guidelines for the dosing of thrombolytics or glycoprotein IIb/IIIa agents in this situation. Empirically, we have administered a dose of 0.125 mg/kg of abciximab, alone or in combination with 5 to 20 mg of tissue plasminogen activator (tPA), given intra-arterially in divided doses at the site of the occlusion. Unfortunately, the efficacy of these maneuvers is unpredictable, which is likely explained by the fact that these emboli are composed of atheromatous debris and generally do not respond to conventional intervention techniques (23). Occlusions of smaller branch vessels (i.e., those of less than 2-mm diameter) are probably best managed noninvasively. If the patient has a significant neurologic deficit, a bolus and infusion of an intravenous glycoprotein IIb/IIIa inhibitor through a peripheral IV system may be administered in an effort to minimize the infarct size.

Strokes beyond the immediate periprocedural period (i.e., but within the first 2 weeks following carotid intervention) are rare and are typically minor in severity (24). The mechanism of these strokes is unclear. Manipulation of atheroma in the aortic arch or CCA may result in delayed embolization of plaque elements or of platelet thrombi that form on the surface of the traumatized atheroma. The stent surface may also serve as a focus for platelet thrombi formation and embolization, and delayed extrusion of plaque elements through the interstices of the stent may also occur.

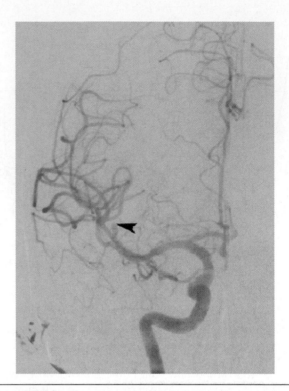

Figure 10.23 • Example of distal embolization to a major branch of the M-2 segment of the right middle cerebral artery (*arrowhead*) in a patient, following carotid stenting.

If a patient presents with a delayed stroke following carotid intervention, the first priority should be to rule out an intracranial hemorrhage. In the absence of hemorrhage, management is typically conservative.

Adverse Cardiac Events

The frequency of myocardial infarction in high-risk patients in the 30 days following CAS is approximately 2% in most series (20,25). Of these, the majority are non-Q wave in type. In the randomized cohort of the SAPPHIRE trial, the 30-day incidence of myocardial infarction in the stent arm was 1.9%, compared with 6.6% in the CEA arm. This difference was statistically significant and suggests a major advantage of CAS over CEA in patients with significant coronary artery disease (25).

Despite these data, caution is recommended in the use of CAS in the subset of patients with critical coronary or cardiac disease awaiting open-heart surgery. This is an extremely high-risk patient subset, with a significant risk of mortality during the typical 3- to 4-week waiting period between CAS and open-heart surgery. Previously, the authors' strategy in this group was to perform carotid intervention using stents. The patient received a minimum of 4 weeks of antiplatelet therapy with aspirin and clopidogrel, followed approximately 5 to 7 days later by open-heart surgery. Using this strategy, the anecdotal experience had been an excess of cardiac mortality in this patient cohort during this waiting period. As a result, the strategy has been revised. Now, the use of stents during the carotid intervention is avoided, and carotid angioplasty is performed alone, using cutting balloons to minimize the risk of dissection.

The goal of therapy is to achieve normal carotid flow, and a moderate residual stenosis is tolerated. Antiplatelet therapy consists of aspirin and one of the short-acting, small-molecule, intravenous GP IIb/IIIa inhibitors. Following the procedure, the patient proceeds within the next 1 to 2 days to open-heart surgery, stopping the glycoprotein IIb/IIIa inhibitor 4 to 6 hours prior to surgery. Postoperatively, the patient receives aspirin therapy, and clopidogrel is added within 48 hours. At 6 to 8 weeks, a carotid ultrasound is performed, and if needed a carotid stent may be placed in an elective procedure, using routine antiplatelet and anticoagulant pharmacotherapy.

Slow-Flow

Delayed antegrade flow in the ICA is frequently observed during CAS procedures using filter-type EPDs and is referred to as slow-flow. This phenomenon is likely explained by excessive distal embolization of plaque elements that block the pores of the filter and thus interfere with antegrade flow through the filter (Fig. 10.24).

The phenomenon is most commonly observed following postdilation of the stent (i.e., ~75%) and stent deployment (i.e., ~25%). Angiographically, the spectrum of slow-flow may vary from mild delay to complete cessation of antegrade flow.

In an analysis of some 420 patients from a carotid intervention registry slow-flow occurred in approximately 10% of patients. Symptomatic status (i.e., stroke or transient ischemic attack within the last 6 months), increased patient age, and larger stent sizes were independently associated with this event. Comparing patients who experienced slow-flow to those with normal flow, there was a significantly increased risk of periprocedural stroke in the slow-flow group (i.e., 9.5% vs. 1.7%), although the majority of these were minor. The mechanism of this increased stroke risk is debatable. The belief is that it results from the accumulation of embolized debris in the column of blood, proximal to the filter, under the conditions of slow-flow (i.e., when the filter pores are blocked). For this reason, it is generally recommended to aspirate the column of blood proximal to the filter when slow-flow is observed. This is achieved using the export catheter of the Percusurge® system. The export catheter is advanced over the filter wire to the level of the filter. It is then withdrawn toward the carotid bifurcation and approximately 20 cc of blood is aspirated. This process is repeated three to four times. This aspiration does not affect the angiographic appearance of flow, since the filter remains obstructed with debris. Failure to aspirate, however, exposes the patient to a potentially large burden of embolized debris at the time of filter retrieval. Filter retrieval universally restores normal antegrade flow.

Postprocedural Care and Follow-Up Monitoring

Patients are admitted overnight to a step-down telemetry care unit following CAS and, typically, are discharged the following day. The major management issue following intervention is blood pressure. Nursing and medical staff should be keenly aware of the importance of this fact and respond appropriately to both hypotension and hypertension. Particular attention should be paid to the reintroduction and titration of blood pressure medications. This process requires a significant investment of time, involving making arrangements for twice-daily blood pressure measurements and daily contact between the patient and the health care professional until a stable blood pressure state has been reached. A stable state is usually reached about 1 week following the procedure, but for some patients, it may take longer.

Secondary risk factor modification is also mandatory. All patients should receive lifelong aspirin therapy unless contraindicated, and clopidogrel therapy is recommended for a minimum of 4 weeks following the procedure. There are currently no data to support more prolonged use of clopidogrel in patients with carotid disease. It is also reasonable to treat all patients with a statin drug.

Long-term follow-up evaluation of patients involves monitoring for evidence of restenosis or progression of disease in the contralateral carotid artery. Fortunately, CAS is associated with a low rate of restenosis (i.e., 2% to 5%). The target lesion

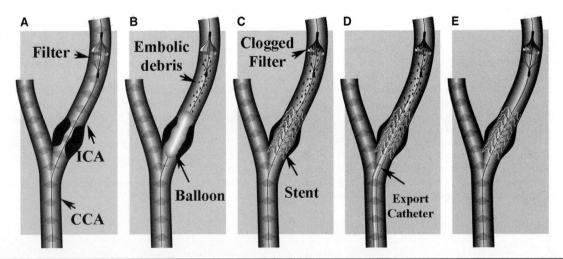

Figure 10.24 • Schematic of proposed mechanism of slow-flow and rationale for aspiration. **A:** Carotid bifurcation lesion with filter placed distally. **B,C:** Balloon angioplasty and stenting result in embolization of debris from atherosclerotic plaque, toward filter, causing occlusion of filter pores and accumulation of debris in column of blood proximal to the filter. **D,E:** Aspiration proximal to filter removes debris from column of blood without affecting debris causing occlusion of filter.

revascularization rate at 1 year in the CAS arm of the randomized SAPPHIRE cohort was 0.7%. Ipsilateral stroke or transient ischemia attack (TIA) beyond the initial 2 weeks following CAS is extremely rare. These data certainly underscore the long-term durability and efficacy of the procedure. There is no consensus regarding the management of severe restenosis following CAS. The risk of stroke from restenosis is poorly defined but is suggested to be low (26). The authors adopt an aggressive approach to the treatment of high-grade restenosis (i.e., greater than 80%). In the past, angioplasty and brachytherapy using γ radiation were the most commonly employed treatment strategy (25). Unfortunately, γ-brachytherapy systems for vascular treatment are rarely available. In the absence of this therapy, angioplasty alone, with peripheral cutting balloons, is a reasonable percutaneous option.

CONCLUSIONS

Carotid intervention using carotid stents and EPDs is now established as the treatment of choice for individuals with significant carotid disease who are at high risk for CAS. The technique has many technical challenges and requires a thorough knowledge of the anatomy, vascular biology, and pathology of the cerebrovascular system. In addition, these procedures are associated with a number of well-recognized complications that require careful management by a multidisciplinary team of endovascular specialists, cardiologists, internists, and neurologists.

References

1. Brown MM. Carotid artery stenting—evolution of a technique to rival carotid endarterectomy. *Am J Med*. 2004;116:273–275.
2. Ansel GM, Hopkins LN, Jaff MR, et al. Safety and effectiveness of the INVATEC MO.MA proximal cerebral protection device during carotid artery stenting: results from the ARMOUR pivotal trial. *Catheter Cardiovasc Interv*. 2010;76:1–8.
3. Stabile E, Salemme L, Sorropago G, et al. Proximal endovascular occlusion for carotid artery stenting. *J Am Coll Cardiol*. 2010;55:1661–1667.
4. Bush RL, Lin PH, Bianco CC, et al. Reevaluation of temporary transvenous cardiac pacemaker usage during carotid angioplasty and stenting: a safe and valuable adjunct. *Vasc Endovascular Surg*. 2004;38:229–235.
5. Mlekusch W, Schillinger M, Sabeti S, et al. Hypotension and bradycardia after elective carotid stenting: frequency and risk factors. *J Endovasc Ther*. 2003;10:851–859; discussion 860–861.
6. Mendelsohn FO, Weissman NJ, Lederman RJ, et al. Acute hemodynamic changes during carotid artery stenting. *Am J Cardiol*. 1998;82:1077–1081.
7. Qureshi AI, Luft AR, Sharma M, et al. Frequency and determinants of postprocedural hemodynamic instability after carotid angioplasty and stenting. *Stroke*. 1999;30:2086–2093.
8. Leisch F, Kerschner K, Hofmann R, et al. Carotid sinus reactions during carotid artery stenting: predictors, incidence, and influence on clinical outcome. *Catheter Cardiovasc Interv*. 2003;58:516–523.
9. Bove EL, Fry WJ, Gross WS, et al. Hypotension and hypertension as consequences of baroreceptor dysfunction following carotid endarterectomy. *Surgery*. 1979;85:633–637.
10. Abou-Chebl A, Yadav JS, Reginelli JP, et al. Intracranial hemorrhage and hyperperfusion syndrome following carotid artery stenting: risk factors, prevention, and treatment. *J Am Coll Cardiol*. 2004;43:1596–1601.
11. Sundt TM Jr, Sharbrough FW, Piepgras DG, et al. Correlation of cerebral blood flow and electroencephalographic changes during carotid endarterectomy: with results of surgery and hemodynamics of cerebral ischemia. *Mayo Clin Proc*. 1981;56:533–543.
12. Sbarigia E, Speziale F, Giannoni MF, et al. Post-carotid endarterectomy hyperperfusion syndrome: preliminary observations for identifying at risk patients by transcranial Doppler sonography and the acetazolamide test. *Eur J Vasc Surg*. 1993;7:252–256.
13. Jansen C, Sprengers AM, Moll FL, et al. Prediction of intracerebral haemorrhage after carotid endarterectomy by clinical criteria and intraoperative transcranial Doppler monitoring: results of 233 operations. *Eur J Vasc Surg*. 1994;8:220–225.
14. McCabe DJ, Brown MM, Clifton A. Fatal cerebral reperfusion hemorrhage after carotid stenting. *Stroke*. 1999;30:2483–2486.
15. Morrish W, Grahovac S, Douen A, et al. Intracranial hemorrhage after stenting and angioplasty of extracranial carotid stenosis. *AJNR Am J Neuroradiol*. 2000;21:1911–1916.
16. Al-Mubarak N, Roubin GS, Vitek JJ, et al. Subarachnoidal hemorrhage following carotid stenting with the distal-balloon protection. *Catheter Cardiovasc Interv*. 2001;54:521–523.
17. Caplan LR, Skillman J, Ojemann R, et al. Intracerebral hemorrhage following carotid endarterectomy: a hypertensive complication? *Stroke*. 1978;9:457–460.
18. Cheung RT, Eliasziw M, Meldrum HE, et al. Risk, types, and severity of intracranial hemorrhage in patients with symptomatic carotid artery stenosis. *Stroke*. 2003;34:1847–1851.
19. Wholey MH, Al-Mubarek N. Updated review of the global carotid artery stent registry. *Catheter Cardiovasc Interv*. 2003;60:259–266.
20. Reimers B, Schluter M, Castriota F, et al. Routine use of cerebral protection during carotid artery stenting: results of a multicenter registry of 753 patients. *Am J Med*. 2004;116:217–222.
21. Yadav JS. Stenting and angioplasty with protection in patients at high risk for endarterectomy: 30-day results. In: *The American Heart Association Scientific Sessions*. Chicago, IL; 2002.
22. Schluter M, Tubler T, Steffens JC, et al. Focal ischemia of the brain after neuroprotected carotid artery stenting. *J Am Coll Cardiol*. 2003;42:1007–1013.
23. Wholey MH, Tan WA, Toursarkissian B, et al. Management of neurological complications of carotid artery stenting. *J Endovasc Ther*. 2001;8:341–353.
24. Endovascular versus surgical treatment in patients with carotid stenosis in the Carotid and Vertebral Artery Transluminal Angioplasty Study (CAVATAS): a randomised trial. *Lancet*. 2001;357:1729–1737.
25. Yadav JS. Stenting and angioplasty with protection in patients at high risk for endarterectomy. In: *The American Heart Association Meeting*. Chicago, IL; 2002.
26. Ansel GM. Treatment of carotid stent restenosis. *Catheter Cardiovasc Interv*. 2003;58:93–94.

CHAPTER 11

Carotid Artery Stenting: Advanced Techniques

Ravish Sachar and Jay S. Yadav

Reducing the risk of stroke during carotid artery stenting requires a combination of proper patient selection and impeccable technique. Each phase of the procedure carries risk, and achieving optimal outcomes involves meticulous attention to detail at each step. It is essential for the interventionalist to have a thorough understanding of cerebrovascular anatomy, vascular biology, and anatomic variations, along with a complete knowledge of the full spectrum of available equipment.

The importance of proper patient selection cannot be overstated. A number of patient characteristics increase the risk of either surgical or percutaneous carotid revascularization (Fig. 11.1). Patients with visible thrombus in the internal carotid artery (ICA) should be avoided and referred for surgical revascularization. However, if absolutely necessary, these patients can be addressed percutaneously with proximal occlusion systems by experienced operators. Similarly, if tortuosity of the ICA precludes the use of distal embolic protection devices (EPDs) (see below), the patient should be referred for endarterectomy unless the operator is comfortable with the use of proximal occlusions systems.

There are several steps during carotid stenting that must be successfully negotiated to achieve procedural success. Figure 11.2 shows the risk of stroke associated with the three main phases of the procedure. Data from the XACT, CAPTURE, and CASES PMS (1,2) postmarket registries indicate that at 30 days, about 10% to 15% of strokes have occurred in the contralateral hemisphere. This suggests that these strokes are due to diagnostic catheter manipulation during angiography or subsequent sheath or guide placement in the common carotid artery (CCA). Assuming that an equal number of strokes that occur in the ipsilateral hemisphere are also due to catheter manipulation, it is likely that about 20% to 30% of strokes at 30 days are likely due to catheter manipulation in the carotid. This number may be slightly inflated as it includes strokes that occurred after discharge that are unrelated to carotid artery disease.

Analyses of data from the CAPTURE registry suggest that approximately 20% of strokes occur post-procedure (2). This figure is questionable, however, given the timing of neurologic follow-up post-procedure. Minor peri-procedural strokes are often missed by operators and not detected until the next day when the patient is seen by the neurologist. Thus, these strokes may be misclassified as post-procedural strokes. It is the authors' experience that a small minority of strokes occur postprocedure (probably less than 5%).

The majority of strokes occur at the time of the stenting procedure itself (Fig. 11.3). Transcranial Doppler (TCD) data

from multiple studies have shown that there are microemboli to the middle cerebral artery (MCA) during all phases of the procedure (3). However, the risk of stroke is not equal in all phases of the procedure. Among the three phases of the procedure, only postdilation has been shown to be an independent predictor of stroke (4).

ANGIOGRAPHY

Reducing the risk of stroke during carotid artery stenting begins with adhering to meticulous technique during diagnostic angiography. There are a few basic tenets that can reduce the risk of stroke with each individual step, thereby contributing to a significantly lower overall risk for the procedure (Table 11.1).

Use of a manifold allows real-time monitoring of hemodynamics throughout the case, and we believe that it is essential to use a manifold during carotid artery stenting. This is especially important in patients with concomitant coronary artery disease or aortic stenosis. It also helps reduce the risk of injecting into plaque by monitoring for dampening of waveforms during catheter positioning.

It is also important not to power inject into the common carotid arteries. In situations where power injection is being used, the physician often leaves the patient's bedside after positioning the diagnostic catheter in the CCA. Patient movement during this time can result in inadvertent angulation of the diagnostic catheter toward the vessel wall, and subsequent power injection can result in carotid dissection. Instead, the authors recommend hand injections with routine use of a manifold. This minimizes the risk of air embolism associated with direct connection of contrast-filled syringes, and also reduces the risk of complications related to power injection.

The vertebral arteries should not be routinely cannulated during carotid angiography, and selective vertebral artery angiography should be reserved for those cases where knowledge of posterior circulation anatomy will help with decision making, or where there is a true concern for vertebrobasilar insufficiency. In such cases, nonselective injection of contrast into the subclavian arteries, while a blood pressure cuff is inflated on the ipsilateral arm, may suffice. If cannulation is truly indicated, then the ostium of the vertebral artery must be visualized prior to selection with a diagnostic catheter as ostial disease of the vertebral arteries is quite common (Fig. 11.4). The contralateral oblique projection is usually best for optimal visualization of the vertebral artery ostium.

Figure 11.1 • **A:** Factors that increase the risk of carotid revascularization. XRT, radiation therapy; CN, cranial nerve; Pulm, pulmonary; Coag, coagulopathy; Ca^{++}, calcification. **B:** Example of carotid stenosis that is high-risk for stenting due to severe calcification of the distal common carotid artery and proximal internal carotid artery. Such severe concentric calcification can preclude optimal stent expansion and there is also a risk of carotid perforation if excessive post-dilatation is performed to try to achieve adequate stent expansion. CCA, common carotid artery; ICA, internal carotid artery; ECA, external carotid artery.

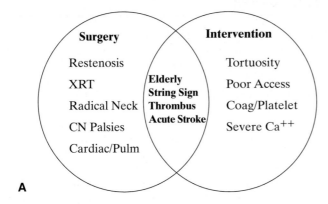

SEVERE TYPE III AORTIC ARCH ANATOMY

The approach to carotid stenting based on arch type has been described in Chapter 10. However, in some patients the angle of origin of the innominate artery or the left CCA is so acute that attempts to advance wires into the CCA or external carotid artery (ECA) through a regular or reverse curve diagnostic catheter result in the catheter being prolapsed into the aorta (Fig. 11.5A, B).

In such cases, the authors recommend using a modification of the telescoping technique. A H1 guide catheter is used to directly engage the innominate artery or the left CCA, as shown in Figure 11.5C. Care must be taken to minimize manipulation of the guide in the aortic arch. Once the guide is

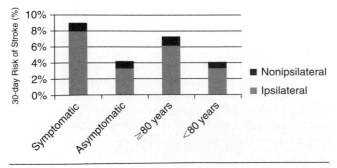

Figure 11.2 • Risk of ipsilateral and contralateral stroke from the CAPTURE registry according to symptomatic status and patient age.

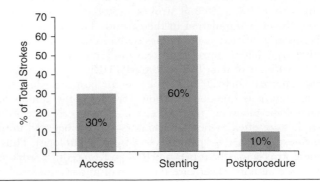

Figure 11.3 • The risk of stroke during the three main phases of carotid artery stenting procedure.

TABLE 11.1 Tips to Reduce the Risk of Stroke During Carotid Angiography

Dos	Don'ts
Use manifold	Use power injections
Pull back on contrast before each injection to reduce risk of air embolus	Routinely selectively cannulate the vertebral artery
Minimize catheter manipulation in the arch	

in position, a long 0.035″ glidewire is carefully advanced into the ECA under roadmap guidance. A 5 Fr. 125-cm diagnostic catheter, such as a JR4, is then advanced into the ECA over the glidewire through the H1 guide. Once in position, the H1 guide can be telescoped over the diagnostic catheter and glidewire into position. Care must be taken to monitor for sudden forward movement of the entire system as the guide is advanced into the CCA, as this can result in plaque dissection or embolization.

Another option is to use a Simmons guide catheter to access the innominate or left CCA. The Simmons catheter can be shaped in the descending thoracic aorta, ascending thoracic aorta, or using the left subclavian artery. Usually a Simmons 1 catheter will not be long enough, and a Simmons 2 will work better (5). However, care must be taken as excessive manipulation of this catheter in the aortic arch can increase the risk of stroke, especially in older patients.

A bovine origin of the left CCA combined with a steep type III arch can be particularly challenging. In such cases, both the Vitek and Simmons 2 diagnostic catheters are useful options, particularly if combined with the telescoping technique. Alternatively, an AL 1 guide catheter can be used to engage the proximal left CCA, and can remain in this position during the procedure. This is also a useful technique in patients with proximal left CCA disease with a bovine aortic arch (Fig. 11.6). When using guides that engage only the proximal part of the carotid, a stiff 0.014″ coronary buddy wire should be positioned in the ECA for support because there is a risk of guide prolapse during stent advancement; guide or sheath prolapse while an EPD is deployed can result in the open EPD being pulled through the lesion with adverse consequences. Guide and sheath position should be monitored during balloon and stent advancement by either panning or using a large field of view.

OSTIAL INNOMINATE ARTERY AND LEFT COMMON CAROTID ARTERY DISEASE

Ostial lesions of the innominate artery and left CCA are challenging to treat, but with the proper technique, can be treated safely and effectively percutaneously. These are complicated cases with multiple steps, and should only be treated by an experienced operator. The key tenet is that the guide or sheath must not cross or touch the lesion at any point, and must remain in the aorta at all times. Patients may present with combined internal carotid and ostial CCA or innominate disease, and both can be treated in the same setting. In these cases, the

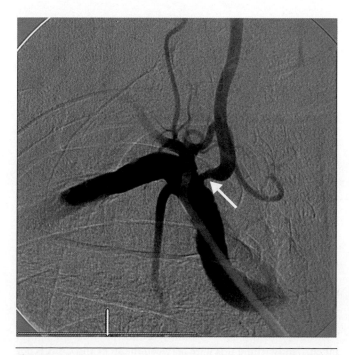

Figure 11.4 • Moderate ostial stenosis of right vertebral artery (*arrow*).

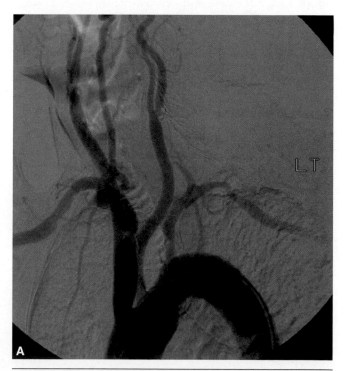

Figure 11.5 • Some patients have such acute angles of origin of the great vessels from the aortic arch **(A)** that advancing a 0.035″ wire into the vessel through a normal or reverse curve diagnostic catheter results in catheter prolapse **(B)**. (*Continued*)

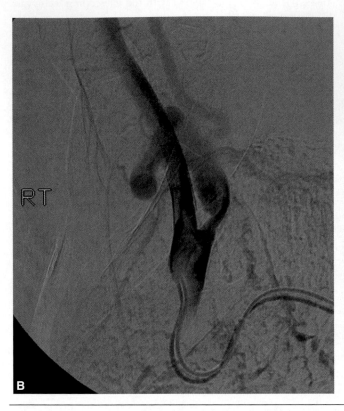

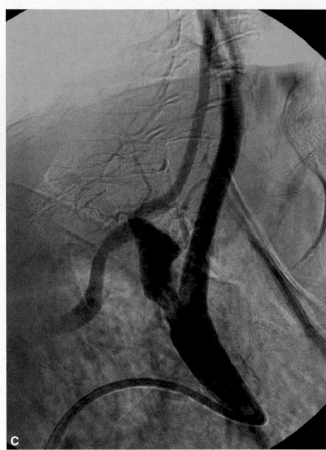

Figure 11.5 • *(Continued)* In such cases, it may be useful to cannulate the ostium of the innominate artery or left common carotid artery directly with an 8 Fr. H1 guide catheter, as shown in this RAO projection angiogram **(C)**.

ICA must be stented before the ostial CCA as it may be difficult to advance a self-expanding stent through a deployed ostial stent. Ostial disease is often calcified and recalcitrant to dilation, and it is therefore preferable to use balloon-expandable stents as compared to self-expanding stents. Balloon-expandable stents offer a further advantage of more precise placement and deployment, which is critical when treating ostial disease. Before beginning, it is important to start with a good quality aortic arch angiogram in the left anterior oblique (LAO) projection to properly evaluate the ostia of the great vessels. A step-by-step method of safely treating ostial lesions of the left CCA and right CCA is described below.

Ostial Left CCA Stenosis

Moderate ostial disease that does not require treatment but is found incidentally in the presence of a severe internal carotid stenosis may be crossed with a diagnostic catheter or sheath. This is one instance in which we prefer a sheath to a guide due to the better transition between the sheath and the dilator that should cause less trauma to the ostial lesion (Fig. 11.7).

For severe lesions of the left carotid ostium that warrant treatment, a "no-touch" technique is highly recommended. The lesion should not be crossed or engaged with diagnostic or guide catheters; sheaths should not be used for these lesions. Guide shapes that will not accidentally engage the CCA

should be chosen. Our preferred guide is the 8 Fr. Multipurpose, which can usually be placed adjacent to the ostium but will typically not engage the ostium (Fig. 11.8).

With the Multipurpose guide adjacent to the ostium, an extra-support 0.014″ wire (e.g., Grand Slam, Abbott Vascular, Menlo Park, CA) should be advanced across the lesion and placed in the ECA. If this proves to be excessively difficult, a Vitek catheter can be advanced through the guide and used to steer the wire across the lesion; if at all possible, the Vitek should not be advanced across the lesion. Once the 0.014″ wire is in the ECA, an EPD should be placed in the ICA. At this point, a 0.014″ compatible balloon is advanced over the EPD wire and the lesion is pre-dilated. A 0.014″ compatible balloon-expandable stent is then advanced over the EPD wire; 7- or 8-mm diameter stents are usually adequate and in smaller patients, 6 mm diameter stents may be adequate. These lesions are typically associated with significant aortic arch disease and calcification, and it is possible to cause dissections and perforations of the aortic arch with aggressive sizing. The approach to these lesions is much more conservative than that with coronary ostial disease. The 0.014″ buddy wire in the ECA should not be removed until the EPD is removed and the final angiogram taken. Sandwiching this wire between the stent and CCA is not a problem and it can easily be removed at the end. Hydrophilic wires should not be used as buddy wires because it is possible to strip the hydrophilic coating during wire removal.

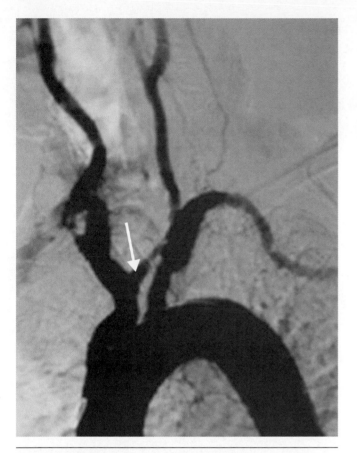

Figure 11.6 • Bovine origin of the left common carotid artery *(arrow)* in a patient with a type III aortic arch. The acute angulation of the left common carotid artery origin makes carotid stenting from the femoral approach challenging. In such cases, right radial or brachial approaches may be useful. This patient has concomitant stenosis of the proximal left and right common carotid arteries, adding to the complexity of the case.

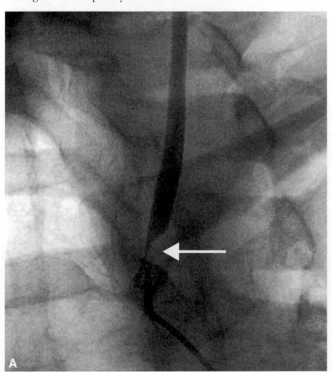

Ostial left CCA lesions with a bovine arch can be particularly challenging. These are best approached with an AL 1 guide; occasionally a H1 guide may be appropriate (Fig. 11.9). The remainder of the procedure is as described above. There is a tendency for the AL 1 guide to engage the left CCA and cross the lesion once the buddy wire is in place; mild forward pressure on the guide will prevent this from occurring.

Ostial Innominate Artery Disease

As with ostial left CCA disease, high-grade stenoses of the innominate artery are challenging to treat due to the location, short length, and highly variable diameter of the vessel, often due to post-stenotic dilation. Furthermore, these lesions are usually heavily calcified. The combination of these factors makes it difficult to find an appropriately sized stent in terms of length, diameter, and radial force. Balloon-expandable stents are most often the correct choice due to the shorter lengths that are available, ability to position precisely, and greater radial force. However, there is a higher risk of size mismatch and malapposition of portions of the stent. This increases the risk of stent migration and dislodgment, which can have disastrous consequences.

The technique for percutaneous revascularization of the innominate artery is similar to that of ostial left CCA stenoses. For true ostial lesions that are severe, every attempt should be made not to cross the lesion with either a diagnostic or guide catheter and the "no-touch" technique described for ostial left CCA disease should be employed.

For less critical lesions, it is permissible to cross the lesion with a 4 or 5 Fr. soft-tipped angled diagnostic catheter, such as a glide catheter or a Bernstein catheter. In cases of severe tortuosity, a JR4 or reverse curve catheter can be used. Ensure that the waveform is not dampened prior to any contrast injections. Use of a manifold is recommended

Figure 11.7 • **A:** Ostial left common carotid artery (CCA) stenosis *(white arrow).* This patient presented with crescendo left hemispheric transient ischemic attacks. Angiography was performed with a 5 Fr. Berenstein catheter (Boston Scientific, MA) positioned near the true ostium. **B:** Schematic illustration of management of moderate ostial left CCA stenosis in setting of treatment of internal carotid artery stenosis. Moderately diseased ostia can be crossed with a sheath; a sheath is preferable to a guide due to the better transition between the dilator and catheter resulting in less trauma to the plaque.

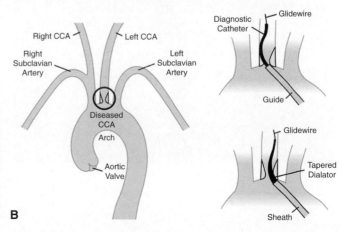

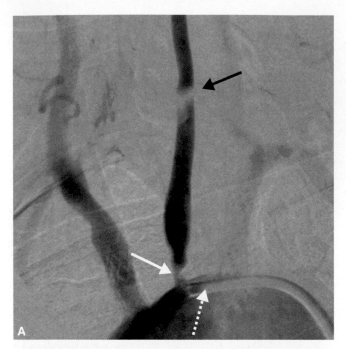

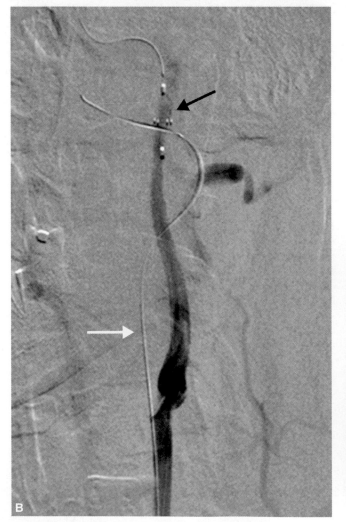

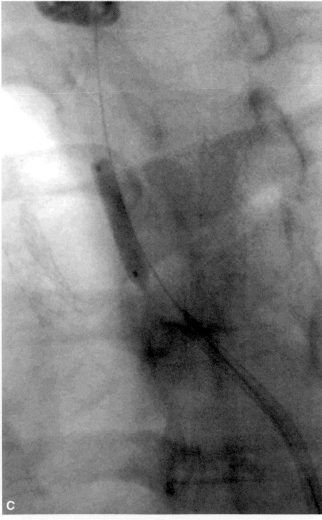

Figure 11.8 • **A:** Severe disease of the ostium *(white arrow)* and proximal *(black arrow)* left common carotid artery (CCA). An 8 Fr. Multipurpose (MP) guide has been positioned adjacent to the ostium (tip of guide indicated by *interrupted white arrow*). Note that the shape of the MP guide makes it unlikely that it will accidentally engage the left CCA. **B:** An extra-support wire *(white arrow)* has been placed in the external carotid artery (ECA) and a filter-type embolic protection device (EPD) *(black arrow)* has been placed in the internal carotid artery (ICA). **C:** Predilation over the EPD wire.

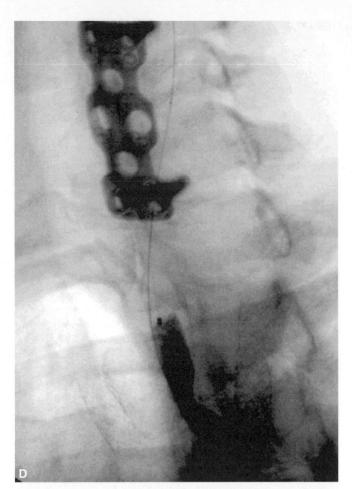

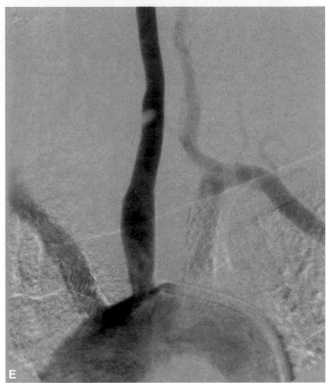

Figure 11.8 • *(Continued)* **D:** Placement of balloon-expandable stent at ostium of left CCA over the EPD wire. Note that the buddy wire has been sandwiched between the stent and artery wall. The buddy wire should be removed at the end of the procedure after removal of the EPD. **E:** Final angiogram of the left CCA.

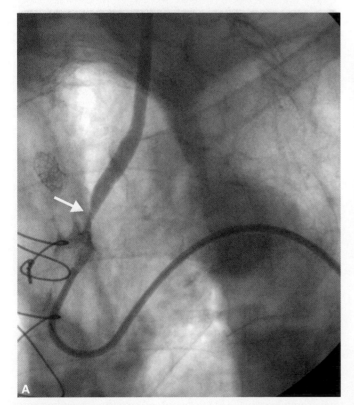

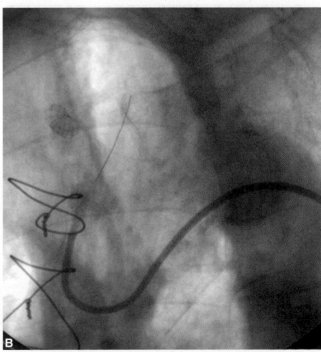

Figure 11.9 • **A:** Bovine origin of the left common carotid artery (CCA) with severe ostial disease *(arrow)*. An AL 1 guide is positioned proximal to the lesion without engaging the artery. **B:** A 0.014″ extra-support wire is passed into the external carotid artery (ECA) prior to placement of embolic protection device (EPD) in the internal carotid artery (ICA). *(Continued)*

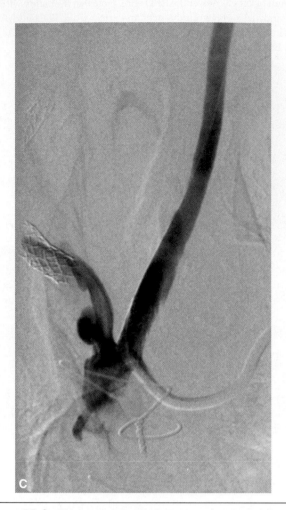

Figure 11.9 • *(Continued)* **C:** Final angiographic result following placement of balloon-expandable stent.

to allow monitoring of hemodynamics throughout the case and prevent inadvertent injection into plaque. Under roadmap guidance, advance a 0.035″ glidewire into the right subclavian artery through the diagnostic catheter in the right anterior oblique (RAO) projection. A stiff glidewire may be used if needed. Advance the diagnostic catheter into the right subclavian artery, and remove the glidewire. Advance a long (i.e., 260 cm) Super Stiff Amplatz wire or equivalent into the subclavian artery through the diagnostic catheter, and then remove the diagnostic catheter. Remove the short sheath from the patient's groin, and advance an 8 Fr. sheath over the Amplatz wire and position if in the aorta, with its tip adjacent to the ostium of the innominate artery. Because of the size of the stents needed to treat the innominate artery and the need for buddy wires, 8 Fr. sheaths are generally preferred. In particularly challenging cases, a 9 Fr. guide may be needed. Care must be taken not to disturb the lesion with the shuttle sheath or its dilator. Leaving the Amplatz wire in place, advance a 0.018″ guidewire into the right subclavian artery, and then remove the Amplatz wire. Advance a 0.014″ filter–type EPD into the right ICA, and deploy it in a suitable position in the cervical segment. Pre-dilate the innominate artery lesion with a

suitably sized balloon over the 0.014″ EPD wire. Take care to ensure that the balloon does not extend into the right CCA or right subclavian artery. Advance a suitably sized 0.014″ balloon-expandable stent over the EPD wire. If a 0.035″ balloon-expandable stent is used, it can be advanced over both the 0.018″ and 0.014″ wires. If it is truly an ostial lesion, then the stent will have to protrude slightly into the aorta to ensure proper coverage of the lesion. In patients with ostial disease, it is a good idea to post-dilate the ostial segment. Gently pull back the stent balloon, so that the distal portion is in the ostium, and post-dilate. The balloon should be pulled back very carefully as this can dislodge the stent. In patients with severe calcification, there is a risk of perforation with aggressive balloon dilation. If the patient complains of pain, stop inflating and deflate the balloon immediately. Once this step is complete, remove the EPD from the cervical ICA using the supplied recovery sheath, and then remove the 0.018″ buddy wire in the subclavian artery after performing final angiography.

For innominate bifurcation lesions, a kissing balloon technique is necessary (Fig. 11.10). This generally necessitates

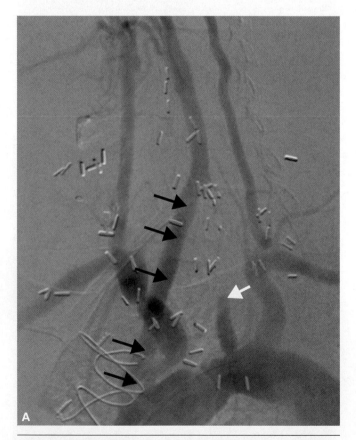

Figure 11.10 • **A:** A 50-year-old man reported right arm claudication and dizziness with upper extremity exertion. An 80-mm Hg pressure difference was noted between both arms. He was not deemed to be a surgical candidate due to the presence of severe three-vessel coronary allograft vasculopathy. Of note, he had a motor vehicle accident in 1992 resulting in occlusion of his left common carotid artery (CCA) *(white arrow)* requiring ascending aorta to left CCA bypass *(black arrows)*.

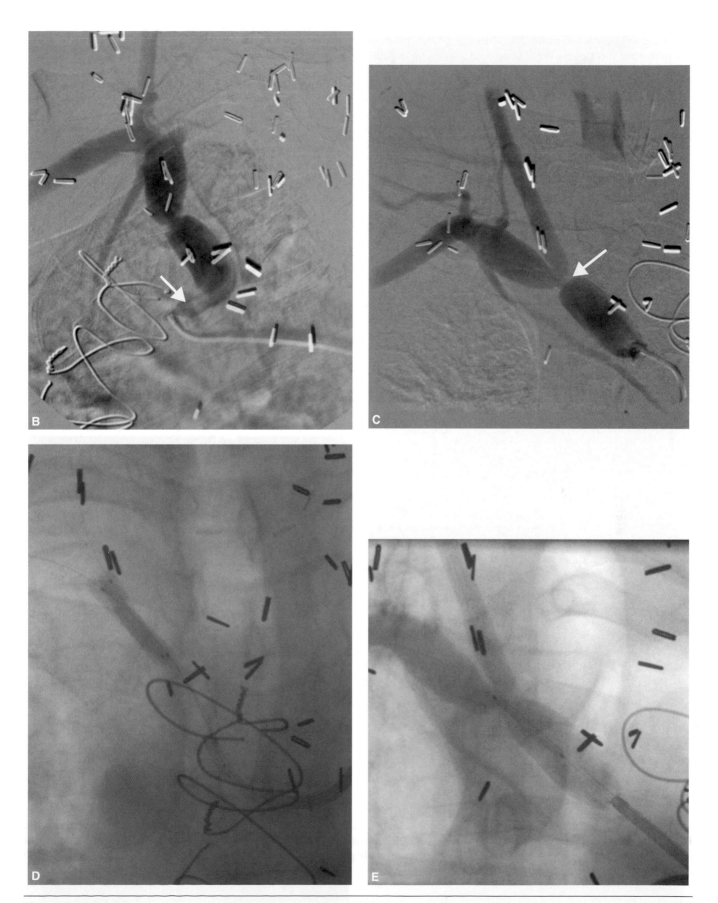

Figure 11.10 • *(Continued)* **B:** LAO view demonstrating a long tubular stenosis at the ostium of the innominate artery *(arrow)* with significant tortuosity. **C:** RAO view demonstrating a critical innominate artery bifurcation stenosis *(arrow)*. **D:** Kissing balloon pre-dilation of innominate artery bifurcation with 3.0 mm diameter balloons. **E:** 8 × 18 mm balloon-expandable stent placed over both wires. *(Continued)*

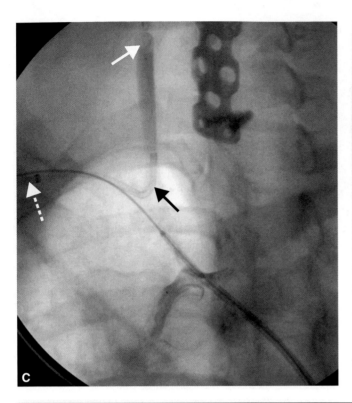
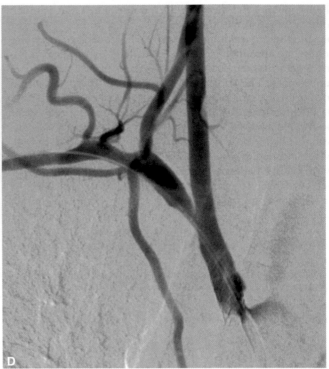

Figure 11.11 • *(Continued)* **C:** A 6 Fr. sheath was placed in the right brachial artery *(interrupted white arrow)*. A 6 Fr. LIMA guide *(black arrow)* and 0.014″ over-the-wire system were used to gain entry to the right CCA. A PercuSurge occlusion balloon *(white arrow)* was placed in the right CCA to protect the right ICA. A 0.035″ wire was advanced from femoral guide into the right SCA and an 8 × 18 mm balloon-expandable stent was advanced into the innominate artery. **D:** Final angiogram with restoration of flow to the carotid, right SCA, and right vertebral artery. Note the moderate lesion of the right SCA ostium that was not treated. The narrow angle of the innominate bifurcation would have necessitated the SCA stent encroach on the right CCA.

PROXIMAL AND OSTIAL RIGHT CCA DISEASE

These lesions represent a challenge due to the proximity of the lesion to the right subclavian artery and the potential for plaque shift. The anatomy must be completely evaluated in multiple projections, but the RAO projection with slight cranial or caudal angulation is usually most suitable to show the innominate artery bifurcation and proximal right CCA.

One option in these cases is to directly cannulate the innominate artery with an 8 Fr. guide catheter, such as a H1 guide (Cordis Corporation, NJ). If the position is felt to be secure, an EPD can be advanced into the ICA, and the lesion in the proximal right CCA can be treated with pre-dilation, stenting, and post-dilation. It is important to use a 300-cm long wire with the filter device, especially if the lesion will require treatment with an over-the-wire 0.035″ compatible over-the-wire stent. If the positioning is not felt to be secure, a buddy wire can be advanced into the right subclavian artery. In such cases, it may be necessary to use a 7 or 8 Fr. sheath as an 8 Fr. guide may not be large enough to support a buddy wire as well as a stent catheter.

A 9 Fr. H1 guide is an alternative in such situations, and has a distinct advantage in facilitating selective wiring of the CCA and right subclavian artery by providing some ability to direct the tip of the catheter. Balloon-expandable stents should be used for ostial lesions of the right CCA due to the need for precise placement. In this regard, if the diameter of the right CCA is approximately 7 mm or less, a balloon-expandable stent on a monorail platform that is designed for use at the ostium of the renal artery (e.g., Express SD) may be used. These stents have the advantage of being designed for delivery over a 0.014″ wire, and being of much lower profile than 0.035″ over-the-wire balloon expandable stents, which can be challenging to delivery over 0.014″ wires. However, these stents typically are only available on a stent delivery platform that is 90 cm in length. Therefore, using a 70-cm sheath or shortening the usual 100 cm H1 guide is necessary to allow delivery of such stents to this location. In treating true ostial CCA lesions it is usually necessary to extend the stent into the innominate artery, and care must be taken to prevent the stent from occluding the origin of the right subclavian artery. If it is necessary to stent across the origin of the subclavian artery, a balloon-expandable stent is mandatory so as to allow access to the subclavian through the stent. The option of surgical revascularization should always be considered and discussed with these patients.

TORTUOSITY OF THE CCA

Tortuosity of the CCA can limit the ability to advance a sheath or guide to the distal segment of the vessel. Attempts to advance through this significant tortuosity can result in vessel dissection. Even if the vessel is successfully negotiated, the resultant straightening of the vessel can translate the tortuosity distally, resulting in kinking of the cervical ICA. While mild-to-moderate tortuosity does not usually present a limiting problem, severe tortuosity (Fig. 11.12A) or diseased common carotid arteries (Fig. 11.12B) may be best addressed by positioning the sheath or guide proximal to the tortuous or diseased segment. As a result, it is usually preferable to use an 8 Fr. coronary guide catheter instead of a sheath. The curve at the distal end of the guide helps anchor the guide against the side of the proximal CCA or in the ostium of the vessel. In some cases, it may be necessary to use a buddy wire to stabilize the system.

DISTAL COMMON CAROTID ARTERY STENOSIS

In most cases, if there is a patent ECA available, then exchanging the diagnostic catheter for the sheath or guide should be done over a wire positioned in the ECA. This has been described in detail in Chapter 10. However, some patients may have high-grade distal CCA stenoses, or a high-grade stenosis or occlusion of the ostial ECA (Fig. 11.13A) limiting or increasing the risk of advancing a wire or diagnostic catheter into the ECA. In such cases, a 5 Fr. diagnostic catheter is advanced under roadmap guidance to the distal CCA over a soft-tipped 0.035″ wire. Leaving the diagnostic catheter in place, a long stiff wire with a short flexible tip, such as a Super Stiff Amplatz with a 1-cm soft tip, or a Supra Core wire, can be positioned in the distal CCA through the diagnostic catheter. The soft 1-cm distal tip of the Super Stiff Amplatz wire does not come with a pre-shaped curve, so a pigtail type curve needs to be created at the distal tip using a hemostat to reduce the risk of plaque disruptions (Fig. 11.13B). The diagnostic catheter is then removed over the stiff wire, the 5 Fr. short sheath in the groin is removed, and the desired sheath or guide can be advanced into the distal CCA. Care must be taken not to advance the sheath dilator into the lesion inadvertently as it is not radiopaque.

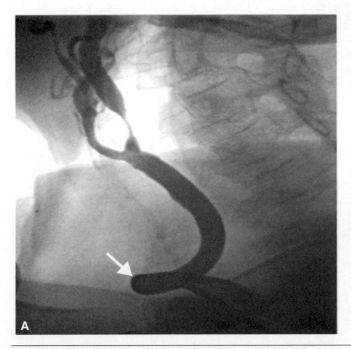
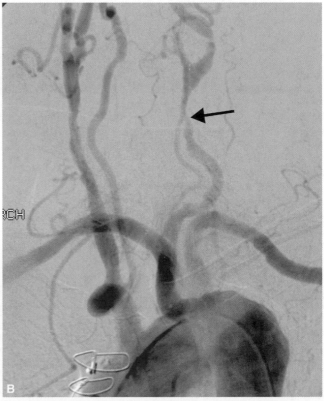

Figure 11.12 • Examples of severe tortuosity (*white arrow* in **A**) and disease (*black arrow* in **B**) of the left common carotid artery (CCA) that make delivery of a sheath or guide to the distal CCA difficult. Advancing a guide or sheath through these anatomic challenges can increase the risk of dissection and translate the tortuosity distally, resulting in kinking of the cervical internal carotid artery. In these cases, it may be useful to position an 8 Fr. H1 guide proximal to the tortuosity or disease.

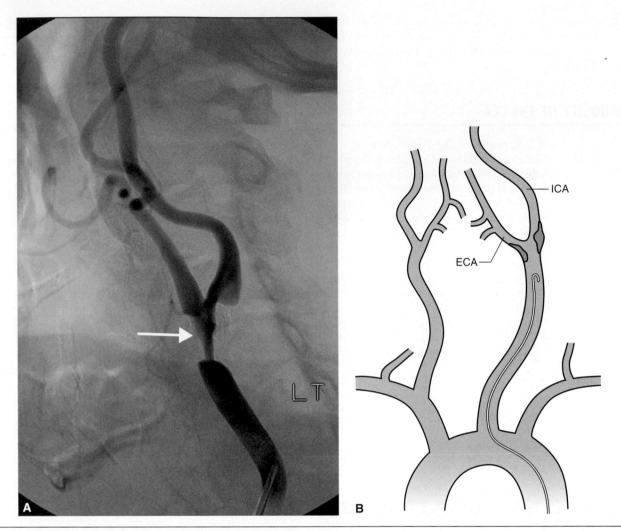

Figure 11.13 • High-grade stenosis in the distal common carotid artery *(arrow)* **(A)**. This makes it difficult to use the external carotid artery for catheter exchanges. As a result, a 1-cm, soft-tipped, Super Stiff Amplatz wire with a pigtail distal curve can be positioned in the distal common carotid artery, proximal to the lesion to facilitate sheath/guide delivery **(B)**.

The remainder of the procedure is performed as per usual techniques. Alternatively, an AL 1 guide can be positioned in the ostium and the risk of placing a guide or sheath into the common carotid avoided.

TORTUOUS INTERNAL CAROTID ARTERIES

Significant tortuosity of the cervical ICA can interfere with the ability to advance and deploy a distal filter–based EPD. However, not all tortuosity is prohibitive, and the ability to tackle patients with tortuous internal carotid arteries increases with experience (Fig. 11.14A,B). Inexperienced operators should avoid vessels that they are uncomfortable approaching. In general, one or two bends that are 90 degrees or less in severity can be readily addressed, as long as there is a suitable disease-free landing zone for the EPD. With more severe angulations, distal filter–type EPDs can become impossible to use (Fig. 11.14C).

The buddy wire technique can help in some situations. A soft or medium-support coronary 0.014″ guidewire is typically used. We prefer wires such as the BMW (Abbott Vascular) or the Runthrough (Terumo Corporation). It is important not to advance the buddy wire all the way into the petrous segment, as this will result in straightening of the cervical tortuosity and risk the creation of pseudostenoses. Once this occurs, it is difficult to advance the EPD. Thus, the buddy wire should first be advanced such that only the soft distal radiopaque tip is around the first bend of the tortuous segment in the cervical ICA. This distal radiopaque tip of the EPD wire is then positioned adjacent and parallel to the buddy wire. The two are then advanced together by gently advancing the buddy wire first, and then immediately following with the EPD. This will result in both wires going across the tortuous segment almost simultaneously. Once through the tortuous segment, the EPD can be advanced to a suitable location and deployed, after which the buddy wire can be removed (Fig. 11.15A,B).

The buddy wire technique is also helpful in cases where there is a sharp angulation of the origin of the ICA from the CCA (Fig. 11.16). In these cases, the EPD tends to prolapse into the ECA. By advancing a buddy wire into the ICA first, the angle of origin of the ICA can be made slightly more favorable for the EPD to enter the ICA.

Proximal balloon occlusion systems, such as the MOMA (Medtronic Invatec, Minneapolis, MN) or GORE Flow Reversal System (W.L. Gore and Associates, Phoenix, AZ), are good choices for patients with anatomy that precludes the use of distal filter–type EPDs. In fact, it can be argued that these systems should be used whenever there are anatomic challenges to placing distal filter–type devices. However, the cumbersome nature of proximal occlusion systems has limited their use thus far.

STRING SIGNS

The angiographic string sign refers to a very high-grade carotid stenosis with a long, thin, barely discernible post-stenotic segment (Fig. 11.17). The apparent stenosis can extend beyond the proximal ICA, into the mid-to-distal cervical segment, and sometimes the petrous segment of the ICA. However, the segment of the carotid artery beyond the proximal high-grade stenosis is often disease free, but has collapsed due to decreased perfusion pressure. In some cases, such as patients with a history of radiation exposure, the disease may truly extend into the distal cervical and petrous segments of the carotid artery. It is important to evaluate the vessel in multiple projections during angiography, with long imaging series to identify early filling and late phase filling.

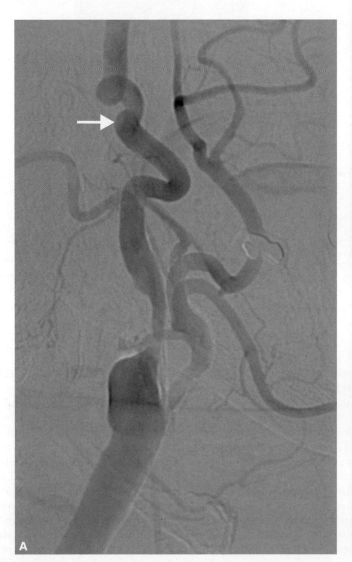
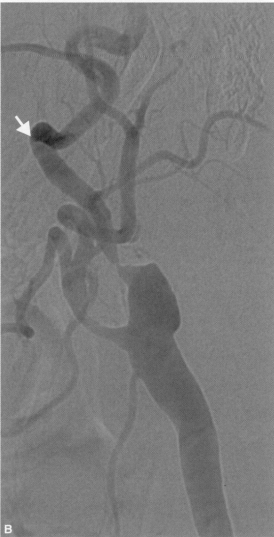

Figure 11.14 • Significant tortuosity (indicated by *white arrows*) of the cervical internal carotid artery can make use of distal filter–type embolic protection devices difficult, even in experienced hands **(A,B)**. *(Continued)*

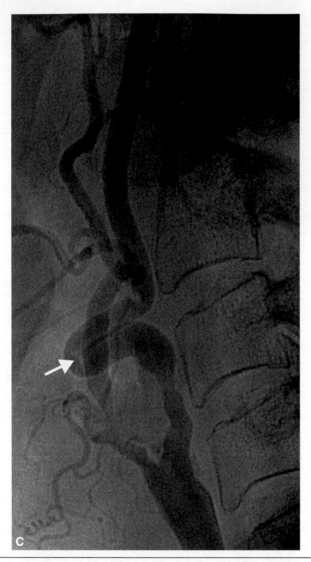

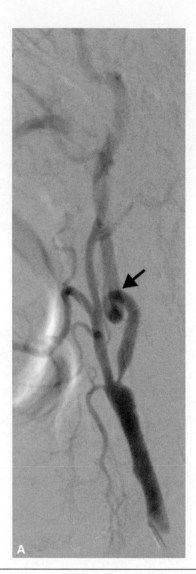

Figure 11.14 • *(Continued)* In some cases, use of a distal filter-type embolic protection device may be impossible **(C)**. In such cases, consideration must be given to surgical revascularization or proximal occlusion-type embolic protection devices.

Figure 11.15 • Use of a buddy wire can help negotiate significant tortuosity *(arrow)* of the cervical internal carotid artery **(A)**

Often what appears to be a very high-grade stenosis is actually a total occlusion with bridging collaterals (Fig. 11.18). Sometimes this may not be apparent until an attempt is made to cross the lesion with a wire.

There does appear to be a benefit after revascularizing string signs in symptomatic patients as compared to medical therapy alone, but the reduction in risk of stroke is not as significant as when high-grade stenoses in symptomatic patients without string signs are revascularized. It is unclear if there is a benefit of revascularizing string signs in asymptomatic patients as the large randomized trials of asymptomatic patients comparing carotid endarterectomy to medical therapy did not require angiographic evaluation prior to revascularization.

Due to the severity of stenosis, lesions with angiographic string signs usually require pre-dilation prior to crossing with a distal filter–type EPD. This is helpful even in lesions

that are not string signs, but are so severe that the EPD may have difficulty crossing (Fig. 11.19). Once the sheath or guide is in place in the distal CCA, the lesion should be evaluated in multiple projections prior to crossing with a 0.014″ coronary guidewire. Hydrophilic wires should be avoided due to the risk of dissection unless absolutely necessary. Once the lesion has been crossed, it may be prudent to advance an over-the-wire coronary balloon beyond the lesion and inject through it to confirm intraluminal position. This will require the use of a long 0.014″ guidewire. Once intraluminal position is confirmed, the lesion can be pre-dilated gently. This is usually done with a 2.0 mm diameter coronary balloon. There is negligible risk of stroke when gently pre-dilating high-grade carotid stenoses with a small-diameter coronary balloon without an EPD.

Once the lesion has been pre-dilated successfully, angiography should be performed to better evaluate the carotid anatomy

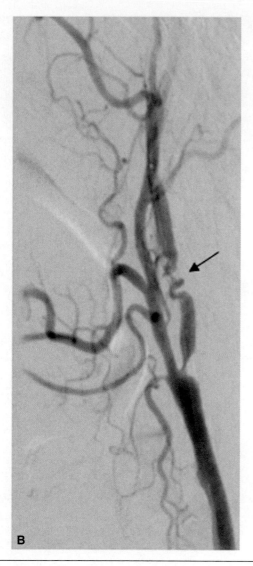

Figure 11.15 • *(Continued)* but can result in the formation of pseudostenoses *(arrow)* **(B)**.

distal to the lesion. Often intra-arterial verapamil or nitroglycerin can help maximally dilate the carotid artery beyond the lesion. If a suitable distal landing zone is present, a filter–type EPD can be advanced through the lesion and deployed. The remainder of the procedure can then be performed routinely. However, if there is significant disease distal to the proximal lesion, a long stent, or two stents, may have to be deployed. If there is insufficient space for a distal filter–based EPD, a proximal occlusion device can be considered. The use of proximal occlusion during the treatment of angiographic string signs has been described (6).

THROMBUS

Asymptomatic patients with an incidental discovery of thrombus or mobile plaque on ultrasound should be managed with anticoagulation and a repeat ultrasound study in

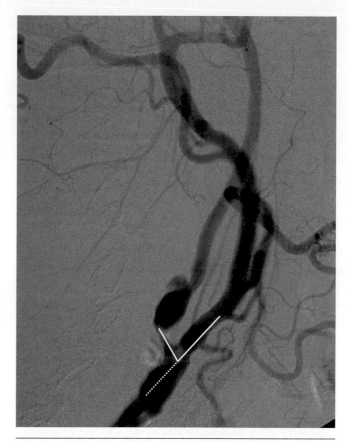

Figure 11.16 • The sharp angle of origin of the internal carotid *(solid white line)* artery from the common carotid artery *(interrupted white line)* can result in prolapse of embolic protection devices into the external carotid artery. The use of a buddy wire can be helpful in such cases.

6 to 8 weeks. Symptomatic patients with thrombus should be initially treated with anticoagulation but if they fail anticoagulation, surgery should be considered. If surgery is not an option, intervention can be performed by experienced operators. The technique is similar to the approach to acute stroke intervention. A proximal occlusion approach should be utilized due to risk of embolization during lesion crossing and treatment as well as the overall thromboembolic burden (Fig. 11.20).

CAROTID ANEURYSMS

Aneurysms and pseudoaneurysms of the extracranial carotid usually occur after trauma, surgery, or spontaneous dissection and may present as a pulsatile neck mass (Fig. 11.21). The primary goal of endovascular therapy is to isolate the aneurysmal sac, pseudoaneurysm, or false lumen in the presence of carotid dissection, from the true lumen while maintaining the long-term patency of the main artery (7,8). Placement of balloon-expandable or self-expanding stents, with or without detachable coils, is the mainstay of treatment. Self-expanding stent grafts are available from a number of companies and are used in the cervical portion of the carotid (Fig. 11.22). Balloon-expandable stent grafts (Jostent, Abbott Vascular) are

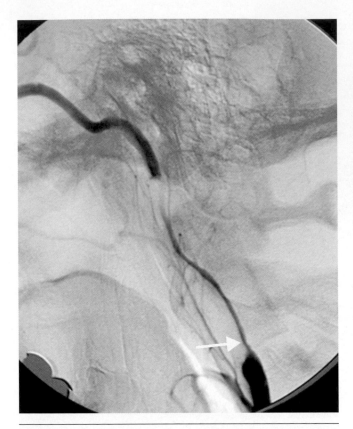

Figure 11.17 • The angiographic string sign: a very high-grade internal carotid artery stenosis *(arrow)* with disease that appears to extend into the mid and distal cervical segments. However, the vessel may be angiographically normal once the proximal cervical segment is treated and flow is restored into the mid and distal cervical segments.

preferred in the noncervical carotid due to precision of placement (Fig. 11.23). If the stent graft has to be placed across the external carotid, coil embolization of the external carotid is necessary prior to stent graft placement. Patency of the contralateral ECA must be established prior to coil embolization.

Intravascular ultrasound (IVUS) is frequently necessary for proper sizing and occasionally for discrimination of the true lumen. Significant guide support is necessary when placing these devices (due to increased caliber and stiffness of covered stents), and care has to be taken to prevent common carotid injury. There is also some risk of embolization of thrombus from within the aneurysm sac during wire and device placement. EPDs are typically not used due to the low risk of embolization and the need for good wire support. High-pressure (8 to 12 atm) dilation of the stent graft is mandatory to assure full expansion of the graft fabric. A residual contrast blush may be present through the stent graft but it typically resolves after reversal of anticoagulation.

CAROTID DISSECTION

Carotid dissections are broadly divided into traumatic (e.g., following motor vehicle accident, blunt injury, iatrogenic injury) and nontraumatic categories (i.e., spontaneous

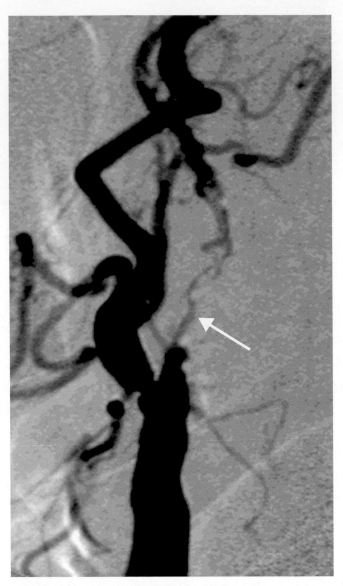

Figure 11.18 • Total occlusion of the internal carotid artery *(arrow)* with subsequent recanalization via bridging collaterals. These vessels should not be revascularized unless truly symptomatic.

carotid dissection). Within the latter category, the predisposing pathology may include fibromuscular dysplasia or collagen vascular disorders (e.g., Ehlers–Danlos syndrome), but is often not defined. Although more than 85% of medically treated patients with spontaneous carotid dissection improve clinically and angiographically, it can have a catastrophic presentation (Fig. 11.24), and there are at least four circumstances under which medical management may be insufficient: patients with recurrent symptoms despite anticoagulation, patients in whom anticoagulation is contraindicated because of the risk of bleeding, patients with an expanding or symptomatic pseudoaneurysm, and patients with significantly compromised cerebral blood flow due to the involvement of multiple vessels, poor collateral vessels, or both (9).

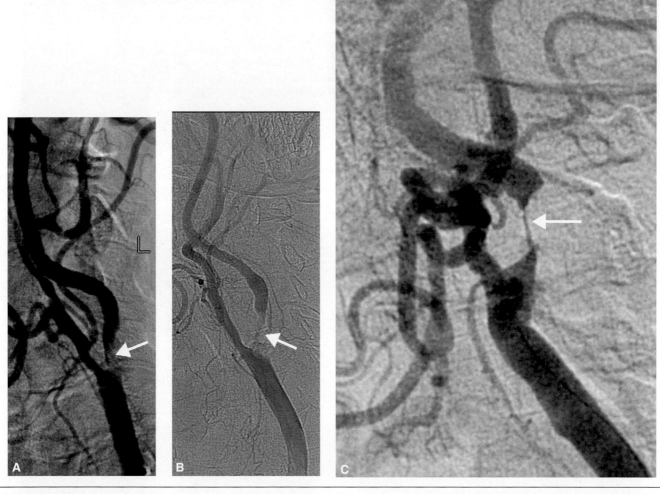

Figure 11.19 • A–C: Very high-grade stenoses of the proximal internal carotid artery *(arrows)*. All of these lesions are readily treatable by stenting, and do not constitute angiographic string signs. However, in each case, pre-dilation with a small coronary balloon before advancing an embolic protection device may be helpful.

It is critical to identify the true lumen of the dissected vessel using high-resolution angiography with high frame rates (5 to 10 frames/sec) and multiple projections. It is often helpful to perform nonsubtracted angiograms to better visualize the thin luminal flaps, which can be subtracted out with digital subtraction techniques. When there is doubt about the true lumen, a soft, nonhydrophilic 0.014″ wire should be passed distal to the lesion into the presumed true lumen; a microcatheter or 1.5 mm over-the-wire balloon should then be inserted distal to the lesion and aspirated for blood return. If there is blood return, a very gentle manual injection of 0.25 to 1 mL of contrast should be injected through the microcatheter or central balloon lumen to confirm that the tip is in the true lumen. It should be noted that simply obtaining a blood return is not sufficient, since the false lumen may have some degree of blood flow.

IVUS is often helpful for proper sizing since angiography is often misleading in the presence of severe vessel disruption. IVUS with agitated saline injections is also helpful in the identification

of the true lumen (Fig. 11.25). Cervical lesions may be treated with self-expanding stents. Previously, noncervical lesions were treated with coronary balloon-expandable stents. More recently, the availability of self-expanding stents specifically designed for use in the intracranial circulation (e.g., Neuroform—Boston Scientific, Enterprise—Codman, formerly Cordis Endovascular) has changed this paradigm. Although the latter stents are designed for use in the treatment of intracranial aneurysms, they are highly deliverable and are very effective in sealing carotid dissections that extend into the petrous portion of the carotid artery. Expanding pseudoaneurysms are treated with covered stents, either self-expanding or balloon-expandable, depending on the location. Excellent results are achievable in these patients but it should be kept in mind that arteries prone to spontaneous dissection are very fragile and it is easy to make the patient's situation worse. A very careful, precise technique is essential.

Some patients may have such severe redundancy and tortuosity of the carotid artery that a combined surgical and

Figure 11.20 • **A:** Patient with multiple transient ischemic attacks on intravenous heparin with mobile filling defect in a severely stenosed left internal carotid artery (ICA). **B:** Proximal occlusion is obtained with concentric balloon-tipped guide catheter and external carotid artery (ECA) is occluded with a PercuSurge GuardWire prior to crossing lesion with a 0.014″ wire. **C:** Final angiogram. The ICA stent was not aggressively dilated due to the risk of distal embolization. The distal ICA is small but will increase in caliber with increased perfusion pressure.

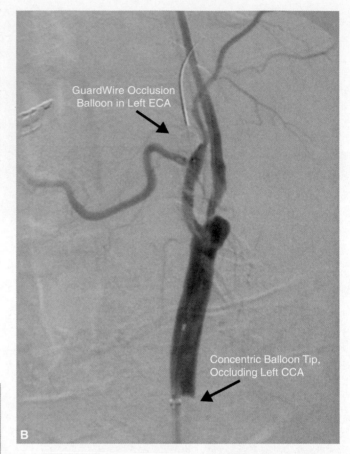

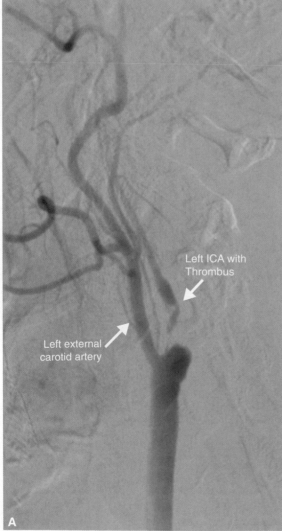

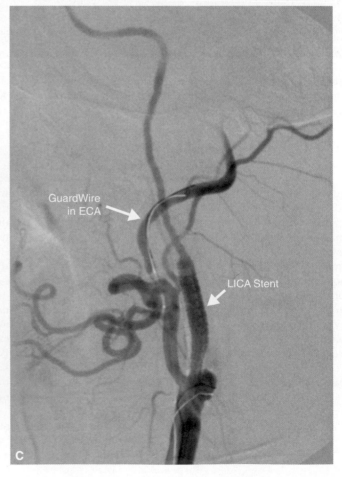

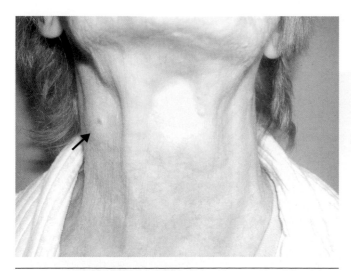

Figure 11.21 • Pulsatile cervical mass (location indicated by *arrow*) due to internal carotid artery aneurysm.

endovascular approach is necessary (Fig. 11.26). A portion of the common carotid is resected to reduce the redundancy of the ICA that can then be stented. It is helpful to perform abdominal angiography to visualize the renal arteries to help make the diagnosis of fibromuscular dysplasia (FMD).

POST-DILATION

Despite advances in procedural technique, use of EPDs, stringent patient selection, and increasing operator experience, there remains a risk of procedural stroke among patients undergoing carotid stenting (1,10–14). This risk appears to be especially high among octogenarians and symptomatic patients (15).

During carotid artery stenting (CAS) performed using filter-based EPDs, interrogation of the middle cerebral artery (MCA) by transcranial Doppler (TCD) has shown that embolic particles reach the MCA despite the use of embolic protection (16–19). Embolic signals are detected during all phases of the procedure. Some strokes can occur while the ipsilateral CCA is being accessed, due to manipulation of catheters and wires in the aortic arch and ostia of the great vessels. Such strokes can often be in the contralateral hemisphere, especially in patients with atheromatous disease of the aortic arch. The risk of a stroke during this phase is higher among patients with challenging anatomy requiring a longer and more aggressive manipulation of catheters and equipment in the aortic arch. Strokes occurring during this phase of the procedure likely account for 20% to 30% of all strokes that occur during carotid stenting.

However, the majority of strokes that occur during carotid stenting tend to occur during the post-dilation phase when a large balloon forces the stent struts into plaque at high pressure. This leads to a massive release of embolic particles when the balloon is deflated, a phenomenon that has been documented by TCD (Fig. 11.27). Such emboli result in new ischemic lesions on diffusion-weighted MRI (20–22), and embolization specifically during the post-dilation phase has been shown to be an independent predictor of adverse outcomes (23–25). Theoretically, the presence of an EPD should eliminate the risk of stroke during stenting and post-dilation. However, TCD data show us that despite the use of EPDs, emboli reach the MCA in almost every case.

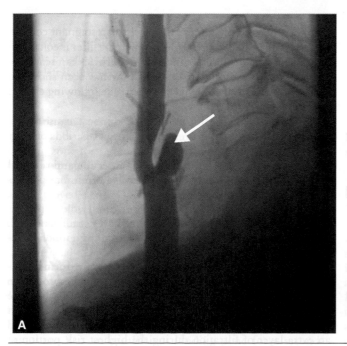
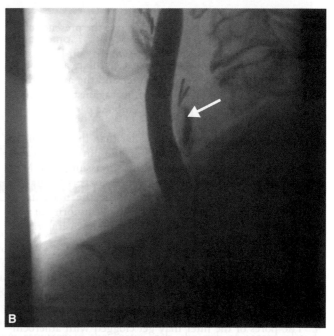

Figure 11.22 • **A:** Postsurgical pseudoaneurysm of left common carotid artery *(arrow)*. **B:** After placement of a covered self-expanding stent (Wallgraft), a small residual contrast blush is still noted *(arrow)*. This will resolve after reversal of anticoagulation.

Figure 11.25 • **A:** Patient with an expanding pseudoaneurysm after spontaneous carotid dissection due to fibromuscular dysplasia. Angiogram revealed a true and a false lumen. A 0.014″ BMW wire was placed across the presumed true lumen of the aneurysmal segment *(arrow)*. **B:** Intracarotid ultrasound across the lesion demonstrated simultaneous filling of both chambers with agitated saline contrast (* denotes the false lumen). **C:** The Jostent *(arrowheads)* was placed across the distal part of the aneurysm over the Synchro™ Neuro guidewire. **D:** Angiography after the first stent placement revealed residual leak into the false lumen through the proximal segment of the lesion.

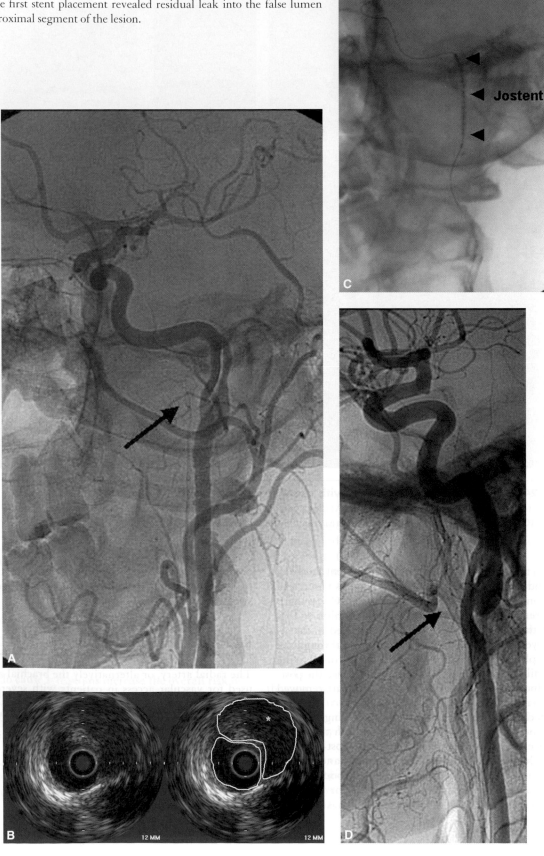

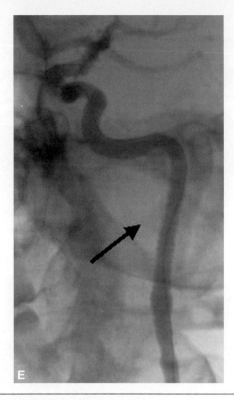

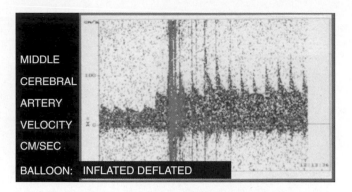

Figure 11.27 • Interrogation of the middle cerebral artery by transcranial Doppler shows a large number of embolic particles on deflation of the post-dilation balloon after stent implantation.

Figure 11.25 • *(Continued)* **E:** Placement of a second stent resulted in complete coverage of the false lumen.

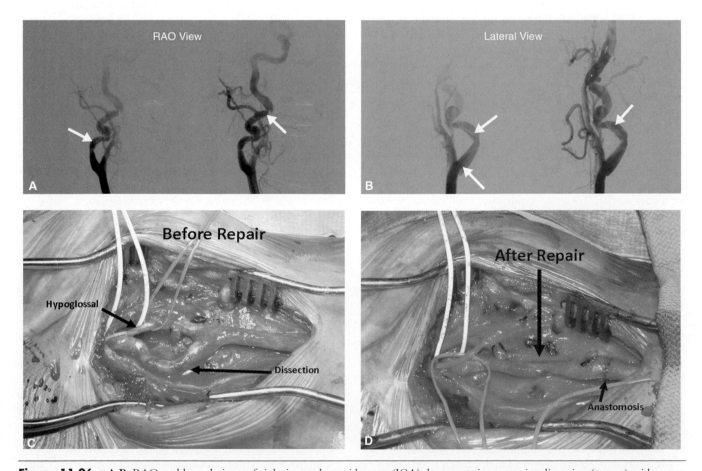

Figure 11.26 • **A,B:** RAO and lateral views of right internal carotid artery (ICA) demonstrating extensive dissection *(arrows)* with severe redundancy due to fibromuscular dysplasia. **C:** Intraoperative view demonstrating intramural hematoma at site of dissection. **D:** After resection of a segment of the common carotid, ICA redundancy is markedly reduced. The patient subsequently had successful right ICA stenting.

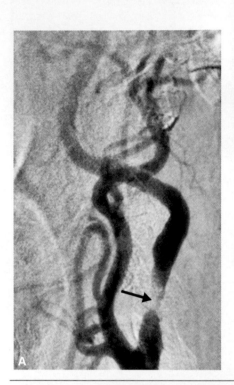 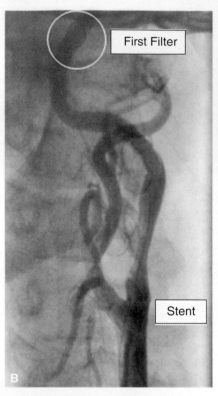 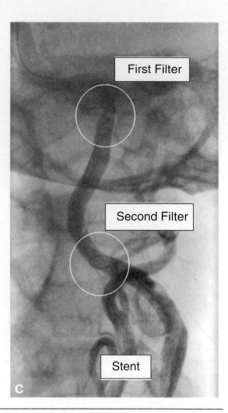

Figure 11.28 • Double filtration during carotid artery stenting. High-grade symptomatic left internal carotid artery stenosis *(arrow)* in a patient with crescendo transient ischemic attacks **(A)**. A distal filter is deployed in the internal carotid artery and the lesion is stented **(B)**. Prior to post-dilation, a second filter is deployed in the internal carotid artery, positioned proximal to the first filter and distal to the stent **(C)**. The lesion is then post-dilated, and the filters are sequentially removed.

For right internal carotid lesions, a Vitek or Simmons 1 diagnostic catheter is advanced from the left radial artery access site into the aortic arch over a wire, and then pulled back to engage the right CCA (Fig. 11.29A). If necessary, a 0.025″ glidewire can be used. Once the right CCA has been accessed, an extra-support coronary guidewire, such as a Mailman (Boston Scientific), or Grand Slam (Abbott Vascular), is advanced into the ECA under roadmap guidance. The Simmons 1 catheter is then advanced into the ECA over the extra-support wire (Fig. 11.29B). The 0.014″ wire is removed, and a 260-cm, 0.035″ J-wire is advanced through the diagnostic catheter into the ECA. In cases where the ECA is occluded or the ostium is severely diseased, the J-wire can be positioned in the distal CCA. This must be done meticulously and deliberately under roadmap guidance to prevent sudden jumping of the system into the ICA. Once the diagnostic catheter is removed, a 6 Fr. sheath is advanced over the J-wire and positioned in the distal CCA (Fig. 11.29C). The remainder of the procedure is done in the usual manner.

Approaching the left ICA via the right radial approach is slightly more difficult as there is no innominate artery to act as a support. An exception is in patients with a bovine origin of the left CCA from the innominate artery, which is very readily accessed via the right radial approach (Fig. 11.30) as the innominate artery provides support. In cases where the

left CCA arises from the aortic arch, the technique is similar. A Vitek or Simmons 1 diagnostic catheter is placed in the aortic arch and used to access the left CCA. An extra-support coronary guidewire is then advanced into the left ECA under roadmap guidance. Care must be taken to prevent prolapse of the Vitek or Simmons 1 catheter into the aorta. Once the diagnostic catheter is in the ECA, the 0.014″ wire is removed and replaced with a 260-cm, 0.035″ J-wire or a 260-cm Super Stiff Amplatz wire. A 6 Fr. sheath can then be advanced to the distal left CCA. In most cases, the shuttle sheath will rest against the contralateral wall of the aortic arch during the procedure.

Other combinations of catheters and guides can be used. While we have found the above technique to be reliable, reproducible, and safe, the risk of an unsuccessful case is higher when treating a left carotid lesion as compared to a right carotid lesion (27).

CONCLUSIONS

With proper patient selection, extensive training and experience, and a thorough knowledge of anatomy and equipment, the majority of ICA lesions can be treated successfully using percutaneous means. It is essential to be deliberate

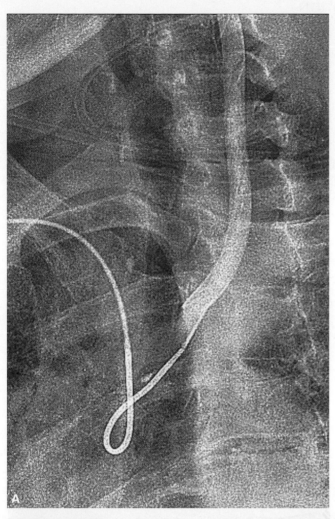

Figure 11.29 • Radial artery access for treatment of a right internal carotid artery lesion. A Simmons 1 diagnostic catheter is used to cannulate the right common carotid artery **(A)**. It is then advanced into the right external carotid artery over a stiff 0.014″ coronary guidewire **(B)**. A 0.035″ exchange length J-wire is advanced into the external carotid artery, and a 6 Fr. sheath is then positioned in the distal right common carotid artery **(C)**.

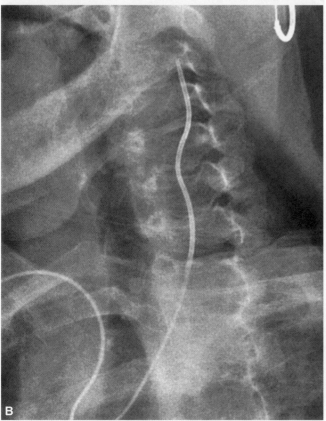

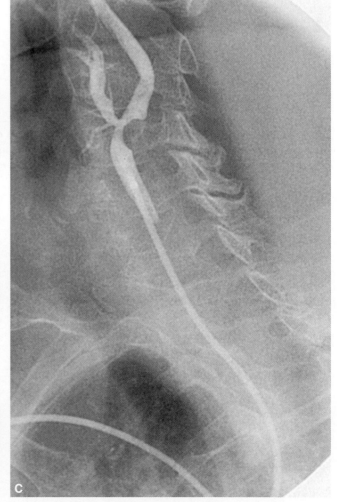

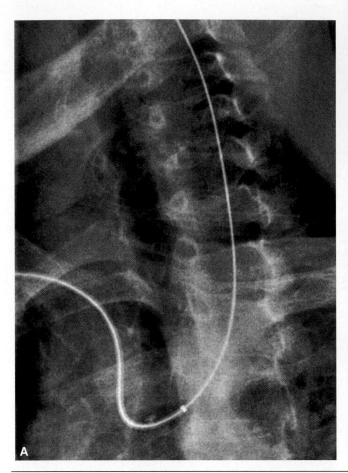

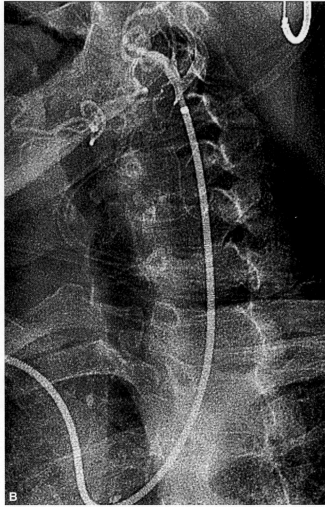

Figure 11.30 • Radial artery access with a bovine origin of the left common carotid artery. The ostium of the bovine left common carotid artery is accessed with a 6 Fr. AL 1 coronary guide **(A)**. A 0.035″ guidewire is advanced to the distal segment, and a 6 Fr. sheath is advanced over the wire to the distal common carotid artery **(B)**.

with each step, have meticulous technique, and not to cut corners. It is equally important to recognize one's limitations and know when to say no. One must keep in mind that the goal is not to prove the superiority of one technique over another, but to revascularize the patient with as low a risk as possible.

References

1. Gray WA, Yadav JS, Verta P, et al. The CAPTURE registry: results of carotid stenting with embolic protection in the post approval setting. *Catheter Cardiovasc Interv.* 2007;6:341–348.
2. Katzen BT, Criado FJ, Ramee SR, et al., CASES-PMS Investigators. Carotid artery stenting with emboli protection surveillance study: thirty-day results of the CASES-PMS study. *Catheter Cardiovasc Interv.* 2007;70(August):316–323.
3. Rubartelli P, Brusa G, Arrigo A, et al. Transcranial Doppler monitoring during stenting of the carotid bifurcation: evaluation of two different distal protection devices in preventing embolization. *J Endovasc Ther.* 2006;13:436–442.
4. Ackerstaff RG, Suttorp MJ, van den Berg JC, et al. Prediction of early cerebral outcome by transcranial Doppler monitoring in carotid bifurcation angioplasty and stenting. *J Vasc Surg.* 2005;41:618–624.
5. Chang FC, Tummala RP, Jahromi BS, et al. Use of the 8 French Simmons-2 guide catheter for carotid artery stent placement in patients with difficult aortic arch anatomy. *J Neurosurg.* 2009;110(March):437–441.
6. Nikas DN, Ghany MA, Stabile E, et al. Carotid artery stenting with proximal cerebral protection for patients with angiographic appearance of string sign. *JACC Cardiovasc Interv.* 2010;3(March):298–304.
7. Mukherjee D, Roffi M, Yadav JS. Endovascular treatment of carotid artery aneurysms with stent grafts. *J Invasive Cardiol.* 2002;14:269–272.
8. Chan AW, Yadav JS, Krieger D, et al. Endovascular repair of carotid artery aneurysm with Jostent covered stent: initial experience and one-year result. *Catheter Cardiovasc Interv.* 2004;63:15–20.
9. Edgell R, Abou-Chebl A, Yadav J. Endovascular management of spontaneous carotid artery dissection. *J Vasc Surg.* 2005;42:854–860.

10. Yadav JS, Wholey MH, Kuntz RE, et al. Protected carotid-artery stenting versus endarterectomy in high-risk patients. *N Engl J Med.* 2004;351:1493–1501.
11. White CJ, Iyer SS, Hopkins LN, et al. Carotid stenting with distal protection in high surgical risk patients: the BEACH trial 30 day results. *Catheter Cardiovasc Interv.* 2006;67:503–512.
12. Gray WA, Hopkins LN, Yadav S, et al. Protected carotid stenting in high-surgical-risk patients: the ARCHeR results. *J Vasc Surg.* 2006;44:258–268.
13. Safian RD, Bacharach JM, Ansel GM, et al. Carotid stenting with a new system for distal embolic protection and stenting in high-risk patients: the carotid revascularization with ev3 arterial technology evolution (CREATE) feasibility trial. *Catheter Cardiovasc Interv.* 2004;63:1–6.
14. Macdonald S. Is there any evidence that cerebral protection is beneficial? Experimental data. *J Cardiovasc Surg (Torino).* 2006;47:127–136.
15. Mathur A, Roubin GS, Iyer SS, et al. Predictors of stroke complicating carotid artery stenting. *Circulation.* 1998;97:1239–1245.
16. Ribo M, Molina CA, Alvarez B, et al. Transcranial Doppler monitoring of transcervical carotid stenting with flow reversal protection: a novel carotid revascularization technique. *Stroke.* 2006;37:2846–2849.
17. Powell RJ, Alessi C, Nolan B, et al. Comparison of embolization protection device-specific technical difficulties during carotid artery stenting. *J Vasc Surg.* 2006;44:56–61.
18. Chen CI, Iguchi Y, Garami Z, et al. Analysis of emboli during carotid stenting with distal protection device. *Cerebrovasc Dis.* 2006;21:223–228.
19. Schmidt A, Diederich KW, Scheinert S, et al. Effect of two different neuroprotection systems on microembolization during carotid artery stenting. *J Am Coll Cardiol.* 2004;44:1966–1969.
20. Pinero P, Gonzalez A, Mayol A, et al. Silent ischemia after neuroprotected percutaneous carotid stenting: a diffusion-weighted MRI study. *Am J Neuroradiol.* 2006;27:1338–1345.
21. du Mesnil de Rochemont R, Schneider S, Yan B, et al. Diffusion-weighted MR imaging lesions after filter-protected stenting of high-grade symptomatic carotid artery stenoses. *Am J Neuroradiol.* 2006;27:1321–1325.
22. Cosottini M, Michelassi MC, Puglioli M, et al. Silent cerebral ischemia detected with diffusion-weighted imaging in patients treated with protected and unprotected carotid artery stenting. *Stroke.* 2005;36:2389–2393.
23. Hammer FD, Lacroix V, Duprez T, et al. Cerebral microembolization after protected carotid artery stenting in surgical high-risk patients: results of a 2-year prospective study. *J Vasc Surg.* 2005;42:847–853 [discussion 853].
24. Schluter M, Tubler T, Steffens JC, et al. Focal ischemia of the brain after neuroprotected carotid artery stenting. *J Am Coll Cardiol.* 2003;42:1007–1013.
25. van Heesewijk HP, Vos JA, Louwerse ES, et al. New brain lesions at MR imaging after carotid angioplasty and stent placement. *Radiology.* 2002;224:361–365.
26. Casserly IP, Abou-Chebl A, Fathi RB, et al. Slow-flow phenomenon during carotid artery intervention with embolic protection devices: predictors and clinical outcome. *J Am Coll Cardiol.* 2005;46:1466–1472.
27. Folmar J, Sachar R, Mann T. Transradial approach for carotid artery stenting: a feasibility study. *Catheter Cardiovasc Interv.* 2007;69:355–361.

CHAPTER 12

Extracranial Vertebral Artery Disease

Debabrata Mukherjee, Pareena Bilkoo, and Ken Rosenfeld

Compared with anterior cerebral circulation ischemia, our knowledge regarding ischemia of the posterior cerebral circulation is more rudimentary. With improved technology that allows imaging of the brain and vascular lesions causing vertebrobasilar ischemia (VBI), this gap has closed and many misconceptions have been challenged.

Based on data from a well-characterized group of patients with signs and symptoms of posterior circulation ischemia ($n = 407$), the causes of VBI have been defined (1). Embolism is the dominant mechanism, accounting for approximately 40% of cases. Emboli may arise from the heart (usually thrombus), aorta (usually atheroma), or proximal vessel thrombus (predominantly the vertebral artery). Large artery disease, predominantly involving the vertebral artery, is the second most common mechanism accounting for approximately 32% of cases, with ischemia being produced on a hemodynamic basis or by occlusion of important penetrating or circumferential branches arising from the diseased vessel. The remaining cases are caused by a variety of conditions such as dissection, fibromuscular dysplasia, migraine, and rare arteriopathies that often involve the vertebral artery. These data highlight the importance of vertebral artery disease in causing posterior cerebral circulation ischemia, a phenomenon that has previously been underappreciated in clinical practice.

Atherosclerosis is the dominant pathology seen in the vertebral artery and has a predilection for the origin and proximal section of the extracranial (i.e., termed the V1 segment) and the intracranial portion of the vessel. The focus of this chapter will be on the interventional management of patients with proximal extracranial vertebral artery (ECVA) disease. Management of intracranial artery disease is discussed in Chapters 13A and 13B. Although it has generally been considered that ECVA disease has a more benign outcome compared to intracranial vertebral artery disease, significant occlusive disease of the proximal vertebral artery was present in 20% of patients who presented with VBI at a tertiary referral center and was felt to represent the primary cause of ischemia in 9% of patients (2).

ANATOMY

The vertebral artery typically arises from the superoposterior aspect of the first part of the subclavian artery and is usually the first branch of this vessel. In approximately 5% of patients, the left vertebral artery arises directly from the aortic arch, between the origin of the left common carotid and left subclavian arteries (Fig. 12.1).

Other rare anomalies have been described including origin directly from the aortic arch distal to the left subclavian artery, origin distal to the thyrocervical branch of the subclavian artery, origin of the right vertebral from the right common carotid artery, and duplication of the vertebral artery that may occur at any level of the artery (3).

The vertebral artery is arbitrarily divided into four anatomic parts (Fig. 12.2)

- V1—The portion extending from the origin to the point at which it enters the transverse foramina of either the fifth or sixth cervical vertebra.
- V2—The course within the intervertebral foramina until exiting at the level of the atlas (i.e., C2).
- V3—The extracranial segment between the transverse process of the C2 and the base of the skull, as it enters the foramen magnum.
- V4—The final intracranial portion that begins as it pierces the dura and arachnoid mater at the base of the skull and ends as it meets its opposite vertebral artery to form the midline basilar artery at the level of the medullopontine junction.

The intracranial part gives off major anterior and posterior spinal arteries to the medulla and spinal cord, minute penetrating vessels to the medulla, and the largest branch, the posterior inferior cerebellar artery (PICA), to a portion of the dorsal medulla and cerebellum. One of the vertebral arteries is often larger (i.e., left more frequently than right) and provides most of the blood supply to the posterior circulation (i.e., dominant artery). Stenosis of the dominant artery is more likely to cause symptoms.

CLINICAL PRESENTATION OF EXTRACRANIAL VERTEBRAL ARTERY DISEASE

Extracranial vertebral artery (ECVA) disease causing hemodynamic compromise typically produces dizziness accompanied by other signs of hind-brain ischemia (e.g., diplopia, hemiparesis, bilateral leg weakness, numbness) consistent with global ischemia of the posterior circulation (4,5). The nonspecific nature of a number of these symptoms, particularly in an elderly population, has contributed to the failure to associate vertebral artery disease and VBI.

Embolization from proximal vertebral atherosclerosis produces a variety of syndromes based on the site of distal embolization. The typical sites of embolization include the PICA, superior cerebellar artery (SCA), and posterior cerebral artery. Obstruction

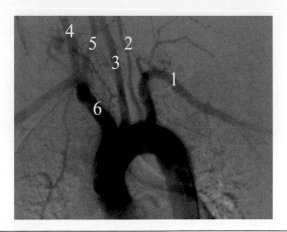

Figure 12.1 • Left vertebral artery arising directly from the aortic arch. 1. Left subclavian; 2. Left vertebral; 3. Left common carotid; 4. Right common carotid; 5. Right vertebral; 6. Innominate.

of circumferential arteries (e.g., PICA, SCA) results in typical lateral syndromes that affect cerebellar function, sensation, and lateral cranial nerves. In contrast, the clinical presentation following obstruction of midline perforator branches is highly variable. In general, midline syndromes tend to affect the pyramidal system, consciousness, and midline cranial nerves.

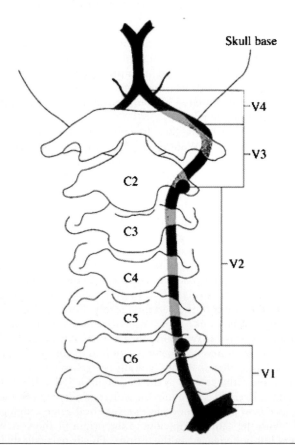

Figure 12.2 • Schematic of the four parts of the vertebral artery. (From Cloud GC, Markus HS. Diagnosis and management of vertebral artery stenosis. *QJM.* 2003;96(1):27–54, by permission of Oxford University Press.)

PATIENT SELECTION

Considerable controversy surrounds the indications for endovascular intervention for occlusive disease of the ECVA. The reasons for this have been well described and are multiple (6). Relatively inexpensive, noninvasive testing with ultrasonography has been unreliable in this location. CT and MR angiography also have significant limitations, often resulting in the need for routine invasive angiography to help make a reliable anatomic diagnosis of disease. In contrast to the treatment of carotid bifurcation disease, there is an absence of an effective and safe surgical therapy for the treatment of proximal ECVA disease. These factors have contributed to a knowledge gap, with respect to vertebral artery disease and the potential for revascularization to alter the natural history of the disease.

Endovascular approaches to proximal ECVA disease have transformed approaches to therapy. In contrast to surgical revascularization, where surgical accessibility is particularly demanding and likely contributes to the very high morbidity and mortality rates for these procedures (i.e., approximately 20%) (7), endovascular access is straightforward, and the techniques of angioplasty and stenting are readily applied to the treatment of proximal ECVA stenoses. Although endovascular ECVA revascularization has been practiced at multiple centers for over two decades, the techniques continue to evolve, and currently available data are still derived from relatively small registries. Therefore, appropriate decisions regarding patient management remain hampered by a lack of data.

Despite these limitations, it is generally accepted that intervention is indicated in patients with symptomatic vertebral artery stenosis who fail or are intolerant of medical therapy. Intervention in patients with symptomatic disease without a trial of medical therapy is also probably justified, in view of the outcomes reported from observational studies. Decisions regarding intervention in asymptomatic patients are more uncertain. A thorough review of the clinical history and angiographic findings by a neurologist, together with the interventionist, is recommended. Factors that will influence the decision include the severity of the stenosis, the angiographic appearance of the stenosis (i.e., friability, presence of ulceration), the adequacy of collateral flow, and the age of the patient. A severe, ulcerated stenosis without good collateral flow, in a relatively young, asymptomatic patient may be approached after appropriate discussion with the patient.

ENDOVASCULAR INTERVENTION FOR ECVA DISEASE

Arterial Access

The choice of an appropriate arterial access site is crucial to performing safe and successful angiography, and intervention of the vertebral artery (4). Access is typically obtained using the retrograde common femoral artery (CFA) approach. Ipsilateral brachial artery access is considered in individuals with bilateral, severe, iliac artery stenosis or distal aortic occlusions. Brachial access may also be indicated in patients with severe tortuosity or stenosis of the proximal subclavian artery, Type III aortic arch anatomy, or an acute angulation of the origin and proximal segment of the vertebral artery. If brachial or radial artery access is used, 3000 to 5000 U of unfractionated heparin should be injected through the sidearm of the sheath immediately following sheath insertion to minimize the risk of thrombosis, and liberal use of intra-arterial vasodilators such as nitroglycerin (in 100 μg boluses), verapamil (100 to 200 μg boluses), or nitroprusside (100 to 200 μg boluses) is recommended to prevent spasm.

DIAGNOSTIC ANGIOGRAPHY

Arch Aortogram

Where possible, an arch aortogram should be performed prior to attempts at selective cannulation of the vertebral arteries (4). Arch aortography is typically performed in the LAO 30° to 45° projection, using an injection rate of 20 cc/sec for a total of 40 cc and a PSI limit of 1000. This allows an assessment of the complexity of the aortic arch, the origin of the great vessels from the arch, and some information about the origin of the vertebral arteries (Fig. 12.3).

Typical arch anatomy with separate origin of the brachiocephalic, left carotid, and left subclavian arteries is seen in more than 70% of cases. A shared origin of the brachiocephalic trunk and left common carotid artery is seen in 15% of cases, while a bovine arch (i.e., origin of the left common carotid artery from the brachiocephalic trunk) is seen in 8% to 10% of cases (Fig. 12.4).

Selective Vertebral Artery Angiography

When using femoral access, the initial goal of vertebral artery angiography is engagement of the innominate or left subclavian artery angiography. One should start with a catheter

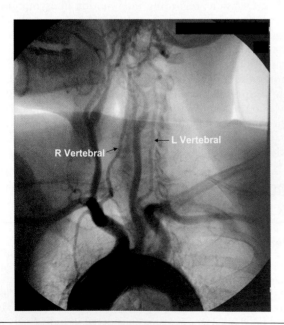

Figure 12.3 • Arch aortogram in left anterior oblique 30° projection visualizing both vertebral arteries.

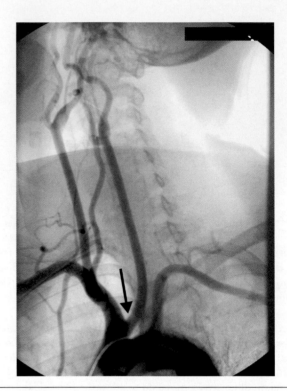

Figure 12.4 • A bovine arch, which defines the origin of the left common carotid artery (*arrow*) from the brachiocephalic trunk.

appropriate to the aortic arch type, rather than repeatedly scraping the arch with an inappropriate catheter that increases the risk of stroke and other procedural complications. In most patients, both the innominate and left subclavian arteries may be cannulated with a Bernstein, JB1, or Judkins® Right (JR4) catheter.

A Vitek® (COOK Inc., Bloomington, IN) or a Headhunter® (Meditech, Watertown, MA) catheter is a reasonable initial catheter choice in individuals with a moderately tortuous arch and Simmons® 1 or 2 catheters (Angiodynamics, Queensbury, NY) are reasonable options in individuals with a severely tortuous arch. Since even small emboli may have devastating consequences if they embolize the cerebral circulation, the use of gentle and meticulous technique is imperative. Following engagement of the appropriate great vessel, an appropriate 0.035 in. wire should be advanced into the axillary artery (typically under roadmap guidance), allowing subsequent delivery of the Bernstein, JB1, or JR4 catheter to a position close to the origin of the vertebral artery. For uncomplicated anatomy, a Wholey or Magic torque wire may suffice, whereas tortuous anatomy may require the use of an angled glidewire. If a Vitek or Simmons catheter is required to engage the great vessel, these catheters should typically be exchanged for a more deliverable catheter such as the Bernstein or JB1 catheter following delivery of a wire into the axillary artery. The authors' practice is to perform nonselective vertebral artery angiography, with the catheter tip close to the origin of the vertebral artery but not engaged in the ostium. This is particularly important where proximal V1 segment disease is suspected. An inflated blood pressure cuff on the ipsilateral arm will help maximize visualization of the vertebral artery during nonselective angiography.

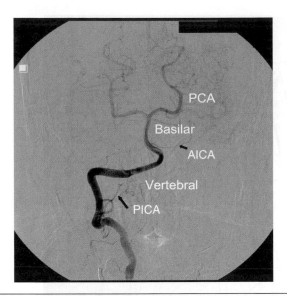

Figure 12.5 • Digital subtraction angiogram of the right vertebral artery in the posteroanterior (PA) projection. AICA, anterior inferior cerebellar artery; PICA, anterior inferior cerebellar artery.

The ostia of the vertebral arteries are typically visualized in the contralateral oblique projection, although some variation should be expected. The remainder of the V1 segment, and the V2 and V3 segments, is visualized using posteroanterior (PA) and lateral views. Alternatively, a single ipsilateral oblique view may suffice. The intracranial posterior circulation is best visualized in steep (i.e., approximately 40°) PA cranial (i.e., Townes view) (Fig. 12.5) and cross-table views (Fig. 12.6).

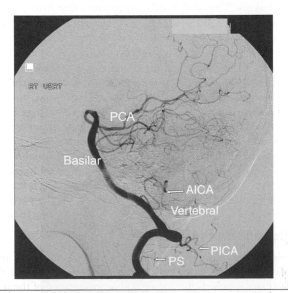

Figure 12.6 • Digital subtraction angiogram of the right vertebral artery in the lateral projection. AICA, anterior inferior cerebellar artery; PICA, posterior inferior cerebellar artery; PS, posterior spinal artery.

INTERVENTION

Anticoagulation/Antithrombotics

All patients should have received aspirin (i.e., 325 mg daily) and clopidogrel (i.e., 300 to 600 mg loading dose, followed by 75 mg daily) for at least 2 days prior to the procedure. A baseline activated clotting time (ACT) is obtained prior to the interventional procedure. The patient then receives a weight-adjusted bolus of unfractionated heparin of 60 U/kg body weight, to ensure a value greater than twice baseline ACT, or longer than 250 seconds. The role of glycoprotein IIb/IIIa inhibitors during vertebral artery intervention is not well defined and therefore, currently, is not recommended.

Guide/Sheath

Vertebral artery intervention may be performed using either a sheath or guide system. When using brachial access, a long (i.e., 35 cm length) 5 or 6 Fr. sheath may be used, with newer stent systems (e.g., Cobalt Blue, Cordis Corporation) being deliverable through a 5 Fr. sheath. Minimization of sheath size is important in minimizing ischemic complications associated with brachial access. When using the retrograde CFA approach, an 80-cm long 6-Fr. Shuttle sheath or 100 cm long 8 Fr. guide (e.g., JR4, H1, or Multipurpose) may be used. The use of the sheath is favored in patients with severe PVD or ostial subclavian artery disease because of the lower profile (4).

When using a guide, the telescoping technique employed for carotid intervention may be employed to facilitate safe delivery of the guide to the region of the vertebral artery ostium (Fig. 12.7). With this technique, a long 125-cm diagnostic catheter (e.g., JR 4, JB 1) is telescoped through the guide and used to engage the ostium of the subclavian/innominate artery. A wire (e.g., Wholey® or stiff-angled glidewire) is then advanced into the axillary artery, and the diagnostic catheter is advanced over the wire into the distal subclavian artery. The guide is then advanced over the wire–catheter combination into the proximal subclavian artery, near the vertebral artery origin. A useful option is to leave an 0.035 in. Wholey wire in place in the axillary or brachial artery, to stabilize the guide during the intervention. This may be particularly useful in patients with marked proximal tortuosity of the subclavian or innominate arteries.

When using a sheath, one may similarly telescope the long 125-cm diagnostic catheter through the sheath, engage the subclavian with the catheter, advance the 0.035 in. wire (Wholey or angled glidewire) distally as before, and advance the diagnostic catheter into the axillary artery. At this point, the authors typically exchange the 0.035 in. wire for a stiff wire (e.g., stiff Amplatz wire, SupraCore wire), remove the diagnostic catheter, and advance the sheath with its dilator, such that the sheath is positioned proximally to the vertebral artery. The sheath tip is placed very close to the ostium of the vertebral artery, without actually intubating it.

Wires

Once the ACT is longer than 250 seconds, the lesion is traversed with a 0.014 in. exchange length wire (e.g., BMW® wire, Asahi soft, Abbott Vascular). Hydrophilic wires should generally be avoided, to minimize the risk of dissection or perforation, which could have devastating consequences in this area. Some vertebral arteries are very tortuous and a hydrophilic wire may be necessary, initially, to wire the vessel (e.g., Whisper®, Pilot® 50).

occlusive device has a lower crossing profile than filter devices and may be used for severe stenoses in which occlusion of ipsilateral vertebral flow does not produce symptoms. Qureshi et al. demonstrated the feasibility of performing stent placement for vertebral artery origin stenosis using a distal protection device (Filter EX; Boston Scientific, Natick, MA) in 12 patients with symptomatic vertebral artery origin stenosis (12). Technical success was achieved in 11 of the 12 patients in whom distal protection device placement was attempted (12). Further studies are indicated to assess the safety and effectiveness of emboli-protection devices during vertebral artery intervention.

Potential Complications

Potential major complications include posterior circulation distribution strokes and transient ischemic attacks (TIAs). These events are generally embolic and occur in approximately 1% of interventions. Most other complications are related to access site issues and include hematomas, pseudoaneurysms, and arteriovenous fistulas at the CFA access site, and ischemic complications at the brachial access site.

POSTPROCEDURAL CARE

Patients are generally observed overnight following the procedure, with frequent neurologic checks. Hypertension should be treated, to minimize the risk of reperfusion hemorrhage, and hypotension should also be avoided. The optimum blood pressure range is 110 to 130 mm Hg systolic and over 70 to 85 mm Hg diastolic. Patients are discharged on lifelong aspirin therapy and clopidogrel 75 mg daily for a minimum of 1 month. Long-term appropriate follow-up monitoring is extremely important in detecting potential recurrence of symptoms and restenosis. It is also imperative that these patients be treated with adequate secondary prevention agents such as beta-blockers, statins, and angiotensin-converting enzyme (ACE) inhibitors, which in turn translates into improved clinical outcomes (13).

CLINICAL OUTCOMES

In patients with significant stenosis involving the vertebral or basilar artery territories, transluminal angioplasty may be of significant benefit in alleviating symptoms and improving blood flow to the posterior cerebral circulation. However, adequate dilation of the origin of the vertebral artery with balloon angioplasty, alone, has resulted in high restenosis rates of 10% in one series (14) and up to 75% in another series (15). Arterial spasm and dissection may occur in some instances, with subsequent hemodynamic compromise (6,11). These data have encouraged the use of stents for vertebral artery lesions.

Several case series and one small trial of patients treated with vertebral artery stenting have been reported (Table 12.1) (8,10,16–18). The trial of 16 patients was underpowered and failed to show a benefit of endovascular treatment of vertebral artery stenosis over medical therapy.

The data show that stent placement for symptomatic stenosis involving the vertebral artery is safe and effective for alleviating symptoms of VBI, with good long-term results. Overall technical success is greater than 90%, with less than 1% risk of procedural complications including stroke. Late stroke is uncommon (i.e., less than 1%) and restenosis is seen in 8% to 10% of patients. The use of drug-eluting stents may further reduce restenosis rates in the future as suggested by one retrospective case series (22).

FUTURE PERSPECTIVES

Future advances using MR technology to delineate plaque composition/characteristics may help better define the indications for intervention, particularly in asymptomatic patients. Randomized trials with, and without, the use of filter devices will better define the risks and benefits of intervention compared to medical therapy. As mentioned before, drug-eluting stents may further improve long-term outcomes in patients undergoing vertebral

TABLE 12.1 Studies of Vertebral Artery Stenting

	n	Technical Success	Procedural Complications	Improvement in Symptoms	Mean Follow-Up (Months)	Late Stroke	Restenosis
Mukherjee et al. (10)	12	100%	None	12/12	6.4	0	1/12
Malek et al. (18)	13	100%	1 TIA	11/13	20.7	0	N/A
Jenkins et al. (19)	32	100%	1 TIA	31/32	10.6	0	1/32
Chastain et al. (8)	50	98%	None	48/50	25	1	5/50
Levy (20)	8	88%	1 TIA	7/8	6	0	N/A
Cloud et al. (21)	10	100%	None	14/14	33.6	0	1/10
Coward et al. (16)	8*	100%	2 TIA	N/A	56.4	0	3/7†
Lin et al.‡ (22)	11	100%	NONE	11/11	18.7	0	0/11

*6/8 (75%) of the patients underwent balloon angioplasty alone without stenting.
†3/6 patients treated with angioplasty had restenosis, one patient who was treated with primary stenting did not have follow-up imaging.
‡Drug-eluting stents are implanted.
TIA, transient ischemic attack; N/A, not available.

artery intervention by reducing restenosis. Continued innovation and refinement of endovascular devices and techniques, together with optimization of pharmacologic regimens, will improve technical success rates, reduce complications, and broaden the applications of endovascular therapy for cerebrovascular diseases.

References

1. Caplan L. Posterior circulation ischemia: then, now, and tomorrow. The Thomas Willis Lecture-2000. *Stroke*. 2000;31:2011–2023.
2. Wityk RJ, Chang HM, Rosengart A, et al. Proximal extracranial vertebral artery disease in the New England Medical Center Posterior Circulation Registry. *Arch Neurol*. 1998;55:470–478.
3. Koenigsberg RA, Pereira L, Nair B, et al. Unusual vertebral artery origins: examples and related pathology. *Catheter Cardiovasc Interv*. 2003;59:244–250.
4. Mukherjee D, Pineda G. Extracranial vertebral artery intervention. *J Interv Cardiol*. 2007;20:409–416.
5. Caplan LR. Vertebrobasilar disease. *Adv Neurol*. 2003;92:131–140.
6. Rocha-Singh K. Vertebral artery stenting: ready for prime time? *Catheter Cardiovasc Interv*. 2001;54:6–7.
7. Phatouros CC, Higashida RT, Malek AM, et al. Endovascular treatment of noncarotid extracranial cerebrovascular disease. *Neurosurg Clin N Am*. 2000;11:331–350.
8. Chastain HD, Campbell MS, Iyer S, et al. Extracranial vertebral artery stent placement: in-hospital and follow-up results. *J Neurosurg*. 1999;91:547–552.
9. Jain S, Ramee S, White C. Treatment of atherosclerotic vertebral artery disease by endoluminal stenting: results from a multicenter registry. *J Am Coll Cardiol*. 2000;35:86A.
10. Mukherjee D, Roffi M, Kapadia SR, et al. Percutaneous intervention for symptomatic vertebral artery stenosis using coronary stents. *J Invasive Cardiol*. 2001;13:363–366.
11. Piotin M, Spelle L, Martin JB, et al. Percutaneous transluminal angioplasty and stenting of the proximal vertebral artery for symptomatic stenosis. *Am J Neuroradiol*. 2000;21:727–731.
12. Qureshi AI, Kirmani JF, Harris-Lane P, et al. Vertebral artery origin stent placement with distal protection: technical and clinical results. *Am J Neuroradiol*. 2006;27:1140–1145.
13. Mukherjee D, Lingam P, Chetcuti S, et al. Missed opportunities to treat atherosclerosis in patients undergoing peripheral vascular interventions: insights from the University of Michigan Peripheral Vascular Disease Quality Improvement Initiative (PVD-QI2). *Circulation*. 2002;106:1909–1912.
14. Higashida RT, Tsai FY, Halbach VV, et al. Transluminal angioplasty for atherosclerotic disease of the vertebral and basilar arteries. *J Neurosurg*. 1993;78:192–198.
15. Crawley F, Brown MM, Clifton AG. Angioplasty and stenting in the carotid and vertebral arteries. *Postgrad Med J*. 1998;74:7–10.
16. Coward LJ, McCabe DJ, Ederle J, et al. Long-term outcome after angioplasty and stenting for symptomatic vertebral artery stenosis compared with medical treatment in the Carotid And Vertebral Artery Transluminal Angioplasty Study (CAVATAS): a randomized trial. *Stroke*. 2007;38:1526–1530.
17. Jenkins JS, White CJ, Ramee SR, et al. Vertebral insufficiency: when to intervene and how? *Curr Interv Cardiol Rep*. 2000;2:91–94.
18. Malek AM, Higashida RT, Phatouros CC, et al. Treatment of posterior circulation ischemia with extracranial percutaneous balloon angioplasty and stent placement. *Stroke*. 1999;30:2073–2085.
19. Jenkins JS, White CJ, Ramee SR, et al. Vertebral artery stenting. *Catheter Cardiovasc Interv*. 2001;54:1–5.
20. Levy EI, Hanel RA, Bendok BR, et al. Staged stent-assisted angioplasty for symptomatic intracranial vertebrobasilar artery stenosis. *J Neurosurg*. 2002;97:1294–1301.
21. Cloud GC, Crawley F, Clifton A, et al. Vertebral artery origin angioplasty and primary stenting: safety and restenosis rates in a prospective series. *J Neurol Neurosurg Psychiatry*. 2003;74:586–590.
22. Lin YH, Hung CS, Tseng WY, et al. Safety and feasibility of drug-eluting stent implantation at vertebral artery origin: the first case series in Asians. *J Formos Med Assoc*. 2008;107:253–258.

Acute Ischemic Stroke

Alex Abou-Chebl and Vincent V. Truong

Acute ischemic stroke (AIS) is the leading cause of adult disability and the third leading cause of death in the United States. Despite these facts, AIS was considered to be untreatable until recently. Major advances in endovascular therapy in the past 10 to 15 years have now made treatment a reality with the potential for remarkable recovery. Although intravenous (IV) thrombolysis with tissue plasminogen activator (tPA) has been approved by the Food and Drug Administration (FDA) since 1996, it has been used in only 3% to 4% of ischemic stroke patients due to major limitations and a narrow 3-hour treatment window (1,2). In addition, IV-tPA is often ineffective, particularly in the treatment of large vessel occlusions (3,4), the most common cause of severe and fatal AIS. Fortunately, large vessel occlusions are amenable to endovascular therapy, analogous to acute coronary syndromes presenting as ST elevation myocardial infarction (STEMI). However, unlike acute coronary artery syndromes, which are most often caused by atherosclerotic plaque rupture, AIS and transient ischemic attacks may be caused by several different mechanisms including (1) cardiac embolism, (2) extracranial arterial atherosclerosis complicated by thrombosis or artery-to-artery embolism, (3) intracranial arterial atherosclerosis leading to thrombosis or hypoperfusion, (4) embolism from aortic atheroma, (5) perforator occlusion due to lipohyalinosis, arteriosclerosis, or embolism, (6) spontaneous or traumatic arterial dissection, (7) vasculitis, (8) venous thrombosis, and (9) miscellaneous other causes. Therefore, no single specific therapy will be effective for all cases, particularly when the multitude of factors (see below) affecting neurologic outcome are considered. These factors determine the risk of intracerebral hemorrhage (ICH), the most feared and devastating complication associated with all treatments for the treatment and prevention of ischemic stroke (5,6). This risk of ICH is the single limiting factor in almost all aspects of AIS treatment including recanalization therapy. The reality is that there is no effective treatment for ICH; moreover, when it complicates a revascularization intervention, the risk of mortality is 80%.

The heterogeneity of AIS and the specter of ICH mandate that stroke specialists have a thorough understanding of all clinical, anatomic, pathologic, and radiologic aspects of AIS. In this chapter, the authors will attempt to present a cursory discussion of these issues along with a detailed description of the current endovascular treatment techniques and devices.

CEREBRAL VASCULATURE— ANATOMIC CONSIDERATIONS

There are many similarities between atherosclerotic stroke and atherothrombotic events in other vascular territories, particularly in the coronary circulation. The vessels of the circle of Willis, most often associated with severe AIS, are comparable in size to the coronary arteries. These vessels include the paired internal carotid arteries (ICAs, 3 to 4 mm), middle cerebral arteries (MCAs, 2 to 3 mm), anterior cerebral arteries (ACAs, 1.5 to 2 mm), vertebral arteries (VAs, 2 to 3 mm), posterior cerebral arteries (PCAs, 1.5 to 2 mm), and the singular basilar artery (BA, 2.75 to 3.5 mm) (Figs. 13A.1–13A.4). The atherosclerotic process affecting the coronary arteries is the same process affecting the cerebral vessels with similar propensity for plaque progression and regression, and rupture. Furthermore, the fundamental principle of ACS treatment that early revascularization leads to reduced tissue injury and mortality also applies to the brain. Additionally, vessel revascularization to improve flow, treat thrombosis, and prevent embolization is the most effective means of preventing recurrent events. The same effective medical and interventional approaches for the treatment of CAD, both symptomatic and asymptomatic, are also effective for AIS and intracranial atherosclerotic disease.

Despite these similarities, there are major differences between the cerebral vessels and the coronary and other muscular arteries. First, the cerebral vessels are histologically different: they have no external elastic lamina, a thinner tunica media, and trivial adventitia, making them quite fragile. They also differ from the coronary arteries in being surrounded, in part, by bone (e.g., the petrous and cavernous carotids) or rigid and fibrous tissue (e.g., the dura matter). This, combined with the significant tortuosity in their proximal segments, makes the navigation of endovascular devices to the intracranial vessels extremely difficult if not impossible at times, which greatly increases the risk of vessel injury and perforation during endovascular therapy. The petrous and cavernous segments of the ICAs are the most tortuous and rigid, making access to the MCAs difficult. This is very problematic because approximately 80% of large vessel AIS involve the MCAs.

When vessel perforation or dissection occurs, catastrophic complications (i.e., fatal in up to 80% of cases) usually follow because the vessels course in the subarachnoid space, which is surrounded by the noncompliant skull. As a result, there is often a rapid increase in intracranial pressure leading to cessation of cerebral blood flow (CBF) and death. Neurosurgical rescue is rarely if ever beneficial, and in the presence of anticoagulants, antiplatelet agents, or fibrinolytics, surgery is often contraindicated. Another unique characteristic of the brain is that it is very sensitive to embolic debris, even if nearly microscopic in size.

The circle of Willis is another unique anatomic characteristic of the cerebral vasculature. This potentially robust source of collateral blood flow can completely restore flow to the territory of an occluded ICA or VA. The circle of Willis consists of

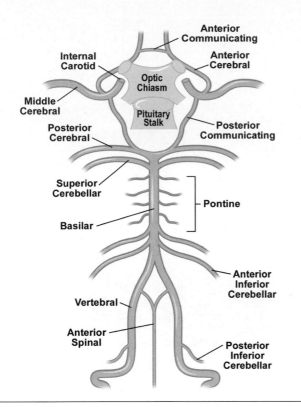

Figure 13A.1 • Schematic illustration of the anatomy of the circle of Willis demonstrating the location of the anterior communicating (ACOM) and posterior communicating (PCOM) arteries. Note that the ACOM artery links the right and left anterior cerebral arteries, and the PCOM links the ipsilateral distal internal carotid artery with the ipsilateral posterior cerebral artery.

the two posterior communicating arteries (PCom) connecting the terminal ICAs (arising posteriorly) and the PCAs and the anterior communicating artery (ACom) connecting the two ACAs (Figs. 13A.1 and 13A.2). Unfortunately, the circle of Willis is fully developed in only 25% of humans with numerous anatomic variants. Pial collaterals, which are connections between the distal branches of the MCAs, ACAs, and PCAs and the cerebellar arteries over the surface of the brain, provide a less robust potential collateral pathway.

Neurointerventionists must also be aware of the presence of multiple small perforating branches from both the MCAs and BA, which originate superiorly and posteriorly, respectively, to avoid their inadvertent cannulation. These are end arteries, have poor collaterals, and their ostia can potentially be occluded following angioplasty and stenting leading to ischemia. Other essential branches to be aware of include the ophthalmic artery arising anteriorly just distal to the cavernous ICA (Fig. 13A.2) and the very small anterior choroidal artery arising from the terminal ICA just distal to the PCom. Occlusion of this vessel causes infarction of the internal capsule with a resultant severe contralateral hemiplegia. The VA has several muscular branches in its distal cervical segments, and the posterior inferior cerebellar artery (PICA) can often arise extracranially at the C1 level. Intracranially, the VA gives off the PICA dorsally and just before the vertebrobasilar (VB) junction, each VA gives off the very small anterior spinal artery dorsomedially to the spinal cord (Figs. 13A.1 and 13A.3).

INDICATIONS

The indications for endovascular treatment (also referred to as intra-arterial therapy [IAT]) of AIS are evolving. Since there is no FDA-approved IAT for stroke, there is a great deal of variability between experts in the field with regard to the indications for treatment. In general, any patient with AIS presenting under 3 hours should be offered IV-tPA if they meet the appropriate clinical criteria. IAT may be offered to these patients with a clear understanding that the standard of care in AIS presenting less than 3 hours from symptom onset is IV-tPA administration. Those patients who do not meet the criteria for IV-tPA due to presentation beyond the 3-hour time window or some other factor(s) may be offered IAT. The traditional time window for IAT is up to 6 hours and that for mechanical embolectomy is 8 hours from stroke onset or the last time the patient was known to be neurologically intact. The authors and their colleagues have treated highly selected patients well beyond these time limits with excellent success, but such treatment does not represent the standard of care and is considered experimental (data in press).

All patients should be evaluated clinically, with laboratory tests and cerebral imaging before an intervention is contemplated. The duration of ischemia is a leading predictor of neurologic outcome (6,7). The patient must also have a clinical deficit severe enough to warrant intervention, both to justify the risk of the procedure and to ensure that an intervention is likely to be associated with a clinically significant benefit, since patients with mild strokes (National Institutes of Health Stroke Score [NIHSS] < 4) are unlikely to have a visible arterial occlusion and typically have a good outcome without endovascular therapy (8). In contrast, patients with the most severe strokes (NIHSS > 20) are less likely to benefit from treatment (7).

There are several contraindications to AIS intervention, with the primary consideration being any history or propensity for ICH (Table 13A.1). Therefore, all patients being considered for a cerebrovascular intervention must have a baseline computerized tomography (CT) scan of the brain to differentiate ischemic from hemorrhagic stroke. This is the current standard of care and no stroke revascularization therapy may be initiated without a baseline CT of the brain to exclude ICH or other contraindication(s).

Patients are best selected for IAT with the help of perfusion imaging. This technique permits the assessment of the ischemic penumbra (brain tissue that is ischemic but not irreversibly injured) and thus helps define any salvageable brain tissue and the size of the necrotic, irreversibly injured, core of the stroke. The ideal patient is one with little or no necrotic core and a large area of penumbra. These patients have the most to gain with the least risk, whereas patients with a large necrotic core, even with a concurrent large penumbra, have a high risk for ICH because revascularization of necrotic tissue is the presumed mechanism of hemorrhagic transformation. Those patients with no penumbra, even with no necrotic core, in general, have nothing to gain by interventional therapies. The penumbra and ischemic core can be assessed noninvasively with MR and CT imaging. With the former, diffusion-weighted images (DWI) generally predict the areas of infarct tissue, and perfusion-weighted images (PWI) indicate the hypoperfused regions. CT perfusion provides several possible types of images including cerebral blood volume (CBV) maps (Fig. 13A.5A), best predicting the

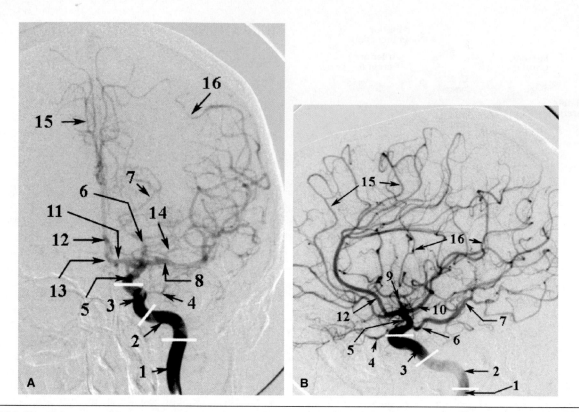

Figure 13A.2 • AP (**A**) and lateral (**B**) cerebral digital subtraction angiograms following selective left internal carotid artery (ICA) injection. 1, Cervical ICA; 2, petrous ICA; 3, cavernous ICA; 4, ophthalmic artery; 5, supraclinoid ICA (ICA terminus); 6, posterior communicating artery (PCom); 7, posterior cerebral artery (PCA); 8, middle cerebral artery, main trunk or M1 segment; 9, superior division of MCA; 10, inferior division of MCA; 11, anterior cerebral artery, precommunicating/A1 segment; 12, anterior cerebral artery, postcommunicating/A2 segment; 13, region of the anterior communicating artery (ACom); 14, lenticulostriate arteries; 15, distal ACA branches; 16, distal MCA branches.

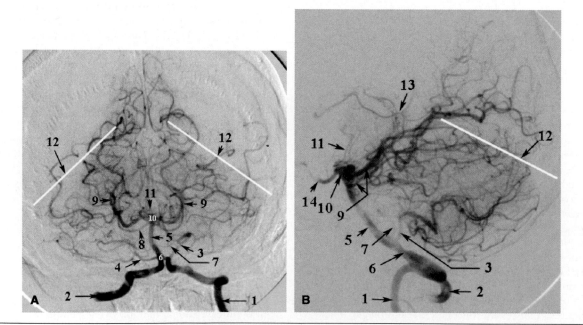

Figure 13A.3 • AP (**A**) and lateral (**B**) cerebral digital subtraction angiograms following selective left vertebral artery (VA) injection. 1, Left VA; 2, right VA; 3, left posterior inferior cerebellar artery (PICA), high but normal origin off left VA; 4, right PICA, anomalous origin from vertebrobasilar junction; 5, basilar artery (BA); 6, vertebrobasilar junction (VBJ); 7, left anterior inferior cerebellar artery (AICA); 8, right superior cerebellar artery (SCA); 9, bilateral posterior cerebral arteries (PCA); 10, top of the basilar; 11, thalamoperforators; 12, approximate location of the tentorium cerebelli that separates the cerebral hemispheres from the cerebellum (*white lines*); 13, posterior choroidal artery; 14, left posterior communicating artery (PCom).

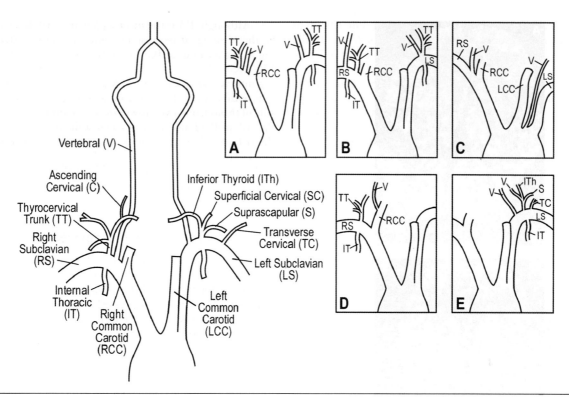

Figure 13A.4 • Normal and variant anatomy of the origin of the vertebral artery. **A:** Normal origin of the right and left vertebral artery as the first branch from the proximal subclavian artery. **B:** Origin of the right vertebral artery lateral to or as common trunk with thyrocervical trunk. **C:** Origin of the left vertebral artery from the aortic arch between the origin of the left common carotid and left subclavian arteries. **D:** Origin of the right vertebral artery from right common carotid artery, typically in patients with anomalous origin of the right subclavian artery. **E:** Dual or accessory origin of the vertebral artery from the thyrocervical trunk.

TABLE 13A.1 Contraindications to Acute Ischemic Stroke Intervention

Intracerebral hemorrhage (lobar, subdural, intraventricular)

Subarachnoid hemorrhage

History of ICH

Cerebral arteriovenous malformation or giant thrombosed cerebral aneurysm*

Computerized tomography evidence of > 1/3 MCA territory

Acute infarct or large ischemic core on perfusion imaging

Absence of ischemic penumbra

Uncontrolled hypertension > 185/110 mm Hg

Unknown stroke duration or duration > 6 hours

Thrombocytopenia < 100,000

Bleeding diathesis

International normalized ratio >1.7 (if fibrinolysis planned)

History of Alzheimer disease or amyloid angiopathy

*Unruptured, incidental, nonthrombosed aneurysms are not a contraindication.

necrotic core, cerebral blood flow (CBF) maps (Fig. 13A.5B), mean contrast transit time, and time-to-peak contrast density (a very sensitive marker for delayed flow but not a specific marker of tissue viability) (Fig. 13A.5C). There are controversies regarding these techniques and the exact definition of the penumbra. A full discussion of these issues is beyond the scope of this chapter. Interested readers should refer to the many publications on these matters, and nonstroke specialists should seek the assistance of stroke specialists to decide on which modalities to use and how to select patients appropriately.

CLINICAL ASPECTS

It is valuable to determine the likely etiology of the stroke prior to the intervention. For example, a lesion thought to be due to atherothrombosis may be approached differently than the one due to cardioembolism (9). A CT scan of the brain is mandatory in all patients and it is the standard means of differentiating AIS from ICH. Any sign(s) of ICH is an absolute contraindication to intervention, regardless of the size or severity of the deficit. Other modalities such as diffusion- and perfusion-weighted MR imaging may be useful in selecting the optimal patients for intervention since those with a large penumbra and a small ischemic core are the most likely to benefit from revascularization therapy with a lower risk of hemorrhagic transformation (10,11). Other factors such as patients' age, duration of ischemia, presence of early infarct signs, presenting blood pressure (BP), serum glucose level, and the presence of collaterals are also considered.

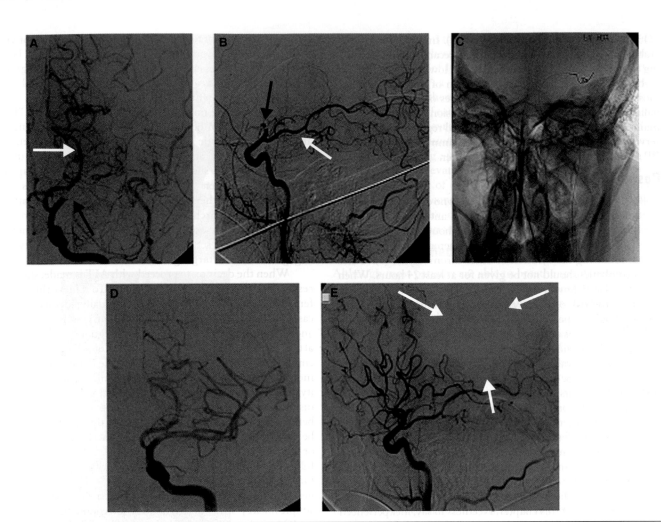

Figure 13A.6 • A 29-year-old woman presented 14 hours after the onset of a left middle cerebral artery (MCA) syndrome with a severe neurologic deficit. A CT scan showed subtle early changes in the insula and basal ganglia consistent with MCA trunk occlusion, and CT perfusion revealed a large penumbra throughout the MCA territory. **A,B:** AP and lateral cerebral angiography confirmed the presence of a terminal left internal carotid occlusion and MCA trunk occlusion *(black arrows).* Fetal posterior cerebral artery is shown by *white arrows.* **C:** A MERCI™ device was deployed in the left MCA truck with retrieval of two thrombus fragments and recanalization of the ICA but with residual MCA occlusion. **D,E:** PA and lateral cerebral angiography following angioplasty of the MCA trunk with a 1.5-mm balloon showing partial recanalization of the MCA trunk but with persistent occlusion of the inferior division of the MCA (note the wedge of absent arterial and capillary filling posterioraly marked by the arrows). Because of the prolonged duration of ischemia, evidence of an early infarct on CT, further treatment (particularly fibrinolysis), was not performed. The patient began recovery almost immediately and survived with a moderate deficit and nearly independent function.

have been used) over 0.5 to 2 hours (7,17,18). In the authors' opinion, waiting 2 hours for a fibrinolytic to take effect is too long; more rapid recanalization techniques such as multimodal therapy or mechanical clot extraction should be considered, particularly if the thrombus burden is high in large-caliber vessels such as the M1 segment of the MCA and the BA. If distal branch occlusions are the problem, microcatheter fibrinolytic infusions are appropriate. Depending on the clinical circumstances (see below), the dosage and rate of infusion can be adjusted, but based on personal experience and preference, a 30- to 45-minute duration of infusion is appropriate. The total dose of fibrinolytic is generally one fourth to one fifth of the IV dose (e.g., 5 to 20 mg of tPA, 1 to 4 U reteplase, etc.) (18–21) and infused primarily within and just proximal to the thrombus; however, some advocate infusion of a small amount of lytic immediately distal to the thrombus.

Multimodal Approach

Increasingly, the combination of both thrombolytic agents and GPIIb/IIIa antagonists has been described (9,17,22). The use of these agents seems to make sense in cases of atherosclerotic occlusions or artery-to-artery emboli, but less so in the setting of cardioembolism in which fibrin-rich clots are expected. However, the fundamental principle of AIS therapy is rapid and timely revascularization with the least risk of ICH. Therefore, when adding GPIIb/IIIa receptor antagonists to either fibrinolytics or angioplasty and stenting procedures, the neurointerventionist must weigh the definite increased risk of ICH versus the potential benefit. There are no randomized or large trial data available to guide the choice, route, and dosage of GPIIb/IIIa receptor antagonists but the same guidelines for fibrinolytic use also apply to GPIIb/IIIa receptor antagonists:

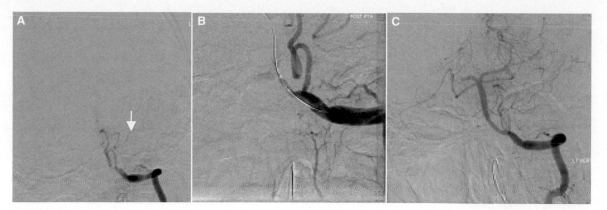

Figure 13A.7 • A 35-year-old male smoker with a family history of premature coronary artery disease presented with progressive dysarthria, left greater than right hemiparesis, horizontal gaze palsy, and sleepiness. He was outside of the IV-tPA window and underwent emergent angiography. Bilateral vertebral artery (VA) angiography revealed bilateral distal VA occlusions with no filling of the basilar artery (BA). **A:** Left VA angiogram showing distal occlusion of the left VA and filling of the posterior inferior cerebellar (PICA) only *(white arrow)*. The Penumbra™ 032 catheter was used to aspirate thrombus from the vertebrobasilar junction revealing an underlying critical atherosclerotic stenosis. **B:** Angioplasty was then performed followed by placement of a balloon expandable stent in the proximal BA and the distal VA. **C:** Final left VA angiography showing complete recanalization of the distal left VA and the BA but persistent occlusion of the right VA. The stent was intentionally undersized because the distal left VA could not accommodate a larger stent. The patient had complete recovery over the following 2 days.

use the smallest possible dose of the shortest acting agent (e.g., eptifibatide) and avoid them in the high-risk patients (see clinical aspects). The authors will typically begin with one fourth to one fifth of the usual loading dose of GPIIb/IIIa receptor antagonist (e.g., abciximab 5 to 15 mg, eptifibatide 4 to 12 mg) given directly within the thrombus alternating with small aliquots of fibrinolytic (e.g., tPA 1 to 4 mg, reteplase 0.5 to –1 U). Although the maximum dose of GPIIb/IIIa receptor antagonist is unknown, one half to three fourths of the usual weight-based bolus dose appears to be effective in most cases and certainly no more than the usual IV loading dose should be used. There is no indication for continuous infusion of these agents, or any fibrinolytic, or antithrombotic (even heparin) for that matter, following the procedure. The brain is not like the peripheral vasculature and prolonged infusions are associated with very high rates of ICH and death (23).

Mechanical Clot Disruption and Extraction

Purely mechanical approaches using balloons, snares, or embolectomy devices have been described (24–26). Angioplasty, especially of underlying atherosclerotic or stenotic lesions, has been highly effective in several large Japanese series (27,28). Recanalization rates of 91% have been described with lower risks of ICH compared with fibrinolysis (3% vs. >10%). Such high success with angioplasty may be unique to the Japanese population, which has a very high incidence of intracranial atherosclerosis causing ischemia, compared with an incidence of 8% to 10% in the United States (29–32). Although angioplasty is sometimes effective even in the absence of an underlying stenosis, stenting of an underlying stenosis or occlusion is almost always effective and should be considered in selected patients (9,21,33).

Stenting of the intracranial vessels is associated with very high recanalization rates. It is particularly effective for atherosclerotic, acute cervical ICA origin occlusions, but comes at a cost of potentially increased risk of complications and the need for dual antiplatelet therapy (34,35). The latter is potentially hazardous in

individuals who have large infarcts or receive therapy because of the increased risk of ICH; also if the patient were to develop a complete MCA infarct with brain swelling and herniation, the use of dual antiplatelet therapy may increase the risk of complications with potentially lifesaving decompressive hemicraniectomy. Acute stenting appears to be associated with high rates of early in-stent restenosis (unpublished data). Also, stenting at bifurcations, where emboli tend to lodge, can result in recanalization of one branch but not other (Fig. 13A.7). For these reasons, the author prefers angioplasty/stenting as a first-line strategy for the treatment of atherosclerotic occlusions. The authors also have low threshold for angioplasty/stenting in patients with cardioembolism who are able to tolerate potent platelet inhibition (i.e., patients who have no or minimal ischemic changes on initial CT) and who are deemed to be at high risk for malignant MCA syndrome or brainstem infarction; these two situations are associated with 40% to 90% mortality and less than 10% probability of a good outcome, so desperate measures may be justifiable even if they would mandate dual antiplatelet therapy.

All balloons must be undersized for the smallest segment in which they are to be placed, and stents should be slightly undersized or sized one to one if focal type A lesions are encountered. Oversizing a balloon or stent is associated with a high rate of vessel rupture and death and should never be performed in any cerebral vessel.

Mechanical embolectomy with the MERCI (Mechanical Embolus Removal in Cerebral Ischemia) Clot Retriever™ (Concentric Medical Systems Inc.) was approved by the FDA in August 2005 for the removal of "blood clots from the brain in patients experiencing an ischemic stroke" (Figs. 13A.8–13A.10) (36). With the aid of negative pressure applied through a balloon occlusion guide catheter, the device can be used to extract clots with a 45% to 58% efficacy (25). The single arm study of the device showed feasibility and safety but failed to show efficacy in terms of stroke outcomes or mortality compared with historical controls; this has been used by many

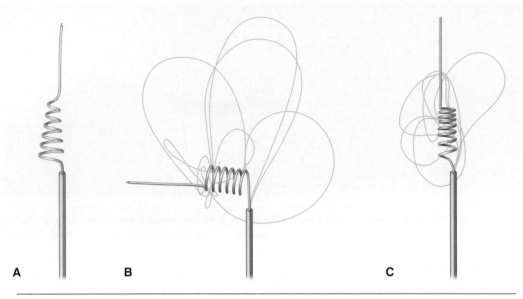

Figure 13A.8 • The MERCI™ devices.   Illustration of X6 **(A)**, L5 **(B)**, and V-series **(C)** devices.

as an argument that mechanical embolectomy is not an effective stroke treatment. None of the studies conducted with the MERCI™ retriever, nor its recent competitor the Penumbra™ (Penumbra Medical Inc.) system, was intended or powered to show efficacy. Therefore, it is a valid argument that these devices are not proven effective in stroke treatment. However, it is clear that recanalization, when appropriately timed, is the most effective treatment for stroke and these devices do recanalize vessels (Fig. 13A.7). Therefore, clinical benefit will be dependent on appropriate patient selection and safe endovascular technique. The main disadvantages of the MERCI™ and Penumbra™ clot retrieval devices are that they can cause vessel injury (<5%) and lesion wire access is lost with each clot extraction attempt (with the MERCI™ device) potentially requiring multiple wire passes through the lesion. Nevertheless, this approach may be the preferred therapeutic option in patients with presumed cardioembolic stroke or those in whom thrombolytics may be contraindicated or have failed.

The MERCI™ retrieval technique begins with placing a wire distal to the occlusion as described above. The

microcatheter is then removed and the appropriate MERCI™ microcatheter (as the X series of devices is phased out, the newer generations of retrievers are all compatible with the 18L microcatheter) is then advanced over the wire just past the site of occlusion. The site of occlusion can be found in several ways. The safest way is to simply film late when injecting the parent vessel and observe for retrograde pial collateral flow that often reaches the distal aspect of the occlusion. If collateral flow is so poor that no retrograde pial flow is seen, the interventionist should reconsider treating the patient since the complete absence of collaterals on angiography is a good predictor of inevitable infarction with little chance of neurologic recovery (37). The other technique is to place the microcatheter past the typical site of occlusion—in the MCA, it is usually the MCA bifurcation and in the BA, it is usually the proximal PCA—and then withdraw the wire to allow a gentle microcatheter contrast injection with digital subtraction angiography. This technique clearly defines the distal face of the thrombus, but it carries the risk of causing distal embolization as well as vessel perforation and ICH (38). Once the distal aspect of vessel occlusion is defined, the MERCI™ microcatheter is advanced just beyond it. The microguidewire is removed and the appropriate MERCI™ retriever is then slowly deployed by unsheathing it from the microcatheter, with the first one to two loops just distal to the thrombus and the remainder of the loops within the thrombus. The retriever should be sized for the smallest segment in which it will be placed. The stiff retrievers should be reserved for ICA occlusions, proximal thrombi in straight MCA trunks, and BA occlusions. The soft devices are safer for vessels <2.5 mm in diameter and MCA branch occlusions or where there is significant tortuosity or a bifurcation. After complete deployment and documenting the retriever has assumed its fully deployed configuration, the microcatheter is readvanced until it reaches the proximal loop. Both devices are then slowly withdrawn as a unit over 2 to 4 minutes while making sure not to pull back too quickly so that the retriever does not stretch and lose its shape, which it often does. When the retriever reaches

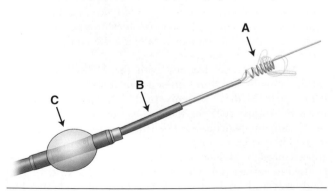

Figure 13A.9 • Illustration of Triaxial system with the MERCI™ microcatheter **(A)**, DAC™ **(B)**, and balloon occlusion guide catheter **(C)**.

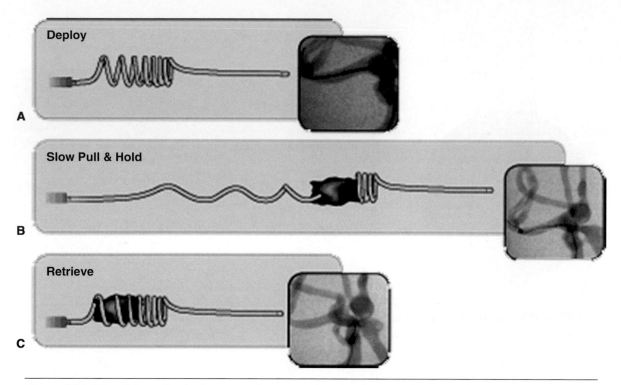

Figure 13A.10 • Schematic of technique used to extract clot using the Merci clot retrieval system. See text for details.

the terminal ICA or comes proximal to the VB junction, the balloon on the guide catheter should be inflated and gentle suction applied on the guide catheter central lumen. The retriever and microcatheter are continuously withdrawn under suction until they exit the guide catheter. The latter is then vigorously back-bled and control angiography is performed. If the first pass is unsuccessful, which is typical, the lesion is recrossed with the microguidewire and microcatheter, which are then exchanged for the MERCI™ system and the process is repeated. On average, three passes are needed for clot retrieval. Multiple retrievers are often needed, frequently requiring downsizing as the thrombus moves distally.

The Penumbra™ clot-extraction system is the second FDA-approved device for the removal of clots from the brain (Fig. 13A.11). It was tested in much the same way as the MERCI™ system in a single arm registry (26). A total of 125 patients were treated with a recanalization rate of 82% (39). The advantage of this system is that complete access to the lesion is not always lost, although it often is if the clot involves a bifurcation. Like the MERCI™ system, the Penumbra™ microcatheter of choice (i.e., the largest catheter that will fit in the occluded segment) is advanced into the lesion with an exchange-length wire. The MERCI™ and Penumbra™ microcatheters are typically too stiff to be navigated primarily with the microguidewire, except in younger patients with straight arteries. Once the Penumbra™ microcatheter is placed at the proximal aspect of the thrombus—the authors have actually found that it is best to advance the microcatheter to the distal aspect which is contrary to the instructions for use and company literature which recommend that the device is to be used from proximal to distal—the microwire is exchanged for the appropriate Separator™ wire chosen to match the size of the

microcatheter. The suction apparatus is activated, applying 1 atm of continuous suction through the microcatheter. The Separator™ wire is then moved in and out of the microcatheter as the microcatheter is advanced forward. In this way, the thrombus is removed one small fragment at a time. The Separator™ wire acts to break up any thrombus sucked into the microcatheter to maintain flow within the catheter. The drawback of proximal to distal motion is that neither the Separator™ wire nor the microcatheter are shaped and as a result, they often cannot be advanced beyond the straight segments of the MCA or BA. Unfortunately, most emboli tend to lodge at the MCA bifurcation or BA apex. By starting distal to proximal, the catheter and separator "fall back" into the straight segment, hopefully after removing the distal thrombus. In reality, multiple passes and devices are required per case. The largest Penumbra™ catheter, the 054 device, has the highest efficacy but is too large for most MCA trunks and all MCA and BA branches.

Both the MERCI™ and Penumbra™ devices have been associated with SAH and vessel perforation. In most cases, the perforations occur at the M2 and M3 branches of the MCA and the P1 and P2 segments of the PCA. Great care must be taken when smaller branches are cannulated with these devices, and it is reasonable to assume that in general, these devices have poor efficacy and should be avoided in any branch less than 2 mm in diameter. Neither device is compatible with vessels ≤ 1.5 mm.

In clinical practice, there are significant differences in technique for recanalization, and until a randomized trial shows benefit of one approach over another, the interventional treatment of AIS is likely to remain variable between institutions.

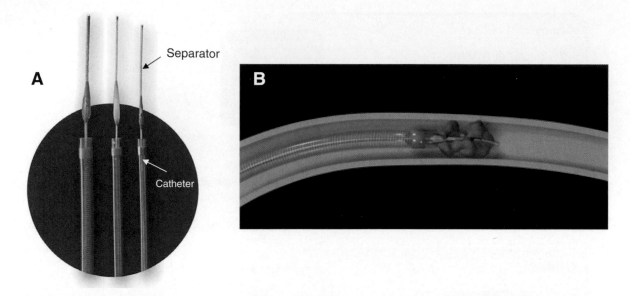

Figure 13A.11 • The Penumbra™ system. **A:** Picture of catheters and Separator™ wires in all three sizes: 026, 032, and 041. **B:** Schematic illustration of the Penumbra™ system proximal to a thrombus with the Separator™ wire engaging the thrombus. (Used with permission from Penumbra Medical Inc.)

EQUIPMENT

In selecting equipment for AIS intervention, the operator must be aware that the majority of devices used do not have FDA labeling for intracranial use and in the discussion that follows, the majority of devices described by the authors are used off-label. Therefore, a frank and honest discussion with everyone involved, from administrators and institutional review board members to patients and their families regarding the off-label use of the devices, is mandatory. AIS interventions are typically performed with 6-Fr. guide catheter–compatible equipment, with the exception of the MERCI™ clot-extraction devices, which are typically performed with 8- or 9-Fr. guide catheters. The most common guide catheter used is a Cordis Inc. Envoy™ 6-Fr. guide catheter with a multipurpose shaped tip (e.g., MPD). A 90-cm length is usually sufficient but in taller individuals or those with severe tortuosity, longer guide catheters in the 100-cm range are preferred. There are many other guide catheters on the market that have exceptional trackability (e.g., Neuron™ guide catheter by Penumbra Inc.), but the authors have more experience with the Envoy™. These devices come in various lengths up to 125 cm, allowing intracranial placement of the guide catheter tip to facilitate the navigation of devices.

Numerous microcatheters are also available and most interventions are performed with 2.3-Fr. endhole microcatheters; the authors' workhorse is a Rapid Transit™ by Cordis Inc. In general, smaller catheters are easier to navigate, but their inner lumen size makes microcatheter injections difficult. The authors perform all cases with 0.014″ microwires. Smaller wires have less support and a greater risk of artery perforation, and larger wires are not as steerable through the tortuous cerebral vessels. As a rule, hydrophilic wires are needed to access the branches of the MCA or PCA, and due to vessel fragility, the wire should have the softest tip possible. Middleweight wires

may rarely be placed intracranially by microcatheter exchange to give support, but they are not used primarily and stiff wires are never used. The risk of perforation is simply too high to permit anything but the softest tipped wires to be navigated to the brain. There are numerous microwires available, each with different purported benefits. The best wire is often the one that the interventionist has the most experience with. Examples of good wires include the Whisper™ (Abbott Vascular), Transcend Floppy or Extra-Floppy™ (Boston Scientific Inc.), and Synchro (Boston Scientific Inc.).

For balloon angioplasty, the best balloons are the coronary balloon systems, particularly the Maverick™ (Boston Scientific Inc.). Over-the-wire systems should be used for several reasons. First, rapid exchange (Rx) devices are difficult to navigate to the brain. Second, if wire or catheter exchanges are needed, they are not possible with Rx systems. Third, an over-the-wire balloon may be used as a microcatheter if needed to inject contrast, lytics, or exchange equipment. Therefore, the authors exclusively use exchange-length wires for all acute stroke interventions.

In some cases, acute stenting is indicated. For extracranial ICA stenoses leading to occlusion, the same devices used for elective carotid stenting should be used including emboli prevention devices (EPDs), if possible. The authors perform all emergent carotid stenting procedures with an EPD (either the filter type devices or the proximal flow arrest devices). The latter are preferred because they can facilitate clot extraction if needed. For intracranial stenting, the same devices used for elective stenting are preferred. The more flexible cobalt–chromium stent platforms are the ideal stents (e.g., Vision™ [Abott Vascular Inc.] or Driver™ [Medtronic Inc.]). The stainless steel devices are often very difficult to deliver and greatly increase the risks of complications. In the acute setting, the authors prefer not to use drug-eluting stents because of the need for prolonged dual antiplatelet therapy and the increased risk of stent thrombosis associated with off-label use (25,26,31–43).

The only other devices typically used are the clot-extraction devices approved by the FDA, namely, the MERCI™ and the Penumbra™ systems. Each of these systems consists of several sizes of microcatheter and wire combinations, and the MERCI™ system also includes a balloon occlusion guide catheter. The MERCI™ clot-extraction device is a corkscrew-shaped nitinol wire that has four configurations (X, L, V, and K-mini) (Fig. 13A.8), different stiffness (soft vs. stiff), and sizes (2, 2.5, and 3 mm). Depending on the wire chosen, one of two microcatheters is required to deploy the device. With this system, clot extraction is most efficient if proximal occlusion can be achieved. Concentric Medical Inc. manufactures three balloon occlusion guide catheter sizes: 7, 8, or 9 Fr. Larger guides are less likely to be occluded by extracted clot but at the cost of greater risk of vessel injury and access sheath size. In addition, Concentric Medical has recently made available a Distal Access Catheter (DAC™) that serves as a guide within a guide (Fig. 13A.9). It is advanced through the 6-Fr. guide over the microcatheter in a triaxial (i.e., "telescoping" setup) and is withdrawn with the microcatheter during clot-extraction attempts. Anecdotally, it appears to improve clot-extraction efficacy.

The Penumbra™ system currently consists of four microcatheter sizes (2.6, 3.2, 4.1, and 5 Fr.), each with its own Separator™ wire and universal suction apparatus (Fig. 13A.11). The devices are chosen based on vessel size and tortuosity (i.e., the largest catheter that will safely fit in the smallest target branch should be used, but this must be balanced against the increased stiffness of the larger devices and for thrombi at bifurcations, the two smaller-sized catheters are safer choices). The larger catheters are more efficient at clot extraction but are more difficult to deliver and have a tendency to kick back at genus, especially the MCA bifurcation and BA apex.

LIMITATIONS

There has been only one randomized trial of an endovascular acute stroke treatment. Although the study was positive, the drug tested (recombinant prourokinase [r-proUK]) is not commercially available (7). In addition, although there are now FDA-approved devices for mechanical clot removal from the cerebral vessels, clinical efficacy has not been demonstrated (25). As a consequence, AIS interventions remain essentially "investigational" and unregimented. Much of the above discussion and much of the literature represent little more than anecdotal experience despite the scientific integrity of the investigators.

Another major limitation is that recanalization efficacy with traditional intra-arterial fibrinolysis is relatively poor compared with that achieved during ACS interventions during coronary intervention. However, stenting, mechanical embolectomy, and multimodal approaches are able to achieve nearly complete recanalization. This technical success has not been associated with equivalent improvement in clinical outcomes. In the best series, including the authors' experience, only about 50% of patients have major neurologic improvement to the point of having no disability or minimal disability (5,9,44). The remainder of patients either have minimal or no recovery or die as a result of the stroke, brain edema, symptomatic ICH, or as a direct complication of the procedure. The latter occurs less frequently in contemporary series but still occurs in 10% to 15% of procedures. Complete recanalization itself may be responsible for the poor outcomes, either due to

ICH or due to reperfusion injury and cytotoxicity. Some patients are better off not receiving recanalization therapy. Currently, there are no effective treatments or preventative measures for reperfusion injury other than appropriate patient selection through penumbral imaging and BP control. Neuroprotectant drugs and hypothermia in particular are promising potential therapies but remain investigational at this time. The selection of patients plays a crucial role in preventing ICH and reperfusion injury, and an experienced stroke neurologist is essential in this process.

Factors such as patient age over 80 years, elevated serum glucose above 200 mg/dL, profound or difficult-to-control hypertension > 185/110 mm Hg, active treatment with warfarin, heparin, or heparinoids, therapy with high-dose aspirin and clopidogrel or platelet GPIIb/IIIa receptor antagonists, other coagulopathies or thrombocytopenia < 100,000 should be considered as potential contraindications for interventional therapy (5). Those patients with an early infarct area measuring more than one third of the MCA territory are generally not candidates for intervention because they tend to have very poor collateral flow and poor neuronal viability with a high propensity for hemorrhagic transformation following intervention (37). Underlying poor neuronal reserve (e.g., dementia, especially Alzheimer's type with or without known amyloid angiopathy) should be considered a strong contraindication for pharmacologic recanalization because of a very high risk of ICH and such patients tend not to do well even with successful recanalization.

CONCLUSIONS

A variety of endovascular therapies are available for AIS. The choice of therapy should be based on probable stroke etiology and the known factors that predispose to ICH. Mechanical embolectomy is ideal when thrombolytics are contraindicated and for embolic occlusion, angioplasty and stenting should be considered early for atherosclerotic occlusion, and multimodal treatment should be considered in all cases. Clinical success requires appropriate patient selection to avoid catastrophic ICH and reperfusion injury.

References

1. Albers GW, Olivot JM. Intravenous Alteplase for ischemic stroke. *Lancet.* 2007;369:249–250.
2. Rosamond W, Flegal K, Friday G, et al. Heart disease and stroke statistics—2007 update: a report from the American Heart Association Statistics Committee and Stroke Statistics Subcommittee. *Circulation.* 2007;115:e172.
3. Wolpert SM, Bruckmann H, Greenlee R, et al. Neuroradiologic evaluation of patients with acute stroke treated with recombinant tissue plasminogen activator. The rt-tPA Acute Stroke Study Group. *Am J Neuroradiol.* 1993;14:3–13.
4. Saqqur M, Uchino K, Demchuk AM, et al. Site of arterial occlusion identified by transcranial Doppler predicts the response to intravenous thrombolysis for stroke. *Stroke.* 2007;38:948–954.
5. Adams HP Jr, Brott TG, Furlan AJ, et al. Guidelines for thrombolytic therapy for acute stroke: a supplement to the guidelines for the management of patients with acute ischemic stroke. A statement for healthcare professionals from a Special Writing Group of the Stroke Council, American Heart Association. *Circulation.* 1996;94:1167–1174.
6. Hacke W, Ringleb P, Stingele R. How did the results of ECASS II influence clinical practice of treatment of acute stroke. *Rev Neurol.* 1999;29:638–641.

7. Furlan A, Higashida R, Wechsler L, et al. Intra-arterial prourokinase for acute ischemic stroke. The PROACT II study: a randomized controlled trial. Prolyse in acute cerebral thromboembolism. *JAMA*. 1999;282:2003–2011.

8. Adams HP Jr, Davis PH, Leira EC, et al. Baseline NIH Stroke Scale score strongly predicts outcome after stroke. A report of the Trial of Org 10172 in Acute Stroke Treatment (TOAST). *Neurology*. 1999;23:126–131.

9. Abou-Chebl A, Bajzer CT, Krieger DW, et al. Multimodal therapy for the treatment of severe ischemic stroke combining GPIIb/IIIa antagonists and angioplasty after failure of thrombolysis. *Stroke*. 2005;36:2286–2288.

10. Albers GW. Expanding the window for thrombolytic therapy in acute stroke. The potential role of acute MRI for patient selection. *Stroke*. 1999;30:2230–2237.

11. Jovin TG, Yonas H, Gebel JM, et al. The cortical ischemic core and not the consistently present penumbra is a determinant of clinical outcome in acute middle cerebral artery occlusion. *Stroke*. 2003;34:2426–2433.

12. Figueroa BE, Keep RF, Betz AL, et al. Plasminogen activators potentiate thrombin-induced brain injury. *Stroke*. 1998;29:1202–1207.

13. Adams HP Jr, del Zoppo G, Alberts MJ, et al. Guidelines for the early management of adults with ischemic stroke: a guideline from the American Heart Association/American Stroke Association Stroke Council, Clinical Cardiology Council, Cardiovascular Radiology and Intervention Council, and the Atherosclerotic Peripheral Vascular Disease and Quality of Care Outcomes in Research Interdisciplinary Working Groups: the American Academy of Neurology affirms the value of this guideline as an educational tool for neurologists. *Stroke*. 2007;38:1655–1711.

14. Adams HP Jr, Brott TG, Crowell RM, et al. Guidelines for the management of patients with acute ischemic stroke. A statement for healthcare professionals from a special writing group of the Stroke Council, American Heart Association. *Circulation*. 1994;90:1588–1601.

15. Bershad EM, Feen ES, Hernandez OH, et al. Impact of neurointensive care team on outcomes of critically ill acute ischemic stroke patients. *Neurocrit Care*. 2008;9:287–292.

16. Varelas PN, Schultz L, Conti M, et al. The impact of neurointensivist on patients with stroke admitted to a neurosciences intensive care unit. *Neurocrit Care*. 2008;9:293–299.

17. Qureshi AI, Ali Z, Suri MF, et al. Intra-arterial third-generation recombinant tissue plasminogen activator (reteplase) for acute ischemic stroke. *Neurosurgery*. 2001;49:41–48.

18. Arnold M, Schroth G, Nedeltchev K, et al. Intra-arterial thrombolysis in 100 patients with acute stroke due to middle cerebral artery occlusion. *Stroke*. 2002;33:1828–1833.

19. del Zoppo GJ, Ferbert A, Otis S, et al. Local intra-arterial fibrinolytic therapy in acute carotid territory stroke. A pilot study. *Stroke*. 1988;19:307–313.

20. del Zoppo GJ, Sasahara AA. Interventional use of plasminogen activators in central nervous system diseases. *Med Clin North Am*. 1998;82:545–568.

21. Gupta R, Vora NA, Horowitz MB, et al. Multimodal reperfusion therapy for acute ischemic stroke: factors predicting vessel recanalization. *Stroke*. 2006;37:986–990.

22. Lee DH, Jo KD, Kim HG, et al. Local intra-arterial urokinase thrombolysis of acute ischemic stroke with or without intravenous abciximab: a pilot study. *J Vasc Interv Radiol*. 2002;13:769–774.

23. Adams HPJr., Effron MB, Torner J, et al. Emergency administration of abciximab for treatment of patients with acute ischemic stroke: results of an international phase III trial: Abciximab in emergency treatment of stroke trial (AbESTT-II). *Stroke*. 2008;39:87–99.

24. Chopko BW, Kerber C, Wong W, et al. Transcatheter snare removal of acute middle cerebral artery thromboembolism: technical case report. *Neurosurgery*. 2000;46:1529–1531.

25. Smith WS, Sung G, Starkman S, et al. Safety and efficacy of mechanical embolectomy in acute ischemic stroke: results of the MERCI trial. *Stroke*. 2005;36:1432–1438.

26. Bose A, Henkes H, Alfke K, et al. The Penumbra system: a mechanical device for the treatment of acute stroke due to thromboembolism. *Am J Neuroradiol*. 2008;29:1409–1413.

27. Nakano S, Iseda T, Yoneyama T, et al. Direct percutaneous transluminal angioplasty for acute middle cerebral artery trunk occlusion: an alternative option to intra-arterial thrombolysis. *Stroke*. 2002;33:2872–2876.

28. Yoneyama T, Nakano S, Kawano H, et al. Combined direct percutaneous transluminal angioplasty and low-dose native tissue plasminogen activator therapy for acute embolic middle cerebral artery trunk occlusion. *Am J Neuroradiol*. 2002;23:277–281.

29. Sacco RL, Kargman DE, Gu Q, et al. Race-ethnicity and determinants of intracranial atherosclerotic cerebral infarction. The Northern Manhattan Stroke Study. *Stroke*. 1995;26:14–20.

30. Thijs VN, Albers GW. Symptomatic intracranial atherosclerosis: outcome of patients who fail antithrombotic therapy. *Neurology*. 2000;55:490–497.

31. Wityk RJ, Lehman D, Klag M, et al. Race and sex differences in the distribution of cerebral atherosclerosis. *Stroke*. 1996;27:1974–1980.

32. Feldmann E, Daneault N, Kwan E, et al. Chinese-white differences in the distribution of occlusive cerebrovascular disease. *Neurology*. 1990;40:1541–1545.

33. Lee TH, Choi CH, Park KP, et al. Techniques for intracranial stent navigation in patients with tortuous vessels. *Am J Neuroradiol*. 2005;26:1375–1380.

34. Jovin TG, Gupta R, Uchino K, et al. Emergent stenting of extracranial internal carotid artery occlusion in acute stroke has a high revascularization rate. *Stroke*. 2005;36:2426–2430.

35. Abou-Chebl A, Vora N, Yadav JS. Safety of angioplasty and stenting without thrombolysis for the treatment of early ischemic stroke. *J Neuroimaging*. 2009;19:139–143.

36. Meyers PM, Schumacher HC, Higashida RT, et al. Indications for the Performance of intracranial endovascular neurointerventional procedures. A Scientific Statement from the American Heart Association Council on Cardiovascular Radiology and Intervention, Stroke Council, Council on Cardiovascular Surgery and Anesthesia, Interdisciplinary Council on Peripheral Vascular Disease, and Interdisciplinary Council on Quality of Care and Outcomes Research. *Circulation*. 2009;119:2235–2249.

37. Barr J. Cerebral angiography in the assessment of acute cerebral ischemia: guidelines and recommendations. *J Vasc Interv Radiol*. 2004;15:S57–S66.

38. Khatri R, Khatri P, Khoury J, et al. Microcatheter contrast injections during intraarterial thrombolysis increase parenchymal hematoma risk: registry experience. *Stroke*. 2008;38:454–455.

39. The Penumbra Pivotal Stroke Trial Investigators. *Stroke*. 2009;40:2761–2768.

40. Yeter E, Kurt M, Silay Y, et al. Drug-eluting stents for acute myocardial infarction. *Expt Opin Pharmacother*. 2009;10:19–34.

41. Ong AT, McFadden EP, Regar E, et al. Late angiographic stent thrombosis (LAST) events with drug-eluting stents. *J Am Coll Cardiol*. 2005;45:2088–2092.

42. Park DW, Yun SC, Lee SW, et al. Stent thrombosis, clinical events, and influence of prolonged clopidogrel use after placement if drug-eluting stent data from an observational cohort study of drug-eluting versus bare-metal stents. *JACC Cardiovasc Interv*. 2008;1:494–503.

43. Slottow TL, Steinberg DH, Roy P, et al. Drug-eluting stents are associated with similar cardiovascular outcomes when compared to bare metal stents in the setting of acute myocardial infarct. *Cardiovasc Revasc Med*. 2008;9:24–28.

44. Lin R, Vora N, Zaidi S, et al. Mechanical approaches combined with intra-arterial pharmacological therapy are associated with higher recanalization rates than either intervention alone in revascularization of acute carotid terminus occlusion. *Stroke*. 2009;40:2092-2097.

Intracranial Angioplasty and Stenting

Alex Abou-Chebl and Vincent V. Truong

Intracranial atherosclerosis is a major cause of stroke and accounts for 8% to 10% of ischemic stroke in mixed patient populations (1–4). The vessels involved are mainly those of the circle of Willis. In addition to atherosclerosis, consideration should be given to other etiologies of intracranial disease such as vasculitis, dissection, embolism undergoing recannuliza-tion, moyamoya arteriopathy, postradiation arteriopathy, and infectious vasculitides (5).

The Warfarin-Aspirin for Symptomatic Intracranial Dis-ease (WASID) trial demonstrated that a significant proportion of patients with significant symptomatic intracranial disease (defined as stenosis between 50% and 99%) who are treated medically will experience a recurrent ischemic stroke in the distribution of the stenotic artery (2,6). This is likely related to hypoperfusion from the residual flow-limiting stenosis that is not responsive to antithrombotic therapy. In such patients, res-toration of adequate cerebral blood flow should be the primary goal of intervention. Extracranial-to-intracranial bypass surgery has been essentially abandoned due to near doubling of the risk of stroke in patients receiving bypass for severe middle cerebral artery (MCA) stenosis compared with medical therapy (7). With developments in stent technology, endovascular approaches have emerged as feasible and potentially highly effective therapy for those patients who fail medical treatment.

PREOPERATIVE PATIENT SELECTION

The most crucial indication for intracranial stenting is the presence of a symptomatic intracranial atherosclerotic steno-sis despite optimal medical therapy. Results from the WASID trial show that in patients with a high-grade stenosis (>70%), the risk for subsequent stroke in the territory of the stenotic artery is 23% at 1 year and 25% at 2 years (6,8,9). Although pa-tients with stenoses of less than 70% are also at increased risk of stroke, the risk is relatively low compared with the risk of en-dovascular intervention; therefore, patients with greater than 70% symptomatic intracranial stenoses are the most likely to benefit from invasive treatment strategies. In addition, patients must be able to tolerate dual antiplatelet therapy for 30 days or longer and their symptoms should be attributable to the ter-ritory distal to the stenotic segment. This last point is critical since the basilar artery (BA) and MCA have many important perforators that originate from their main trunks that often cause clinical syndromes due to parent vessel atherosclerosis. Angioplasty or stenting in such circumstances (i.e., recurrent perforator ischemia) has a high probability of causing perfora-tor occlusion and stroke (10).

ENDOVASCULAR APPROACH

The endovascular approach for intracranial angioplasty and stenting is similar to that of acute stroke intervention, but pretreatment with dual antiplatelet agents is critical. A femoral approach is preferred especially for MCA and in-ternal carotid artery (ICA) procedures. Heparin is given to achieve an activated clotting time (ACT) between 250 and 300 seconds. Treatment for vasospasm should be considered during the procedure although there are no data to support this practice. In defense of this practice, cerebral vessels are particularly prone to spasm, and since proper stent sizing is essential, antispasm treatment may help improve the accuracy of device sizing. A long sheath (6- to 8-Fr. 80-cm Shuttle™ [Cook Medical Inc.]) should be advanced into the common carotid artery (CCA) or subclavian artery (except in the rare patients with no tortuosity and a relatively proximal stenosis where a short sheath may be used) and a 6-Fr. guide (Envoy™ [Cordis Inc.] or Neuron™ [Penumbra Inc.]) should be placed distally in the cervical ICA or vertebral artery (VA). The le-sion should then be crossed with a hydrophilic, soft microwire with an atraumatic tip (e.g., Synchro™ or Transcend Floppy™ [Boston Scientific Inc.], among others). The tip of the guide-wire should be positioned distal to the stenosis with great care to avoid placing the wire in small branches or perfora-tors. For terminal ICA and MCA treatment, the wire should be passed into the second or proximal third-order branches of the MCA (Fig. 13B.1A). In the posterior circulation, the wire should be placed in a posterior cerebral artery (PCA) if possible (Fig. 13B.1B). The authors' approach is to always predilate the lesion with an undersized, over-the-wire bal-loon (e.g., Maverick™ or Gateway™ [Boston Scientific Inc.], among others) keeping in mind that vessel rupture or dissec-tion with subarachnoid hemorrhage are often fatal in this set-ting (Fig. 13B.1C). This practice permits adequate sizing of the vessel and observation of lesion response to angioplasty. Postangioplasty angiography should then be done and unless an excellent result with <30% residual stenosis is seen, stent-ing should be performed with a stent size no larger than the smallest normal reference vessel segment proximal and distal to the lesion. The length of the stent should be kept to the minimum needed to cover the lesion or the angioplasty seg-ment since longer stents are more difficult to deliver. Post-stenting dilation is rarely needed unless a self-expanding stent is used; this last point is controversial and based on anecdotal experience with the Wingspan™ stent system (see below). If a large branch or perforator emanates from the lesion, then the increased risk of branch occlusion and consequent stroke

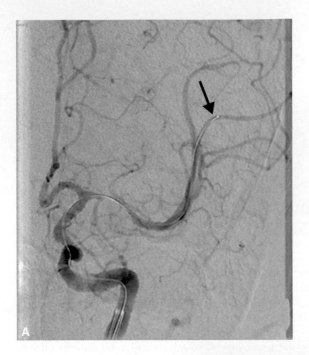
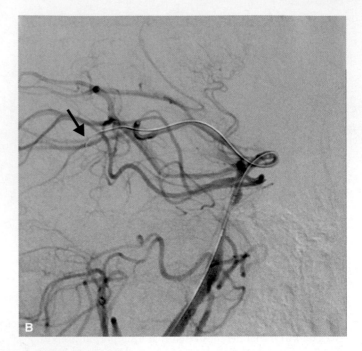
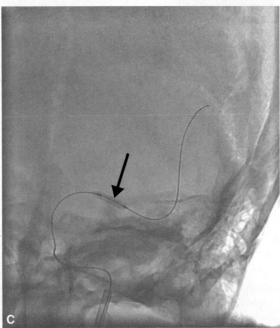

Figure 13B.1 • **A:** Middle cerebral artery (MCA) intervention with the wire tip *(arrow)* in M2 branch of the MCA. **B:** Basilar artery intervention with a wire *(arrow)* in the left posterior cerebral artery (PCA). **C:** Predilation of the MCA lesion in **(A)** with the Gateway™ balloon (Boston Scientific Corporation) *(arrow)* before MCA stenting.

should be discussed with the patient preprocedure. If this occurs, the authors have found, anecdotally, that intra-arterial infusion of glycoprotein (GP)IIb/IIIa antagonist may recanalize the occluded branch.

Restoration of the normal vessel lumen diameter is not required to significantly improve flow through the stenosis because flow is proportional to the fourth power of the radius. As a result, the angiographic end point of a smooth, normal-caliber lumen, while desirable, must be balanced with the knowledge that the cerebral vessels are very fragile and

persistent attempts to achieve such a goal may easily lead to tragic complications of arterial rupture or dissection and intracerebral hemorrhage (ICH).

PERIOPERATIVE MANAGEMENT

Because of the need for constant neurologic assessment of patients undergoing intracranial intervention, the author recommends that these procedures should not be performed under general anesthesia (10). If there is any clinical deterioration, angiography of the appropriate vessel should be performed immediately. Vasospasm, embolization, and dissection are the most likely etiologies of intraoperative deficits and should be treated appropriately. If angiography is normal but the patient has a clear neurologic deficit, an expanding ICH should be suspected and appropriate measures need to be taken. If there is frank extravasation of contrast on angiography, immediate blood pressure lowering, heparin reversal, and even temporary balloon occlusion should be considered. If there is no angiographic evidence of extravasation but a hematoma is suspected, intraoperative computerized tomography should be performed immediately. Under these circumstances, the authors have seen only a few patients survive despite all of the measures mentioned. If there are no new neurologic deficits, heparin may be discontinued at the end of the procedure but not reversed except in those who are at high risk for hyperperfusion syndrome or ICH. Routine use of GPIIb/IIIa antagonists is discouraged unless patients are inadequately premedicated with antiplatelet agents.

POSTOPERATIVE CARE

Close observation of neurologic status and monitoring of blood pressure are critical. If there is a risk of hyperperfusion syndrome and ICH, blood pressure should be kept in the low normal range for at least 14 days. Dual antiplatelet therapy needs to be continued for at least 30 days but may be continued for 6 to 12 months or until a follow-up angiogram confirms that there is no restenosis. If drug-eluting stents (DES) were placed, prolonged therapy for 1 to 2 years may be necessary. In addition, all patients should have a 30-day follow-up with a transcranial Doppler ultrasound (TCD) and neurologic examination. At 6 months, another follow-up is needed, and unless the stented segment is easily evaluated by TCD, angiography should be

done to assess stent patency. The authors have found it useful to know whether any early, severe neointimal proliferation occurs; in such cases, more frequent clinical assessments and continued dual antiplatelet therapy are warranted.

CLINICAL OUTCOMES

Stent delivery is the most challenging single aspect of intracranial interventions, especially stent delivery to the terminal ICA and MCA. The latest generation of coronary stents (particularly the cobalt–chromium platforms, e.g., Vision™ [Abbott Vascular Inc.] or Driver™ [Medtronic Inc.]) has proven to be highly deliverable, but in 8% to 10% of patients, even these stents cannot be delivered safely through the cavernous carotid artery in particular. The bulk of published series of intracranial angioplasty and stenting has been in series of patients treated with balloon-expandable coronary stents. The reported outcomes with these stents have been highly variable because of differences in patient selection, techniques, and operator experience. Most series have reported 30-day stroke, ICH, and death rates of 8% to 20%, but some have had rates as high as 50%, with an average rate of 10% to 12% (11–14). The author has reported on the use of DES for intracranial stenoses with excellent success, but the ultimate safety of this approach is unclear (15).

The balloon-expandable Neurolink™ Stent System (Guidant Corporation, San Francisco, CA) was the first stent designed specifically for cerebrovascular applications (Fig. 13B.2). It was evaluated in 43 intracranial lesions in a multicenter, nonrandomized, feasibility study, the Stenting of Symptomatic Atherosclerotic Lesions in the Vertebral or Intracranial Arteries (SSYLVIA) study (16). The investigators reported a high procedural success rate of 95% and a low stroke rate of 6.6% at 30 days and 14% at 1-year follow-up. However, in-stent restenosis of more than 50% occurred in 32.4% of the patients in the stent group. Unfortunately, although the stent

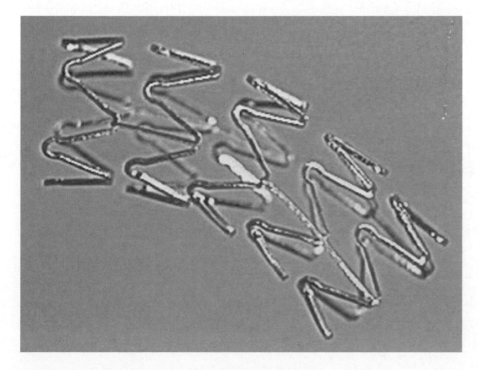

Figure 13B.2 • The Neurolink™ (Guidant Corp.) stent, no longer commercially available in the United States.

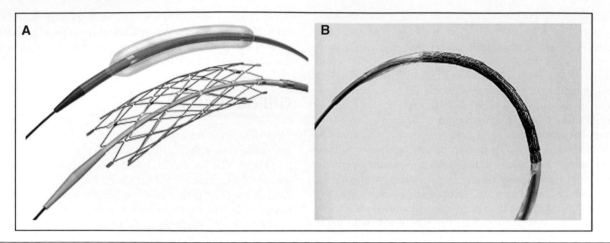

Figure 13B.3 • Two brain-specific stent systems. **A:** Wingspan™ self-expanding stent system with Gateway™ balloon Catheter (Boston Scientific Inc.). **B:** The Pharos Vitesse™ stent (Micrus Endovascular Inc.).

received a humanitarian device exemption (HDE) from the FDA, it is no longer commercially available.

In 2005, a novel, nitinol, self-expanding stent system (Wingspan™ Stent System and Gateway percutaneous transluminal angioplasty [PTA] balloon catheter; Boston Scientific Corp.) was released under an HDE for the treatment of symptomatic intracranial stenoses (>50%) refractory to medical therapy (Fig. 13B.3A). The single-arm, multicenter Wingspan study of 45 qualified patients (17) had a procedural success of 97.7%. The rates for the composite end point of ipsilateral stroke or death at 30 days, 6 months, and 1-year follow-up were 4.5%, 7.1%, and 9.3%, respectively. Accepting that angiographic follow-up in this study was inadequate, none of the 7.5% of patients with angiographically proven in-stent restenosis of ≥50% were symptomatic.

Currently, the ongoing randomized, controlled SAMMPRIS (Stenting vs. Aggressive Medical Management for Preventing Recurrent Stroke in Intracranial Stenosis) trial is comparing the Wingspan stent and best medical therapy in patients with symptomatic intracranial stenosis of 70% or more who have stroke or TIA within 30 days (18). In addition, there are two prospective, multicenter Wingspan stent registries established in the United States. The National Institute of Health Multicenter Wingspan Intracranial Stent Registry enrolled 129 patients with stenosis of 70% to 99% (19). The initial analysis showed a technical success of 96.7% and stroke or death rate of 9.6% and 14% at 30 days and 6 months, respectively. Restenosis of 50% or more was found in 25% of 52 patients who underwent follow-up angiography. In the U.S. Wingspan Registry supported by a research grant from Boston Scientific Corporation, there were 78 patients with 82 intracranial stenoses of ≥50% (20). The stent was successfully placed in 98.8% of the patients. Major periprocedural complications were reported in 6.1% of treatments. In-stent restenosis ≥50% within or adjacent to the implanted stents and absolute luminal loss of more than 20% was seen in 34.5% of patients, 76% of whom were asymptomatic (21). The major limitation of this stent system is the instructions for use, which prohibit poststenting angioplasty, often resulting

in significant residual stenoses, which in vessels measuring less than 3 mm would be expected to have a high risk of early restenosis. The self-expanding nature of the stent, despite high hopes, does not appear to be useful in maintaining vessel patency but has been of great benefit in improving safety and stent delivery compared with balloon-expandable stents (Fig. 13B.4).

The Pharos™ stent (Micrus Endovascular Corporation, Sunnyvale, CA), derived from one of the most flexible balloon-expandable monorail coronary stents, has been initially evaluated in a German prospective, single-center study that enrolled 21 patients with symptomatic intracranial stenosis of 50% or more (22). A technical success rate of 90.5% was achieved with a stroke rate of 9.5% at 30 days. However, there was a stent thrombosis rate of 9.5%. The second-generation Pharos Vitesse™ balloon-expandable stent (Fig. 13B.3B), already authorized by the CE for commercial distribution in the European Union, is being investigated in the United States, Europe, and Asia in the Vitesse Intracranial Stent Study for Ischemic Therapy (VISSIT) study, a prospective, randomized, multicenter study (23). This stent has a cobalt–chromium platform with a silicon carbide coating, which is purported to have improved biocompatibility and decreased thrombocyte activation.

Long-term follow-up of intracranial stenting has generally been lacking. There has been only one series with long-term follow-up, which included 53 patients with 69 arterial lesions who were followed for up to 7 years with a median follow-up of 24 months (24). The technical success rate was 98.6% with a reduction of the median percent stenosis from 85% to 0%. Stents, all balloon-expandable, were implanted in 76.8% (53/69) of the procedures. The 30-day death/stroke rate was 10.1% with only one death. During the follow-up period, the transient ischemic attack or stroke rate was 5.8% (4/69) giving a 2-year stroke/death/TIA rate of 15.9%, which is less than the 23% annual rate of stroke expected with medical therapy. The restenosis rate at 1 year was 15.9% (note: treatment included a mix of angioplasty, bare-metal stents, and DES) and was symptomatic in 18.2%. The restenosis rate was 50% for angioplasty (8/16) and 7.5% (4/53) for stenting (hazard

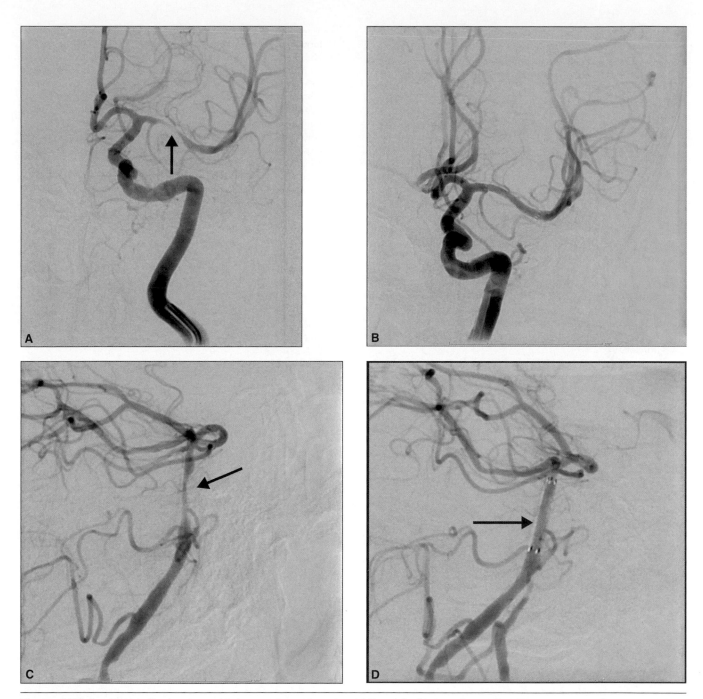

Figure 13B.4 • **A:** Baseline angiographic image of symptomatic middle cerebral artery stenosis *(arrow)*. **B:** Angiographic image following placement of Wingspan stent. **C:** Baseline angiographic image of symptomatic basilar artery stenosis *(arrow)*. **D:** Angiographic image following placement of Wingspan stent.

ratio = 5.02; 95% CI = 1.22 to 20.68). Factors that were associated with restenosis were vessel size < 2.5 mm (hazard ratio = 4.78; 95% CI = 1.35 to 16.93) and interventions performed in the setting of an acute stroke (hazard ratio = 6.36; 95% CI = 1.78 to 22.56).

All of the published retrospective series and prospective device studies have differed markedly in techniques and outcome definitions. They all share a lack of adequate angiographic follow-up and most have poor clinical follow-up. Therefore, no firm conclusions regarding long-term safety, efficacy, and durability can be drawn from the available data.

CONCLUSION

Because of the lack of efficacy and durability data from prospective, randomized, multicenter trials, intracranial stenting remains investigational and should be used only in carefully selected patients after thorough evaluation of their clinical and anatomic factors. The authors do not recommend stenting of chronic occlusions, asymptomatic lesions and generally do not advocate stenting in very old patients, especially those with underlying dementia and severe calcification of their vessels.

However, symptomatic patients with angiographically documented >70% stenoses who have failed medical therapy are appropriate candidates for intracranial angioplasty and stenting and should be enrolled in clinical trials when possible.

References

1. Sacco RL, Kargman DE, Gu Q, et al. Race-ethnicity and determinants of intracranial atherosclerotic cerebral infarction. The Northern Manhattan Stroke Study. *Stroke.* 1995;26:14–20.
2. Thijs VN, Albers GW. Symptomatic intracranial atherosclerosis: outcome of patients who fail antithrombotic therapy. *Neurology.* 2000;55:490–497.
3. Wityk RJ, Lehman D, Klag M, et al. Race and sex differences in the distribution of cerebral atherosclerosis. *Stroke.* 1996;27:1974–1980.
4. Feldmann E, Daneault N, Kwan E, et al. Chinese-white differences in the distribution of occlusive cerebrovascular disease. *Neurology.* 1990;40:1541–1545.
5. Yadav JS, Abou-Chebl A. Intracranial angioplasty and stenting. *J Interven Cardiol.* 2009;22:9–15.
6. Chimowitz MI, Lynn MJ, Howlett-Smith H, et al. Comparison of warfarin and aspirin for symptomatic intracranial arterial stenosis. *N Engl J Med.* 2005;352:1305–1316.
7. The EC/IC Bypass Study Group. *N Engl J Med.* 1985;313:1191–1200.
8. Kasner SE, Chimowitz MI, Lynn MJ, et al. Predictors of ischemic stroke in the territory of a symptomatic intracranial arterial stenosis. *Circulation.* 2006;113:555–563.
9. Kern R, Steinke W, Daffertshorfer M, et al. Stroke recurrences in patients with symptomatic vs. asymptomatic middle cerebral artery disease. *Neurology.* 2005;65:859–864.
10. Mazighi M, Abou-Chebl A. Stenting and prevention of ischemic stroke. *Curr Drug Targets.* 2007;8:867–873.
11. Abou-Chebl A, Krieger WD, Bajzer CT, et al. Intracranial angioplasty and stenting in the awake patient. *J Neuroimaging.* 2006;16:216–223.
12. Lylyk P, Vila JF, Miranda C, et al. Endovascular reconstruction by means of stent placement in symptomatic intracranial atherosclerotic stenosis. *Neurol Res.* 2005;27(suppl 1):S84–S88.
13. Marks MP, Wojak JC, Al Ali F, et al. Angioplasty for symptomatic intracranial stenosis: clinical outcomes. *Stroke.* 2006;37:1016–1020.
14. Gupta R, Schumacher HC, Mangla S, et al. Urgent endovascular revascularization for symptomatic intracranial atherosclerotic stenosis. *Neurology.* 2003;61:1729–1735.
15. Abou-Chebl A, Bashir Q, Yadav JS. Drug-eluting stent for the treatment of intracranial atherosclerosis: initial experience and midterm angiographic follow-up. *Stroke.* 2005;36:e165–e168.
16. The SSYLVIA Study Investigators. Stenting of symptomatic atherosclerotic lesions in the vertebral or intracranial arteries (SSYLVIA). *Stroke.* 2004;35:1388–1392.
17. Bose A, Hartmann M, Henkes H, et al. A novel, self-expanding, nitinol stent in medically refractory intracranial atherosclerotic stenoses: the Wingspan study. *Stroke.* 2007;38:1531–1537.
18. Anonymous. Stenting vs. Aggressive Medical Management for Preventing Recurrent Stroke in Intracranial Stenosis (SAMMPRIS) trial. Available at: www.clinicaltrials.gov [NCT 00576693].
19. Zaidat OO, Klucznik R, Alexander MJ, et al. The NIH registry on use of the Wingspan stent for symptomatic 70–99% intracranial arterial stenosis. *Neurology.* 2008;70:1518–1524.
20. Fiorella D, Levy E, Turk AS, et al. US multicenter experience with the Wingspan stent system for the treatment of intracranial atheromatous disease: periprocedural results. *Stroke.* 2007;38:881–887.
21. Levy EL, Turk AS, Albuquerque FC, et al. Wingspan in-stent restenosis and thrombosis: incidence, clinical presentation, and management. *Neurosurgery.* 2007;67:644–651.
22. Kurre W, Berkefeld J, Sitzer M, et al. Treatment of symptomatic high-grade intracranial stenoses with the balloon-expandable Pharos stent: initial experience. *Neuroradiology.* 2008;50:701–708.
23. Anonymous. VISSIT Intracranial Stent Study for Ischemic Therapy. Available at: www.clinicaltrials.gov [NCT 00816166].
24. Mazighi M, Yadav JS, Abou-Chebl A. Durability of endovascular therapy for symptomatic intracranial atherosclerosis. *Stroke.* 2008;39:1766–1769.

SECTION V

Lower Extremity Intervention

CHAPTER 14

Acute Limb Ischemia: Overview, Thrombolysis, and Mechanical Thrombectomy

Brian G. Hynes, Ronan J. Margey, Kenneth Rosenfield, Kenneth Ouriel, Samir R. Kapadia, and Ivan P. Casserly

Acute limb ischemia (ALI) refers to the sudden or rapid reduction (i.e., typically <14 days) in arterial extremity perfusion wherein its viability is threatened. Although epidemiologic data are limited, ALI is reported to have an annual incidence of 4 to 17 cases per 100,000 population (1–4). ALI continues to be associated with an extremely grave prognosis, with amputation rates varying from 5% to 30%, and mortality rates as high as 14% to 18% in some series (5–7). This chapter is divided into four sections: (1) A general discussion of ALI, detailing the etiology and pathophysiology of ALI, and the initial clinical assessment, medical management, and general treatment strategies for patients with ALI (2). The role of catheter-directed thrombolysis in the treatment of ALI (3). The role of percutaneous mechanical thrombectomy in the treatment of ALI (4). Case examples of ALI are presented that reinforce the concepts discussed in the earlier sections.

PART I: OVERVIEW OF ALI

Etiology and Pathophysiology of ALI

ALI may result from extrinsic or intrinsic vascular processes leading to sudden compromise of limb perfusion. Acute arterial occlusion secondary to trauma is beyond the remit of this chapter. Classically, intrinsic ALI may result from embolic or thrombotic interruption of arterial blood flow (Table 14.1). Differentiating an occlusion due to embolism from an occlusion due to local thrombosis is frequently challenging (Table 14.2). However, a thorough history and clinical evaluation often yield incisive data, which may help direct patient management.

Arterial embolic occlusion precipitating ALI is cardiogenic in origin in over 80% of cases (8). Intracardiac thrombus formation is most commonly found in the left atrial appendage in the setting of atrial fibrillation (9) and within hypokinetic/akinetic areas of the left ventricle in the setting of a cardiomyopathy or prior myocardial infarction (10). Artery-to-artery embolization may also occur. Aneurysms within the aorta and iliac, femoral, or popliteal arteries may give rise to in situ thrombus formation, which can then embolize, blocking the downstream arterial system. Other potential causes of embolism are listed in Table 14.1. Emboli tend to lodge at bifurcation points within the arterial tree such as at the distal common femoral, iliac, and popliteal arteries in order of decreasing incidence (Fig. 14.1). Similarly, the distal brachial artery is the most common site of embolic occlusion in the upper limb, which together with the renal and mesenteric vascular beds receive approximately 15% of all systemic emboli (11,12).

Acute peripheral arterial occlusion may also result from abrupt thrombus formation at the site of pre-existing atherosclerotic plaque or prior endovascular intervention or within surgical bypass grafts (native vein or prosthetic). Spontaneous plaque rupture complicated by thrombotic occlusion appears to be a rare event in the periphery and occurs most commonly within the superficial femoral artery (13) (Fig. 14.2). While the key event in the vast majority of acute coronary syndrome (ACS) presentations appears to be related to acute disruption of a pre-existing thin fibrofatty plaque with subsequent thrombosis of the coronary artery (14), less is known about spontaneous plaque rupture precipitating ALI. A recent study demonstrated a very high incidence of plaque rupture (~42%) as determined by intravascular ultrasound in the iliofemoral segment of patients undergoing angioplasty, the majority of which were confined to the proximal segment of each artery, where the greatest atherosclerotic burden was found (15). This suggests that plaque rupture may be more frequent than previously believed in the periphery, even if it is not as frequently complicated by thrombotic occlusion as coronary plaque rupture.

Clinical Approach to the Patient with Suspected ALI

The key determinants of the clinical presentation of ALI include the vascular distribution of the occluded artery, the extent of pre-existing atherosclerotic disease, and the degree of prior collateral development. Typically, embolic occlusion of a peripheral artery with no pre-existing peripheral artery disease (PAD) or collateral network results in the acute onset of the classical ALI findings: pain, pallor, poikilothermia (cold), pulselessness, paresthesia, and paralysis. Physical findings consistent with ALI are usually found one joint level distal to the site of arterial occlusion.

The clinical presentation of acute arterial thrombosis may involve less of the classic signs and symptoms of ALI, which may delay the initial diagnosis. The precise duration of symptoms may also be more difficult to discern, and often the vascular exam of the contralateral limb reveals evidence of significant PAD. Table 14.2 lists the clinical characteristics that may aid differentiation of embolic from thrombotic ALI.

Irreversible limb injury is thought to occur in a limb after about 6 hours of complete interruption of arterial inflow. However, clinically, complete interruption of arterial inflow is rare, due to the presence of collaterals. Hence, the ischemic window is typically considerably longer than 6 hours (16). Muscle cells and subcutaneous tissue are less vulnerable to progressive ischemia compared with neurons and skin. During ischemia, the acute reduction in oxygen impairs mitochondrial production

TABLE 14.1   List of Embolic and Thrombotic Causes of Acute Peripheral Arterial Occlusion

Embolic	Thrombotic
Cardiogenic	Plaque rupture within pre-existing atherosclerosis
Atrial fibrillation	Hypercoagulable states
Left ventricular dysfunction	Hypoperfusion secondary to cardiogenic failure/shock

Valvular heart disease
    Prosthetic
    Endocarditis
    Rheumatic
	Inotrope-induced peripheral vasospasm
	Trauma
	Arterial dissection

Vascular	
Aneurysms Aortic, iliac, popliteal	
Iatrogenic Distal embolism related to endovascular intervention	
Paradoxical embolism	
Right-to-left shunting through ASD or PFO	
Other	
Air, amniotic fluid, tumor, intra-arterial drugs, etc.	

(Modified from O'Connell JB, Quinones-Baldrich WJ. Proper evaluation and management of acute embolic versus thrombotic limb ischemia. *Semin Vasc Surg.* 2009;22:10–16.)
ASD, atrial septal defect; PFO, patent foramen ovale.

of normal energy products such as ATP and cell contraction ceases. In an attempt to maintain cell integrity, a switch to anaerobic glycolysis is initiated. However, a resultant accumulation of lactic acid limits this salvage pathway and a paradoxical energy production situation occurs, known as the "oxygen wastage phenomenon," with a buildup of intracellular hydrogen ions and a reduction of pH. The ensuing processes of lipid breakdown and beta oxidation expends more ATP, culminating in failure of cell membrane integrity and elevated systemic levels of potassium, creatinine kinase, and myoglobin (17,18). Ischemic reperfusion injury may have harmful contributory effects enhancing the systemic inflammatory response (19,20).

The Society of Vascular Surgery/International Society of Cardiovascular Surgery (SVS/ISCVS) classification provides an important aid to classify the severity of ALI and guide clinical management. The critical components of this assessment in determining the severity of extremity hypoperfusion include the sensory and motor function of the limb, and the condition of the arterial and venous Doppler signals. Based on the constellation of the clinical findings observed, ALI may be divided into one of three categories, as described in Table 14.3. Category I describes a viable limb that is not under threat. These patients have no motor or sensory symptoms, and have audible arterial and venous Doppler signals. Category II describes a

TABLE 14.2   Characteristic Clinical Features of Acute Limb Ischemia due to Embolic and Thrombotic Causes

Clinical Feature	Embolic Occlusion	Thrombotic Occlusion
Symptom onset	Sudden and severe	More gradual, less severe initially
Prior intermittent claudication	Infrequent	Common
Contralateral limb	Often normal	Frequent coexistent PAD
Coexistent cardiac disease	Frequent (especially AF)	May or may not be present

(Adapted from O'Connell JB, Quinones-Baldrich WJ. Proper evaluation and management of acute embolic versus thrombotic limb ischemia. *Semin Vasc Surg.* 2009;22:10–16.)
IC, intermittent claudication; AF, atrial fibrillation; PAD, peripheral arterial disease.

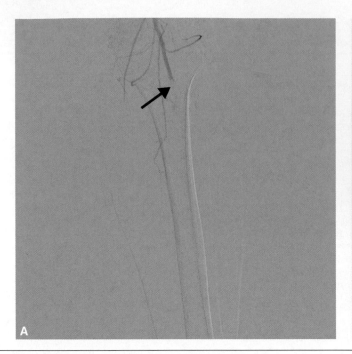
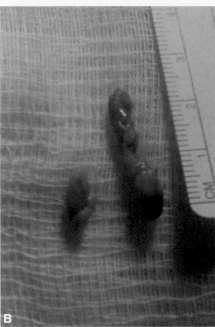

Figure 14.1 • Embolic arterial occlusion. A: Angiographic appearance of embolic occlusion in distal popliteal artery *(arrow)*. **B:** Extracted embolic material removed following left superficial femoral artery cut-down and Fogarty balloon thromboembolectomy.

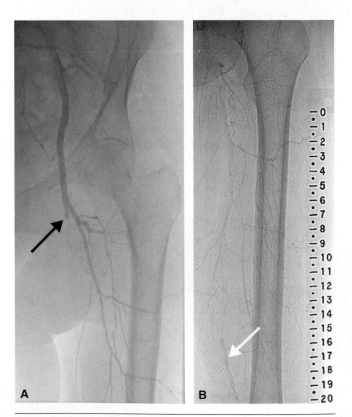

Figure 14.2 • Thrombotic arterial occlusion. Angiogram from patient with thrombotic occlusion of the length of the superficial femoral artery (SFA) extending from the proximal segment *(black arrow, A)* to the distal SFA *(white arrow, B)*, with reconstitution of the distal SFA via collaterals from the profunda femoral artery.

threatened limb that requires revascularization to salvage the limb. This category is distinguished from category I by the loss of arterial Doppler signals in the limb and the onset of sensory and motor dysfunction. Category II is subdivided into marginally (category IIa) and immediately (category IIb) threatened groups. Patients with category IIa ALI have mild sensory symptoms, usually localized to the forefoot. Patients with category IIb have more extensive sensory symptoms extending above the level of the forefoot, and have signs of motor weakness. Category III describes a nonviable limb that has profound sensory loss (typically anesthetic) and significant limb paralysis. Loss of venous Doppler signals is typical. If patients present late, muscle rigor and marbling of the skin may be observed. The limb in these patients has experienced irreversible injury that is not salvageable, even if successful revascularization is performed. Approximately 45% of patients with ALI present with category I ischemia, with 10% having a category III nonviable limb on initial evaluation (21).

Initial Medical Assessment and Therapy

ALI constitutes a vascular emergency that requires rapid diagnosis and prompt management to reduce the substantial risk to both life and limb. In addition to thorough examination of the affected extremity, clinical examination should focus on the cardiovascular system. Features suggestive of high procedural (especially surgical) risk include the presence of left ventricular failure as evidenced by pulmonary edema, hypotension, or arrhythmia. Clinical signs of other potential diagnoses that may mimic ALI should be looked for such as severe cardiac failure, acute deep venous thrombosis, and acute compressive neuropathy. Baseline metabolic and hematologic laboratory profiles should be obtained, and basic resuscitation measures such as intravenous fluids and continuous cardiac monitoring should be instigated. Fluid and electrolyte replacement

TABLE 14.3 Rutherford SVS/ISCVS Classification of Acute Limb Ischemia

	Category	Description	Sensory Loss	Muscle Weakness	Arterial Doppler	Venous Doppler
I	Viable	Not immediately threatened	None	Absent	Audible	Audible
IIa	Threatened marginally	Salvageable if promptly revascularized	Minimal or none	Absent	Often inaudible	Audible
IIb	Immediately threatened	Salvageable if revascularized immediately	More than toes associated with rest pain	Mild, moderate	Usually inaudible	Audible
III	Irreversible	Major tissue loss or permanent nerve damage	Profound deficit	Profound paralysis	Inaudible	Inaudible

(Adapted from Katzen BT. Clinical diagnosis and prognosis of acute limb ischemia. *Rev Cardiovasc Med.* 2002;3(suppl 2):S2–S6.)

requires careful consideration, given the severe metabolic derangements frequently encountered with ALI. Furthermore, mechanical thrombectomy devices resulting in intravascular hemolysis may lead to acute renal failure secondary to nonimmune hemoglobinuria. Due to the significant morbidity and mortality of ALI, further management of the patient often requires the input of multiple specialists and can be best achieved in a critical care setting. In particular, where surgery appears to be the most likely treatment path, immediate consultation should be sought prior to the administration of anticoagulation so as not to preclude spinal anesthesia.

Specific guidelines to aid the physician managing the ALI patient remain extremely limited in comparison with those governing care for patients with an ACS. The Trans-Atlantic Inter-Society Consensus Document on Management of Peripheral Arterial Disease (TASC) II guidelines recommend immediate anticoagulation with intravenous unfractionated heparin (UFH) unless a specific contraindication exists (21). Difficulties with UFH administration include reduced bioavailability at low doses, in addition to marked interpatient variability in anticoagulation, necessitating activated partial thromboplastin time measurement. Low-molecular-weight heparins (LMWHs) (mean molecular weight 4000 to 5000 Da) have a number of advantages over UFH largely due to their more predictable anticoagulation response. They act predominately by enhancing antithrombin activity, but unlike UFH they exhibit reduced thrombin-inactivating properties. Also they have higher ratios of anti-Xa to anti-IIa activity, and lead to lower rates of platelet activation and heparin-induced thrombocytopenia (HIT) (22,23). However, the ease of reversing the anticoagulant effect of UFH with protamine sulfate, and its short half-life compared with that of LMWHs, ensure its continued usefulness in clinical practice. Where heparin is contraindicated (due to the presence of HIT), direct thrombin inhibitors such as bivalirudin or argatroban that bind directly to the active site on thrombin, and the selective factor Xa inhibitor fondaparinux, may be used (14,24). In a retrospective review of 48 patients with suspected or confirmed HIT undergoing lower extremity revascularization, the use of the direct thrombin inhibitor argatroban has been shown to be safe and

feasible (25). Major bleeding and the composite end point of death, urgent revascularization or amputation occurred in 6% and 25% of patients, respectively.

Although no specific recommendations exist concerning antiplatelet therapy in ALI, it seems reasonable to administer aspirin (ASA) as soon as possible, given the high burden of cardiovascular disease in this patient cohort (21). The Antithrombotic Trialists' Collaboration found that ASA and other antiplatelet agents reduced the risk of vascular death, stroke, or myocardial infarction by 22% in high-risk ACS patients (26). PAD patients are known to have higher levels of platelet reactivity and exhibit a lesser response to aspirin (27,28). General guidelines for PAD, such as the 2006 ACC/AHA guidelines for PAD, stipulate that antiplatelet therapy should be initiated where possible (29). Aspirin at a dose of 75 to 325 mg/day is recommended primarily as the drug of choice, with clopidogrel considered an effective alternative therapy in the general management of PAD (30).

Imaging

Following the initial medical assessment and stabilization of the patient with suspected ALI, a decision with regard to further vascular imaging to anatomically define the arterial obstruction and the arterial inflow and outflow needs to be made. Imaging options include computed tomographic angiography, magnetic resonance angiography, arterial duplex ultrasonography, and invasive contrast arteriography. Ultimately, the choice should be individualized based on patient variables (e.g., clinical stability of the patient, the severity of ALI, and comorbidities such as renal dysfunction) and system variables that influence the availability of the different imaging modalities. In general, invasive angiography allows the minimal delay between diagnosis and potential endovascular revascularization. As such, patients with Category IIb ALI should routinely proceed directly to invasive angiography as immediate revascularization is vital to preserve limb viability. For patients with Category I ALI, noninvasive evaluation is generally recommended, as there is typically sufficient time to allow such studies to be performed. Since Category IIa ALI represents the intermediate group, clinical judgment will determine whether noninvasive imaging is performed prior to invasive angiography. For example, where complex anatomic issues are anticipated that might influence the choice of arterial access of the revascularization strategy, preprocedural noninvasive imaging is clearly of benefit. Noninvasive or invasive imaging is futile if the limb is nonviable.

Primary Management Strategies in Patients with ALI

The clinical categories of ALI described above form the basis for broad recommendations regarding the primary management strategy for ALI (31).

For patients with category I ALI (i.e., viable limb), medical therapy with heparin and careful assessment regarding the need for revascularization are appropriate. Indications for proceeding to revascularization include the anticipation of symptoms of limb ischemia based on the functional status and activity level of the patient. The threshold for offering revascularization should reflect the balance between the likelihood of achieving a successful revascularization with the anticipated complication rate based on the patient age, comorbidities, and vascular anatomy (e.g., vascular access, anatomy of occlusion, and quality of arterial inflow and outflow). Therefore, in older sedentary patients who have severe comorbidities and complex arterial anatomy, medical therapy alone may be a reasonable option.

The management of patients with category IIa ALI is similar to that of patients with category I ALI. In this patient cohort, there is typically sufficient time to anatomically define the arterial anatomy while medical therapy is instituted. In general, the threshold for offering revascularization in this cohort is low, with the expectation that reasonably active individuals will experience significant limb ischemia in the absence of revascularization. Since the limbs of these individuals are marginally threatened, there is sufficient time to allow the typical 10- to 24-hour duration of catheter-directed thrombolysis (CDT) therapy. Percutaneous mechanical thrombectomy (PMT) may also reasonably be offered by trained operators with access to a range of thrombectomy technologies, assuming the vascular anatomy is appropriate. If either of these modalities is contraindicated, surgical revascularization should be offered.

The most critical decision making relates to the management of patients with category IIb ALI. In these patients, immediate restoration of flow is essential to maximize the chance of limb salvage. Therefore, the use of traditional methods of CDT that require prolonged infusion of thrombolytic agents to achieve resolution of thrombus is not appropriate. The options, therefore, include the use of surgical revascularization or PMT as the dominant strategy to achieve reperfusion to the limb. In the past, there was a bias toward offering surgical revascularization for this group. For patients who present late (i.e., >14 days), surgical revascularization may remain a better option, given the difficulty in dealing with more chronic clot using endovascular techniques. However, there is an increasing shift toward PMT for the treatment of category IIb ALI, which is driven by an increasing array of thrombectomy technologies and increased operator experience. The use of adjunctive thrombolysis with PMT using bolus dosing rather than infusions may facilitate the aim of restoring limb perfusion quickly.

In general, patients with category III ALI are best managed with a major amputation of the limb. Attempts to revascularize such a limb may actually result in harm, since reperfusion of a limb with extensive muscle necrosis can result in severe metabolic disturbance, including myoglobinemia, which can precipitate acute renal failure. The exception to this generalization is the patient who presents acutely (i.e., within 1 to 2 hours) with signs of category III ALI. These patients have typically experienced an embolic event. In such cases, rapid revascularization of the limb (using surgical revascularization or PMT) should be attempted. Careful observation of such patients following revascularization is clearly critical, understanding that such patients have a significantly increased likelihood of metabolic disturbances and development of compartment syndrome (see below).

PART II: CATHETER-DIRECTED THROMBOLYSIS

Choice of Candidates for Catheter-Directed Thrombolytic Therapy

Decisions regarding the use of thrombolytic therapy for a patient with ALI are founded upon a fundamental knowledge base and the personal experiences that a clinician gains over the course of his or her clinical practice. There exist some data in the literature to suggest which patients do best with thrombolytic therapy, in comparison to other options (e.g., open surgical revascularization), but much of the decision-making process must be intuitive and based on something less than objective information.

Most importantly, thrombolytic therapy is contraindicated in patients with bleeding diatheses. Thus, patients with a history of gastrointestinal bleeding, recent major surgery, or stroke should normally not be considered for pharmacologic thrombolysis (Table 14.4). In addition, patients with contraindications to the angiographic procedures inherent in thrombolytic therapy may represent poor candidates for thrombolysis. Specifically, patients with impaired renal function should be treated with caution. Open surgery, mechanical thrombectomy, or anticoagulation alone (if the ischemia is not severe) may be more appropriate options.

Certain clinical variables have been identified as predictors of outcome with thrombolytic therapy. In a series of 80 patients undergoing arterial thrombolysis, success was defined by the complete (i.e., >80% volume) dissolution of thrombus and the absence of the need for open surgical intervention (32). Success was more frequent in prosthetic graft (78%) and native arterial (72%) occlusions than in vein graft occlusions (53%, $P = 0.017$) and in nondiabetics than in diabetics (80% vs. 52%, $P = 0.031$). Lysis was dependent on placement of the catheter into the substance of the thrombus (85% vs. 0% success, $P = 0.004$) and passage of a guidewire through the occlusive process (92% vs. 10% success, $P = 0.001$). The only parameter independently predictive of successful outcome, without the use of adjuvant procedures, was the location of the occlusion; additional procedures were necessary in 88% of aortoiliac and 82% of infrainguinal occlusions versus only 17% of upper extremity occlusions ($P = 0.005$).

The Surgery or Thrombolysis for the Ischemic Lower Extremity (STILE) trial randomized 393 patients with lower

TABLE 14.4 Contraindications for Pharmacologic Thrombolysis*

Absolute contraindications	
Cerebrovascular accident	Within 6 months
Intracranial surgery	Within 6 months
Gastrointestinal hemorrhage	Within 10 days
Major surgical procedure or trauma	Within 10 days
Uncontrolled hypertension	>180/110 mmHg
Puncture of a noncompressible site	Within 48 hours
Intracranial neoplasm, aneurysm, AVM	
Relative contraindications	
Renal insufficiency (contrast load)	Creatinine >2.5**
Hepatic insufficiency	Enzymes >3 × normal
Transient ischemic attack	Within 3 months
Diabetic retinopathy	
Pregnancy	
Thrombocytopenia	<100,000/dL
Elevated prothrombin time	INR > 1.5

* The table is not complete, and many of the contraindications and time-frames are not based on objective clinical data; rather, each represents the standard of care.
** Unless patient is on dialysis
AVM, arteriovenous malformation; INR, international normalized ratio.

extremity ischemia to thrombolysis (i.e., urokinase [UK] or alteplase [rt-PA], 1:2 ratio) or primary surgical intervention (33). Subsequent to the primary publication, two subgroup analyses were published. These studies confirmed the finding that patients with bypass graft occlusions had improved outcome with thrombolysis, compared with results of primary surgical intervention (34). The amputation rate at 1 year was significantly lower in patients treated with thrombolysis, compared with those treated with primary surgical revascularization (P = 0.02). By contrast, patients with native artery occlusions had better outcomes with surgical treatment, with a 1-year amputation rate of 0% versus 10% (P = 0.002) (35). While these data do not exclude the appropriate use of thrombolysis for native artery occlusions, the threshold for using a percutaneous means of restoring arterial perfusion in these cases should be higher than for bypass graft occlusions. Specifically, surgical management should be the primary consideration in patients with more chronic native artery occlusions (i.e., older than 14 days) and those with a reasonable, open surgical option (e.g., those patients with an adequate autogenous saphenous vein conduit).

In a multivariable analysis of the 544 patients randomized to thrombolytic therapy or open surgery in the Thrombolysis

or Peripheral Arterial Surgery (TOPAS) trial, 28 variables predictive of amputation-free survival were evaluated (36). Among these, eight main effects were predictive of amputation-free survival. These included two demographic factors: white race (risk ratio [RR] = 1.75; P = 0.003) and younger age (RR = 1.015; P = 0.046). Comorbidities comprised four of the eight main effects: history of central nervous system disease (RR = 1.726; P = 0.005), history of malignancy (RR = 1.615; P = 0.024), congestive heart failure (RR = 2.202; P < 0.001), or low body weight (RR = 1.007 per pound; P = 0.006). The severity of the process was also predictive, as gauged by the presence of skin color changes (RR = 1.585; P = 0.007) or pain at rest (RR = 0.503; P = 0.003). All eight effects were similar in the two treatment groups; none of these variables predicted improved outcome with one form of initial therapy over the other (i.e., there was no therapy-by-variable interaction). The length of occlusion, however, predicted whether a patient would fare better with thrombolysis or operation. With a threshold occlusion length of 30 cm, the relative risk for longer occlusions to shorter occlusions was 43% better in patients who received thrombolysis, whereas the situation was reversed for those who were randomized to surgery.

Choice of the Thrombolytic Agent

There exist four clinically available thrombolytic agents: streptokinase (SK), urokinase (UK), alteplase (rt-PA), and reteplase (r-PA). Of interest, SK is the only agent to have been approved for peripheral vascular indications by the U.S. Food and Drug Administration (FDA), although it is rarely used in clinical practice today. UK holds FDA indications for pulmonary embolism, rt-PA for coronary occlusion and pulmonary embolism, and r-PA for coronary occlusion alone. Nevertheless, each agent has been used with success for peripheral artery occlusions, despite this use being off-label for UK, rt-PA, and r-PA (37).

The history of the development of pharmacologic thrombolysis began over 70 years ago. In 1933, Tillett and Garner at the Johns Hopkins School of Medicine discovered that filtrates of broth cultures of certain strains of hemolytic *streptococcus* bacteria had fibrinolytic properties (38). This streptococcal byproduct was originally termed *streptococcal fibrinolysin*. The purity of this agent was poor, however. Clinical use, of necessity, awaited adequate purification. Tillett and Sherry administered SK intrapleurally, to dissolve loculated hemothoraces, in the late 1940s (39), but intravascular administration was not attempted until the following decade. Tillett et al. first reported intravascular administration of a thrombolytic agent in an article published in 1955 (40). A concentrated and partially purified SK was injected into 11 patients. This investigation was performed with the intent to gain data on the safety of the agent in volunteers; in no case was the SK administered to dissolve pathologic thrombi. Fever and hypotension developed as the amount of SK approached therapeutic levels. Whereas fever was generally mild and controllable with antipyretics, hypotension was sometimes prominent. The mean fall in systolic pressure was 31 mm Hg, and three of the patients manifested systolic pressures below 80 mm Hg. These untoward reactions were more likely a result of contaminants in the preparation, rather than in the SK itself. Despite these reactions, systemic proteolysis was observed, with a decrease in fibrinogen and plasminogen, concurrent with a mild increase in the prothrombin time.

These early studies were followed by reports on the use of SK in patients with occlusive vascular thrombi. In 1956, E. E. Cliffton, at the Cornell University Medical College in New York, was responsible for the first brief description of the clinical effectiveness of intravascular thrombolytic administration (41). The following year, Cliffton published his results for 40 patients with occlusive thrombi treated with a SK–plasminogen complex (42). The locations of the thrombi were diverse, and included peripheral arterial thrombi, venous thrombi, pulmonary emboli, retinal occlusions, and in two patients, occlusive carotid thrombi. The Cliffton clinical results were far from exemplary; recanalization was not uniform and bleeding complications were frequent. Nevertheless, he must be credited with the first use of thrombolytic agents for the treatment of pathologic thrombi, as well as with the first use of catheter-directed administration of a thrombolytic agent.

Several schemes may be used to classify thrombolytic agents. The agents may be grouped by their mechanisms of action (i.e., those that directly convert plasminogen to plasmin vs. those that are inactive zymogens and require transformation to an active form before they may cleave plasminogen). Thrombolytic agents may be grouped by their mode of production (i.e., those manufactured via recombinant techniques and those of bacterial origin). Of interest, recombinant agents harvested from a bacterial-expression system, such as *Escherichia coli*, do not contain carbohydrates, while products of mammalian hybridoma (e.g., recombinant prourokinase [r-ProUK] from mouse hybridoma SP2/0 cells) are fully glycosylated. Thrombolytic agents may be classified by their pharmacologic actions (i.e., those that are fibrin specific, binding to fibrin but not to fibrinogen, vs. nonspecific, as well as those that have a great degree of fibrin affinity, binding avidly to fibrin, vs. those that do not). It is most efficient to divide the agents into four groups: the SK compounds, the UK compounds, the tissue-plasminogen activators, and then an additional, miscellaneous group, consisting of novel agents distinct from agents in the three other groups.

STREPTOKINASE COMPOUNDS

Streptokinase (SK), originating from the streptococcus bacteria, was the first thrombolytic agent to be described. SK is a 50-kDa molecule with a biphasic half-life comprising a rapid $t\frac{1}{2}$ of 16 minutes, and a second, slower $t\frac{1}{2}$ of 90 minutes (43). Whereas the initial half-life is accounted for by the complex of the molecule with SK antibodies, the second half-life represents the actual biologic elimination of the protein. SK differs from other thrombolytic agents with respect to the stoichiometry of plasminogen binding. Whereas other agents directly convert plasminogen to plasmin, SK must form an equimolar stoichiometric complex with a plasmin or plasminogen molecule, to gain activity. Only then may this SK–plasmin(ogen) complex activate a second plasminogen molecule to form active plasmin; thus, two plasminogen molecules are used in SK-mediated plasmin generation. Unfortunately, SK suffers from the limitation of antigenic potential. Preformed antibodies exist, to a certain extent, in all patients who have been infected with the streptococcus bacterium. Similarly, patients with exposure to SK may have high antibody titers on repeat exposure. These neutralizing antibodies inactivate exogenously

administered SK. SK antibodies may be overwhelmed through the use of a large, initial bolus of drug, and a large, initial SK loading dose may be employed in this regard. Some investigators have recommended measurement of antibody titers prior to beginning SK therapy, gauging the loading dose on the basis of this titer (44).

SK administration is complicated by allergic reactions in approximately 2% of patients treated with the development of urticaria, periorbital edema, and bronchospasm. Pyrexia may also occur, but is usually adequately treated with acetaminophen. The major untoward effect associated with SK is hemorrhage. SK-associated hemorrhage may be no different than bleeding associated with any thrombolytic agent. The primary cause is likely the actions of the systemic agent on the thrombi, sealing the sites of vascular disintegrity. The generation of free plasmin, however, may contribute to the problem, with degradation of fibrinogen and other serum clotting proteins, as well as the release of fibrin(ogen)-degradation products that are potent anticoagulants and exacerbate the coagulopathy.

Recognizing potential limitations with SK, anisoylated plasminogen–SK activator complex (APSAC) was developed by pharmacologists at Beecham Laboratories (45). APSAC has a longer half-life than SK, since acylation rendered the complex less susceptible to degradation. Owing to this property, it was anticipated that APSAC would be associated with a reduced risk of rethrombosis. Contrary to expectations, APSAC offered little clinical benefit over other agents, and at present, is not used to treat thrombi in the peripheral vasculature.

UROKINASE COMPOUNDS

MacFarlane first described the fibrinolytic potential of human urine in 1947 (46). The active molecule was extracted, isolated, and named urokinase (UK) in 1952 (47). This UK-type plasminogen activator is a serine protease composed of two polypeptide chains, occurring in low-molecular-weight (32 kDa) and high-molecular-weight (54 kDa) forms. The high-molecular-weight form predominates in UK isolated from urine, while the low-molecular-weight form is found in UK obtained from tissue cultures of kidney cells. Unlike SK, UK directly activates plasminogen to form plasmin; prior binding to plasminogen or plasmin is not necessary for activity. Also in contrast to SK, preformed antibodies to UK are not observed. The agent is nonantigenic, and untoward reactions of fever or hypotension are rare. Presently, the most commonly employed UK in the United States is of tissue-culture origin, manufactured from human neonatal kidney cells. UK has been fully sequenced, and a recombinant form of UK (r-UK) was tested in two multicenter trials of patients with peripheral arterial occlusion (48,49). r-UK is fully glycosylated, since it is derived from a murine hybridoma cell line. r-UK differs from UK in several respects. First, r-UK has a higher molecular weight than UK. Second, r-UK has a shorter half-life than its low-molecular-weight counterpart. Despite these differences, however, the clinical effects of the two agents have been quite similar.

A precursor of UK was discovered in urine in 1979 (50). ProUK was characterized and subsequently manufactured by recombinant technology, using *E. coli* (nonglycosylated) or mammalian cells (fully glycosylated) (51). This single-chain form is an inactive zymogen, inert in plasma, but may be activated by kallikrein or plasmin, to form active two-chain UK. This property accounts for amplification of the fibrinolytic process; as plasmin is generated, more ProUK is converted to active UK, and the process is repeated. ProUK is relatively fibrin specific; that is, its fibrin-degrading (*fibrinolytic*) activity greatly outweighs its fibrinogen-degrading (*fibrinogenolytic*) activity. This feature is explained by the preferential activation of fibrin-bound plasminogen found in a thrombus over free plasminogen found in flowing blood. Nonselective activators, such as SK and UK, activate free and bound plasminogen equally, and induce systemic plasminemia with resultant fibrinogenolysis and degradation of factors V and VII. Given the potential advantages of ProUK over UK, Abbott Laboratories produced a recombinant form of ProUK (r-ProUK) from a murine hybridoma cell line. This recombinant agent is converted to active two-chain UK by plasmin and kallikrein. r-ProUK has been studied in the settings of myocardial infarction, stroke, and peripheral arterial occlusion. To date, it appears that r-ProUK offers the advantages associated with an agent that does not originate from a human cell source. Fibrin specificity, however, may be lost at the higher-dose levels necessary to effect more rapid thrombolysis.

TISSUE-PLASMINOGEN ACTIVATORS

Tissue-plasminogen activator (t-PA) is a naturally occurring fibrinolytic agent produced by endothelial cells and intimately involved in the balance between intravascular thrombogenesis and thrombolysis. Wild-type t-PA is a single-chain (527 amino acid) serine protease with a molecular weight of approximately 65 kDa. Plasmin hydrolyzes the Arg275–Ile276 peptide bond, converting the single-chain molecule into a two-chain moiety. In contrast to most serine proteases (e.g., UK), the single-chain form of t-PA has significant activity. t-PA has potential benefits over other thrombolytic agents. The agent exhibits significant fibrin specificity (52). In plasma, the agent is associated with little plasminogen activation. At the site of the thrombus, however, the binding of t-PA and plasminogen, to the fibrin surface, induces a conformational change in both molecules, greatly facilitating the conversion of plasminogen to plasmin and resulting in dissolution of the clot. t-PA also manifests the property of fibrin affinity; it binds strongly to fibrin. Other fibrinolytic agents, such as ProUK, do not share this property of fibrin affinity. Recombinant t-PA (rt-PA, alteplase) was produced in the 1980s after molecular cloning techniques were used to express human t-PA DNA (53). A predominantly single-chain form of rt-PA was eventually approved in the United States for the indications of acute myocardial infarction and massive pulmonary embolism. rt-PA has been studied extensively in the setting of coronary occlusion. In the GUSTO-I study of approximately 41,000 patients with acute myocardial infarction, rt-PA was more effective than SK in achieving vascular patency (54). Despite a slightly greater risk of intracranial hemorrhage with rt-PA, overall mortality was significantly reduced.

In an effort to lengthen the duration of bioavailability of t-PA, the molecule was systematically bioengineered. Initial investigations identified regions in kringle 1 and the protease portion of t-PA that mediated hepatic clearance, fibrin specificity, and resistance to plasminogen-activator inhibitor. Three sites were modified to create TNK-tPA (tenecteplase), a novel molecule with a greater half-life and fibrin specificity (55). The longer half-life of TNK-tPA allowed successful administration as a single bolus, in contrast to the requirement for an infusion with rt-PA. In addition, TNK-tPA manifests greater fibrin specificity than rt-PA, resulting in less fibrinogen depletion. In studies of acute coronary occlusion, TNK-tPA performed at least as well as rt-PA, concurrent with greater ease of administration (56).

RETEPLASE

Similar to TNK-tPA, the novel recombinant plasminogen activator, reteplase, comprises the kringle 2 and protease domains of t-PA. Reteplase was developed with the goal of avoiding the necessity of a continuous intravenous infusion, thereby simplifying ease of administration (57). Reteplase, produced in *E. coli* cells, is nonglycosylated, demonstrating a lower fibrin-binding activity and a diminished affinity to hepatocytes (58). This latter property accounts for a longer half-life than that of rt-PA, potentially enabling bolus injection versus prolonged infusion. The fibrin affinity of reteplase was only 30% of that exhibited with t-PA, similar to UK. The decrease in fibrin affinity was hypothesized to reduce the incidence of distant bleeding complications, in a manner similar to that of SK over rt-PA, in the GUSTO trial. In fact, several properties of reteplase may account for a decreased risk of hemorrhage, including poor lysis of platelet-rich, older clots. Reteplase has demonstrated some benefit over rt-PA in the RAPID 1 and RAPID 2 studies, as well as in GUSTO-III (59). To date, a handful of peripheral arterial and venous studies have been published using this agent (60–63).

Comparison of the Agents in Studies of Peripheral Vascular Disease

To date, there have been few well-designed clinical comparisons of various thrombolytic agents in the peripheral vasculature. There exist a variety of in vitro studies and retrospective clinical trials, most pointing to improved efficacy and safety of UK and rt-PA over SK (64–66). In an analysis of data collected in a prospective, single institution registry at the Cleveland Clinic Foundation, UK demonstrated a diminished rate of bleeding complications when compared with rt-PA (67). Efficacy was not evaluated in this trial.

There have been two prospective, randomized comparisons of UK and rt-PA. Neither was blinded. Meyerovitz and associates from the Brigham and Women's Hospital (Massachusetts) randomized 32 patients with peripheral artery or bypass graft occlusions, of less than 90 days' duration, to rt-PA (10 mg bolus, 5 mg/h for a maximum of 24 hours) or UK (60,000 IU bolus, 4000 IU/min for 2 hours, 2000 IU/min for 2 hours, and then 1000 IU/min to a maximum of 24 hours, total administration) (68). There was significantly greater systemic-fibrinogen degradation in the rt-PA group ($P = 0.01$), indicating that the fibrin specificity of rt-PA was lost at this dosing regimen. rt-PA patients achieved more rapid initial thrombolysis, but efficacy was identical in the two groups, by 24 hours. The trade-off to more rapid thrombolysis was a trend toward a higher rate of bleeding complications in the rt-PA-treated patients ($P = 0.39$). The second, randomized comparison of UK and rt-PA was the STILE trial, a three-armed, multicenter comparison of UK (250,000 IU bolus, 4000 IU/min for 4 hours, and then 2000 IU/min for up to 36 hours), rt-PA (0.05 to 0.1 mg/kg/h, for up to 12 hours), and primary operation (33). There was one intracranial hemorrhage in the UK group (0.9%) and two in the rt-PA group (1.5%, no significant difference). Although actual rates of overall bleeding complications and efficacy were not reported for the two thrombolytic groups, the authors remarked that there were no significant differences detected in any of the outcome variables. In a subsequent reanalysis of the data, reported in 1999, the frequency of complete clot lysis was similar with UK and rt-PA, at the time of the early arteriographic study (69). These recent data suggest that the rate of thrombolysis may be quite similar, in direct contradiction to the popularly held view that rt-PA is a much more rapidly acting agent.

A multicenter, blinded trial compared the results of thrombolysis with UK versus r-UK in 300 patients with peripheral arterial occlusion (70). Despite a shorter half-life for r-UK, there were no significant clinical differences noted between the two agents. A North American multicenter trial compared three different doses of r-ProUK to UK in 241 patients with lower extremity arterial occlusions of less than 14 days' duration (71). While the higher r-ProUK dose was associated with a slightly greater percentage of patients with complete (>95%) clot lysis at 8 hours, there was a mild increase in the rate of bleeding complications in this group, compared with either the UK or the lower-dose r-ProUK group. The fibrinogen levels fell in the higher r-ProUK group, suggesting that fibrin specificity is lost at the higher-dose regimens for this compound.

Technique for Thrombolysis of Peripheral Arterial Occlusions

Once the determination to implement thrombolytic therapy has been made, and the particular agent has been selected, several procedural issues must be resolved. Each of these issues plays an important role in achieving a therapeutic success. Precise attention to every clinical detail is imperative to accomplish reasonably rapid dissolution of the thrombus and normalization of arterial blood flow, without complications that may result in the loss of limb or life.

MANAGEMENT OF THE ANTICOAGULATED PATIENT

At the outset, one must be cognizant of coagulation abnormalities that are frequent in patients with acute arterial occlusions. Many patients are on aspirin or clopidogrel, potentially increasing the risk of puncture site bleeding complications. A significant proportion of patients will be fully anticoagulated with warfarin at the time of presentation, prescribed and administered as a result of cardiac arrhythmia or a previous occlusive event. As well, patients with a distal bypass conduit, such as a prosthetic femoral-tibial graft, may be on long-term anticoagulation. There are two choices in such patients; either correct the international normalized ratio (INR) to acceptable levels (e.g., 1.5 or below) or proceed, using a micropuncture technique. In cases of severe ischemia, a micropuncture technique is elected, using a 4-Fr. system and, if necessary, ultrasound guidance, to ensure a single anterior wall puncture. In cases where an additional period of several hours between presentation and treatment may be tolerated, fresh frozen plasma is given to restore a normal INR. In general, it is recommended to refrain from the use of vitamin K to reverse anticoagulation, since the administration of more than trivial amounts of vitamin K makes subsequent re-anticoagulation extremely difficult.

CHOICE FOR ARTERIAL ACCESS

The choice for the arterial access site is of great importance and is one of the primary determinants of complications associated with thrombolytic therapy. The peripheral pulse examination, preprocedural anatomic assessment (i.e., using preprocedural imaging), and the location of the arterial occlusion guide this decision. In most circumstances, access is attempted using a retrograde approach through the contralateral common femoral artery (e.g., occluded femoral–popliteal graft with normal iliac anatomy) or an ipsilateral antegrade approach through the common femoral artery (e.g., ipsilateral popliteal artery occlusion with diseased contralateral iliac artery). If the contralateral femoral pulse is weak or absent, or in patients with an aortofemoral-bypass graft, a left brachial approach may be more appropriate. For femoral access, a single-wall puncture technique is important. For brachial access, one should maintain a low threshold for an open exposure of the artery. Direct cannulation of the brachial artery, just above the antecubital crease, may prevent complications such as brachial sheath hematoma and peripheral nerve palsies or brachial artery thrombosis.

Irrespective of the site of access, a complete diagnostic arteriogram is necessary in all patients with adequate renal function, obtaining full views of the runoff vessels in the affected limb. A complete interrogation of the lower extremity vessels will allow one to make an accurate assessment of whether or not the event is secondary to thrombosis or embolization, and to provide some indication of the chronicity of the problem. Lastly, it is important to image the ipsilateral outflow vessels adequately to provide baseline distal views should subsequent distal embolization occur during thrombolysis.

PLACEMENT OF THE INFUSION SYSTEM

Just as gaining uncomplicated arterial access is the most important determinant of local bleeding complications (safety), accurate placement of the infusion system into the occluding thrombus is the primary determinant of successful and efficacious clot dissolution.

In the case of occlusion of the superficial femoral artery or a bypass graft that originates from proximal femoral inflow, the contralateral femoral approach is the best. The 5-Fr. short sheath is exchanged for a 6-Fr. crossover sheath. When possible, it is best to place the distal tip of the sheath within the external iliac artery (EIA), to minimize contrast agent loss into the hypogastric (i.e., internal iliac) system.

Next, attempts are made to cannulate the occluded artery or bypass graft. Oblique views are helpful to find the orifice. One useful method is to use a 5-Fr. angled catheter (e.g., Bernstein or glide catheter) and an angled 0.035″ hydrophilic wire, placing the catheter just proximal to the expected occluded ostium with careful manipulation of the wire to gain access to the occlusion. Once access has been achieved, the wire is advanced well into the occlusion, so that the catheter may be advanced into the occluded artery or bypass graft.

At this point, the guidewire may be exchanged for a stiffer wire. A sturdy wire is necessary to advance the thrombolytic infusion catheter into the occlusion, since the infusion catheters do not track as well as other, more flexible catheters. After estimating the length of the occlusion, an infusion catheter with an appropriate length of side holes is chosen and advanced into position. Typically, the infusion catheter should be long

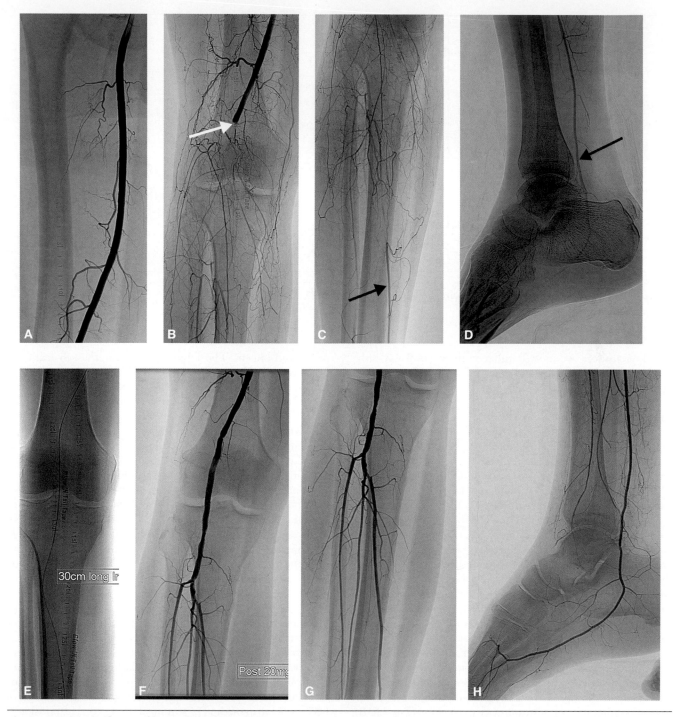

Figure 14.3 • Catheter-directed thrombolysis. A–D: Baseline angiography in 50-year-old male who presented with category IIa acute limb ischemia due to thrombotic occlusion of a previously placed Viabahn stent in the popliteal artery (for treatment of popliteal artery aneurysm). Note abrupt occlusion of the above-knee popliteal artery *(white arrow)*. The posterior tibial artery *(black arrows)* filled faintly via collaterals and provided the main arterial inflow to the foot. **E:** A 30 cm long infusion catheter was placed across the length of the occlusion, and t-PA was administered at 1 mg/h. **F–H:** Angiographic appearance following 20 hours of t-PA infusion.

enough to cover the length of the occlusion plus a 2 to 5 cm margin at either end of the occlusion (Fig. 14.3).

An infusion wire will be necessary in cases when the thrombus is discontinuous (e.g., an occluded femoral–popliteal bypass graft, with an open popliteal artery but with thrombotic occlusion of the tibioperoneal trunk) or when the occlusion

length is longer than the longest infusion length (i.e., usually 50 cm) of the infusion catheter. The infusion wire may come with the particular thrombolytic infusion catheter, or if not, a Tuohey-Borst connector needs to be applied to the end of the infusion catheter through which the infusion wire can be inserted.

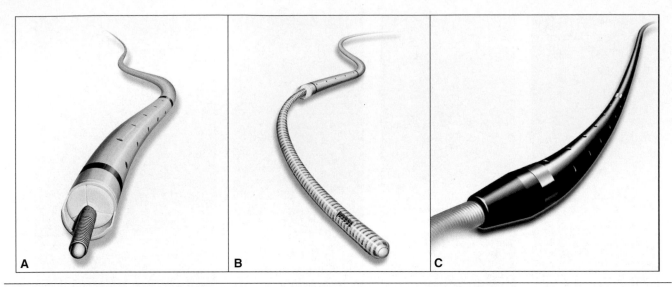

Figure 14.4 • Infusion catheters and wires. **A:** Cragg–McNamara infusion catheter. **B:** ProStream® infusion wire. **C:** MicroMewi® infusion catheter.

The authors are most familiar with the infusion catheters (Cragg–McNamara and MicroMewi®) and wire (The ProStream®) provided by ev3 (Fig. 14.4). The Cragg–McNamara infusion catheter is available in 4-Fr. and 5-Fr. sizes that are compatible with 0.035″ and 0.038″ wires, respectively (Fig. 14.4A). They are available in a variety of catheter lengths varying from 40 to 135 cm. The choice of catheter length will depend on the anticipated distance from the arterial access to the target treatment site. For lower extremity work, the 100 and 135 cm lengths are most commonly used. The actual infusion length (i.e., the length over which the catheter has side holes) varies from 5 to 50 cm to accommodate the range of treatment lengths required, and is indicated by proximal and distal markers on the catheter. In general, the Cragg–McNamara catheters are suited for use in the above-knee and popliteal arteries in the lower extremity and for the subclavian, axillary, and brachial arteries in the upper extremity. One important feature of the Cragg–McNamara catheter is that there is a valve at the catheter tip that is designed to maximize the delivery of active thrombolytic agent through the side holes of the catheter. This valve must be overcome during wire exchanges of the catheter. If significant resistance is met that cannot be overcome with a conventional wire, a stiff-angled glidewire will have sufficient body at the tip to overcome the valve. When it is used in combination with an infusion wire (see below) (Fig. 14.4B), the authors usually adopt the following strategy: the 5-Fr. (not the 4-Fr.) Cragg–McNamara catheter is delivered to the distal end of the target site for the infusion wire. The infusion wire is then advanced through the Tuohey-Borst connector at the end of the infusion catheter until it reaches the tip of the infusion catheter. At this point, the infusion catheter is withdrawn over the infusion wire to its desired location. These maneuvers are necessary because of the valve at the distal end of the infusion catheter and the fact that the infusion wire is not steerable.

The MicroMewi® infusion catheter has been designed for use in smaller caliber vessels (e.g., infrapopliteal and forearm arteries) (Fig. 14.4C). It is deliverable over a 0.018″ wire and is available in a single 2.9-Fr. size with catheter lengths of 150 and 180 cm. The active infusion length of the catheter is either 5 or 10 cm. In contrast with the Cragg–McNamara catheter, this catheter does not have a valve at the catheter tip, and cannot be used in combination with an infusion wire.

The ProStream® infusion wire is a single-lumen 0.035″ wire with a closed end and multiple side holes. It is available in two lengths (145 and 175 cm) and three infusions lengths (6, 9, and 12 cm). It is typically used in combination with the Cragg–McNamara catheter (as described above).

Some clinicians prefer to lace the thrombus with thrombolytic agent prior to instituting a slow infusion. There are several methods to accomplish this. The most common merely involves the use of the multi-side-hole infusion catheter, manually injecting a dose of agent in a rapid, pulsed fashion into the thrombus. If the length of the thrombotic occlusion exceeds the length of the side-hole region of the catheter, the catheter may be repositioned one or more times to achieve an adequate distribution of thrombolytic agent throughout the thrombus. Other clinicians use a pulse-spray infusion, where a console and catheter (i.e., Angiojet, Medrad Interventional-Possis) are used to provide rapid pulses of agent in attempts to provide better distribution into the thrombus, as well as some element of mechanical disruption (72,73). The authors and others have not found the pulse-spray technique to offer significant advantages over a slow-drip method of administration (74). The infusion is begun once the catheter is in position. If an infusion wire is used, the dose of thrombolytic agent may be split between the catheter and the wire, in a ratio that is appropriate for the volume of thrombus addressed by the two systems. The authors use t-PA exclusively, and typically use a total dose of 1 mg/h divided between the infusion catheter and the wire. Concomitant heparin therapy, is administered at a low dose—usually 500 to 800 hundred units per hour based on patients' weight—through the side arm of the arterial access sheath (62). Importantly, the heparin may never be mixed with the thrombolytic agent, as the low pH of the heparin solution may cause precipitation of the agent.

Once the infusion has begun, the patient is sent to an intensive care unit or step-down unit for monitoring.

The determination of when the patient is returned for a lytic checkup test is based on the severity of ischemia and the practicalities of the clinical schedule. In cases of severe ischemia, it is important to obtain an early angiogram, usually within 4 to 8 hours, with repositioning of the catheter if necessary. In less severely ischemic cases, the patient may be returned for a check at 12 hours, or even the next morning.

When distal embolization is heralded by the sudden development of worsening distal ischemia, continued upstream infusion usually suffices and the ischemia improves over an hour or two. This represents the single example of when regional thrombolysis may be effective in dissolving a peripheral arterial thrombus, presumably because the embolized clot contains thrombolytic agent that provides active, ongoing thrombolysis. If improvement does not occur within a few hours, the patient should be returned to the angiography suite for repositioning of catheters and wires, in attempts to address the embolized fragments directly. Mechanical thrombectomy should also be considered when distal embolization is not resolved.

The decision to terminate thrombolytic therapy is not as simple as it may seem. One must often strike a risk–benefit balance between complete clot lysis and the risk of hemorrhagic complications. Although a longer infusion duration produces a more pristine angiographic appearance, the risk of hemorrhage rises over time. Traditionally, the cutoff time for discontinuation of thrombolytic administration has been 48 hours (75,76). The risk of hemorrhagic complications is said to increase dramatically beyond this time point, but there exist no objective data on which to base this contention. Some clinicians measure fibrinogen levels and terminate thrombolysis when the levels decline below 100 mg/dL (77). Fibrinogen, however, has been disappointing as a predictor of bleeding (48,78).

In practice, thrombolytic therapy should be terminated when there is antegrade flow through the target artery or bypass graft, when the amount of residual mural thrombus does not appear to be flow limiting, and when there is no significant thrombus in the outflow bed. Thrombolytic administration should be terminated earlier if hemorrhagic complications arise. Consideration should be made to lower the infusion rate or to discontinue thrombolytic administration transiently, when precipitous fibrinogen decrements are noted, but this remains controversial. In most cases, thrombolysis should be terminated after no more than 48 hours of infusion, irrespective of the clinical course. Careful attention to these details will diminish the frequency of hemorrhagic complications.

Treatment after Thrombolysis

The objective of thrombolytic therapy is to dissolve the majority of intravascular thrombus and unmask any underlying arterial lesions that were responsible for the occlusive event. Thrombolysis, in and of itself, should never be considered the sole therapy. Studies where thrombolysis was not routinely followed by correction of the underlying lesion, expectedly, found the therapy to be of little use (79). In fact, despite complete thrombolytic dissolution of clot, the failure to find and correct an underlying culprit lesion is tantamount to failure. In a study of thrombolyzed infrainguinal grafts, when a flow-limiting lesion was identified and corrected by angioplasty or surgery, the patency rate was significantly improved over those grafts without such lesions (79.0% vs. 9.8% at 2 years, $P = 0.01$) (80).

Fortunately, most lesions may be addressed with contemporary percutaneous techniques. In the TOPAS trial, 46% of subjects treated with thrombolytic therapy left the hospital with nothing more than a percutaneous procedure (48). In the more recent study of r-ProUK for ALI, this percentage had increased to approximately 66% (71). The use of newer stents, and other percutaneous techniques with improved effectiveness for infrainguinal disease, will only increase the number of patients that may be treated with a fully percutaneous strategy. In this manner, it is hoped that the excessive morbidity and mortality associated with acute peripheral arterial occlusion may be lowered, dramatically.

Complications of CDT: Compartment Syndrome

In addition to the bleeding complications associated with thrombolytic therapy (intracranial, access site, retroperitoneal, gastrointestinal, and genitourinary), an awareness and early recognition of ischemic reperfusion injury leading to acute limb compartment syndrome is vital to prevent further morbidity and mortality (81). Prompt vascular surgery evaluation during ALI treatment is an important part of the patient's ongoing care. Acute compartment syndrome is thought to arise from a complex local inflammatory response upon restoration of blood flow involving polymorphonuclear leukocytes, oxygen-derived free radicals, and a multitude of cytokines such as tumor necrosis factor, which enhances endothelial cell permeability culminating in the accumulation of fluid within the lower limb compartments (82). Elevation of pressure impinges venous return, capillary flow, and eventually arterial blood supply to the limb. Normal resting intramuscular pressure is 0 to 8 mm Hg and many use the cutoff of an intracompartment pressure (ICP) of more than 30 mm Hg to perform a decompression fasciotomy (83). Acute compartment syndrome has been reported to occur in up to 21% of cases of ALI, after restoration of arterial flow. Risk factors include increasing duration of ischemia, age, systemic hypotension, and an abrupt onset of ischemia. Symptoms and signs are outlined in Table 14.5. A limb may become nonviable when an ICP of 30 mm Hg is exceeded for only 6 to 8 hours. To ensure satisfactory decompression, fasciotomy of all three thigh (anterior, posterior, and medial) and four leg (anterior, peroneal, deep, and superficial posterior) compartments may be necessary.

TABLE 14.5 Signs and Symptoms of Acute Compartment Syndrome

Symptoms	Signs
Worsening pain	Pain on passive movement, which progress rapidly
Paresthesia	Pallor
Paralysis	Swelling (wood hard) of limb
	Loss of distal pulses

(Adapted from Tiwari A, Haq AI, Myint F, et al. Acute compartment syndromes. *Br J Surg.* 2002;89:397–412.)

TABLE 14.6 Mechanical Thrombectomy Devices

Aspiration devices
- Export® XT/AP Catheter (Medtronic, Inc.)
- Pronto® V3/LP/0.035″/Short Extraction Catheter (Vascular Solutions, Inc.)
- Xtract Aspiration Catheter (Volcano)
- QuickCat Extraction Catheter (Spectranetics)
- Diver CE Extraction Catheter (Invatec Inc.).
- Fetch Aspiration Catheter (Medrad Interventional/Possis)
- Aspire Aspirator (Control Medical Technology)
- Xtract Aspiration Catheter (Lumen Biomedical)

Hemodynamic recirculation devices
- AngioJet® (Medrad Interventional/Possis)
- Hydrolyzer® (Cordis Corporation)

Rotational devices
- HELIX® Clot Buster Thrombectomy device (ev3)

Ultrasonic devices
- EkoSonic Endovascular System (peripheral) (Ekos Corporation)
- EkoSonic SV Endovascular System (small vessel) (Ekos Corporation)

Miscellaneous group
- X-SIZER® Catheter (ev3 Inc, Plymouth, MN)
- Trellis® Thrombectomy System (Covidien)

PART III: PERCUTANEOUS MECHANICAL THROMBECTOMY

Percutaneous mechanical thrombectomy (PMT) evolved in an attempt to overcome the main limitations of CDT, namely, the need for prolonged lytic infusion (with the associated rise in hemorrhagic complications) and the slow rate of reperfusion. The following section provides the functioning and technical specifications of the array of devices currently available in the United States for the percutaneous mechanical treatment of arterial thrombus. Table 14.6 lists these devices.

Simple Aspiration Catheters

The simplest thrombectomy devices are catheters with a large distal port for application of suction. Currently, there are eight commercially available aspiration catheters for use in the coronary and peripheral circulations including Export XT and AP, Pronto V3 and LP, Fetch, Xtract, Diver CE, and QuickCat (Fig. 14.5). All of these catheters have a monorail design, and are delivered over a 0.014″ guidewire. The suction lumen is large (Fig. 14.5), and extends from the tip of the catheter to the hub, where a syringe is attached for aspiration. There is some variation in the outer diameter, extraction lumen area, and aspiration speed across the range of these catheters. The clinical consequence of these variations is uncertain.

These catheters work most effectively when there is no flow in the artery. In the presence of flow, the catheter aspirates blood instead of thrombus. In the authors practice, the catheter is advanced to the proximal level of the thrombotic occlusion and aspiration is applied. The catheter is then advanced slowly along the length of the occlusion. A new syringe is then used to apply aspiration as the catheter withdrawn over the interventional wire. This process may be repeated several times until no further thrombotic material is removed or flow is restored. If the catheter gets clogged, it should be removed outside of the body and flushed. In small vessels (i.e., up to 3 to 4 mm) these catheters seem to work well. When the thrombus burden is large, other mechanical devices are generally required to remove the remaining thrombus. These catheters may be used as a pretreatment, in some cases, prior to using more bulky devices for thrombectomy (see below), in an effort to minimize distal embolization at the time of insertion of the latter devices.

Hydrodynamic Aspiration Devices

This group of devices exploits the use of high-speed saline jets to create a Venturi effect at the catheter tip, which results in

Figure 14.5 • Schematic illustration of Pronto® aspiration catheter with a magnified cross-sectional view and magnified view of the catheter tip.

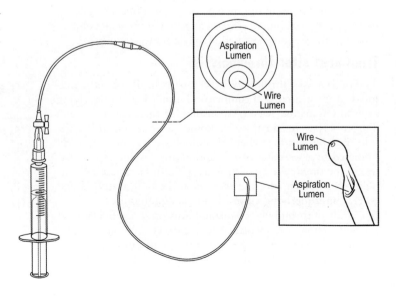

TABLE 14.7 *AngioJet® Catheters*

Catheter	XMI	Spiroflex	XVG	Spiroflex VG	Xpeedior	DVX	AVX
Minimal vessel diameter	≥2 mm	≥2 mm	≥3 mm	≥3 mm	≥3 mm	≥3 mm	≥3 mm
Optimal vessel range	2–5 mm	2–5 mm	3–8 mm	3–8 mm	4–12 mm	4–12 mm	4–12 mm
Working length	135 cm	135 cm	140 cm	135 cm	120 cm	90 cm	50 cm
Delivery	OTW	Rx	OTW	Rx	OTW	OTW	OTW
Wire	0.014″	0.014″	0.014″	0.014″	0.035″	0.035″	0.035″
Minimum guide	6 Fr.	7 Fr.	7 Fr.	6 Fr.	8 Fr.	8 Fr.	8 Fr.
Minimum sheath	4 Fr.	5 Fr.	5 Fr.	8 Fr.	6 Fr.	6 Fr.	6 Fr.

lysis and aspiration of thrombus. Saline is injected through a narrow injection lumen toward the catheter tip. Using a variety of designs, the jet(s) is (are) then directed backward, toward the proximal portion of the catheter. A low-pressure zone is thus created around these high-speed jets, which has the effect of fragmenting and aspirating the thrombus through the hole(s) that are present in the catheter tip. A large export lumen then carries the aspirated thrombus toward a collection area. Various designs of the fluid delivery, pressure generation, and suction provide specific advantages and disadvantages to these systems. The specific design features of the two representatives of this class of thrombectomy device are outlined in the following section.

ANGIOJET

The AngioJet® has three components: a drive unit that monitors the performance of the system and a pump set that is responsible for delivery and removal of equal volumes of fluid from the final component of the system, the catheter. The drive unit and pump set are housed in a console whose platform accommodates an array of catheters that have been developed for use in vessels of different caliber (Table 14.7).

It is important to be aware of the appropriate wire and guide/sheath compatibilities of the various devices. The Xpeedior®, DVX, and AVX® catheters are specifically marketed for use in the peripheral circulation. They are each delivered over a 0.035″ wire, and their outer diameters mandate the use of an 8-Fr. guide or 6-Fr. sheath. They differ only in the catheter length (i.e., 50 cm vs. 90 cm vs. 120 cm). In smaller vessels in the periphery, it is appropriate to use the XVG® and XMI® catheters, or their monorail equivalents (i.e., Spiroflex and Spiroflex VG), which are specifically marketed for use in saphenous vein grafts and native coronary arteries, respectively.

All catheters share the same basic technology. At the tip of the catheter, the fluid that is delivered into the catheter by the pump is directed backward toward the operator from the tip in six high-velocity jets (Fig. 14.6). These jets create a low-pressure zone at the catheter tip, producing a vacuum

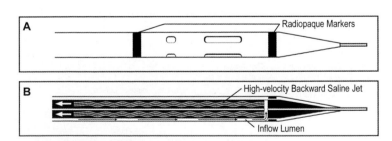

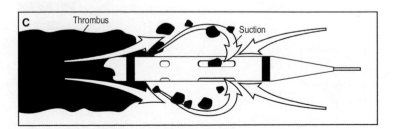

Figure 14.6 • Schematic illustration of the distal portion of the AngioJet® catheter. A: Intact distal portion of the catheter showing the site of the radiopaque markers and entry holes. **B:** Cross-sectional view through the distal portion of the catheter, showing the location and backward direction of the high-speed saline jets. **C:** Activation of the saline jets results in aspiration of thrombus through the holes in the distal portion of the catheter.

that draws thrombus through holes located between the two radiopaque markers in the distal portion of the catheter. Once captured in the hole, the thrombus is fragmented by the saline jets and returned to the pump set. Calculations of pressure at the tip of the AngioJet catheter show it to be an almost perfect vacuum (i.e., negative 760 mm Hg). If one considers that the normal pressure inside an artery is approximately 100 mm Hg, one may begin to appreciate the pressure difference (i.e., 860 mm Hg) that drives thrombotic debris through the openings at the catheter tip (84).

Prior to insertion in the patient, the catheter is flushed outside the body, by activating the pump (using a pedal), for a duration of approximately 20 seconds, while keeping the catheter tip under water. There is continued debate over the best strategy for the initial activation of the device in the patient; some operators activate the pump when advancing the catheter into the thrombus, while others activate while withdrawing the catheter from the thrombus. The manufacturer recommends the latter approach. Following the initial activation, the pump is activated during both advancement and withdrawal of the catheter. This is repeated several times until the bulk of the thrombus burden is removed, as determined by angiography.

A number of potential complications are associated with the use of the AngioJet device. The large size of the catheter may cause distal embolization while traversing the thrombus. Some operators employ an adjunctive distal-emboli prevention device to minimize the risk of this complication. Significant vessel dissection may also occur following AngioJet use. This is more commonly seen with the larger catheter sizes, and emphasizes the need to use the appropriately sized catheter, based on vessel size.

HYDROLYZER SYSTEM

The Hydrolyzer® device is marketed for use in the treatment of thrombus in hemodialysis fistulas and acute arterial thrombosis below the inguinal ligament, in either native arteries or synthetic grafts. This device is delivered through a 6-Fr. sheath, over a 0.018″ wire, and is available in working lengths of 65 and 100 cm.

The device functions as follows (Fig. 14.7): heparinized saline is injected through a narrow injection lumen, using a conventional power injector. The recommended maximum flow and pressure settings on the power injector are 5 mL/sec

and 750 psi, respectively. A total of 100 to 150 mL of saline is typically injected during passage of the catheter through the thrombus. At the catheter tip, the injection lumen makes a 180° loop and terminates just distal to an oval side hole located 4 mm proximal to the distal smooth tip. The proximally directed jet of saline creates a pressure reduction at the site of the oval hole, which aspirates and fragments thrombus from around the catheter into a larger exhaust lumen that empties into a collection bag. With a guidewire in place, the device performs isovolumetrically. The eccentric location of the hole in this device is a potential disadvantage in that the suction vortex created is less than 360°. This raises the potential for asymmetric suction on the vessel wall, increasing the risk for vessel trauma.

COMPLICATIONS WITH HYDRODYNAMIC ASPIRATION DEVICES

Macroembolization

All of these devices are relatively bulky and are potential causes of distal macroembolization during manipulation of the catheters in thrombus-laden vessels. While hemodialysis fistulas usually tolerate this downstream embolization into the large capacitance venous system, this event is typically poorly tolerated in the peripheral arterial circulation (85).

Vessel Trauma

In theory, these devices exert their effect without making contact with the vessel wall. However, in practice, the negative suction effect created at the tip of these catheters has the potential to draw the vessel wall into the openings in the catheter tip. Angiographically, it is rare to observe evidence of vessel trauma (i.e., frank vessel dissection), but angioscopic and histologic studies commonly demonstrate evidence of endothelial denudation (86). The asymmetry in the opening of the Hydrolyzer device may increase the risk of this complication compared to that associated with the AngioJet. Reducing the flow rate of the saline solution is likely to reduce the risk of this complication.

Hemolysis and Anemia

Hemolysis resulting in anemia may occur during the mechanical disruption of red blood cells in the path of the high-velocity saline jets. Long activation runs of these devices, together with larger amounts of applied saline, increase the risk of this

Figure 14.7 • Hydrolyzer® thrombectomy system. Inset shows magnified view of the tip of the catheter.

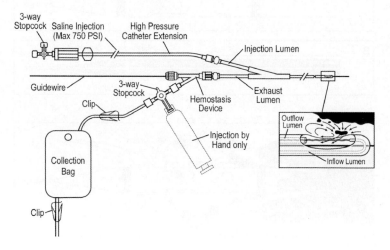

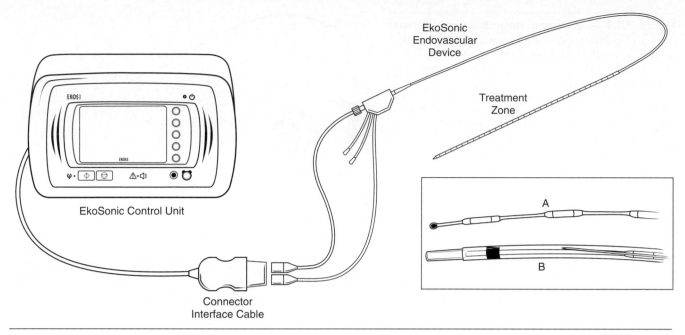

Figure 14.8 • Ekosonic endovascular system. Inset shows distal portions of drug delivery catheter (**A**) and ultrasound core catheter (**B**).

complication. One of the effects of hemolysis is the release of adenosine, which may cause significant heart block in some patients. This is very commonly seen during coronary artery intervention, but has been observed in peripheral arterial and venous interventions also.

Fragmentation Devices

This group of thrombectomy devices exerts its actions by mechanically fragmenting the thrombus, and then dispersing the dissolved thrombus. In theory, these devices are more likely to be associated with distal embolization, since there is no attempt to aspirate the thrombus from the vessel.

HELIX CLOT BUSTER THROMBECTOMY DEVICE

The HELIX® Clot Buster Thrombectomy Device (formerly known as Amplatz Thrombectomy Device) is the only current member of this group of thrombectomy devices. The device has a 7-Fr. outer lumen and is delivered, without the use of a guidewire, to the desired location within the vessel (i.e., has no guidewire lumen). It is available in catheter lengths of 75 and 120 cm.

A compressed gas–driven turbine (i.e., using air or nitrogen) activates a drive shaft that runs the length of the catheter. This causes rotation of an encapsulated impeller housed at the distal end of the device, at approximately 100,000 rpm. The miniature impeller creates a recirculating vortex that draws thrombus to the catheter tip, where it is macerated into microscopic fragments and dispersed into the bloodstream. A Turbo Wash™ Hydraulic fluid is injected through the catheter to facilitate removal of adherent mural thrombus, without allowing contact between the device and the vessel wall.

Ultrasound-Induced Thrombolysis

The use of ultrasound for purposes other than diagnostic imaging has evolved considerably over the last decade. One currently available device in the United States has been developed that exploits the tissue effects of low-frequency (i.e., 20 to

40 kHz), high-energy ultrasound waves. In liquid media such as blood, these energy waves create tiny microvacuums by a process known as cavitation. When these bubbles contract, they release a focused shock wave of acoustic energy that may cause the disintegration of surrounding tissue, such as thrombus, into microemboli of subcapillary size, while sparing the normal tissue of the vessel wall. The effect is therefore to achieve thrombus lysis without causing macroembolization.

EkoSonic ENDOVASCULAR SYSTEM

The EkoSonic Endovascular System (EKOS) consists of a reusable control unit and a single-use infusion catheter system (87) (Fig. 14.8). The latter includes a 5.2-Fr. multilumen drug delivery catheter (DDC) that is delivered through a 6-Fr. sheath over a 0.035″ guidewire through its central lumen. There are three small lumens arranged radially around the central lumen through which drug (i.e., thrombolytic) is delivered. The thrombolytic agent leaves through side holes along the treatment length at the distal end of the DDC (ranging from 6 to 50 cm in length). Once the DDC has been positioned across the thrombotic occlusion, the guidewire is removed and an ultrasound core catheter (USCC) is delivered through the central lumen of the DDC. This catheter has up to 50 encapsulated radiopaque ultrasound transducers along its distal length. Saline is infused through the central lumen (70 mL/h) to cool the USCC. The USCC delivers high-frequency (2.2 MHz) low-power (0.45 W) ultrasound that serves to mechanically break up the thrombus, exposing the fibrin to the thrombolytic agent, thus facilitating thrombolysis. Clinical experience suggests that the rate of complete lysis achieved with this device may be superior to conventional thrombolytic delivery systems, and the total dose of lytic required is reduced, which reduces bleeding complications (88).

A small vessel (EkoSonic SV Endovascular System) version of this system also exists. It is deliverable through a 6-Fr. guide, over a 0.014″ wire, and has a 150 cm working length. The catheter delivers drug through the end hole, and the

Figure 14.9 • X-Sizer® thrombectomy system.
A: Low magnification view of entire system. **B:** High magnification view of the helical cutter at the tip of the catheter. **C:** High magnification view of the helical cutter at the tip of the catheter in cross section.

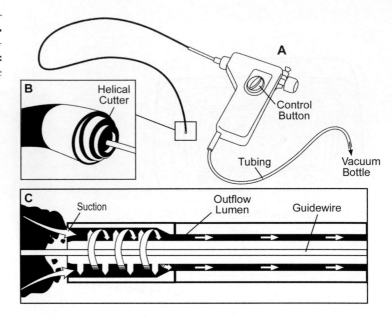

ultrasound element is located on the catheter tip. This system has been used in the neurovasculature.

Miscellaneous Group

A number of other devices have been developed that do not fit neatly into any specific category of thrombectomy device.

X-SIZER CATHETER SYSTEM

The X-Sizer® Catheter is a novel device that functions as both a fragmentation and an aspiration device (89,90). It is FDA approved for use in the mechanical removal of thrombus in synthetic hemodialysis grafts, but has found a clinical application in the periphery. Available in 6-Fr. and 7-Fr. sheath compatible sizes, it is delivered over a 0.014″ wire and has a working length of 135 cm.

The device contains a hand-held control unit that houses a battery-powered motor. When activated, a motor-driven drive shaft runs the length of the catheter and rotates a stainless steel helical cutter at 2100 rpm. The cutter extends approximately 1 mm beyond a protective housing at the catheter tip (Fig. 14.9). The rotating helix entrains and macerates the thrombus and allows its aspiration through the vacuum port. The vacuum mechanism, which generates a negative pressure of approximately 700 mm Hg, is activated simultaneously with the helical cutter by the motor unit.

TRELLIS THROMBECTOMY SYSTEM

The Trellis® catheter is a further example of a novel device for the treatment of arterial thrombus. Using a unique design and technology, it allows both localized mechanical lysis and pharmacologic fibrinolysis of thrombus in the arterial circulation. Currently, the FDA has approved the device only for the administration of fibrinolytic agents.

The device is available in two sizes (6-Fr. and 8-Fr. sheath compatible) and working lengths (80 and 120 cm), and is delivered over a 0.035″ wire. Near the distal end of the catheter, there are two compliant balloons with infusion holes located in between (Fig. 14.10). When inflated, the compliant balloons isolate a treatment zone that effectively maintains the concentration of the infused fluid. Depending on the length of

Figure 14.10 • Trellis® thrombectomy catheter showing major components of system.

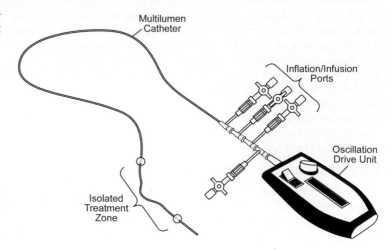

thrombus to be treated, catheters with a 10- or 20-cm distance between the balloons may be chosen. The device also has a central through-lumen that is compatible with a 0.035″ guidewire, to allow delivery of the device. The mechanical thrombectomy component of the system requires that the guidewire be exchanged for the dispersion wire component, which is a shape-set nitinol cable. Once placed, the shape-set region of the dispersion wire resides between the two balloons of the catheter. The dispersion wire is connected to an integral drive unit that oscillates the dispersion wire within the isolated region, to further disperse the infused fluid and mechanically lyse the thrombus.

Clinical Outcomes With Mechanical Thrombectomy For Acute Peripheral Arterial Occlusive Disease

There is a relative paucity of clinical data comparing the effectiveness of the various forms of mechanical thrombectomy, and an absence of randomized data comparing mechanical thrombectomy with surgical or pharmacologic therapies. The result is that any assessment of the efficacy of the various methods of mechanical thrombectomy is currently based largely on case reports, and single and multicenter registry experiences with these devices, without any comparison control group (summarized in Table 14.8).

The largest amount of data is available for the AngioJet system. Initial thrombus extraction rates have ranged from 52% to 95%. Most of the studies have used adjunctive therapy, including thrombolytic agents, balloon angioplasty, and stenting, to achieve adequate reperfusion. When mechanical therapy with the AngioJet is used in isolation, the results are only moderately good.

In a study reported from the Cleveland Clinic involving 83 patients, the initial success rate was 61% with the AngioJet as stand-alone therapy. Adjunctive thrombolytic therapy was used in 50 patients, the majority for angiographic evidence of distal small vessel occlusion (i.e., beyond the reach of the device). Müller-Hülsbeck et al. reported the use of the AngioJet thrombectomy catheter in 112 patients with occluded arterial or bypass grafts. Overall angiographic success (i.e., greater than 75% thrombus removal) was seen in 88.4% of patients, and adjunctive thrombolytic therapy was required in 29% of these patients. Mild elevation in plasma-free hemoglobin was noted for 24 hours postprocedure, with no adverse clinical sequelae. Immediate amputations were required in two patients and the 2-year amputation-free survival rate was 75%.

Rilinger et al. reported the largest experience in the use of the HELIX Clot Buster thrombectomy system for acute peripheral arterial ischemia. A majority of the patients had an embolic occlusion ($n = 32$) with a mean duration of ischemia of 2 days. Complete thrombus extraction with the device, as stand-alone therapy, was seen in 75% of the patients, which is impressive. No clinically relevant distal embolization was reported in this series. There were no in-hospital deaths, adjunctive thrombolytic therapy was used in eight patients, and two patients required early amputation. Of particular concern, however, was the reported inability to remove the device percutaneously in 7.5% of patients. In a smaller study involving 14 patients, a similar initial success of 71% was reported with 6-month patency rate of 43%.

Clinical information for acute leg ischemia with the Hydrolyzer catheter has been limited. In two clinical trials the initial success rate was high at 82% and 83%. Reekers et al. reported higher success rates for procedures performed on grafts (88%) compared to those performed on native vessels (73%). They noted a mean catheter activation time of only 3 minutes, and the avoidance of thrombolytic drugs in 58% of patients. Angiographic evidence of embolization was noted in seven patients, of which six underwent successful management with percutaneous aspiration or thrombolysis; the remaining patient required an amputation.

Although data for the Trellis infusion catheter system for local fibrinolytic therapy have been encouraging, the data on the mechanical catheter are relatively sparse (91,92).

Lessons Learned

A number of lessons have been learned from the experience with mechanical thrombectomy devices (MTDs). First, mechanical thrombectomy does not eliminate the need for pharmacologic thrombolysis or surgical therapies. When distal small vessel occlusion is present, the current generations of MTDs are too bulky to allow treatment at these sites. Second, MTDs are less successful when treating older adherent thrombus; in these cases, pharmacologic thrombolysis has an advantage. These considerations likely explain the high use of adjunctive thrombolysis in almost all series using MTDs to treat acute peripheral arterial occlusive disease (range 10% to 66%). Finally, MTDs do not treat the culprit lesion underlying the cause of acute vessel occlusion. This requires the use of adjunctive endovascular or surgical therapies, to prevent recurrences.

Despite these shortcomings, mechanical thrombectomy does have a number of distinct advantages in the treatment of arterial thrombosis. It rapidly debulks thrombus, and therefore minimizes the duration of tissue ischemia in the area supplied by that arterial segment. There is clearly an advantage of using mechanical thrombectomy in patients who are either high risk for open surgery or have contraindications to pharmacologic thrombolysis. In patients with a relative contraindication to thrombolysis, mechanical thrombectomy may enhance the effectiveness of pharmacologic thrombolysis by exposing a greater surface area of thrombus to the agent. The dose and duration of pharmacologic therapy may therefore be minimized, reducing the risk of bleeding.

PART IV: CASE EXAMPLES

In this section, we describe four cases of ALI that illustrate aspects of the multiple approaches employed in the endovascular management of ALI.

Case 1

A 67-year-old female presented with a progressively cold and weak left leg over the course of 5 days. On examination, her left common femoral artery (CFA) pulse was not palpable. She was deemed to have ALI category IIa.

Access was obtained in the contralateral CFA using a 5-Fr. 23 cm sheath advanced over a 0.035″ Versacore wire. Digital subtraction angiography (DSA) of the aortic bifurcation was performed using an Omni flush catheter (AngioDynamics) and

TABLE 14.8 Literature on the Use of the Mechanical Catheters for Limb-Threatening Ischemia

Study	Device	Trial Design	N	Native Vessel (%)	Adjunctive Lysis (%)	Complications (%)				Primary Patency (%)
						Emboli	Bleeding	Amputation	Death	
Wagner 1997 (93)	AngioJet	Prospective multicenter	50	78	30	6	2	8	0	30 d: 76 1 y: 69
Silva 1998 (84)	AngioJet	Prospective	21	62	–	9	10	5	14	6 mo: 89
Müller-Hülsbeck 2000 (94)	AngioJet	Prospective	112	86	18	10	N/A	2	7	6 mo: 68 2 y: 60 3 y: 58
Kasirajan 2001 (85)	AngioJet	Retrospective	86	63	58	2	11	12	9	3 mo: 90 6 mo: 79
Hopfner 1999 (95)	Oasis	Prospective	51	86	10	5	N/A	18	8	1 mo: 64 6 mo: 54
Reekers 1996 (96)	Hydrolyzer	Prospective	28	39	39	18	0	11	0	1 mo: 50
Henry 1998 (97)	Hydrolyzer	Prospective	41	68	24	2.4	N/A	0	0	1 mo: 73
Tadavarthy 1994 (98)	Amplatz	Retrospective	14	14	28	14	14	0	0	6 mo: 43
Rilinger 1997 (99)	Amplatz	Prospective	40	100	22	0	2.5	5	0	N/A
Görich 1998 (100)	Amplatz	Retrospective	18	100	66	N/A	6	6	N/A	N/A

(Adapted from The STILE Investigators. Results of a prospective randomized trial evaluating surgery versus thrombolysis for ischemia of the lower extremity. The STILE trial. *Ann Surg.* 1994;220:251–266; discussion 266–268.)

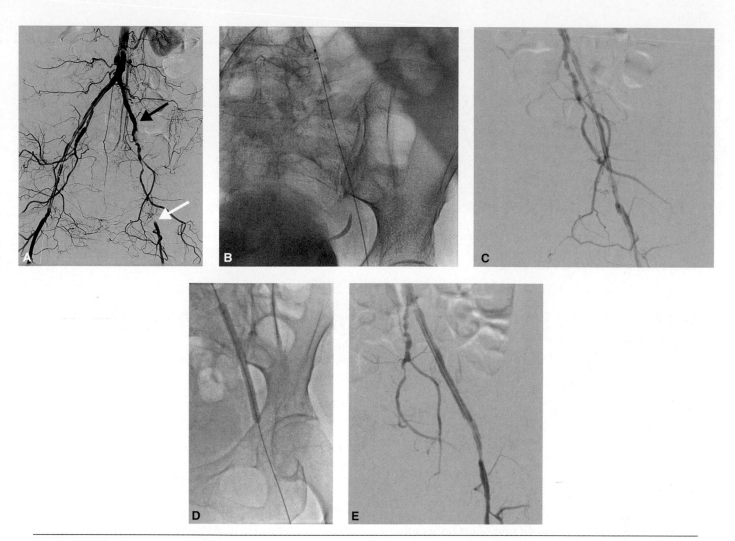

Figure 14.11 • Treatment of thrombotic occlusion of left external iliac artery using catheter-directed thrombolysis and adjunctive percutaneous mechanical therapies. See text for details.

revealed a thrombotic occlusion of the left EIA (black arrow) with reconstitution of the left CFA via collaterals (white arrow) (Fig. 14.11A). Both the right and left superficial femoral artery (SFA) were noted to be occluded. Given the progressive nature of her symptoms, the presence of bilateral PAD, and the absence of an obvious cardiac or noncardiac source of embolus, it was felt her occlusion was secondary to localized thrombosis superimposed on pre-existing severe atherosclerotic disease.

The Omni flush catheter was then retracted to the bifurcation to engage the left common iliac artery (CIA) allowing advancement of the Versacore wire into the left EIA. The Omni flush catheter was then exchanged for a 4-Fr. straight tip glide catheter. The Versacore wire was manipulated across the thrombotic occlusion into the profunda femoral artery (PFA) (Fig. 14.11B).

The short 5-Fr. sheath was exchanged over a 0.035″ Rosen wire for a 5-Fr. 45 cm Ansel 1 sheath. Sheath size was kept to a minimum as there was concern regarding the potential for occlusion of the right CFA and EIA using a 6-Fr. sheath. A 4-Fr. Fountain infusion catheter (Merit Medical Systems, Inc.) with a 20 cm infusion length was then positioned across

the occlusion into the left PFA. A t-PA infusion at 1mg/h was commenced, and the patient was transferred to the coronary care unit (CCU). Intravenous UFH was administered through the side arm of the right CFA sheath to maintain an APTT of 40 to 50 seconds. In addition, the patient was treated with 325 mg of aspirin daily. Close hemodynamic and lower extremity perfusion monitoring in addition to regular evaluation for bleeding complications was observed during CDT.

The following day (10 hours later), the patient returned to the catheterization lab where the indwelling CDT catheter and 5-Fr. sheath were exchanged over a Versacore wire for a 6-Fr. 45 cm Ansel 1 sheath. A significant improvement in flow was noted in the left EIA and CFA (Fig. 14.11C). Percutaneous transluminal angioplasty (PTA) of the residual stenoses in the EIA and proximal CFA was performed with a 5.0 × 60 mm balloon (Fig. 14.11D). Due to elastic recoil and a CFA dissection, a 7.0 × 80 mm self-expanding nitinol stent was deployed and postdilated, yielding a satisfactory result (Fig. 14.11E). Finally, the Ansel sheath was exchanged for a short 5-Fr. sheath, which was later removed using manual pressure to achieve hemostasis.

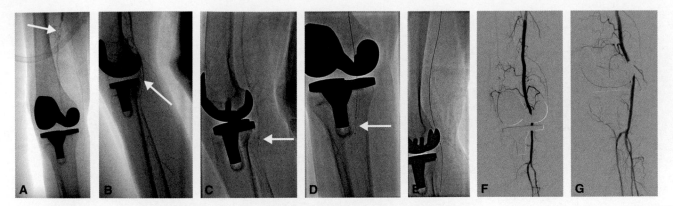

Figure 14.12 • Thrombotic occlusion of distal superficial femoral, popliteal, and tibial arteries following iatrogenic-induced arterial dissection following recent knee replacement surgery. Successful treatment using combined catheter-directed thrombolysis and percutaneous mechanical therapies. See text for details.

Case 2

An 80-year-old female presented with an 8-hour history of right lower extremity pain, parsethesia, coldness, and progressive weakness. She had undergone a right total knee replacement 12 days prior to presentation. A bedside duplex arterial ultrasound examination showed a patent right CFA and SFA to the level of the mid-thigh.

Antegrade access was obtained in the right CFA using a micropuncture technique and a 5-Fr. sheath was placed. Angiography demonstrated thrombus in the distal SFA (Fig. 14.12A-arrow) and a thrombotic occlusion of the popliteal artery (Fig. 14.12B-arrow). The inciting event appeared to be dissection of the SFA with superimposed thrombus formation and distal embolization to the popliteal artery resulting from tourniquet-induced trauma at the time of her orthopedic surgery. The SFA thrombus and popliteal occlusion were crossed with a 0.035″ angled glidewire. The 5Fr sheath was then upsized to a 7Fr 45cm Ansel 1 sheath. The glidewire was then exchanged for a 0.014″ Whisper wire using a 0.035″ Quickcross catheter. A 6-Fr. Export aspiration catheter was advanced over the Whisper wire, and aspiration thrombectomy of the SFA and popliteal artery was performed. Due to significant residual thrombus, additional aspiration using a 7-Fr. MP1 guide advanced over the Whisper wire was performed (Fig. 14.12C-tip of guide indicated by arrow) (aspiration was achieved by applying suction to a 20 cc syringe attached to the side arm of the Tuohy-Borst adapter at the hub of the MP1 guide). The posterior tibial (PT) artery was then wired using a 0.014″ Whisper wire. A 0.014″ Quickcross catheter was advanced over this wire and the Whisper wire was removed. Two milligrams of t-PA was then injected through the catheter end hole as the catheter was withdrawn into the popliteal artery. This strategy was repeated for the peroneal and anterior tibial (AT) arteries. Rheolytic thrombectomy (RT) of the SFA, popliteal artery, and each of the tibial arteries was performed using an AngioJet Ultra Spiroflex Rapid Exchange catheter system (Fig. 14.12D-distal portion of catheter indicated by arrow.). PTA of the AT, PT, and peroneal arteries was performed with a 2.0 × 120 mm balloon at low pressure. PTA of the SFA and popliteal stenoses was performed with a 5.0 × 20 mm balloon. Final angiography demonstrated a

significant reduction in the thrombotic burden in the SFA and popliteal arteries with one vessel runoff (via the PT) to the foot. The Quickcross catheter was then readvanced to the popliteal artery and t-PA was infused at a rate of 0.66 mg/h overnight (Fig. 14.12E).

The patient was evaluated regularly for possible compartment syndrome by vascular surgery upon completion of the procedure. She required fasciotomy of each of the three compartments approximately 8 hours postrevascularization. Repeat angiography was performed the following day and revealed complete resolution of thrombus in the SFA and popliteal arteries with three vessel tibial runoff (Fig. 14.12F and G).

Case 3

A 63-year-old female was transferred to the catheterization lab with a 4-hour history of sudden onset left lower extremity pain with an ipsilateral cold foot. Physical examination revealed atrial fibrillation (new diagnosis), and nonpalpable popliteal and distal left lower extremity pulses. The leg was noted to be cold from the knee distally, with intact sensation and preserved muscle power (ALI category IIa). No contraindication to CDT was present. Retrograde contralateral CFA arterial access was obtained using a 5-Fr. 23 cm sheath. Distal abdominal aortography was obtained using a 5-Fr. Omni flush catheter (Fig. 14.13A). The Omni flush catheter was used to engage the left CIA and a 0.035″ Versacore wire was advanced into the left CFA. The Omni catheter was exchanged for a 4-Fr. 65 cm straight glide catheter, which was used to perform angiography of the left lower extremity. This revealed thrombus in the PFA (Figure 14.13B, white arrow) and an acutely occluded popliteal artery (Figure 14.13C, black arrow), suggestive of an embolic event. The popliteal occlusion was crossed with a 0.014″ wire (Asahi Prowater, Abbott Vascular) that was advanced distally into the AT artery. A 2.0 × 15 mm OTW coronary balloon catheter was advanced into the proximal AT, and angiography showed a patent AT artery to the level of the foot (Fig. 14.13D). A 4-Fr. infusion CDT catheter (Fountain, Merit Medical) with a 20 cm long infusion length was positioned across the entire length of the popliteal occlusion (Fig. 14.13E), with its distal tip in the mid-AT (arrow). Intravenous UFH was commenced through the side arm of the

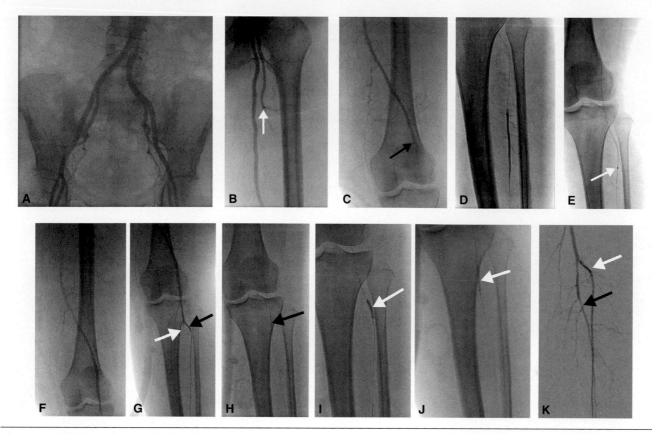

Figure 14.13 • Embolic occlusion of left popliteal artery. Successful treatment using catheter-directed thrombolysis and percutaneous mechanical therapies. See text for details.

CFA sheath with a target APTT of 40 to 50 seconds. A bolus of 2 mg of t-PA was administered into the infusion catheter and an infusion of 1 mg/h was administered for 10 hours while the patient was in the CCU. She was also given aspirin 325 mg and clopidogrel 300 mg orally.

Repeat angiography was performed the following day. Significant clot resolution in the popliteal artery (Fig. 14.13F) enabled the severe stenosis in the AT (Fig. 14.13G, black arrow) and occlusion of the tibioperoneal trunk (TPT) (Fig. 14.13G, white arrow) to be appreciated. Rheolytic thrombectomy using an AngioJet catheter was performed in the AT and TPT (Figure 14.13I—distal portion of catheter indicated by arrow) prior to angioplasty with 2.0 × 15 mm and 3.0 × 20 mm OTW balloons (Voyager, Abbott Vascular) (Figs. 14.13I,J). Final angiography revealed resolution of the popliteal thrombus and restoration of two-vessel tibial runoff (Fig. 14.13K, AT—white arrow, peroneal—black arrow).

Case 4

A 61-year-old male presented with rapidly worsening left calf claudication culminating in rest pain, coolness, and paresthesia over the course of 7 days. Clinical assessment revealed ALI category IIa. He had undergone bilateral femoral–popliteal artery bypass grafting 5 years previously. He had required PTA to the inflow segment of the left graft 1 year prior to presentation. Contralateral retrograde CFA access was obtained and a 5-Fr. sheath was placed. Distal abdominal aortography and runoff angiography revealed diffuse bilateral EIA atherosclerotic disease with an occlusion of the left CFA to popliteal venous bypass graft at its origin (arrows in Figs. 14.14A and B). Selective left lower extremity angiography using a 4-Fr. glide catheter was then performed to the foot. The popliteal artery distal to the bypass graft insertion site was patent with filling from bridging collaterals from the PFA (Fig. 14.14C—point of reconstitution indicated by arrrow.). The infrapopliteal run-off is shown in Figs 14.14D and E.

A 5-Fr. 45 cm Ansel sheath was delivered to the left CFA from the right CFA access site. The occluded left femoral–popliteal graft was wired easily using the 0.035″ angled glidewire supported by a 4-Fr. 110 cm long straight glide catheter. A 5-Fr. 135 cm long Ekos CDT infusion catheter was delivered to the level of the patent popliteal artery spanning the length of the occluded graft (proximal and distal ends of drug delivery portion of the DDC indicated by white and black arrows in Figs 14.14F and G, respectively).

CDT was commenced using 2 mg/h of t-PA for the first 2 hours and then 1 mg/h thereafter. Intravenous UFH was administered through the side port of the right CFA sheath with a target APTT of 40 to 50 seconds, and the patient was transferred to the CCU overnight. Repeat angiography 10 hours later showed that the bypass graft was now patent but with sluggish flow due to proximal and distal anastomotic stenoses (Figs. 14.14H and I). Following deployment of an embolic protective device (5 mm Spider, ev3) (Fig 14.14J, arrow), PTA of the distal and proximal anastomotic sites was performed with 4 × 40 mm and 5 × 80 mm balloons, respectively (Figs. 14.14J and K). Due

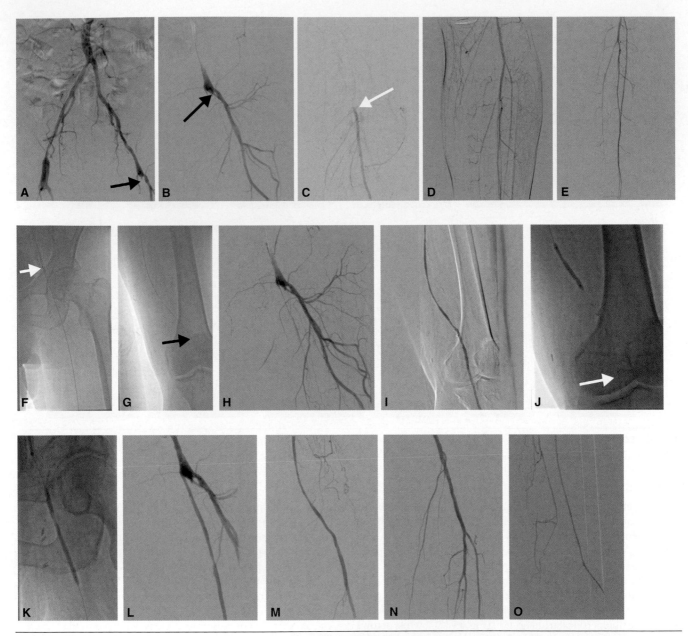

Figure 14.14 • Thrombotic occlusion of left femoropopliteal bypass graft. Successful treatment using catheter-directed thrombolysis and adjunctive percutaneous mechanical therapy. See text for details.

to significant elastic recoil, further PTA using a 5 × 20 mm focal pressure balloon (Angiosculpt, AngioScore, Inc.) was performed proximally. The EPD was retrieved. Examination of the filter revealed captured embolic debris. Final angiography demonstrated successful revascularization of the bypass graft with good distal runoff (Fig. 14.14L–O). Following sheath removal, anticoagulation with heparin was recommenced and the patient was discharged on warfarin and aspirin.

References

1. K. O. Acute limb ischemia. In: Rutherford RB, ed. *Vascular Surgery*. 5th ed. Philadelphia, PA: WB Saunders; 2000:813–821.
2. Dormandy J, Heeck L, Vig S. Acute limb ischemia. *Semin Vasc Surg*. 1999;12:148–153.
3. Bergqvist D, Troeng T, Elfstrom J, et al. Auditing surgical outcome: ten years with the Swedish Vascular Registry--Swedvasc. The Steering Committee of Swedvasc. *Eur J Surg Suppl*. 1998;581:3–8.
4. Davies B, Braithwaite BD, Birch PA, et al. Acute leg ischaemia in Gloucestershire. *Br J Surg*. 1997;84:504–508.
5. Tawes RL Jr, Harris EJ, Brown WH, et al. Arterial thromboembolism. A 20-year perspective. *Arch Surg*. 1985;120:595–599.
6. The STILE Investigators. Results of a prospective randomized trial evaluating surgery versus thrombolysis for ischemia of the lower extremity. The STILE trial. *Ann Surg*. 1994;220:251–266; discussion 266–268.
7. Kuoppala M, Franzen S, Lindblad B, et al. Long-term prognostic factors after thrombolysis for lower limb ischemia. *J Vasc Surg*. 2008;47:1243–1250.

8. Abbott WM, Maloney RD, McCabe CC, et al. Arterial embolism: a 44 year perspective. *Am J Surg.* 1982;143:460–464.

9. Manning WJ, Weintraub RM, Waksmonski CA, et al. Accuracy of transesophageal echocardiography for identifying left atrial thrombi. A prospective, intraoperative study. *Ann Intern Med.* 1995;123:817–822.

10. Fuster V, Gersh BJ, Giuliani ER, et al. The natural history of idiopathic dilated cardiomyopathy. *Am J Cardiol.* 1981;47:525–531.

11. Vrtik L, Zernovicky F, Kubis J, et al. Arterial embolisms in the extremities. *Rozhl Chir.* 2001;80:465–469.

12. Karapolat S, Dag O, Abanoz M, et al. Arterial embolectomy: a retrospective evaluation of 730 cases over 20 years. *Surg Today.* 2006;36:416–419.

13. Cambria RP, Abbott WM. Acute arterial thrombosis of the lower extremity. Its natural history contrasted with arterial embolism. *Arch Surg.* 1984;119:784–787.

14. Anderson JL, Adams CD, Antman EM, et al. ACC/AHA 2007 guidelines for the management of patients with unstable angina/non-ST-Elevation myocardial infarction: a report of the American College of Cardiology/American Heart Association Task Force on Practice Guidelines (Writing Committee to Revise the 2002 Guidelines for the Management of Patients With Unstable Angina/Non-ST-Elevation Myocardial Infarction) developed in collaboration with the American College of Emergency Physicians, the Society for Cardiovascular Angiography and Interventions, and the Society of Thoracic Surgeons endorsed by the American Association of Cardiovascular and Pulmonary Rehabilitation and the Society for Academic Emergency Medicine. *J Am Coll Cardiol.* 2007;50:e1–e157.

15. Okura H, Asawa K, Kubo T, et al. Incidence and predictors of plaque rupture in the peripheral arteries. *Circ Cardiovasc Interv.* 2010;3:63–70.

16. Management of peripheral arterial disease (PAD). TransAtlantic Inter-Society consensus (TASC). *Int Angiol.* 2000;19(suppl 1): I–XXIV, 1–304.

17. Jennings RB, Ganote CE. Structural changes in myocardium during acute ischemia. *Circ Res.* 1974;35(suppl 3):156–172.

18. Buja LM. Myocardial ischemia and reperfusion injury. *Cardiovasc Pathol.* 2005;14:170–175.

19. Smith EF III, Egan JW, Bugelski PJ, et al. Temporal relation between neutrophil accumulation and myocardial reperfusion injury. *Am J Physiol.* 1988;255(5 pt 2):H1060–H1068.

20. Vinten-Johansen J. Involvement of neutrophils in the pathogenesis of lethal myocardial reperfusion injury. *Cardiovasc Res.* 2004;61:481–497.

21. Norgren L, Hiatt WR, Dormandy JA, et al. Inter-society consensus for the management of peripheral arterial disease. *Int Angiol.* 2007;26:81–157.

22. Hirsh J, Bauer KA, Donati MB, et al. Parenteral anticoagulants: American College of Chest Physicians Evidence-Based Clinical Practice Guidelines (8th Edition). *Chest.* 2008;133(6 suppl): 141S–159S.

23. Warkentin TE, Levine MN, Hirsh J, et al. Heparin-induced thrombocytopenia in patients treated with low-molecular-weight heparin or unfractionated heparin. *N Engl J Med.* 1995;332:1330–1335.

24. Maraganore JM, Bourdon P, Jablonski J, et al. Design and characterization of hirulogs: a novel class of bivalent peptide inhibitors of thrombin. *Biochemistry.* 1990;29:7095–7101.

25. Baron SJ, Yeh RW, Cruz-Gonzalez I, et al. Efficacy and safety of argatroban in patients with heparin induced thrombocytopenia undergoing endovascular intervention for peripheral arterial disease. *Catheter Cardiovasc Interv.* 2008;72:116–120.

26. Antithrombotic Trialists' Collaboration. Collaborative meta-analysis of randomised trials of antiplatelet therapy for prevention of death, myocardial infarction, and stroke in high risk patients. *BMJ.* 2002;324:71–86.

27. Walters TK, Mitchell DC, Wood RF. Low-dose aspirin fails to inhibit increased platelet reactivity in patients with peripheral vascular disease. *Br J Surg.* 1993;80:1266–1268.

28. Cassar K, Bachoo P, Ford I, et al. Platelet activation is increased in peripheral arterial disease. *J Vasc Surg.* 2003;38:99–103.

29. Smith SC Jr, Allen J, Blair SN, et al. AHA/ACC guidelines for secondary prevention for patients with coronary and other atherosclerotic vascular disease: 2006 update: endorsed by the National Heart, Lung, and Blood Institute. *Circulation.* 2006;113:2363–2372.

30. Hirsch AT, Haskal ZJ, Hertzer NR, et al. ACC/AHA 2005 Practice Guidelines for the management of patients with peripheral arterial disease (lower extremity, renal, mesenteric, and abdominal aortic): a collaborative report from the American Association for Vascular Surgery/Society for Vascular Surgery, Society for Cardiovascular Angiography and Interventions, Society for Vascular Medicine and Biology, Society of Interventional Radiology, and the ACC/AHA Task Force on Practice Guidelines (Writing Committee to Develop Guidelines for the Management of Patients With Peripheral Arterial Disease): endorsed by the American Association of Cardiovascular and Pulmonary Rehabilitation; National Heart, Lung, and Blood Institute; Society for Vascular Nursing; TransAtlantic Inter-Society Consensus; and Vascular Disease Foundation. *Circulation.* 2006;113:e463–e654.

31. Rutherford RB. Clinical staging of acute limb ischemia as the basis for choice of revascularization method: when and how to intervene. *Semin Vasc Surg.* 2009;22:5–9.

32. Shortell CK, Ouriel K. Thrombolysis in acute peripheral arterial occlusion: predictors of immediate success. *Ann Vasc Surg.* 1994;8:59–65.

33. The STILE Investigators. Results of a prospective randomized trial evaluating surgery versus thrombolysis for ischemia of the lower extremity. The STILE trial. *Ann Surg.* 1994;220:251–266.

34. Comerota AJ, Weaver FA, Hosking JD, et al. Results of a prospective, randomized trial of surgery versus thrombolysis for occluded lower extremity bypass grafts. *Am J Surg.* 1996;172: 105–112.

35. Weaver FA, Comerota AJ, Youngblood M, et al. Surgical revascularization versus thrombolysis for nonembolic lower extremity native artery occlusions: results of a prospective randomized trial. The STILE Investigators. Surgery versus Thrombolysis for Ischemia of the Lower Extremity. *J Vasc Surg.* 1996;24: 513–521.

36. Ouriel K, Veith FJ. Acute lower limb ischemia: determinants of outcome. *Surgery.* 1998;124:336–341.

37. Ouriel K. Urokinase and the US Food and Drug Administration. *J Vasc Surg.* 1999;30:957–958.

38. Tillett WS, Garner RL. The fibrinolytic activity of hemolytic streptococci. *J Exp Med.* 1933;58:485.

39. Tillett WS, Sherry S. The effect in patients of streptococcal fibrinolysin (streptokinase) and streptococcal desoxyribonuclease on fibrinous, purulent, and sanguinous pleural exudations. *J Clin Invest.* 1949;28:173.

40. Tillett WS, Johnson AJ, McCarty WR. The intravenous infusion of the streptococcal fibrinolytic principle (streptokinase) into patients. *J Clin Invest.* 1955;34:169–185.

41. Cliffton EE, Grunnet M. Investigations of intravenous plasmin (fibrinolysin) in humans. *Circulation.* 1956;14:919.

42. Cliffton EE. The use of plasmin in humans. *Ann NY Acad Sci.* 1957;68:209–229.

43. Reddy DS. Newer thrombolytic drugs for acute myocardial infarction. *Indian J Exp Biol.* 1998;36:1–15.

44. Jostring H, Barth U, Naidu R. Changes of antistreptokinase titer following long-term streptokinase therapy. In: Martin M, Schoop W, Hirsh J, eds. *New Concepts of Streptokinase Dosimetry.* Vienna: Hans Huber; 1978:110.

45. Smith RAG, Dupe RJ, English PD, et al. Fibrinolysis with acyl-enzymes: a new approach to thrombolytic therapy. *Nature*. 1981;290:505.

46. MacFarlane RG, Pinot JJ. Fibrinolytic activity of normal urine. *Nature*. 1947;159:779.

47. Sobel GW, Mohler SR, Jones NW, et al. Urokinase: an activator of plasma fibrinolysin extracted from urine. *Am J Physiol*. 1952;171:768–769.

48. Ouriel K, Veith FJ, Sasahara AA. A comparison of recombinant urokinase with vascular surgery as initial treatment for acute arterial occlusion of the legs. *N Engl J Med*. 1998;338:1105–1111.

49. Ouriel K, Veith FJ, Sasahara AA. Thrombolysis or peripheral arterial surgery: phase I results. TOPAS Investigators. *J Vasc Surg*. 1996;23:64–73; discussion 74–75.

50. Husain SS, Lipinski B, Gurewich V. Isolation of plasminogen activators useful as therapeutic and diagnostic agents (single-chair, high-fibrin affinity urokinase). Patent No. 4, 381, 346. 1979.

51. Gurewich V. Pro-urokinase: history, mechanisms of action, and clinical development. In: Loscalzo J, Sasahara AA, eds. *New Therapeutic Agents in Thrombosis and Thrombolysis*. New York: Marcel Dekker; 1997:539–559.

52. Tanswell P, Tebbe U, Neuhaus KL, et al. Pharmacokinetics and fibrin specificity of alteplase during accelerated infusions in acute myocardial infarction. *J Am Coll Cardiol*. 1992;19:1071–1075.

53. Hoylaerts M, Rijken DC, Lijnen HR, et al. Kinetics of the activation of plasminogen by human tissue plasminogen activator: role of fibrin. *J Biol Chem*. 1982;257:2912.

54. The GUSTO Investigators. An angiographic study within the global randomized trial of aggressive versus standard thrombolytic strategies in patients with acute myocardial infarction. *N Engl J Med*. 1993;329:1615.

55. Cannon CP, McCabe CH, Gibson CM, et al. TNK-tissue plasminogen activator in acute myocardial infarction. Results of the Thrombolysis in Myocardial Infarction (TIMI) 10A dose-ranging trial. *Circulation*. 1997;95:351–356.

56. Cannon CP, Gibson CM, McCabe CH, et al. TNK-tissue plasminogen activator compared with front-loaded alteplase in acute myocardial infarction: results of the TIMI 10B trial. Thrombolysis in Myocardial Infarction (TIMI) 10B Investigators. *Circulation*. 1998;98:2805–2814.

57. Martin U. Clinical and preclinical profile of the novel recombinant plasminogen activator reteplase. In: Sasahara AA, Loscalzo J, eds. *New Therapeutic Agents in Thrombosis and Thrombolysis*. New York: Marcel Dekker; 1997:495–511.

58. Meierhenrich R, Carlsson J, Seifried E, et al. Effect of reteplase on hemostasis variables: analysis of fibrin specificity, relation to bleeding complications and coronary patency. *Int J Cardiol*. 1998;65:57–63.

59. Anonymous. A comparison of reteplase with alteplase for acute myocardial infarction. The Global Use of Strategies to Open Occluded Coronary Arteries (GUSTO III) Investigators [see comments]. *N Engl J Med*. 1997;337:1118–1123.

60. Castaneda F, Li R, Young K, et al. Catheter-directed thrombolysis in deep venous thrombosis with use of reteplase: immediate results and complications from a pilot study. *J Vasc Interv Radiol*. 2002;13:577–580.

61. Drescher P, Crain MR, Rilling WS. Initial experience with the combination of reteplase and abciximab for thrombolytic therapy in peripheral arterial occlusive disease: a pilot study. *J Vasc Interv Radiol*. 2002;13:37–43.

62. McNamara TO, Dong P, Chen J, et al. Bleeding complications associated with the use of rt-PA versus r-PA for peripheral arterial and venous thromboembolic occlusions. *Tech Vasc Interv Radiol*. 2001;4:92–98.

63. Ouriel K, Katzen B, Mewissen MW, et al. Initial experience with reteplase in the treatment of peripheral arterial and venous occlusion. *J Vasc Interv Radiol*. 2000;11:849–854.

64. Ouriel K, Welch EL, Shortell CK, et al. Comparison of streptokinase, urokinase, and recombinant tissue plasminogen activator in an in vitro model of venous thrombolysis. *J Vasc Surg*. 1995;22:593–597.

65. Graor RA, Risius B, Denny KM, et al. Local thrombolysis in the treatment of thrombosed arteries, bypass grafts, and arteriovenous fistulas. *J Vasc Surg*. 1985;2:406–414.

66. Gardiner GA Jr, Koltun W, Kandarpa K, et al. Thrombolysis of occluded femoropopliteal grafts. *AJR Am J Roentgenol*. 1986;147:621–626.

67. Ouriel K, Gray B, Clair DG, et al. Complications associated with the use of urokinase and recombinant tissue plasminogen activator for catheter-directed peripheral arterial and venous thrombolysis. *J Vasc Interv Radiol*. 2000;11:295–298.

68. Meyerovitz M, Goldhaber SZ, Reagan K, et al. Recombinant tissue-type plasminogen activator versus urokinase in peripheral arterial and graft occlusions: a randomized trial. *Radiology*. 1990;175:75–78.

69. Comerota AJ. A re-analysis of the STILE data presented at the Annual VEITH symposium; November 17, 1999; New York, NY.

70. Credo RB, Burke SE, Barker WM, et al. Recombinant urokinase (r-UK): biochemistry, pharmacology, and clinical experience. In: Sasahara AA, Loscalzo J, eds. *New Therapeutic Agents in Thrombosis and Thrombolysis*. New York, NY: Marcel Dekker, Inc.; 1997:513–537.

71. Ouriel K, Kandarpa K, Schuerr DM, et al. Prourokinase vs. urokinase for recanalization of peripheral occlusions, safety and efficacy: the PURPOSE Trial. *J Vasc Interv Radiol*. 1999;10:1083–1091.

72. Hye RJ, Turner C, Valji K, et al. Is thrombolysis of occluded popliteal and tibial bypass grafts worthwhile? *J Vasc Surg*. 1994;20:588–596.

73. Armon MP, Yusuf SW, Whitaker SC, et al. Results of 100 cases of pulse-spray thrombolysis for acute and subacute leg ischaemia. *Br J Surg*. 1997;84:47–50.

74. Kandarpa K, Chopra PS, Aruny JE, et al. Intraarterial thrombolysis of lower extremity occlusions: prospective, randomized comparison of forced periodic infusion and conventional slow continuous infusion. *Radiology*. 1993;188:861–867.

75. Thomas SM, Gaines P. Avoiding the complications of thrombolysis. *J Vasc Interv Radiol*. 1999;10(suppl):246.

76. Riggs P, Ouriel K. Thrombolysis in the treatment of lower extremity occlusive disease. *Surg Clin Nor Am*. 1995;75:633–645.

77. Berni GA, Bandyk DF, Zierler RE, et al. Streptokinase treatment of acute arterial occlusion. *Ann Surg*. 1983;198:185–191.

78. Sicard GA, Schier JJ, Totty WG, et al. Thrombolytic therapy for acute arterial occlusion. *J Vasc Surg*. 1985;2:65–78.

79. Faggioli GL, Peer RM, Pedrini L, et al. Failure of thrombolytic therapy to improve long-term vascular patency. *J Vasc Surg*. 1994;19:289–296.

80. Sullivan KL, Gardiner GAJ, Kandarpa K, et al. Efficacy of thrombolysis in infrainguinal bypass grafts. *Circulation*. 1991;83(2 suppl):99–105.

81. Tiwari A, Haq AI, Myint F, et al. Acute compartment syndromes. *Br J Surg*. 2002;89(4):397–412.

82. Duran WN, Takenaka H, Hobson RW 2nd. Microvascular pathophysiology of skeletal muscle ischemia-reperfusion. *Semin Vasc Surg*. 1998;11:203–214.

83. Hargens AR, Romine JS, Sipe JC, et al. Peripheral nerve-conduction block by high muscle-compartment pressure. *J Bone Joint Surg Am*. 1979;61:192–200.

84. Silva JA, Ramee SR, Collins TJ, et al. Rheolytic thrombectomy in the treatment of acute limb-threatening ischemia: immediate results and six-month follow-up of the multicenter AngioJet registry. Possis Peripheral AngioJet Study AngioJet Investigators. *Cathet Cardiovasc Diagn*. 1998;45:386–393.

85. Kasirajan K, Haskal ZJ, Ouriel K. The use of mechanical thrombectomy devices in the management of acute peripheral arterial occlusive disease. *J Vasc Interv Radiol*. 2001;12:405–411.

86. Vesely TM, Hovsepian DM, Darcy MD, et al. Angioscopic observations after percutaneous thrombectomy of thrombosed hemodialysis grafts. *J Vasc Interv Radiol*. 2000;11:971–977.

87. Wissgott C, Richter A, Kamusella P, et al. Treatment of critical limb ischemia using ultrasound-enhanced thrombolysis (PARES Trial): final results. *J Endovasc Ther*. 2007;14:438–443.

88. Motarjeme A. Ultrasound-enhanced thrombolysis. *J Endovasc Ther*. 2007;14:251–256.

89. Stone GW, Cox DA, Low R, et al. Safety and efficacy of a novel device for treatment of thrombotic and atherosclerotic lesions in native coronary arteries and saphenous vein grafts: results from the multicenter X-Sizer for treatment of thrombus and atherosclerosis in coronary applications trial (X-TRACT) study. *Catheter Cardiovasc Interv*. 2003;58:419–427.

90. Kornowski R, Ayzenberg O, Halon DA, et al. Preliminary experiences using X-sizer catheter for mechanical thrombectomy of thrombus-containing lesions during acute coronary syndromes. *Catheter Cardiovasc Interv*. 2003;58:443–448.

91. Sarac TP, Hilleman D, Arko FR, et al. Clinical and economic evaluation of the trellis thrombectomy device for arterial occlusions: preliminary analysis. *J Vasc Surg*. 2004;39:556–559.

92. Kasirajan K, Ramaiah VG, Diethrich EB. The trellis thrombectomy system in the treatment of acute limb ischemia. *J Endovasc Ther*. 2003;10:317–321.

93. Wagner HJ, Müller-Hülsbeck S, Pitton MB, et al. Rapid thrombectomy with a hydrodynamic catheter: results from a prospective, multicenter trial. *Radiology*. 1997;205:675–681.

94. Müller-Hülsbeck S, Kalinowski M, Heller M, et al. Rheolytic hydrodynamic thrombectomy for percutaneous treatment of acutely occluded infra-aortic native arteries and bypass grafts: midterm follow-up results. *Invest Radiol*. 2000;35:131–140.

95. Höpfner W, Vicol C, Bohndorf K, et al. Shredding embolectomy thrombectomy catheter for treatment of acute lower-limb ischemia. *Ann Vasc Surg*. 1999;13:426–435.

96. Reekers JA, Kromhout JG, Spithoven HG, et al. Arterial thrombosis below the inguinal ligament: percutaneous treatment with a thrombosuction catheter. *Radiology*. 1996;198:49–53.

97. Henry M, Amor M, Henry I, et al. The Hydrolyser thrombectomy catheter: a single-center experience. *J Endovasc Surg*. 1998;5:24–31.

98. Tadavarthy SM, Murray PD, Inampudi S, et al. Mechanical thrombectomy with the Amplatz device: human experience. *J Vasc Interv Radiol*. 1994;5:715–724.

99. Rilinger N, Görich J, Scharrer-Pamler R, et al. Mechanical thrombectomy of embolic occlusion in both the profunda femoris and superficial femoral arteries in critical limb ischaemia. *Br J Radiol*. 1997;70:80–84.

100. Görich J, Rilinger N, Sokiranski R, et al. Mechanical thrombolysis of acute occlusion of both the superficial and the deep femoral arteries using a thrombectomy device. *AJR Am J Roentgenol*. 1998;170:1177–1180.

CHAPTER 15

Aortoiliac Intervention

Robert Francis Bonvini and Marco Roffi

The infrarenal abdominal aorta and iliac arteries are among the most common sites of chronic obliterative atherosclerosis, accounting for about one third of all peripheral artery disease (PAD) cases. The standard surgical treatment for aortoiliac disease is aortobifemoral bypass, where a Y-shaped graft is attached to the distal abdominal aorta proximally, and each limb of the Y-graft is attached to the common femoral artery (CFA) distally (Fig. 15.1). Occasionally, the distal limb(s) may be anastomosed to the profunda femoral artery (PFA) when the CFA is diseased. Less common surgical procedures for aortoiliac disease include aortoiliac endarterectomy for the treatment of focal iliac disease, and axillofemoral bypass for patients with occlusive disease of the distal abdominal aorta and severe comorbidities (Fig. 15.1). In patients with unilateral iliac disease, additional surgical options include femorofemoral crossover bypass or iliofemoral bypass (Fig. 15.1).

With respect to aortobifemoral bypass, a meta-analysis of 23 series including over 8000 patients operated between 1975 and 1995 reported an aggregated operative mortality of 4.6% in early studies (performed in the 1970s) and 3.3% in later studies (in the 1990s) (1). The aggregated major morbidity was 13% and 8% for each time period, respectively. Limb-based patency rates for patients with claudication were 91% and 87% at 5 and 10 years, respectively; the corresponding patency rates in patients with critical limb ischemia were 87% and 82%, respectively. No difference in patency was detected between older and more recent studies. Aortoiliac endarterectomy has been associated with patency rates in modern series ranging from 88% to 94% at 1 year and from 60% to 80% at 5 years (2,3). However, since best endarterectomy results were obtained in patients with focal iliac disease, this technique has been largely replaced by endovascular intervention. Axillofemoral bypass has been performed with patency rates ranging from 78% to 93% at 1 year and from 50% to 80% at 5 years (4).

This chapter focuses on percutaneous intervention of aortoiliac disease, which has become the treatment of choice for many patients with aortoiliac atherosclerotic disease.

ANATOMY

The iliac vessels originate from the distal abdominal aorta (Fig. 15.2). The common iliac artery (CIA) subsequently divides into the internal iliac artery (IIA) supplying the pelvic organs, and the external iliac artery (EIA), which continues to become CFA at the level of the inguinal ligament. The diameters of the CIA and the EIA range from 8 to 10 mm, and from 6 to 8 mm, respectively. Because of the abundant collateral circulation through the inferior mesenteric artery, lumbar vessels, and the IIA, limb-threatening ischemia is rare, even in the presence of total occlusion of distal abdominal aorta as long as there is no associated severe femoropopliteal or tibial disease.

Three distinct patterns of atherosclerotic involvement of the infrarenal aorta and the iliac vessels have been described (Table 15.1 and Fig. 15.3) (5). Type I refers to exclusive involvement of the distal abdominal aorta and the CIA, is present in about 5% to 10% of patients with PAD, and is more frequently encountered among women. Type II involves the infrarenal aorta, CIA, and EIA and may extend into the CFA; this pattern may be observed in 35% of patients with PAD. Type III is the most common pattern and involves the infrarenal aorta, iliac, femoral, and popliteal arteries as well as the infrapopliteal circulation.

PATIENT SELECTION

Patients with aortoiliac occlusive disease present most frequently with lifestyle-limiting claudication. Whereas calf pain on exertion is the leading symptom in femoropopliteal arterial disease, patients with aortoiliac involvement may have less characteristic symptoms such as ambulatory back, buttock, hip, and thigh pain, in addition to calf pain. These conditions are frequently misinterpreted as representing pathology of the lower back or hip, delaying diagnosis for many years. Since the chronic progressive nature of the disease allows for the development of a robust collateral circulation, associated critical limb ischemia is rare provided the femoropopliteal and tibial vessels are patent. This is true even in the presence of a distal aortic occlusion (Leriche syndrome).

The most important part of the physical exam in a patient with suspected iliac disease includes an assessment of the CFA pulses. An absent CFA pulse usually indicates either an occlusion of the ipsilateral iliac or CFA (Figure 15.4). The routine diagnostic workup of patients with suspected aortoiliac includes a hemodynamic evaluation (including ankle–brachial index [ABI], segmental limb pressures [SLP], pulse volume recordings [PVR], and exercise testing). The typical hemodynamic findings in patients with iliac disease include a decreased ABI and a significant decrement in the SLP between the brachial artery and upper thigh pressure (i.e., diminished thigh–brachial index) that is associated with a drop in the amplitude of the PVR between the brachial artery and upper thigh. Exercise testing is particularly useful in patients with typical claudication symptoms suggestive of iliac disease (e.g., buttock claudication) but with a normal resting hemodynamic assessment.

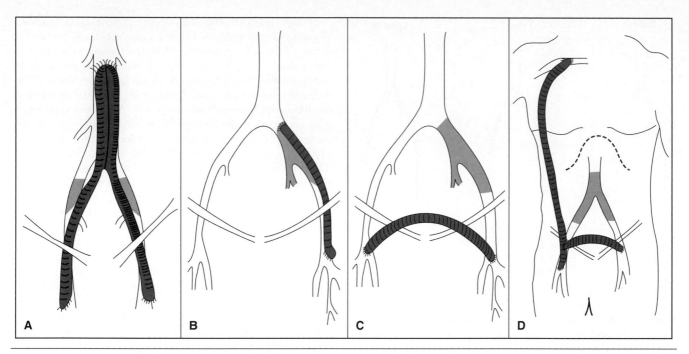

Figure 15.1 • Surgical bypass for aorto-iliac disease. **A:** Aorto-bifemoralbypass. **B:** Ilio-femoral bypass. **C:** Femoral-femoral bypass. **D:** Axillo-femoral bypass combined with femoral-femoral bypass. (Adapted from Neville RF, Deaton, DH. Lower extremity revascularization. *Endovascular Today,* February 2004:49–56.)

Duplex ultrasound imaging is helpful for patients in whom adequate visualization of the iliac arteries is possible. In cases with suboptimal visualization of the pelvic region, assessment of the Doppler flow analysis in the CFA may offer useful information. The presence of a physiologic triphasic waveform in the CFA makes a hemodynamically relevant iliac artery stenosis unlikely.

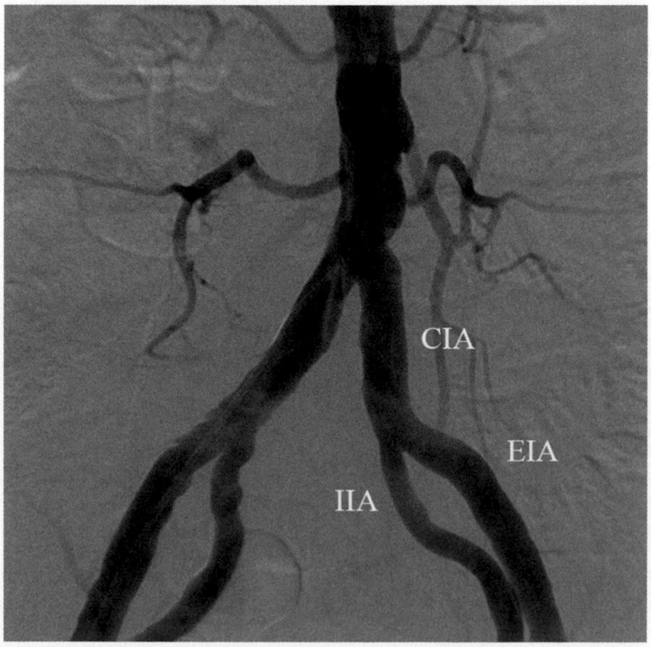

Anatomic assessment of the aortoiliac vessels with computed tomography angiography (CTA) or magnetic resonance angiography (MRA) is highly effective. In addition to having high rates of sensitivity and specificity for the diagnosis of disease, these studies are invaluable in providing information to help guide percutaneous revascularization, if indicated.

An iliofemoral stenosis is generally considered hemodynamically significant if the luminal stenosis on angiography is

Figure 15.2 • Normal anatomy of the distal abdominal aorta, the common iliac arteries (CIA), the internal iliac arteries (IIA), and the external iliac arteries (EIA).

TABLE 15.1 Atherosclerotic Involvement of the Iliac Vasculature

Disease Type	Prevalence (%)	Vascular Beds Involved
Type I	5–10	Infrarenal aorta Common iliac arteries
Type II	35	Infrarenal aorta Common and external iliac arteries Common femoral arteries
Type III	55–60	Infrarenal aorta Common and iliac arteries Common and superficial femoral arteries Popliteal and infrapopliteal circulation

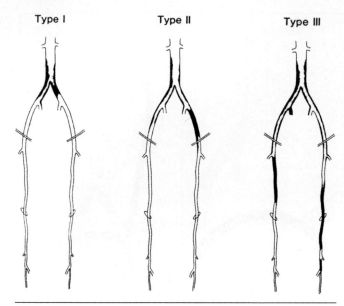

Figure 15.3 • Typical patterns of atherosclerotic involvement of the infrarenal aorta and the iliac vessels, as described also in Table 15.1. (Reproduced with permission from Brewster DC. Clinical and anatomical considerations for surgery in aortoiliac disease and results of surgical treatment. *Circulation.* 1991;83(2 suppl):I42–I52.)

≥70% (6). In borderline cases, assessment of the translesional pressure gradient may be helpful. Although clear-cut pressure gradient thresholds to define the hemodynamic relevance have not been identified, a systolic peak gradient ≥ 10 mm Hg prevasodilation and >15 mm Hg postvasodilatation—as measured with a 4- or 5-Fr. diagnostic catheter—is generally considered significant (7). Appropriate patient selection, taking into consideration the clinical status of the patient, the location, morphology, and physiologic significance of the aortoiliac lesion, as well as the operator's experience, are key factors in determining the appropriateness of endovascular intervention.

The TransAtlantic Inter-Society Consensus (TASC) Working Group published in the year 2000 a comprehensive review of the management of PAD that included classification and management guidelines also of iliac disease (4). Recently, these guidelines and definitions were updated with a new TASC II classification for aortoiliac disease (Fig. 15.5) (7). According to the document, for simple lesions (TASC A–B lesions), endovascular treatment is the therapy of choice and for very complex disease (TASC D lesions), surgery is recommended. There was a lack of consensus regarding TASC C lesions. For this lesion subset, the decision should be made on a case-by-case basis, depending on the clinical presentation, patient comorbidities, the lesion morphology, and operator experience. Despite these general recommendations, the lack of randomized data comparing surgical versus endovascular revascularization and the continuous evolution in revascularization technique and equipment have resulted in marked variation in treatment strategies across institutions. In experienced centers, it is common to adopt an endovascular first approach to even complex aortoiliac disease and to refer only those patients who either fail this endovascular approach or who cannot be approached using endovascular techniques (e.g., complex aneurismal disease, significant CFA disease) to surgery (8–10).

DIAGNOSTIC ANGIOGRAPHY

Access

Generally, diagnostic angiography of the aortoiliac region is performed using retrograde CFA access contralateral to the limb that is more symptomatic and/or demonstrates the worse hemodynamic compromise. If imaging studies (i.e., duplex ultrasound, CTA, or MRA) have already been performed, access can be chosen based on the anatomic findings of these studies. In this circumstance, the location of the lesion(s) to be treated is the most important factor determining the access site. For example, EIA stenoses—especially if located in the distal segment—are treated using a crossover approach from the contralateral CFA, whereas CIA stenoses are typically approached

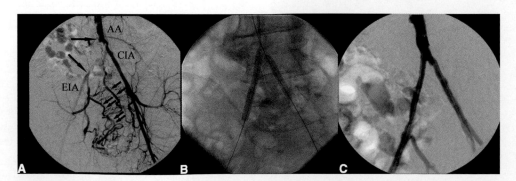

Figure 15.4 • Interventional treatment of right common iliac artery (CIA) occlusion (delineated by large arrows) using antegrade approach. **A:** Baseline pelvic angiography using left brachial access demonstrating occlusion of right CIA and severe stenosis at origin of left CIA. Small arrows demonstrate collateral filling of the right internal iliac artery and subsequently of the right external iliac artery (EIA). AA, abdominal aorta. **B:** Kissing stenting of the aortic bifurcation was performed using dual arterial access from the left brachial artery to treat the right CIA (note the tip of the 90-cm sheath at the aortic bifurcation) and retrograde left common femoral artery access to treat the left CIA stenosis. **C:** Final angiographic result after kissing stenting.

Type A lesions:

• Unilateral or bilateral stenoses of CIA
• Unilateral or bilateral single short (≤3 cm) stenosis of EIA

Type B lesions:

• Short (≤3 cm) stenosis of infrarenal aorta
• Unilateral CIA occlusion
• Single or multiple stenosis totaling 3–10 cm involving the
  EIA not extending into the CFA
• Unilateral EIA occlusion not involving the origins of
  internal iliac or CFA

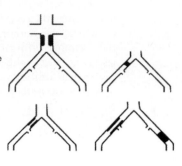

Type C lesions:

• Bilateral CIA occlusions
• Bilateral EIA stenoses 3–10 cm long not extending into
  the CFA
• Unilateral EIA stenosis extending into the CFA
• Unilateral EIA occlusion that involves the origins of
  internal iliac and/or CFA
• Heavily calcified unilateral EIA occlusion with or without
  involvement of origins of internal iliac and/or CFA

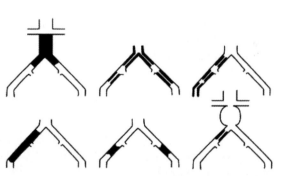

Type D lesions:

• Infrarenal aortoiliac occlusion
• Diffuse disease involving the aorta and both iliac arteries
  requiring treatment
• Diffuse multiple stenoses involving the unilateral CIA,
  EIA, and CFA
• Unilateral occlusions of both CIA and EIA
• Bilateral occlusions of EIA
• Iliac stenoses in patients with AAA requiring treatment
  and not amenable to endograft placement or other
  lesions requiring open aortic or iliac surgery

Figure 15.5 • TransAtlantic Inter-Society Consensus (TASC II) morphologic stratification of iliac lesions. (Reprinted from Norgren L, Hiatt WR, Dormandy JA, et al. Inter-society consensus for the management of peripheral arterial disease (TASC II). *J Vasc Surg.* 2007;45(suppl S):S5–S67, with permission from Elsevier.)

using ipsilateral retrograde CFA access. The choice of access site(s) for the treatment of iliac occlusions requires careful consideration, with some cases requiring bilateral CFA access, and others requiring brachial access, depending on the specific anatomy (see below).

Views and Catheters

Significant tortuosity of the iliac arteries and eccentricity of atherosclerotic involvement in the aortoiliac region is frequent. Therefore, angulated views (30° to 35° right anterior oblique [RAO] and 30° to 35° left anterior oblique [LAO]) are important to optimize the sensitivity of the study. The LAO view will typically provide optimal visualization of the origin of the right CIA and the right CIA bifurcation, whereas the RAO view provides optimal visualization of the left CIA and the left CIA bifurcation. Conversely, the LAO view provides for optimal visualization of the distal left EIA and the left CFA bifurcation and vice versa for the RAO view. In most cases, pelvic diagnostic angiography can be performed using 5- or 6-Fr. pigtail catheter. The catheter is typically positioned at the level of L3, and injection of contrast at 10 to 15 cc/sec for a total of 20 to 30 cc using a mechanical assist device and digital subtraction angiography (DSA) will allow for adequate visualization of the aortoiliac region.

INTERVENTION

Antiplatelet Agents and Anticoagulants

Patients undergoing planned revascularization should preferably be on aspirin for a minimum of 48 hours prior to the procedure. Alternatively, 325-mg oral aspirin may be given prior to gaining femoral access. There is no consensus regarding the use of preprocedural clopidogrel for iliac intervention. However, this practice should be avoided in the treatment of iliac occlusions, where the use of preprocedural clopidogrel might complicate surgical bailout of a significant complication (e.g., perforation). Following successful iliac stenting, the authors' practice is to administer clopidogrel 75 mg/day for at least 1 month, in addition to lifelong aspirin. However, it should be highlighted that in some centers, clopidogrel is not prescribed, especially in the presence of large iliac vessels or in patients at high risk for bleeding events.

The optimal type and level of anticoagulation for peripheral intervention (including aortoiliac intervention) has not been defined. Most investigators use unfractionated heparin for aortoiliac intervention and aim for an activated clotting time (ACT) of between 200 and 250 seconds. Non-Food and

Drug Administration (FDA)-approved alternative anticoagulation agents include direct thrombin inhibitors such as bivalirudin or low-molecular-weight heparins. The use of the latter agents, which do not have a reversing agent available, is discouraged for the treatment of iliac occlusive disease, due to the risk of perforation during these procedures.

Interventional Treatment of Aortoiliac Stenotic Disease

In the current era, the interventional treatment of stenoses in the aortoiliac territory is usually straightforward for appropriately trained endovascular specialists, with a procedural success approaching 100%. These stenoses are easily crossed using 0.035″ wires and treated using 0.035″ balloon and stent systems. Although compelling data supporting stenting in all cases are lacking, most operators have adopted the practice of stenting all iliac lesions because of the predictability of the procedural result achieved with iliac stenting. The major considerations in the interventional strategy in treating stenotic disease of the aortoiliac territory relates to the location of the disease.

OSTIUM OF THE COMMON ILIAC ARTERY AND AORTIC BIFURCATION

Unilateral ostial lesions of the CIA are best approached using ipsilateral retrograde CFA access. In most circumstances, the authors' preference is to perform kissing angioplasty/stenting of the aortoiliac bifurcation, with the goal of preventing plaque shift into the contralateral CIA at the time of stent deployment, which will require bilateral retrograde CFA access. Disease of the aortic bifurcation requires a kissing angioplasty/stenting technique in all cases, using bilateral retrograde femoral access. Stenting at the aortoiliac bifurcation is typically performed using balloon-expandable stents, due to their greater radial strength and ease of accurate positioning (Fig. 15.3). Based on the caliber of most balloon-expandable stents used to treat the typical caliber of the CIA (i.e., 7 to 10 mm), a 7 Fr. is required for most cases.

Following sheath placement, 0.035″ wire(s) (e.g., Wholey, SupraCore) are advanced across one or both CIA into the abdominal aorta. Predilation with an undersized noncompliant balloon is recommended prior to stenting. Stent placement should be performed under road map guidance, using either a pigtail in the distal abdominal aorta or injection through the sidearm of longer CFA sheaths (i.e., 23 cm) prior to insertion of the stent(s) through the sheath(s). With kissing stenting of the aortoiliac bifurcation, the stents are positioned to extend into the distal abdominal aorta. The degree to which the stents are positioned above the aortoiliac bifurcation depends largely on the presence of disease in the distal abdominal aorta, with the goal of covering significant distal aortic disease. In the absence of disease, it is typical to extend the stents about 5 mm above the true bifurcation. Raising the aortic bifurcation in this way clearly compromises and may preclude future attempts at contralateral access. However, one should rarely compromise on the appropriate stent placement based on this concern.

The choice of stent diameter during kissing stenting is an important consideration. This is determined by the diameter of the ipsilateral CIA and the diameter of the distal abdominal aorta. The combined diameter of two circular stents placed in each CIA extending into the distal abdominal aorta is estimated as follows: $0.8(D_1 + D_2) = D_3$ (where D_1 and D_2 represent the effective diameter of both CIA stents, and D_3 represents the diameter of both stents in the distal abdominal aorta). When the distal abdominal aorta is relatively small, the diameter of the CIA stents may be purposely undersized to minimize the risk of aortic rupture. The only circumstance in which the authors have used self-expanding stents at the aortoiliac bifurcation is where both common iliac arteries are of large caliber and the distal abdominal aorta is of insufficient caliber to accommodate the combined diameter of both kissing stents (Fig. 15.6).

NONOSTIAL COMMON ILIAC ARTERY AND PROXIMAL EXTERNAL ILIAC ARTERY

Stenoses of the CIA (excluding the ostium) and the proximal EIA are usually approached using ipsilateral retrograde CFA access (Fig. 15.7). Stenting in these locations may be performed using either balloon- or self-expanding stents. The major determinant of stent choice in this location is related to variations in vessel diameter. For disease with an equivalent proximal and distal reference diameter, a balloon-expandable stent may be used. However, where there is a significant size mismatch between the proximal and distal reference segments, a self-expanding stent is more appropriate, with the stent being sized to be 1 to 2 mm larger than the largest reference diameter.

DISTAL EXTERNAL ILIAC ARTERY STENOSES

In the presence of a stenosis located in the distal portion of the EIA artery, the ipsilateral retrograde CFA approach should not be used due to the immediate proximity between the access site and the lesion. Instead, access should be gained using a crossover technique from the contralateral CFA access site (Figs. 15.8 and 15.9). Stenting in this location is typically performed using self-expanding stents, as the distal EIA is in close proximity to the hip joint and is likely subject to significant conformational changes increasing the risk of stent failure with balloon-expandable stents in this location.

Interventional Treatment of Iliac Artery Occlusions

The interventional treatment of occlusions in the aortoiliac territory presents a fundamentally different set of challenges compared with the treatment of stenoses (Figs. 15.10 and 15.11). The choice and technique of access is more challenging, with a greater requirement for upper extremity access, and dual retrograde CFA access or dual upper extremity and unilateral retrograde CFA access. Often, the CFA distal to the iliac occlusion will need to be accessed, increasing the challenge of gaining successful CFA access.

One of the primary questions that should be addressed prior to attempting the treatment of an iliac occlusion is whether one wishes to approach the occlusion using an antegrade or retrograde approach. The approach will usually be dictated by the anatomy of the occlusion. For example, a flush occlusion of the CIA will dictate a retrograde approach, whereas an occlusion of the CIA with a proximal stump will allow either an antegrade or retrograde approach. The antegrade approach has the potential advantage of minimizing the risk of dissection or perforation of the distal abdominal aorta. However, in

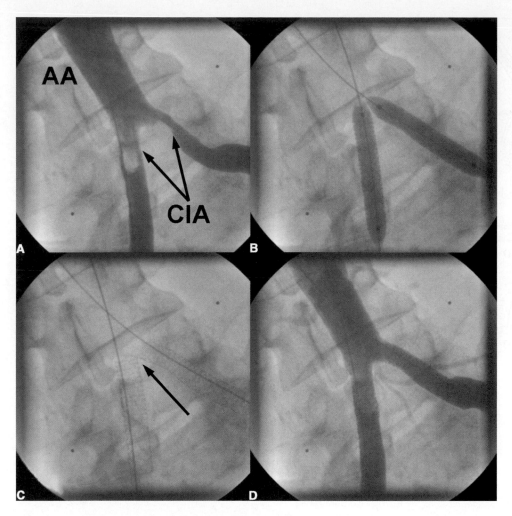

Figure 15.6 • Interventional treatment of aortoiliac bifurcation disease. A: Baseline pelvic angiogram demonstrating significant stenosis of the ostia of both common iliac arteries (CIA) *(arrows)*. AA, abdominal aorta. **B:** Bilateral retrograde CFA access was obtained and 0.035″ wires were advanced into the abdominal aorta from each CFA access site. Simultaneous kissing stenting of both common iliac artery ostia was performed. **C:** The stents were purposely not placed in the distal abdominal aorta due to the absence of plaque in that location. This does allow for future crossover maneuvers. The location of the carina of the CIA stents is indicated by the *arrow*. **D:** Final angiographic result.

the authors' experience, this has not been a significant issue in practice, and there are times when the retrograde approach is technically more straightforward and expedient.

When using an antegrade approach to the treatment of an iliac occlusion, brachial access or contralateral CFA access is required. Using brachial access for these cases is challenging and should be reserved for experienced interventionalists. The left brachial access is preferred because it allows for a more direct access to the descending aorta (i.e., shorter length) and at the same time it minimizes the risk of cerebral embolization since the only cerebral vessel that is crossed is the left vertebral artery. The brachial artery should be punctured in its distal part above the antecubital fossa, where effective hemostasis may be achieved by arterial compression against the humerus. Following initial placement of a short sheath in the left brachial artery, a 0.035″ wire is delivered to the distal abdominal aorta, which is then used to exchange the short sheath for a long 6-Fr. Shuttle sheath whose tip is positioned in the distal abdominal aorta. This approach has the advantage of allowing for a more coaxial alignment of the sheath with the occlusion that improves the ability to cross the occlusion and deliver equipment. The major shortcomings of this approach include the need to manage the brachial access carefully (i.e., monitoring for ischemic complications). In addition, the long length between the brachial artery

and the site of the occlusion may sometimes compromise the pushability of wires and catheters, making it difficult to cross complex calcified occlusions. Finally, treating distal EIA disease in tall individuals may not be possible from the brachial access site due to limitations in the length of balloon and stent delivery catheters.

When using retrograde contralateral CFA access to cross an iliac occlusion in the antegrade direction, there are two broad scenarios that merit description:

1. Treatment of a CIA or CIA/EIA occlusion. In this instance, the authors typically use a Simmons 1 or 2 catheter to engage the contralateral CIA. These catheters should typically be shaped in the thoracic aorta and are withdrawn carefully to engage the contralateral CIA. A 0.035″ glidewire is then used to cross the occlusion that is snared from below using retrograde CFA access. Angioplasty and stenting are then typically performed using the retrograde approach.
2. Treatment of an EIA occlusion (Fig. 15.12). In this instance, a 7-Fr. contralateral sheath can be placed with its tip in the distal CIA, proximal to the EIA occlusion. The authors will use the ipsilateral IIA to provide wire purchase for delivery of the contralateral sheath. Once the contralateral sheath is in position, the occlusion is crossed using 0.035″ glidewires and 0.035″ supportive catheters

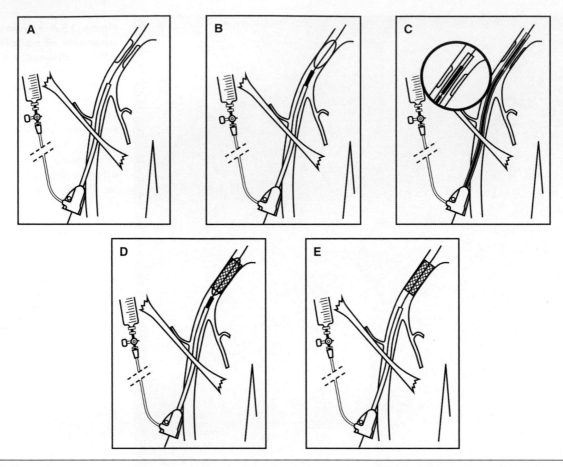

Figure 15.7 • Schematic representation of angioplasty and stenting technique for treatment of right common iliac artery stenosis using ipsilateral retrograde femoral approach. (Reproduced with permission from Scheinert D, Braunlich S, Biamino G. Recanalization of pelvic arteries. In: *The Paris Course on Revascularization Book 14:* Europa Edition; 2003.)

(e.g., glide catheter, Bernstein catheter). Once the wire is in the CFA (using a re-entry device if required), subsequent angioplasty and stenting can be performed using the antegrade approach.

If an iliac occlusion is to be crossed using a retrograde approach, then retrograde CFA access is required. In the authors' experience, access of the CFA distal to an iliac occlusion is greatly facilitated by either using ultrasound guidance or using

a road map to guide the needle puncture following injection of contrast proximal to the occlusion. Once the occlusion is crossed using 0.035″ wires and support catheter, angioplasty and stenting can proceed using the same access.

Regardless of the approach (i.e., retrograde or antegrade), the consideration regarding the choice of which stent type to use in a particular circumstance is similar to that described for the treatment of iliac stenoses and is largely based on the anatomic location of the occlusion.

Figure 15.8 • Interventional treatment of distal right external iliac artery (EIA) stenosis.
A: Using retrograde left common femoral artery (CFA) access, a crossover sheath was placed with its tip in the right common iliac artery (CIA). Baseline angiogram demonstrating severe stenosis in distal portion of right EIA *(arrow).* IIA, internal iliac artery. **B:** Final result after direct stenting of EIA using self-expanding stent.

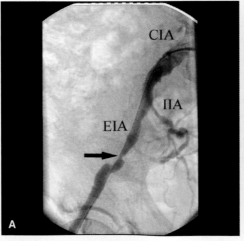

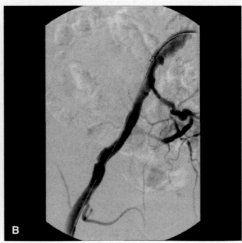

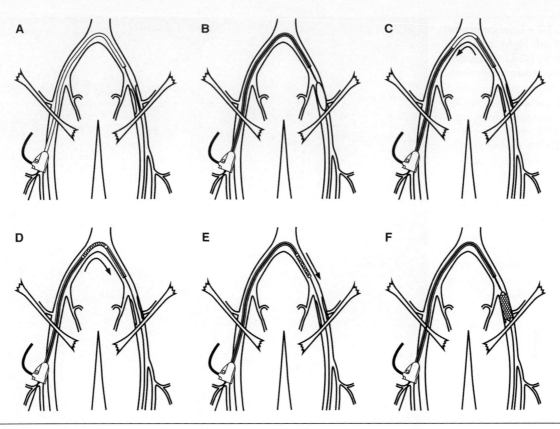

Figure 15.9 • Schematic representation of angioplasty and stenting technique for treatment of a left external iliac artery stenosis using contralateral retrograde femoral access with crossover technique. (Reproduced with permission from Scheinert D, Braunlich S, Biamino G. Recanalization of pelvic arteries. In: *The Paris Course on Revascularization Book 14*: Europa Edition; 2003.)

Interventional Treatment of Distal Abdominal Aortic Disease

Interventional treatment of disease in the distal abdominal aorta is usually achieved using single retrograde CFA approach. On occasion, bilateral retrograde CFA access may be used if balloon dilatation or stent expansion is performed using a double-balloon technique. Following arterial puncture, an 8- to 12-Fr (depending on the aortic diameter) short sheath is inserted and a preprocedural aortogram is obtained. The stenosis of the distal aorta is crossed with a 0.035″ nonhydrophilic (e.g., Magic Torque, Wholey) or hydrophilic (e.g., angled Glide Wire) guidewire. If a balloon-expandable stent is chosen, the authors typically use the Palmaz XL [Cordis] stent, which is hand-mounted onto a large-diameter balloon (e.g., XXL [Boston Scientific] with diameters ranging between 12 and 18 mm or MAXI LD [Cordis] with diameters ranging between 14 and 25 mm). The sheath size required to deliver these devices ranges from 8 to 12 Fr. Since large aortic balloons with diameters between 20 and 25 mm may allow only for low-pressure inflations (i.e., 2 to 4 atm), postinflation using two balloons (e.g., 8 to 12 mm in diameter) should be performed to achieve optimal stent expansion in this location (Fig. 15.13). For the purpose of double-balloon inflation, dual retrograde CFA access is required. The maximum diameter of self-expanding stents does not approach that of hand-mounted balloon-expandable stents (e.g., 16 mm

for the Easy Wallstent [Boston Scientific] or 14 mm for the SMART [Cordis]), and, as such, may only be used to treat disease in the distal aorta where the aortic diameter is 1 to 2 mm smaller than the largest self-expanding stent diameter. However, using the 14-mm SMART stent with postdilatation with a 12-mm balloon (e.g., PowerFlex P3 [Cordis]), the entire procedure can be safely performed through a single 7-Fr. introducer sheath (Fig. 15.14).

Treatment of Occlusion of Infrarenal Aorta

The Leriche syndrome refers to a total occlusion of the abdominal aorta, most commonly in the infrarenal region. Since disease progression is slow, the patient typically presents with bilateral lifestyle-limiting claudication that allows for the development of collateral circulation. In male patients, there is often associated impotence, due to compromise of flow to both internal iliac arteries. Surgery is still regarded as the treatment of choice for infrarenal artery occlusions. However, in dedicated centers, endovascular therapy has been achieved, typically in patients at high risk for surgery. These procedures require an upper extremity access combined with either unilateral or bilateral CFA access (Fig. 15.15).

Stents

The first series on the use of stents in the iliac circulation was published in 1988 and included 15 patients (12). The balloon-expandable Palmaz 308 stent gained FDA approval for iliac

Figure 15.10 • Interventional treatment of right common iliac artery (CIA) occlusion using retrograde approach. **A:** Baseline angiogram using pigtail catheter advanced from left CFA access demonstrating flush occlusion of right CIA and severe stenosis of the left CIA. **B:** Angiography following placement of balloon-expandable stent in the left CIA. **C:** Retrograde right CFA access was obtained and the right CIA occlusion was crossed in a retrograde fashion. Kissing stenting of the aortoiliac bifurcation was performed using balloon-expandable stents (*arrows* indicate position of stents). **D:** Final angiographic result.

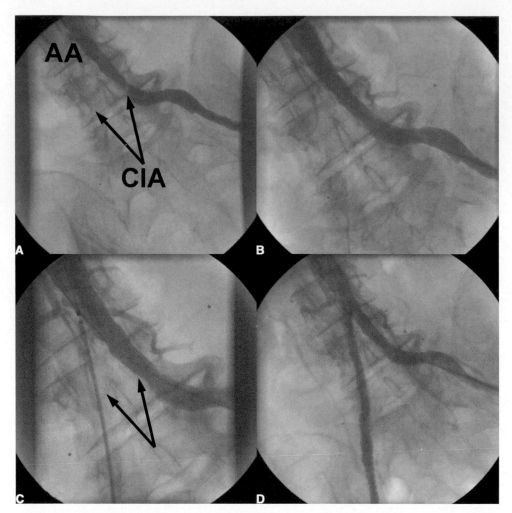

Figure 15.11 • Interventional treatment of right common iliac artery (CIA) occlusion using antegrade approach. **A:** Angiography of right external iliac artery (EIA) obtained following retrograde right common femoral access demonstrating distal end of right CIA occlusion (*arrow*). **B:** Left brachial access was obtained and a 90-cm Shuttle sheath was delivered to the distal abdominal aorta. The right CIA occlusion was crossed using a hydrophilic 0.035″ glidewire supported by a 125-cm long 5-Fr. Judkins right catheter (indicated by *white arrows*) (IIA, internal iliac artery). The intraluminal catheter position is confirmed with contrast injection. **C:** Final result after stenting of the CIA and the proximal part of the external iliac artery (using self-expanding stent).

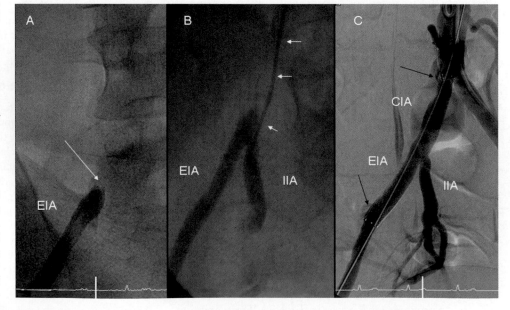

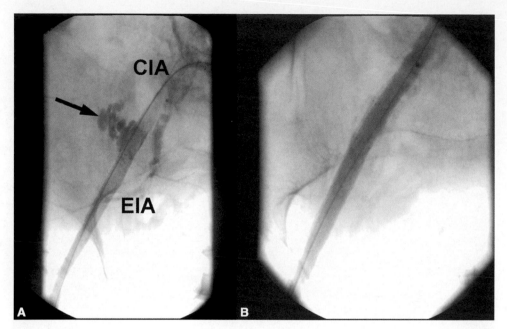

Figure 15.12 • Iliac artery perforation during interventional treatment of right external iliac artery (EIA) occlusion. **A:** Angiogram following successful recanalization and stenting of a chronic total EIA occlusion. Perforation indicated by *arrow*. **B:** Angiogram following immediate balloon occlusion at the level of the perforation, reversal of heparin with protamine, and placement of a covered stent demonstrating effective sealing of the perforation.

interventions in 1991 for suboptimal results following percutaneous transluminal angioplasty (PTA) caused by an extensive dissection or residual pressure gradient, and treatment of total occlusions or restenosis after PTA. Subsequently, three additional devices have gained FDA approval, namely the self-expandable stainless steel Wallstent (Boston Scientific), the self-expandable nitinol SMART stent (Cordis), and the balloon-expandable Express LD stent (Boston Scientific). In addition, numerous other stents that are FDA approved for biliary or tracheobronchial applications have been used "off-label" in the iliac circulation. In clinical practice, the use of these scaffolding devices is far more liberal than the initial FDA label, and stents are abundantly used for ostial, long, or severely calcified lesions (Table 15.2). Frequently, stent placement is considered the default strategy for iliac disease. A meta-analysis including more than 800 patients treated for an iliac occlusive disease showed that the technical success rate of patients' treatment with angioplasty ± stenting was >90% and that the primary and secondary patency rates at 3 years were approximately 80% and 90%, respectively (13).

The value of balloon predilatation prior to planned stenting in aortoiliac interventions remains controversial. While some investigators routinely perform balloon predilatation, others frequently proceed to direct stenting. Predilatation with a slightly undersized balloon may be particularly helpful in ostial or severely calcified lesions, as it may facilitate stent placement and expansion. In addition, balloon inflation may convey important information for proper stent choice, such as lesion length, vessel size, and lesion characteristics.

A theoretical advantage of direct stenting, although not firmly demonstrated, is the reduction of the incidence of dissection and distal embolization. This observation may be particularly important in the case of chronic total iliac occlusions, where it is difficult to predict the amount of organized thrombus present at the occlusion site. In those cases, angioplasty alone with balloon size matching the vessel size and inflated at nominal pressure may be associated with a distal embolization risk of as high as 24% (14). Therefore, we recommend direct stenting whenever feasible in chronic total occlusions,

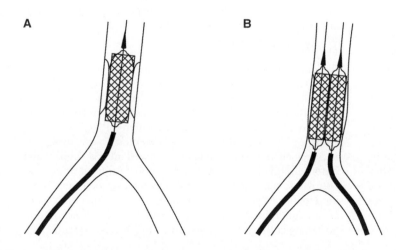

Figure 15.13 • Schematic representation of interventional treatment of stenosis of the distal aorta. **A:** Using retrograde common femoral artery (CFA) access, the distal aortic stenosis is treated with a large balloon-expandable stent. **B:** After contralateral retrograde CFA access is gained, optimal stent expansion is achieved with double-balloon postinflation. (Reproduced with permission from Scheinert D, Braunlich S, Biamino G. Recanalization of pelvic arteries. In: *The Paris Course on Revascularization Book 14*: Europa Edition; 2003.)

Figure 15.14 • Interventional treatment of distal abdominal aorta stenosis. **A:** Baseline angiogram showing distal abdominal aortic stenosis *(arrow)*. **B:** A 0.035″ wire *(arrow)* is advanced into the aorta from retrograde right common femoral artery access. **C:** A self-expanding stent was deployed in the distal abdominal aorta that was postdilated. **D:** Final angiographic result.

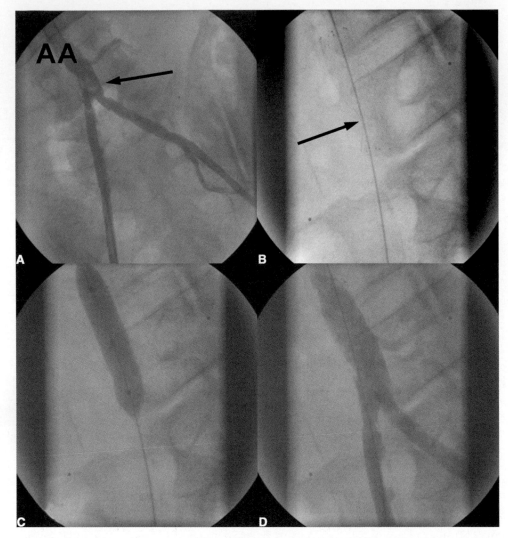

followed by an adequate postdilatation in order to ensure adequate apposition of the stent. This strategy has been shown to be associated with distal embolization in as low as 1% of cases following recanalization of chronic iliac occlusions (15). Current American College of Cardiology/American Heart Association (ACC/AHA) guidelines recommend primary stenting whenever feasible in common iliac arteries (class IB indication) and in external iliac arteries (class IC indication) (6).

BALLOON-EXPANDABLE STENTS

The slotted tube stainless steel Palmaz stent is the prototype for balloon-expandable stents. These devices have several advantages in the aortoiliac circulation compared with self-expanding stents. Their high radial force makes them suitable for heavily calcified lesions. Minimal foreshortening at deployment and good visibility allow for precise placement in the treatment of ostial lesions. Finally, balloon-expandable stents may be further expanded (typically by 1 to 2 mm) after initial deployment by using larger balloons until the desired diameter is achieved. Currently, the vast majority of stents are premounted on a balloon and stent flexibility has improved, allowing for stent delivery using the crossover technique. One of the potential disadvantages of these devices in the iliac circulation is their propensity to

create edge dissections, in particular in heavily calcified vessels or if the stent diameter is oversized. Since balloon-expandable stents are not elastic, they may crush in the presence of extensive compressive forces. Therefore, these devices should not be placed in the CFA and should also be avoided in the distal part of the EIA, where significant conformational change may occur. Since most of the currently available peripheral balloon-expandable stents are made of stainless steel, they cause significant artifacts (i.e., signal loss) on MRA.

SELF-EXPANDING STENTS

The most distinguishing features of self-expanding stents are their elasticity and flexibility. These devices expand to their nominal diameter when released from a constrained state within the delivery system. Typically, a slightly oversized stent (i.e., 1 to 2 mm) is chosen to allow for optimal vessel wall apposition. The flexibility facilitates stent delivery using the crossover technique and allows for excellent trackability and conformability in tortuous iliac vessels. After stent release, postdilatation is usually performed to achieve good stent apposition to the vessel wall. Disadvantages of self-expanding stents include suboptimal radial strength and varying degrees of foreshortening at the time deployment. Therefore, this stent type is

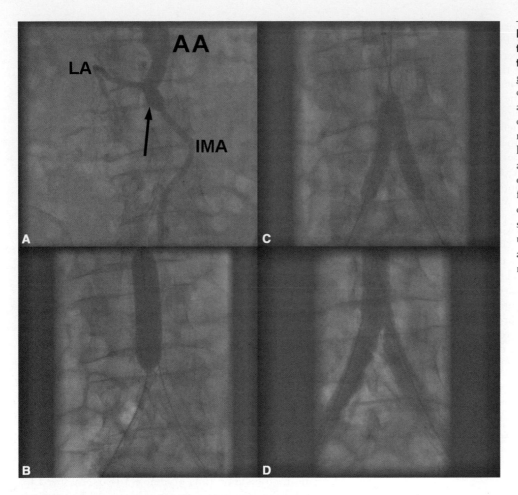

Figure 15.15 • Interventional treatment of infrarenal aortic occlusion. **A:** Baseline angiogram via left brachial artery access demonstrating occlusion of the distal abdominal aorta *(arrow)* with abundant collateralization via the inferior mesenteric artery (IMA) and the lumbar artery (LA). AA, abdominal aorta. **B:** Successful recanalization of occlusion using antegrade approach followed by placement of stent in distal abdominal aorta. **C:** Kissing stenting of the aortoiliac bifurcation using brachial and common femoral artery access. **D:** Final angiographic result.

less suitable for the treatment of ostial lesions. Self-expanding stents should be considered for the treatment of nonostial lesions of the CIA and all EIA lesions.

While the prototype of this stent class (Wallstent) is made of stainless steel, newer-generation devices (e.g., SMART [Cordis], Absolute [Abbott]) are composed of nitinol, an alloy of nickel and titanium. Compared with the stainless steel counterparts, nitinol stents allow for increased radial strength and minimal foreshortening at deployment. The radial strength of nitinol stents has further increased in second-generation devices (e.g., Supera Stent [IDev Tech, TX]), allowing for optimal stent expansion also in severely calcified lesions. In addition, the superior conformability is important in vascular segments with abrupt changes in vessel diameter, as might be encountered at the transition from the common and external iliac arteries. A further advantage of nitinol over stainless steel stents is their magnetic resonance compatibility, achieved however at the cost of a reduced x-ray visibility.

To our knowledge, only one randomized head-to-head comparison between different self-expanding stents in the iliac circulation has been performed. Between 1998 and 2001, the Cordis Randomized Iliac Stent Project (CRISP) trial randomized a total of 203 patients with symptomatic iliac disease and suboptimal results following angioplasty to treatment using a nitinol stent (SMART) or a stainless steel stent (Wallstent) (16). Acute procedural success was significantly higher with the nitinol stent compared with the stainless steel stent (98% vs. 87%, respectively). Primary vessel patency at 12 months was comparable (95% and 91%, respectively).

COVERED STENTS

Covered stents are composite devices consisting of a metallic skeleton covered with synthetic graft material (e.g., Dacron, expanded polytetrafluoroethylene [ePTFE]). Because of the

---

TABLE 15.2	Indications for Stenting in Aortoiliac Disease

Indications

- Provisional stenting for suboptimal result of PTA
  - Extensive dissection
  - Residual translesional pressure gradient ≥ 10 mm Hg
- Total occlusion
- Recurrence after PTA
- Ostial location
- Severe calcification
- Alternatively, primary treatment for all aortoiliac lesions

bulky graft material, these devices require larger delivery systems. They are currently not FDA approved for iliac occlusive disease. Nevertheless, covered stents have been used in this vascular bed, mainly for the treatment of aneurysms but also for bailout of iatrogenic iliac ruptures or arteriovenous fistulas. Isolated aneurysms of the iliac arteries are relatively uncommon, accounting for 2% to 7% of all intra-abdominal aneurysms (17). The most frequently utilized covered stents in the iliac circulation include the self-expanding Wallgraft (Boston Scientific), Viabahn (Gore), and Fluency (Bard) stents, and the balloon-expandable iCAST (Atrium) stent. The self-expanding covered stents are more flexible than the iCAST stent but require larger-caliber access sheaths for delivery. This can be particularly problematic when treating iliac perforations, where the clinical situation may not permit time to change access sheaths. The iCAST balloon-expandable stent consists of a 316L stainless steel stent that is encapsulated with PTFE such that the stainless steel is not exposed to the luminal wall. Although this stent is very stiff, it has the advantage over self-expanding covered stents that stents up to 10 mm in diameter may be delivered through a 7-Fr. sheath. This stent is being used increasingly for the treatment of occlusive iliac disease, and preliminary data suggest that restenosis rates with this stent may be lower than those with uncovered balloon-expandable stents.

RESULTS

Aortoiliac Interventions

PTA VERSUS STENTING

A recent meta-analysis summarized the results of endovascular intervention for aortoiliac occlusive disease stratified for stent use (13). This analysis included six angioplasty studies enrolling a total of 1300 patients and eight stent series enrolling a total of 816 patients. No difference was observed in terms of technical success between PTA and stenting (91% and 96%, respectively). Overall, the systemic complication rate was 1% (ranging from 0% to 3.5%), the local complication rate 9% (ranging from 2.7% to 17.8%), and the rate of major complications necessitating treatment was 4% (ranging from 1.6% to 10.8%). In-hospital mortality ranged from 0% to 2.7%. The mean postprocedural ABI was significantly greater in the stent group compared with the PTA group (0.87 and 0.76, respectively). Among patients treated for claudication, the 4-year primary patency rate following treatment of stenotic lesions was 65% in the PTA group and 77% in the stent group. Corresponding patency rates for the treatment of total occlusions were 54% and 61%, respectively. Among patients presenting with critical limb ischemia, the 4-year patency rate following treatment of stenotic lesions was 53% for PTA and 67% for stent placement. Corresponding patency rates for patients with total occlusions were 44% and 53%, respectively. Despite the limitations of pooling results of series that greatly differ in the patient population enrolled, endovascular technique, and outcome assessment, this analysis suggests that stenting is superior to PTA in terms of acute success and long-term patency.

The Dutch Iliac Stent Trial (DIST) (18) enrolled 279 patients with intermittent claudication, caused by aortoiliac disease, and randomized them to routine stenting or angioplasty with provisional stent use in the presence of a suboptimal result following PTA. In the PTA group, provisional stenting was performed in 43% of cases according to the predefined criteria of a residual mean pressure gradient > 10 mm Hg across the treated site following angioplasty. Initial success and complications did not differ among the groups. Two-year cumulative patency rates (71% in the routine stent group vs. 70% in the provisional stent group) and reintervention rates (7% vs. 4%) were similar. These data demonstrate that PTA alone is unable to deliver an optimal hemodynamic result in the aortoiliac vascular system in a high proportion of patients. Nevertheless, in the absence of a postprocedural gradient or evidence of complications following angioplasty, PTA alone seems a valid alternative to routine stenting.

A European multicenter trial addressed the value of stenting with a flexible balloon-expandable device (Perflex, Cordis) in the iliac circulation in 126 consecutive patients who demonstrated an unsatisfactory angioplasty result (i.e., postdilatation gradient ≥ 10 mm Hg) or had a primary occluded lesion (19). Primary stent patency was 94% at 6 months and 89% at 12 months, supporting the notion that stents are an effective device in the treatment of iliac artery obstructive disease. A recent US series including 365 patients with a total of 505 aortoiliac lesions gives us additional information on the short- and long-term results of stenting (20). Periprocedural success, defined as mean pressure gradient ≤ 5 mm Hg, was achieved in 98% of patients. Major complications (e.g., stent thrombosis, distal embolization, arterial rupture, or acute renal failure) were observed in 7% of cases, in 2% of cases requiring surgery. The 30-day mortality rate was 0.5%. At a mean observation time of almost 3 years, the need for bypass at follow-up was 6% and an additional 1% of patients underwent ipsilateral lower limb amputation. At 8 years, the primary and secondary patency rates were 74% and 84%, respectively (21). The ACC/AHA and the new TASC II guidelines recommend primary stenting in the common iliac artery as a class IB indication and in the external iliac artery as a class IC indication (6,7).

PERCUTANEOUS VERSUS SURGICAL APPROACH

No study has randomized patients with exclusively aortoiliac obstructive disease to surgery versus endovascular intervention. Whereas there is general agreement that simple lesions should be treated percutaneously, it remains a source of debate as to what is the best approach for more complex disease (i.e., TASC C/D lesions). A single-center retrospective analysis addressed the outcomes of stenting (N = 136) and surgery (N = 52) for complex aortoiliac lesions (TASC types B and C) (22). Primary patency rates at 1, 3, and 5 years were 85%, 72%, and 64% after iliac stenting, and 89%, 86%, and 86% after surgical reconstruction, respectively. Although no conclusive recommendation can be made in more complex lesions (TASC C/D lesions), it may be reasonable to attempt percutaneous treatment first, as long as the lesion appears amenable and the operator has the necessary expertise. Should this approach fail, the patient should be referred to vascular surgery. This approach of favoring a first percutaneous attempt and using surgical revscularization in case of failure may be adopted also for complex TASC D lesions. This approach is supported by the technical success and the patency rates achieved in dedicated centers (8–10).

PERCUTANEOUS OUTCOMES IN COMPLEX LESIONS

Recent series have reported long-term results of the endovascular treatment of TASC C/D lesions. Balzer et al. reported a primary technical success rate of 97% and a complication rate of 5.6% in 89 patients with TASC C/D lesions (9). The ABI improved from a mean of 0.51 before the procedure to 0.79 on the day following intervention and to 0.81 at 3 years follow-up. Clinical improvement was observed in 97% of the patients in the TASC C group and in 88% in the TASC D group. Ninety percent of the patients had patent vessels at 3 years follow-up.

Sixt et al. retrospectively compared the acute and long-term outcomes of endovascular therapy for TASC A/B lesions versus TASC C/D lesions in 375 patients with symptomatic aortoiliac disease (8). TASC A/B, C, and D lesions were present in 59%, 26%, and 15% of cases, respectively. Acute treatment success—defined as residual stenosis < 30%—was achieved in all TASC A lesions, in 96% of TASC B lesions, in 93% of TASC C lesions, and in all TASC D lesions. The 1-year primary patency rate was 86% for the entire study cohort with no differences among TASC classes (8). In the TASC C/D and A/B groups, the 5-year event-free survival was comparable (57% vs. 70%; P = NS). The clinical outcome, as measured by Rutherford stage and ABI, improved significantly in all TASC subgroups after successful intervention and was maintained up to 1 year. The placement of one or more stents during the procedure was identified as independent protective factor toward the development of restenosis (HR 0.51, P = 0.008). The authors concluded that, in experienced hands, endovascular therapy of aortoiliac lesions can be successfully performed and is associated with favorable long-term outcomes across the whole spectrum of TASC lesions.

Total Occlusions

The treatment of chronic total occlusions remains a limitation of percutaneous intervention in the iliac circulation. In a series reporting PTA of 82 iliac chronic total occlusions, the procedural success rate was 76% (23). After exclusion of the initial failures, the success rate at 3 years was 59%. Another report involving 59 patients reported a technical success rate of 92% and a primary patency rate at 2 years of 73% (24). Major procedural complications occurred in 6% and included four episodes of distal embolization and one massive bleeding event. Late complications occurred in 12% and included nine stent total occlusions and one severe restenosis.

A recent single-center experience addressed the results of a strategy based on Excimer laser debulking prior to PTA/ stent among 212 consecutive patients with iliac occlusion (15). The rate of major complications was 1.4% and included one arterial rupture and two embolic events. Technical success was achieved in 90% of cases. Primary patency rates were 84% at 1 year, 81% at 2 years, 78% at 3 years, and 76% at 4 years. Secondary patency rates were 88% at 1 year, 88% at 2 years, 86% at 3 years, and 85% at 4 years. Overall stent-supported angioplasty appears to be an effective treatment also for iliac artery occlusion, with favorable morbidity and mortality rates compared to surgery. However, reported long-term patency rates after surgery are generally greater than those observed with interventional treatment. Recently, a retrospective analysis of 66 TASC D iliac lesions has shown a remarkable 100% technical

success rate (defined as residual stenosis <30%) and a 1-year primary patency rate of 85% (8). In this series, stenting was the only independent protective factor identified with respect to restenosis.

Aortoiliac Bifurcation

Several series on kissing stenting for the reconstruction of the aortoiliac bifurcation have been published. A series from Germany documented a technical success of 100% in the absence of major procedure-related complications and a primary patency rate of 87% at 2 years in 48 patients (25). Of note, about half of the patients were treated for total occlusions. An Austrian single-center series including 25 patients reported a technical success rate of 86% and a 2-year primary patency of 65% (26). Periprocedural complications occurred in 20% of cases and included two dissections of the distal aorta that were managed conservatively and three cases of CFA pseudoaneurysm. No death occurred within 30 days of the procedure. A group in Milwaukee described a technical success rate of 100% and a primary patency rate at 20 months of 92% in 50 patients treated with this technique (27). Acute complications occurred in 4% of cases and were all related to distal embolization. One patient required surgery and no procedural death occurred. Amputation-free survival at follow-up was 100% and 92% of patients were free of lifestyle-limiting claudication. Overall, percutaneous reconstruction of the aortic bifurcation appears to be associated with low periprocedural morbidity/mortality and satisfactory mid-term results.

The kissing stent technique offers optimal angiographic results. However, as previously described, it may hamper future crossover maneuvers.

Stenosis of the Infrarenal Aorta

Localized stenosis of the infrarenal abdominal aorta is relatively infrequent and occurs predominantly in younger women who smoke (Fig. 15.6) (28). Until the early 1980s, distal abdominal aortic stenoses were treated surgically with endarterectomy or bypass grafting. Currently, PTA ± stenting has become the treatment of choice for short abdominal aortic stenosis in the absence of significant iliac disease. Failures of angioplasty may be the result of elastic recoil, obstructive intimal dissection, or late restenosis. In a series of 102 patients with mainly isolated distal aortic lesions treated with angioplasty, technical success (defined as residual stenosis <50% or residual mean pressure gradient <10 mm Hg) was achieved in only 76% (29). Stents were placed in a minority of patients (12%) for suboptimal PTA results. No major complications were reported. At 10 years, primary clinical and hemodynamic patency was achieved in 72% and 46% of cases, respectively.

Another series addressed the use of provisional stenting of the distal aorta for failures of angioplasty (30). Outcomes were compared between 55 patients who underwent successful PTA and 19 patients who underwent aortic stenting for angioplasty failure. Three-year clinical and hemodynamic patency rates, respectively, were 85% and 79% for PTA and 69% and 43% for stenting. The difference in outcomes disappeared following multivariate modeling, suggesting that stenting is a valuable option even in patients with poor results following PTA. Nevertheless, the low patency rates achieved with stenting were somehow surprising, because the immediate angiographic and hemodynamic results were described as optimal.

Although no prospective study has addressed routine versus provisional stenting in the distal aorta, primary stenting has been advocated for the treatment of complex lesions (e.g., irregular, eccentric, ulcerated, or calcified) and occlusions. Covering such lesions with a stent before balloon dilatation may minimize the risk of distal embolization by trapping the atheroma between the stent struts and the vessel wall and may reduce the risk of vessel rupture by more evenly distributing the dilating forces against the arterial wall.

It remains a source of debate whether balloon-expandable (e.g., Palmaz) or self-expandable stents (e.g., Wallstent, Smart) are the device of choice for the distal aorta. The advantages of balloon-expandable stents include a more accurate positioning and ability to treat larger aortic diameters. Self-expanding stents may achieve further gradual expansion because of intrinsic radial force, thus allowing the use of smaller balloons and minimizing the risk of acute vessel trauma, and require smaller sheaths for access. In addition, because of smaller cells, a self-expanding device like the Wallstent may more efficaciously trap atheroembolic material at the time of deployment, potentially decreasing the risk of distal embolization.

COMPLICATIONS

Potential complications of aortoiliac interventions include flow-limiting dissection, abrupt vessel occlusion, perforation, and distal embolization. The specific risks vary according to the type of procedure and have been described earlier in the chapter. On a broader perspective, the incidence of complications is greater during recanalization of total occlusions compared with the treatment of nonocclusive lesions. Extensive iliac dissection (Fig. 15.16) can usually be treated successfully with self-expanding stents. In the presence of vessel rupture (Fig. 15.12), immediate balloon occlusion proximal to the perforation, followed by reversal of heparin with protamine and placement of a covered stent, is mandatory. In the meantime, blood should be typed and crossed and vascular surgery notified in case the endovascular salvage fails. If distal embolization is suspected, immediate angiography should be performed and further treatment (e.g., prolonged heparinization, intraarterial lytic therapy, endovascular clot extraction, surgery) should be guided based on the angiographic and clinical findings.

If distal embolization (Fig. 15.17) should occur during an iliac intervention performed with an ipsilateral retrograde approach, it is recommended to access the contralateral CFA and to treat the complication with a crossover approach. Conversion from a retrograde to an antegrade approach through the same access, although technically feasible, should be discouraged because it may seriously damage the CFA at the access site. An alternative approach (i.e., in the absence of acute limb ischemia) is to treat the distal embolization the day after the index procedure using antegrade access. Since large series of aortoiliac PTA with routine follow-up angiography are missing, the true incidence of restenosis in this vascular segment is unknown. Nevertheless, the lower rate of repeat revascularization and data from noninvasive studies suggest that restenosis is a marginal problem. For that reason, drug-eluting stents have not been tested in aortoiliac disease.

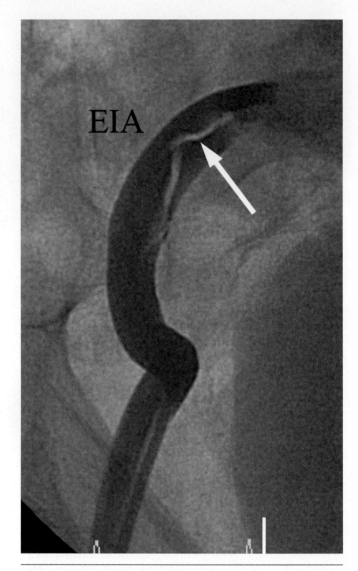

Figure 15.16 • External iliac artery (EIA) dissection *(arrow)* induced by a 0.035" guidewire, which was treated conservatively.

LONG-TERM FOLLOW-UP

Following iliac intervention, all patients should receive lifelong aspirin therapy. Clopidogrel is recommended for at least 4 weeks following stent implantation. Currently, there is no evidence that prolonged dual antiplatelet therapy (i.e., aspirin and clopidogrel) may favorably impact the prognosis of patients with PAD undergoing intervention (31). In follow-up, patients should be screened for evidence of restenosis based on their symptomatology, CFA pulse exam, and ABI measurements. If any of these elements suggests restenosis, then further evaluation is warranted to maintain patency of the treatment site.

KEY PRINCIPLES

The indications for endovascular therapy in the aortoiliac circulation have gradually expanded over the last two decades. While discrete iliac stenosis may be easily treated, the

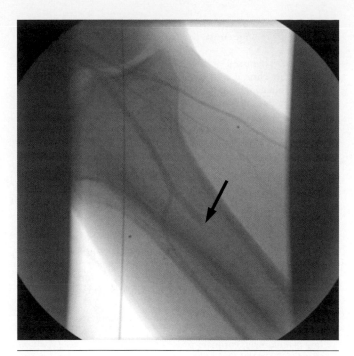

Figure 15.17 • Embolization following iliac artery intervention. Distal embolization at the tibiofibular bifurcation (indicated by *arrow*) occurred during a retrograde recanalization of a chronic total occlusion of the right external and common iliac artery (same patient of Fig. 15.10). The distal embolus, despite being asymptomatic, was successfully aspirated the following day using an ipsilateral right antegrade approach.

endovascular management of long iliac total occlusions or advanced disease of the aortic bifurcation remains challenging. Depending on the location and type of the lesion, as well as the anatomy of the aortic bifurcation, different access techniques may be chosen. The retrograde CFA approach is the easiest and least traumatic and leads to success in the majority of patients with isolated iliac stenosis. In the presence of total occlusions or involvement of the distal EIA, crossover access is preferred. Severe disease of the aortoiliac bifurcation is usually treated with kissing balloon/stenting using a bilateral retrograde femoral access. The brachial approach may be required in a minority of aortoiliac interventions and should only be used by experienced operators.

For discrete, noncalcified, nonstial stenosis, with a good angiographic and hemodynamic result following PTA, stenting may not be necessary. Stenting is recommended for the treatment of long lesions, lesions in an ostial location, total occlusions, and for suboptimal results following PTA. Some investigators consider default stenting the treatment of choice for iliac disease, irrespective of lesion characteristics. Regarding stent type, the high radial strength of balloon-expandable stents and the lack of foreshortening make them suitable in particular for treatment of ostial or severely calcified iliac lesions. The greater flexibility and conformability of self-expanding stents have advantages in the treatment of long lesions in tortuous segments. Based on the low incidence of major complications as well as good long-term results, percutaneous revascularization has replaced surgery for most

aortoiliac occlusive conditions. According to the new TASC II recommendations, TASC A–B lesions should be managed percutaneously, TASC C lesions should be treated percutaneously or surgically according to the anatomic characteristics and the local expertise, and TASC D lesions should be treated surgically. Due to improvements in the equipment and in the expertise of interventionalists, recent reports suggest that even TASC D lesions may be safely and efficaciously treated with an endovascular approach.

ACKNOWLEDGMENT

The authors would like to thank Dr Thomas Zeller for allowing the use of images of patients treated at the Heart Center of Bad Krozingen, Germany.

References

1. de Vries SO, Hunink MG. Results of aortic bifurcation grafts for aortoiliac occlusive disease: a meta-analysis. *J Vasc Surg.* 1997;26:558–569.
2. Vitale GF, Inahara T. Extraperitoneal endarterectomy for iliofemoral occlusive disease. *J Vasc Surg.* 1990;12:409–413; discussion 414–415.
3. van den Dungen JJ, Boontje AH, Kropveld A. Unilateral iliofemoral occlusive disease: long-term results of the semi-closed endarterectomy with the ring-stripper. *J Vasc Surg.* 1991;14:673–677.
4. Dormandy JA, Rutherford RB. Management of peripheral arterial disease (PAD). TASC Working Group. TransAtlantic Inter-Society Consensus (TASC). *J Vasc Surg.* 2000;31(1 pt 2):S1–S296.
5. Brewster DC. Clinical and anatomical considerations for surgery in aortoiliac disease and results of surgical treatment. *Circulation.* 1991;83(2 suppl):I42–I52.
6. Hirsch AT, Haskal ZJ, Hertzer NR, et al. ACC/AHA 2005 practice guidelines for the management of patients with peripheral arterial disease (lower extremity, renal, mesenteric, and abdominal aortic): a collaborative report from the American Association for Vascular Surgery/Society for Vascular Surgery, Society for Cardiovascular Angiography and Interventions, Society for Vascular Medicine and Biology, Society of Interventional Radiology, and the ACC/AHA Task Force on Practice Guidelines (Writing Committee to Develop Guidelines for the Management of Patients With Peripheral Arterial Disease): endorsed by the American Association of Cardiovascular and Pulmonary Rehabilitation; National Heart, Lung, and Blood Institute; Society for Vascular Nursing; TransAtlantic Inter-Society Consensus; and Vascular Disease Foundation. *Circulation.* 2006;113: e463–e654.
7. Norgren L, Hiatt WR, Dormandy JA, et al. Inter-society consensus for the management of peripheral arterial disease (TASC II). *J Vasc Surg.* 2007;45(suppl S):S5–S67.
8. Sixt S, Alawied AK, Rastan A, et al. Acute and long-term outcome of endovascular therapy for aortoiliac occlusive lesions stratified according to the TASC classification: a single-center experience. *J Endovasc Ther.* 2008;15:408–416.
9. Balzer JO, Gastinger V, Ritter R, et al. Percutaneous interventional reconstruction of the iliac arteries: primary and long-term success rate in selected TASC C and D lesions. *Eur Radiol.* 2006;16:124–131.
10. Leville CD, Kashyap VS, Clair DG, et al. Endovascular management of iliac artery occlusions: extending treatment to TransAtlantic Inter-Society Consensus class C and D patients. *J Vasc Surg.* 2006;43:32–39.

11. Scheinert D, Braunlich S, Biamino G. Recanalization of pelvic arteries. In: *The Paris Course on Revascularization Book 14*: Europa Edition; 2003.
12. Palmaz JC, Richter GM, Noeldge G, et al. Intraluminal stents in atherosclerotic iliac artery stenosis: preliminary report of a multicenter study. *Radiology.* 1988;168:727–731.
13. Bosch JL, Hunink MG. Meta-analysis of the results of percutaneous transluminal angioplasty and stent placement for aortoiliac occlusive disease. *Radiology.* 1997;204:87–96.
14. Leu AJ, Schneider E, Canova CR, et al. Long-term results after recanalisation of chronic iliac artery occlusions by combined catheter therapy without stent placement. *Eur J Vasc Endovasc Surg.* 1999;18:499–505.
15. Scheinert D, Schroder M, Ludwig J, et al. Stent-supported recanalization of chronic iliac artery occlusions. *Am J Med.* 2001;110:708–715.
16. Ponec D, Jaff MR, Swischuk J, et al. The Nitinol SMART stent vs Wallstent for suboptimal iliac artery angioplasty: CRISP-US trial results. *J Vasc Interv Radiol.* 2004;15:911–918.
17. Nachbur BH, Inderbitzi RG, Bar W. Isolated iliac aneurysms. *Eur J Vasc Surg.* 1991;5:375–381.
18. Tetteroo E, van der Graaf Y, Bosch JL, et al. Randomised comparison of primary stent placement versus primary angioplasty followed by selective stent placement in patients with iliac-artery occlusive disease. Dutch Iliac Stent Trial Study Group. *Lancet.* 1998;351:1153–1159.
19. Reekers JA, Vorwerk D, Rousseau H, et al. Results of a European multicentre iliac stent trial with a flexible balloon expandable stent. *Eur J Vasc Endovasc Surg.* 2002;24:511–515.
20. Murphy TP, Ariaratnam NS, Carney WI Jr, et al. Aortoiliac insufficiency: long-term experience with stent placement for treatment. *Radiology.* 2004;231:243–249.
21. Klein WM, van der Graaf Y, Seegers J, et al. Long-term cardiovascular morbidity, mortality, and reintervention after endovascular treatment in patients with iliac artery disease: the Dutch Iliac Stent Trial Study. *Radiology.* 2004;232:491–498.
22. Timaran CH, Prault TL, Stevens SL, et al. Iliac artery stenting versus surgical reconstruction for TASC (TransAtlantic Inter-Society Consensus) type B and type C iliac lesions. *J Vasc Surg.* 2003;38:272–278.
23. Johnston KW. Iliac arteries: reanalysis of results of balloon angioplasty. *Radiology.* 1993;186:207–212.
24. Reyes R, Maynar M, Lopera J, et al. Treatment of chronic iliac artery occlusions with guide wire recanalization and primary stent placement. *J Vasc Interv Radiol.* 1997;8:1049–1055.
25. Scheinert D, Schroder M, Balzer JO, et al. Stent-supported reconstruction of the aortoiliac bifurcation with the kissing balloon technique. *Circulation.* 1999;100(19 suppl):II295–II300.
26. Greiner A, Dessl A, Klein-Weigel P, et al. Kissing stents for treatment of complex aortoiliac disease. *Eur J Vasc Endovasc Surg.* 2003;26:161–165.
27. Mouanoutoua M, Maddikunta R, Allaqaband S, et al. Endovascular intervention of aortoiliac occlusive disease in high-risk patients using the kissing stents technique: long-term results. *Catheter Cardiovasc Interv.* 2003;60:320–326.
28. Jernigan WR, Fallat ME, Hatfield DR. Hypoplastic aortoiliac syndrome: an entity peculiar to women. *Surgery.* 1983;94:752–757.
29. Audet P, Therasse E, Oliva VL, et al. Infrarenal aortic stenosis: long-term clinical and hemodynamic results of percutaneous transluminal angioplasty. *Radiology.* 1998;209:357–363.
30. Therasse E, Cote G, Oliva VL, et al. Infrarenal aortic stenosis: value of stent placement after percutaneous transluminal angioplasty failure. *Radiology.* 2001;219:655–662.
31. Bhatt DL, Flather MD, Hacke W, et al. Patients with prior myocardial infarction, stroke, or symptomatic peripheral arterial disease in the CHARISMA trial. *J Am Coll Cardiol.* 2007;49:1982–1988.
32. Kannel WB, Skinner JJ Jr, Schwartz MJ, et al. Intermittent claudication. Incidence in the Framingham Study. *Circulation.* 1970;41:875–883.
33. Patti G, Colonna G, Pasceri V, et al. Randomized trial of high loading dose of clopidogrel for reduction of periprocedural myocardial infarction in patients undergoing coronary intervention: results from the ARMYDA-2 (Antiplatelet therapy for Reduction of MYocardial Damage during Angioplasty) study. *Circulation.* 2005;111:2099–2106.
34. Nikolsky E, Mehran R, Halkin A, et al. Vascular complications associated with arteriotomy closure devices in patients undergoing percutaneous coronary procedures: a meta-analysis. *J Am Coll Cardiol.* 2004;44:1200–1209.
35. Scheinert D, Schroder M, Steinkamp H, et al. Treatment of iliac artery aneurysms by percutaneous implantation of stent grafts. *Circulation.* 2000;102(19 suppl 3):III253–III258.
36. Schroeder RA, Flanagan TL, Kron IL, et al. A safe approach to the treatment of iliac artery aneurysms. Aortobifemoral bypass grafting with exclusion of the aneurysm. *Am Surg.* 1991;57:624–626.
37. Richardson JW, Greenfield LJ. Natural history and management of iliac aneurysms. *J Vasc Surg.* 1988;8:165–171.
38. Wilson SE, Wolf GL, Cross AP. Percutaneous transluminal angioplasty versus operation for peripheral arteriosclerosis. Report of a prospective randomized trial in a selected group of patients. *J Vasc Surg.* 1989;9:1–9.
39. Holm J, Arfvidsson B, Jivegard L, et al. Chronic lower limb ischaemia. A prospective randomised controlled study comparing the 1-year results of vascular surgery and percutaneous transluminal angioplasty (PTA). *Eur J Vasc Surg.* 1991;5:517–522.
40. Mukherjee D, Inahara T. Endarterectomy as the procedure of choice for atherosclerotic occlusive lesions of the common femoral artery. *Am J Surg.* 1989;157:498–500.
41. Springhorn ME, Kinney M, Littooy FN, et al. Inflow atherosclerotic disease localized to the common femoral artery: treatment and outcome. *Ann Vasc Surg.* 1991;5:234–240.
42. Silva JA, White CJ, Quintana H, et al. Percutaneous revascularization of the common femoral artery for limb ischemia. *Catheter Cardiovasc Interv.* 2004;62:230–233.

CHAPTER 16

Endovascular Therapy for Femoropopliteal Artery Disease

Ivan P. Casserly and Jeffrey A. Goldstein

The femoropopliteal (FP) artery is the term used to describe the composite of the superficial femoral (SFA) and popliteal (PA) arteries. In an average adult, this artery measures approximately 50 cm in length. Atherosclerosis of the FP artery is characterized by diffuse involvement, a high incidence of progression to occlusion, a propensity for superimposed calcification, and a large plaque burden (1,2). In addition, the FP artery is flanked by two major flexion points at the hip, proximally, and knee joint, distally and courses through the muscular portion of the thigh (i.e., adductor canal). As a result, the FP artery is subject to significant torsion, bending, and both axial and longitudinal compression forces that produce significant conformational change in the vessel. These factors present a significant challenge for endovascular therapies in this artery.

Despite these challenges, there has been a dramatic increase in percutaneous revascularization procedures in the FP artery. In the period from 1996 to 2006, there has been a rise in FP interventions from 69 to 184 per 100,000 Medicare beneficiaries (Fig. 16.1) (3). This represents nearly 55% of all lower extremity endovascular interventions, demonstrating the frequency of involvement of this artery in patients with peripheral artery disease (PAD). The major driving force behind the increased numbers of FP intervention is the increasing array of interventional tools that allow safe and successful treatment of increasingly complex disease anatomies. It is interesting that the rise in the overall number of FP procedures is paralleled by the increased use of atherectomy (i.e., a term used to describe a group of technologies that allow either ablation or removal of plaque (see Chapter 8). However, continued development of newer generations of bare-metal and covered self-expanding stents together with refinements in technique have also made a significant contribution toward the growth in FP interventional volume.

This chapter provides an overview of the approach to the interventional management of FP disease, including a description of the most commonly used technologies, and a summary of the outcomes following FP intervention.

ANATOMIC CONSIDERATIONS

The SFA represents the direct continuation of the common femoral artery (CFA) following the origin of the profunda femoral branch (PFA) in the femoral triangle (Figs. 16.2 and 16.3). This transition from CFA to SFA usually occurs at the level of the inferior margin of the femoral head. At its origin, the SFA lies medial, and anterior, to the PFA. Proximally, it courses through the femoral triangle to reach the adductor canal. In the adductor canal, the SFA is surrounded by the muscles of the thigh: the adductor longus and magnus muscles, posteriorly, the sartorius muscle, anteriorly, and the vastus medialis muscle, medially. The SFA exits the adductor canal through the tendinous opening in the adductor magnus muscle (i.e., adductor hiatus) to reach the popliteal fossa, located in the distal portion of the posterior surface of the femur. At this point, the SFA changes its name to the popliteal artery. The popliteal artery initially runs in the popliteal fossa posterior to the distal third of the femur (Fig. 16.3), and subsequently along the posterior surface of the tibial plateau. It typically terminates by bifurcating into the anterior tibial artery and tibioperoneal trunk.

One of the distinguishing features of the SFA is the absence of significant branches throughout its course. This explains the constant diameter of this vessel, typically about 5 to 7 mm. A number of small, muscular branches may be seen, and prominent collateral branches are seen in the presence of stenotic or occlusive disease of the SFA. The only named branch of the SFA is the descending genicular branch, which usually arises in the region of the adductor canal, and contributes to the collateral circulation at the knee.

The popliteal artery provides articular branches to the capsule and ligaments of the knee joint, and genicular/sural branches that supply the calf muscles. These genicular branches are important sources of collaterals to the tibial vessels in the presence of significant PA and/or tibial artery disease.

A brief description of the anatomy of the PFA is also pertinent in a discussion of FP intervention, since it makes an important contribution to collateral flow in the presence of FP disease, and also impacts decision-making during intervention to the ostium of the SFA. The PFA arises from the lateral aspect of the CFA and runs posteriorly, and laterally, to the SFA. It gives off two major branches, proximally, the medial and lateral-circumflex femoral branches. One or both of these branches may occasionally (i.e., about 15% to 20%) arise directly from the CFA. In its mid portion and distal portion, the PFA typically gives off three or four perforating branches to the muscles of the thigh. Proximally, the medial and lateral-circumflex branches and the first perforating branch have connections with branches of the internal iliac artery (i.e., superior and inferior gluteal, and obturator branches). Distally, the lateral circumflex artery and the perforating branches have important connections with the collateral network at the knee joint, which connect with the popliteal and tibial vessels. Through these proximal and distal connections,

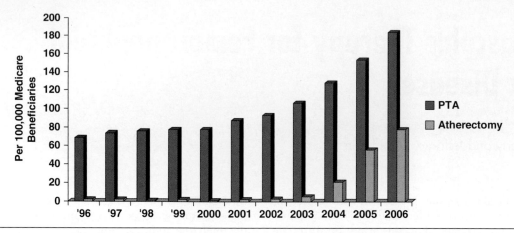

Figure 16.1 • Trends in frequency of femoropopliteal artery intervention among Medicare beneficiaries between 1996 and 2006. (Modified from Goodney PP, Beck AW, Nagle J, et al. National trends in lower extremity bypass surgery, endovascular interventions, and major amputations. *J Vasc Surg.* 2009;50:54–60).

the PFA provides an important source of collateral flow to the leg and foot in patients with significant FP disease.

NONINVASIVE EVALUATION

All details regarding the noninvasive evaluation of patients with lower extremity ischemia are outlined in Chapters 2, 3, and 4.

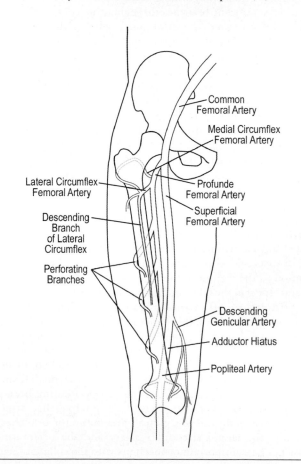

Figure 16.2 • Schematic illustration of anatomy of femoropopliteal artery (right leg).

CLASSIFICATION OF FEMOROPOPLITEAL ARTERY ATHEROSCLEROTIC DISEASE

The TransAtlantic Inter-Society Consensus (TASC II) has classified FP disease into four types (i.e., A to D) based on lesion length, the number of lesions, and the presence of stenosis or occlusion (Fig. 16.4) (4).

This classification has been developed in an attempt to reach consensus regarding the optimal approaches to the revascularization of various lesions, and is useful when performing and comparing investigational studies of FP intervention.

INDICATIONS

Revascularization of the FP artery has traditionally been reserved for only a subset of patients with symptomatic disease, including those with severe lifestyle-limiting claudication, ischemic resting pain, or ischemic tissue loss (4). These indications reflect the approach adopted by vascular surgeons who appropriately balanced the high risk of surgical revascularization in a population with significant comorbidities, with the potential benefit to the patient. For example, the operative mortality rate for femoropopliteal bypass ranged from 1.3% to 6%, with a perioperative risk of myocardial infarction of 1.9% to 3.4%, and a wound complication rate of 10% to 30%. The conservative approach to surgical revascularization was also supported by the recognition that 75% of patients with symptomatic peripheral vascular disease experience stabilization or improvement of their symptoms, and that conservative measures such as exercise therapy, pharmacologic therapy, and risk factor modification may provide significant improvements in walking distances and symptoms.

With the advent of endovascular techniques, the safety of FP artery revascularization even in high-risk patients was dramatically transformed, with a major complication rate with the endovascular approach of less than 1%. This has led to a major shift toward percutaneous revascularization as the therapy of choice for the indications outlined above. The superior safety of the endovascular approach has overridden the continued controversy regarding the long-term efficacy of endovascular versus surgical revascularization.

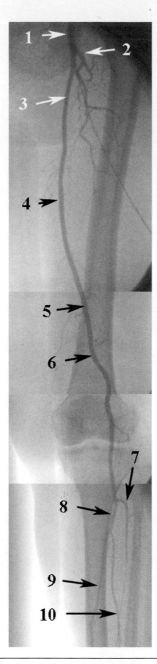

Figure 16.3 • Angiogram of left lower extremity.
(1) Common femoral artery. *(2)* Profunda femoral artery. *(3)* Superficial femoral artery in femoral triangle. *(4)* Superficial femoral artery in adductor canal. *(5)* Adductor hiatus. *(6)* Popliteal artery. *(7)* Anterior tibial artery. *(8)* Tibioperoneal trunk. *(9)* Posterior tibial artery. *(10)* Peroneal artery.

Understandably, the shift in the risk-versus-benefit ratio provided by percutaneous revascularization of the FP artery has resulted in a broader population of patients, with less severe symptomatic disease, being treated. This practice is supported by nonrandomized data from this population showing that revascularization is associated with improved functional capacity, leg symptoms, and quality of life compared with medical therapy (5). However, randomized data would provide more reassuring evidence of the appropriateness of the

broader application of FP intervention in patients with less severely symptomatic disease.

FEMOROPOPLITEAL ARTERY INTERVENTION

Diagnostic Angiography

Quality angiography of the lower extremity is an important component of the evaluation of patients with suspected FP disease. Assessment of the inflow and outflow from the FP artery determines the suitability of the patient for FP intervention and the most appropriate interventional strategy. With modern noninvasive angiographic techniques (i.e., Duplex ultrasound, computed tomography [CT], or magnetic resonance [MR] angiography), invasive angiography is no longer required to make this assessment.

If these noninvasive techniques are not available, or are suboptimal, invasive angiography remains essential. For diagnostic studies, the most common access site chosen is the CFA contralateral to the leg with the worst symptoms (i.e., assuming symptoms are bilateral and asymmetric), since this allows for a subsequent attempt at endovascular revascularization at the same sitting if an intervention is required. A pigtail catheter is advanced over a wire and placed in the distal abdominal aorta, and a static pelvic angiogram (in ipsilateral and contralateral oblique views) spanning the aortic bifurcation to the CFA is performed (i.e., power injector settings: 15 mL/sec for a total of 30 mL). If the CFA bifurcation is not clearly visualized, ipsilateral oblique views are usually helpful in displaying the origins of the SFA and PFA.

At this point, visualization of the infrainguinal arteries may be performed using one of the two methods: (1) sequential static overlapping digital subtraction angiography (DSA) at multiple levels. The authors prefer this method and perform it by placing a multiple side-holed diagnostic catheter (e.g., straight flush) in the ipsilateral (i.e., lower extremity of interest) external iliac artery (EIA) or CFA from the contralateral CFA access. Ipsilateral oblique imaging of the lower extremity is then performed (3 to 4 cc/sec for total of 9 to 12 cc/sec). If the other limb needs to be imaged, selective angiography through the side arm of the CFA sheath is performed using the same method; and (2) the bolus-chase technique. With this technique, a contrast bolus is injected and continually imaged as it progresses distally. Both limbs may be visualized with a pigtail catheter placed in the distal abdominal aorta (i.e., power injector settings: 15 mL/sec for a total of 90 mL), or an individual limb may be visualized with a multiple side-holed, straight flush catheter in the ipsilateral EIA or CFA (i.e., power injector settings: 15 mL/sec for a total of 45 mL). A 15″ image intensifier (minimum) is required for visualization of both lower extremities. With smaller image intensifiers, each leg must be visualized separately.

With modern imaging systems, the need for a central wedge placed between the legs and lateral wedges placed lateral to each leg is rare. Placing either a rigid radiopaque ruler or flexible radiopaque tape in the field of view during diagnostic angiography of the lower extremities provides a useful landmark for the analysis of lesion lengths and positioning of equipment during endovascular procedures and is strongly recommended.

Type A Lesions
- Single stenosis ≤ 10 cm in length
- Single occlusion ≤ 5 cm in length

Type B Lesions
- Multiple lesions (stenoses or occlusions), each ≤ 5 cm
- Single stenosis or occlusion ≤ 15 cm not involving the infrageniculate popliteal artery
- Single or multiple lesions in the absence of continuous tibial vessels to improve inflow for distal bypass
- Heavily calcified occlusion ≤ 5 cm in length
- Single popliteal stenosis

Type C Lesions
- Multiple stenosis or occlusions totaling > 15 cm with or without heavy calcification
- Recurrent stenoses or occlusions that need treatment after two endovascular interventions

Type D Lesions
- Chronic total occlusions of CFA or SFA (> 20 cm, involving the popliteal artery)
- Chronic total occlucion of popliteal artery and proximal trifurcation vessels

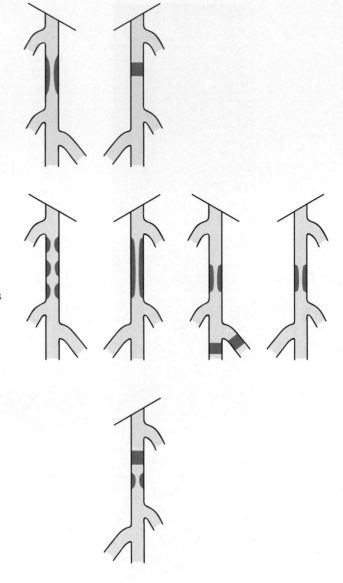

Figure 16.4 • TASC II classification of femoropopliteal artery disease. (Adapted from Norgren L, Hiatt WR, Dormandy JA, et al. on behalf of the TASC II Working Group. Inter-Society Consensus for the Management of Peripheral Arterial Disease (TASC II). *J Vasc Surg* 2007;45:S5–S67.)

Pharmacology

The adjunctive pharmacologic therapies administered during FP artery intervention are similar to those used in most other peripheral vascular procedures. In clinical practice, patients receive aspirin preprocedurally. Unfractionated heparin is the anticoagulant of choice, with a target activated clotting time (ACT) of approximately 250 seconds. In complex FP intervention involving the treatment of long occlusive disease, the authors often aim for an ACT of 250 to 300 seconds. Low molecular-weight heparins or direct thrombin-inhibitors may be used in specific circumstances, but there are no data to support their routine use. Most operators reserve glycoprotein (GP) IIb/IIIa inhibitors for cases complicated by thrombosis.

Access for Intervention

The success and ease with which any endovascular procedure may be performed rely on the platform constructed to perform the procedure (Fig. 16.5). This begins with the choice of arterial access (Table 16.1).

CONTRALATERAL CFA RETROGRADE ACCESS

When approaching an FP lesion, the most commonly chosen and technically simple access is the contralateral CFA, approached in a retrograde manner (Fig. 16.6). The modified Seldinger technique is used to gain access in the contralateral CFA.

A catheter (e.g., IM, Sos, Simmons) is then advanced over a wire into the distal aorta and used to selectively engage the ostium of the contralateral common iliac artery. A stiff-angled glidewire is then advanced with care into the CFA, and the diagnostic catheter is then advanced over the wire into the CFA. The glidewire is then exchanged for a supportive guidewire (e.g., SupraCore, Superstiff Amplatz wire with 1 cm soft tip). The catheter and short femoral sheath are then

removed over the stiff wire, and a long kink-resistant sheath approximately 40 to 50 cm in length (e.g., Balkin Contralateral, Pinnacle Destination, Ansel, Raabe) is advanced into the contralateral CFA. The sheath should always be advanced in combination with the dilator, to avoid trauma to the iliac vessels.

IPSILATERAL CFA ANTEGRADE ACCESS

An antegrade, ipsilateral CFA access may be desirable in patients with specific anatomic issues involving the iliac arteries, including: severe tortuosity or disease in either iliac, or acute angulation of the native or reconstructed (i.e., surgical [e.g., aortobifemoral bypass]) or percutaneous (e.g., kissing stenting) aortoiliac bifurcation (Fig. 16.7).

Although antegrade access provides improved back-up support, compared with the contralateral CFA approach, it is uncommon for this to be a significant issue during FP intervention. In patients with ostial or proximal SFA disease, the antegrade approach may be contraindicated, owing to insufficient room in the CFA to allow a sufficient length of sheath for stable sheath placement (Fig. 16.8).

Particular caution should be exercised in using the antegrade CFA approach in obese patients, and this approach is relatively contraindicated in the morbidly obese, owing to the increased risk of bleeding.

The technical aspects of obtaining antegrade CFA access are outlined in Chapter 6.

IPSILATERAL POPLITEAL RETROGRADE ACCESS

The ipsilateral popliteal retrograde approach is rarely used for FP artery intervention. However, in situations in which both the contralateral CFA and ipsilateral CFA approaches are contraindicated (e.g., severe iliac tortuosity and ostial/

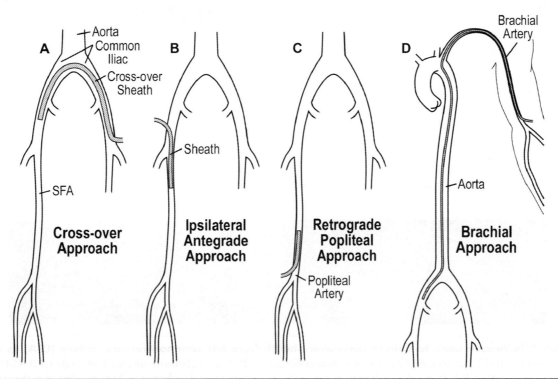

Figure 16.5 • Illustration of array of access-site strategies for femoropopliteal artery intervention.

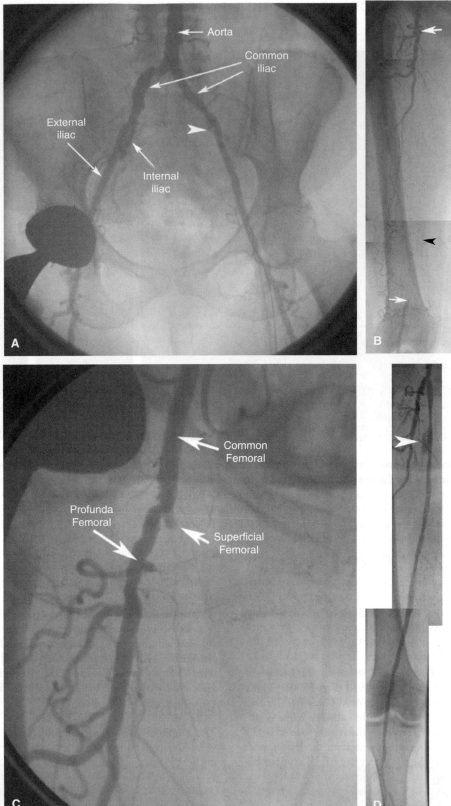

Figure 16.8 • Treatment of complicated right superficial femoral artery (SFA) occlusion.   A: Pelvic angiogram showing benign aortic bifurcation and iliac vessels allowing contralateral access and cross-over technique. B: Angiogram of SFA showing long occlusion of the right SFA extending from the origin to the mid-popliteal artery *(arrows)*. Note the previously placed stent in the distal SFA *(arrowhead)*. The extension of the occlusion into the mid-popliteal artery makes access to the true lumen just distal to the occlusion critical. C: RAO oblique view of the common femoral artery (CFA) bifurcation clearly delineating the stump of the SFA. Access was obtained in the left CFA, and a cross-over sheath was placed in the right CFA. The occlusion was crossed with a stiff-angled glidewire dissected through the subintimal place. Access to the true lumen distally was obtained using the Pioneer catheter. Angioplasty of the occlusion was performed using a 6.0 mm × 10-mm balloon, and the entire occlusion sequentially stented using 7.0 mm diameter nitinol self-expanding stents. The stents were postdilated with the 6.0 mm diameter balloon. D: Angiogram following angioplasty and stenting shows minor perforation in the proximal SFA that was treated by prolonged balloon inflation and reversal of anticoagulation.

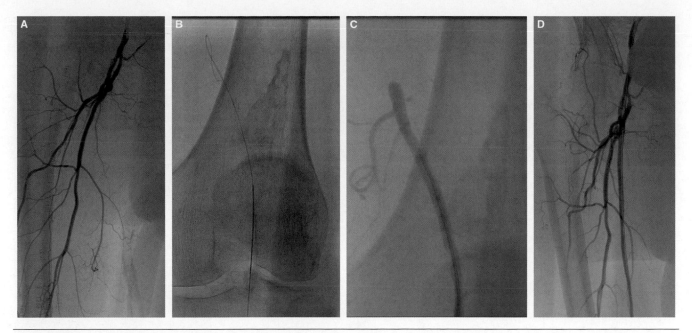

Figure 16.9 • Flush occlusion of right superficial femoral artery (**A**) requiring retrograde popliteal artery access (**B,C**) to achieve successful revascularization (**D**).

commonly seen, but are not usually flow-limiting. DSA tends to underestimate the severity of dissection, which emphasizes the importance of carefully examining the unsubtracted fluoroscopic images. Evaluating the lesion for the presence of a hemodynamically significant gradient is a crucial part of evaluating the lesion after angioplasty. Regardless of the angiographic appearance, if the lesion is not associated with a residual gradient (assessed using a 4-Fr. endhole catheter or pressure wire (e.g., FloWire, Volcano or PressureWire, St Jude—formerly RADI medical system)), consideration should be given to accepting the angioplasty alone result. For focal disease, angioplasty usually provides a reasonable acute

result that is durable. However, for diffuse disease, angioplasty is often associated with a significant residual gradient across the length of the diseased segment, and long-term durability is extremely poor.

STENTING—BARE NITINOL SELF-EXPANDING STENTS

There remains considerable controversy regarding the utility of adjunctive stenting in the FP artery. The initial experience with balloon-expandable Palmaz stents and the stainless steel Wallstent was disappointing (see "FP Artery Intervention – Clinical Efficacy Outcomes"). This led to the development and application of nitinol self-expanding stents in this

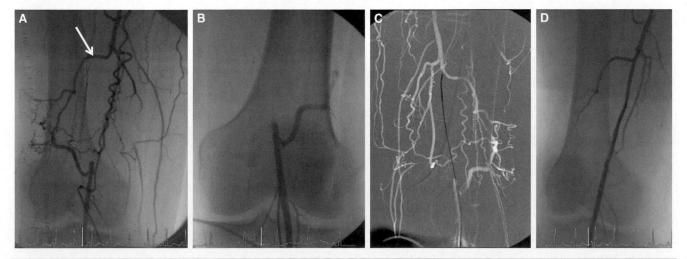

Figure 16.10 • **A:** Occlusion of distal superficial femoral artery with the absence of proximal stump and presence of large collateral *(arrow)* preventing antegrade approach to recanalization. **B:** Retrograde popliteal artery access was obtained. **C:** The lesion was crossed in a retrograde fashion with a glidewire supported by an angled glide catheter. **D:** Revascularization was achieved from the antegrade approach using a Silverhawk LX-M device and balloon angioplasty (5 mm × 10 cm balloon).

Figure 16.11 • Treatment of a superficial femoral artery stenosis. **A:** Angiogram of the left superficial femoral artery shows a focal severe lesion in the mid-portion of the vessel *(arrowhead)*, with moderate diffuse disease proximal and distal to the lesion. The focal lesion was dilated with a 4.0 × 40-mm balloon, and the treatment site stented with a 7.0 × 100-mm nitinol self-expanding stent that was postdilated with a 5.0 × 80-mm balloon. **B:** Final angiogram of the treatment site following intervention.

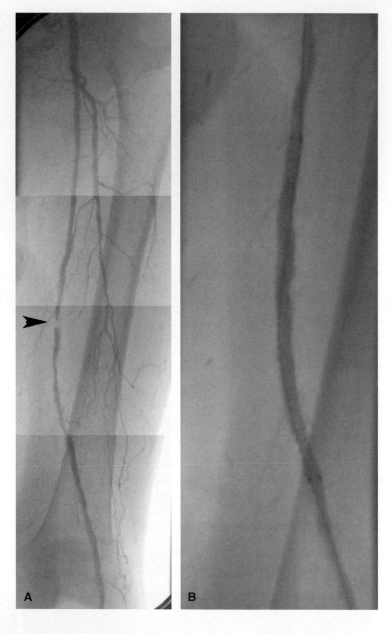

location. There is no doubt that current generation nitinol self-expanding stents are remarkably safe and easy to use, and provide a very predictable and effective acute angiographic result compared with angioplasty, particularly for longer and more complex lesions. The major limitation of stents is the poor long-term patency associated with stenting (see "FP Artery Intervention – Clinical Efficacy Outcomes"). Despite this, four randomized trials comparing current generation nitinol self-expanding stents with angioplasty appear to demonstrate a significant benefit for stenting over angioplasty in the treatment of intermediate length lesions (5 to 10 cm) (6–9) (Fig. 16.12). Unfortunately, these studies are relatively limited in the duration of follow-up (i.e., 12 to 24 months), and there appears to be continued decline in patency rates of stents out to 4 to 5 years where patency rates may drop to 40%. Longer lesions have not been studied in a randomized controlled trial, and it is felt that stenting does not provide a significant benefit over angioplasty in shorter lesions (i.e., <5 cm). Perhaps more problematic than

the high rates of restenosis associated with stenting is the lack of an effective treatment for in-stent restenosis. Recurrence rates of over 70%, regardless of the treatment modality, have been reported (10).

These data have important implications for the clinical indication for using stents in the treatment of FP disease. Clearly, where angioplasty or other interventional technique does not provide an adequate acute result (i.e., residual gradient, flow-limiting dissection, abrupt closure, severe residual stenosis), then stenting is appropriate. In younger patients with claudication, the implications of the high rate of restenosis and need for repeated intervention need to be discussed prior to treatment. In patients with critical limb ischemia, stenting is a reasonable strategy as stenting provides a very reliable and effective hemodynamic result in the initial 6 to 9 months, which is typically sufficient to allow complete wound healing. Since the amount of blood flow required to maintain tissue integrity is exponentially less than that required to heal a wound,

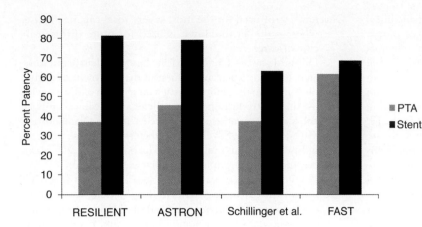

Figure 16.12 • Primary patency rates at 12 months (by Duplex ultrasound) in the four currently published trials of balloon angioplasty versus bare-metal nitinol self-expanding stents in the treatment of femoropopliteal artery disease.

restenosis in this circumstance is often asymptomatic. The exception is the patient who presents with ischemic rest pain, where restenosis is more likely to be symptomatic.

There are a wide variety of bare-metal nitinol self-expanding stents currently used during FP intervention. Only two are FDA approved for this indication—the IntraCoil and Life Stent. The former is rarely used in current practice. Other self-expanding stents used in FP intervention are used off-label. All of these stents are delivered over 0.035″ wires, but may be delivered over supportive 0.014″ wires (provided the anatomy of disease permits). The most common stent diameters used in the FP location range from 5 to 7 mm. In this regard, males generally have significantly larger FP diameters compared with females. Stent diameters are chosen to be at least 1 mm larger than the reference vessel diameter. Since lesion lengths are often long, stent lengths are typically long (up to 150–200 mm). It is generally believed that using a single long stent is preferable to using overlapping stents. Although some operators perform primary stenting (i.e., no predilatation) in the FP artery, the authors routinely perform predilatation prior to stenting. Stents are postdilated with a balloon sized to the reference vessel diameter. If in doubt, the authors would recommend a conservative approach to postdilatation balloon sizing, as these stents continue to exert significant outward force over time. Many stents that acutely appear to be inadequately expanded appear perfectly cylindrical in follow-up. Achieving sufficient postdilatation to remove any pressure gradient with brisk antegrade flow should be the desired endpoint. Overaggressive postdilatation does increase the risk for perforation, which should be avoided at all costs.

Most operators have a preference for a particular bare-metal nitinol self-expanding stent that they use in the FP artery. Having multiple different stent types available is not practical in most laboratories. However, in the authors' opinion, having one stent that has high radial strength (e.g., SMART, Cordis) and another that is highly flexible (e.g., LifeStent, Bard) makes some sense. High radial strength is needed for the treatment of heavily calcified disease, and highly flexible stents are useful when stenting the distal SFA and popliteal artery that appears to be subject to greater physical forces than the proximal/mid-SFA.

STENTING—COVERED SELF-EXPANDING STENTS

The high rates of restenosis associated with bare-metal nitinol self-expanding stents in the FP artery have spurred interest in the use of covered self-expanding stents (see Chapter 7) in this location. In theory, the material covering these stents should prevent the ingrowth of neointima, which is the mechanism of failure for bare-metal nitinol self-expanding stents. This has been borne out in clinical practice, with the main mechanism of failure for covered stents being the development of edge restenosis at the stent margins. Since the Viabahn stent is the covered self-expanding stent with FDA approval in this location, the remaining discussion will relate to this stent only. A randomized comparison of the Viabahn stent versus femoropopliteal bypass using prosthetic conduit showing reasonable patency data at 2-year follow-up that was equivalent to the surgical group (11,12) together with a series of observational studies has lent some credibility to this strategy (13,14).

There are a number of very important practical issues when using these covered self-expanding stents in the treatment of FP disease. Case selection is of the utmost importance and largely relates to the risk of stent thrombosis. There should be adequate run-off distal to the treated segment. A minimum of straight-line flow in one tibial vessel is required. In addition, the proximal and distal margins of the stent should be placed in relatively nondiseased segments. This often results in stenting to the level of the ostium of the SFA, and the use of multiple overlapping stents. Use in FP segments of less than 4 mm diameter is not recommended, and ideally the vessel diameter should be ≥5 mm. Lesions that are noncompliant and that do not respond to predilation or other treatment strategy (e.g., atherectomy—see below) should not be treated. The result of these restrictions is that the spectrum of disease that may be treated with these stents is limited. Finally, patients who are unable to tolerate dual antiplatelet therapy (with aspirin and clopidogrel) for at least 3 months following the procedure should not be treated using these stents.

One of the major drawbacks of covered stenting in the FP artery is that important collateral channels adjacent to the diseased segment of the FP artery are occluded during stent deployment. In the proximal and mid-SFA, this is not usually of a major concern, as there is an adequate length of remaining SFA and popliteal artery to provide connection with collaterals from the profunda femoral artery in the event of stent failure. However, as one moves more distally in the SFA and particularly in the PA, this is of particular concern. If the covered stent fails, the loss of these collateral communications may increase the chance that the patient may present with a more severe degree of chronic limb ischemia than the initial clinical presentation. In addition, acute thrombosis of the covered stent may result in a clinical presentation with acute limb ischemia, although preliminary data from the recent VIBRANT trial suggested that presentation with acute limb ischemia from stent failure with the Viabahn stent is no more frequent than with stent failure using a bare-metal nitinol self-expanding stent. In summary, the decision to use a covered stent in the FP artery requires a careful assessment of the patient and disease anatomy with a thorough understanding of the implications of treatment.

From a practical standpoint, the Viabahn stent should always be delivered over a stiff-bodied 0.035″ wire (e.g., SupraCore, Stiff Amplatz wire). The choice of stent diameter is much more critical with the Viabahn stent compared with bare-metal nitinol self-expanding stents, which can be generously oversized with little consequence. The Viabahn stent diameter should never be more than 1 mm larger than the reference diameter. Oversizing of the Viabahn stent can result in the creation of folds in the stent lining, which is felt to increase the risk of stent thrombosis. Some operators use intravascular ultrasound (IVUS) to accurately measure the lumen diameter and avoid errors in this assessment. Given the need to cover from relatively normal segment proximally to normal segment distally, the stent length chosen should be adequate to meet this requirement. Following careful positioning of the stent, the stent delivery system is immobilized by having an assistant hold the system near the entrance to the access sheath and the primary operator holds the system near the hub of the stent. Deployment by pulling on the string from the side arm at the hub of the stent should be slow. If these maneuvers are implemented, the stent will remain very stable, and very accurate stent placement is possible. It is important to be aware that once the stent is seen to deploy, it cannot be repositioned. The stent does not foreshorten like bare-metal self-expanding stents, a feature that is very helpful when treating ostial SFA disease. Postdilation is recommended using a noncompliant balloon that is sized to the reference vessel diameter.

ATHERECTOMY

The range of plaque removal and plaque ablation devices used in the treatment of infrainguinal disease is described in detail in Chapter 8. Only a brief comment related to their use in the FP artery is provided here.

Few technologies have engendered such polar opinions in the peripheral space as atherectomy devices. However, there is no doubt in the authors' minds that these devices allow for the treatment of a broader range of disease anatomies in the FP artery than is possible using conventional balloon and stent technologies and reduce the need for stenting to achieve an acceptable angiographic and hemodyamic result (15).

The specific disease subsets in which these technologies are useful in the FP artery include:

1. Ostial disease of the SFA—Debulking at the SFA ostium reduces the risk of plaque shift into the PFA. Given the directionality of the Silverhawk catheter, this catheter is favored for this indication.
2. Severe calcific disease—The two systems favored by the authors for this indication include the Diamondback 360° and TurboHawk catheter. The Diamondback tends to be used for the most severe focal calcific disease, whereas the TurboHawk is used for more diffuse calcific disease.
3. Diffuse disease—The Turbo Elite Laser and Jetstream® catheters have particular application in the treatment of diffuse disease due to the ability to treat a long length of disease with the single introduction of the catheter and the lower embolic risk with these catheters compared with the Diamondback 360° device. The Silverhawk catheters can be used to treat diffuse disease, but multiple introductions of the catheter can become time-consuming and lead to catheter failure.
4. Popliteal artery disease. Since stenting with bare-metal nitinol self-expanding stents in this location is contraindicated, any of the plaque removal or ablation devices that can achieve a successful angiographic and hemodynamic result in this location without the need for a stent represent an important advance over angioplasty alone.

There are no randomized comparative studies of atherectomy versus conventional balloon/stent treatments in the FP artery. It is widely believed that long-term restenosis rates with these technologies are unlikely to differ significantly from angioplasty or stenting. These technologies do have complications associated with their use (see "Complications of FP artery intervention"). In particular, the risk of distal embolization needs to be acknowledged. The authors have a very low threshold for using distal embolic protection with these devices using the characteristics of the lesion (e.g., length of disease, presence of thrombus), the quality of the distal runoff, and the clinical indication for the procedure (i.e., claudication vs. critical limb ischemia) to help stratify those patients at greatest risk from embolization. In the authors' experience, there is often evidence of embolization following the use of atherectomy devices (evidenced by filling defects in the filter) that is further exacerbated following angioplasty (± stenting), sometimes to the point of having no flow in the vessel. In such situations, the authors are careful to only partially collapse the filter, ensnaring only the proximal loop of the filter within the recovery sheath, followed by removal of the filter. The intention is to try to prevent loss of embolic material into the distal circulation during filter retrieval.

When EPDs are used, the authors prefer to use either the Emboshield® Nav[6] (Abbott Vascular) or Spider (ev3) filters. The Emboshield® Nav[6] filter can be used with its own BareWire or with the 0.023″ Viper wire (with the 0.023″ distal tip serving as the brake for the filter). This makes it the ideal filter for use with the Diamondback 360° device. Either filter can be used with the remaining atherectomy devices.

TREATMENT OF OCCLUSIONS

Occlusions of the FP artery represent a significantly greater technical challenge compared with stenoses. These occlusions are typically very long, beginning in the proximal third of the SFA and extending to the level of the adductor hiatus and sometimes beyond into the PA (Fig. 16.13). In crossing these occlusions, there are three tasks that need to be accomplished:

1. *Break through the proximal cap*: In most circumstances, the proximal cap is easily breached using a straight-tipped stiff-bodied glidewire supported by a 4 or 5 Fr. angled glide catheter. If the occlusion extends beyond the distal SFA, it is important to use a 125 cm length glide catheter to facilitate wire exchanges. Our practice is to engage the

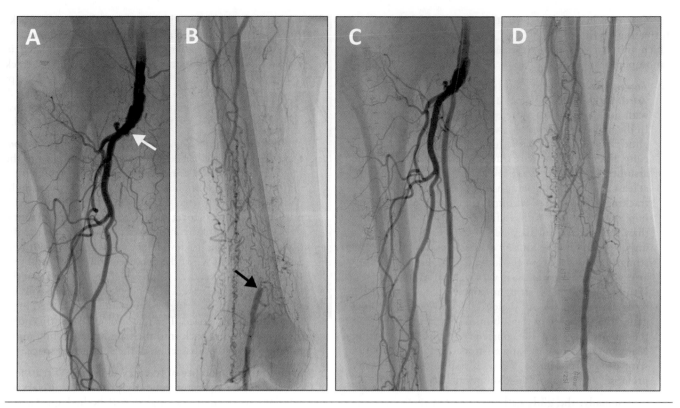

Figure 16.13 • Femoropopliteal (FP) artery occlusion. **A,B:** Baseline angiogram showing long occlusion extending from the origin of the superficial femoral artery *(white arrow)* to the above-knee popliteal artery *(black arrow)*. **C,D:** Angiography following placement of overlapping bare-metal nitinol stents in the FP artery.

proximal stump directly with the angled glide catheter, and then tap the proximal stump with the straight-tipped-stiff-bodied glidewire. Once the proximal cap is breached, the glide catheter is advanced over the glide-wire into the proximal segment of the occlusion to establish the channel for recanalization.

Where this technique fails, there are a couple of options available. One option is to build a better support for the glide-wire/glide catheter combination. This is done by minimizing the distance between the cross-over sheath and the proximal stump, and if needed, telescoping a 6 Fr. guide catheter (usually a multipurpose) through the cross-over sheath into the proximal stump to add a further layer of support (Fig. 16.14).

The second option is to attempt to disrupt the proximal cap using the Frontrunner catheter (Cordis) supported by its dedicated Microglide catheter. This is a blunt dissection tool that is embedded into the proximal cap with the jaws in the closed position. Applying forward pressure to the Frontrunner catheter and the supporting Microglide catheter, the jaws are then opened with the goal of disrupting the cap. This process may have to be repeated several times until the cap is breached. It is helpful to put a curve on the Microglide catheter, so that the Frontrunner catheter can be maneuvered to engage different locations in the proximal cap to achieve the initial breach. In the authors' experience, the Frontrunner catheter is a very useful tool in the most complex cases, but is not required for routine use. In addition, the catheter tends to find the subintimal space quickly, and hence the operator should be prepared to perform subintimal recanalization of the occlusion if this device is required.

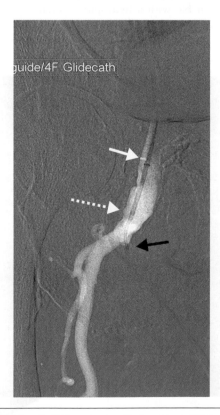

Figure 16.14 • Building support for femoropopliteal artery intervention. Three layers of support for glidewire provided by glide catheter in the proximal stump of the occlusion *(black arrow)*, multipurpose guide *(dashed arrow)*, and cross-over sheath *(solid white arrow)*.

hollow curved 22-guage nitinol needle that is activated by a control knob at the proximal end of the catheter (Fig. 16.17). Similar to the method described above for the Pioneer catheter, the Outback catheter (with the needle in the retracted position) is tracked over a 0.014″ wire whose tip is in the subintimal space adjacent to the true lumen, just inferior to the distal margin of the occlusion. Using radiopaque markers located in the tip of the catheter distal to the point where the needle is deployed, the catheter is oriented with respect to the adjacent true lumen as follows: the view in which the catheter tip lies adjacent to

the true lumen is determined. In this view, the catheter it rotated to achieve an "**L**" shape by the radiopaque markers at the catheter tip (Fig. 16.18). An orthogonal view is then acquired in which the catheter is overlies the true lumen, where a "**T**" shape by the radiopaque markers at the catheter tip should be seen (Fig. 16.18). The view in which the "**L**" shape at the catheter tip is seen is then used to **D**eploy the needle (this technique is referred to as the LTD technique). A new 0.014″ wire is then advanced from the hub of the catheter and exits the nitinol needle into the true lumen. The needle is then withdrawn, the catheter

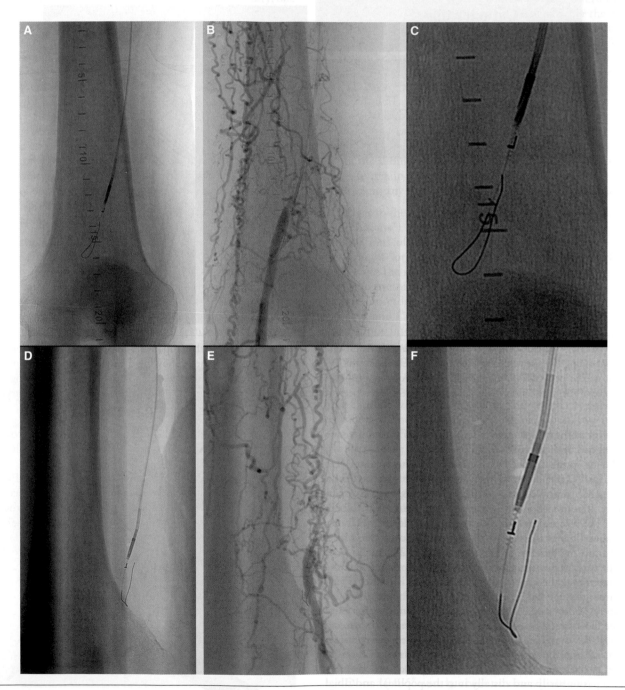

Figure 16.18 • Use of LTD technique to align needle of Outback catheter with true lumen of reconstituted vessel distal to femoropopliteal occlusion (same case as Fig. 16.13). A–B: Low magnification images with and without contrast showing Outback catheter adjacent to the true lumen. **C:** High magnification image showing the 'L' shape by the radiopaque markers at the catheter tip. 'L' shape at the tip of Outback catheter aligned adjacent to the true lumen. **D,E:** Low magnification images with and without contrast showing Outback catheter overlying the true lumen. **F:** High magnification image showing the 'T' shape by the radiopaque markers at the catheter tip.

removed, the 0.014″ wire exchanged for the interventional wire of choice, and the remainder of the procedure completed.

While the description of the use of these re-entry tools sounds straightforward and these devices work very well in the real-world setting, there are some challenges:

1. It is important to assess how deep one is in the subintimal plane prior to using these devices. On rare occasions, one can be too deep in the subintimal plane. When using the Pioneer catheter, this can be suspected when chromoflow in the true lumen cannot be easily seen. With the Outback catheter, the needle may not be able to reach the true lumen despite multiple attempts (Fig. 16.19). Regardless,

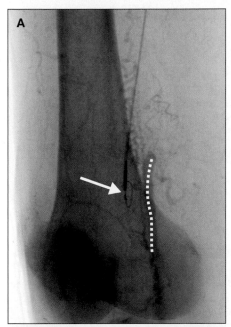

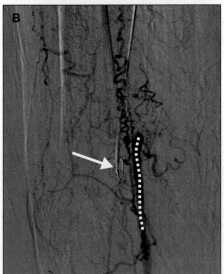

Figure 16.19 • Example of case where the Outback catheter is too deep in the subintimal space. A: Unsubtracted angiogram. B: Subtracted angiogram. Tip of Outback catheter indicated by *white arrow*, and true lumen of vessel indicated by *interrupted line*. The distance between the two is too long for the needle to penetrate into the true lumen.

it seems intuitive that the risk of perforation is increased with excessively deep subintimal recanalization, and in this circumstance, the authors would recommend that the occlusion be reinterrogated more proximally in an attempt to arrive at a location in the subintimal plane that is in closer proximity to the true lumen. Alternatively, one can bring the patient back in 2 to 3 weeks after the initial subintimal plane has healed and reattempt the subintimal recanalization.

2. When using both of these devices, it is important to apply significant forward pressure (by an assistant) during deployment of the needle, as the heavily calcified plaque through which the needle must penetrate offers significant resistance to needle penetration.

3. One of the major drawbacks of the Outback catheter is that the depth of the needle cannot be accurately controlled. If the needle is fully deployed and the wire does not advance easily into the true lumen, slowly withdraw the needle while applying gentle forward pressure to the 0.014″ wire. This will occasionally result in the wire finding the true lumen due to an excessive depth of deployment during the initial needle deployment.

4. Although the LTD technique of the Outback catheter does work in most cases, there are occasions when it is impossible to achieve a perfect L and T shape in orthogonal views. In this situation, one has to do ones best to optimize the L and T shapes, and through some trial and error, vary the rotation of the catheter to gain entry to the true lumen.

INTERVENTIONAL TREATMENT OF FP OCCLUSIONS

Once the lesion is successfully crossed, the length of the occlusion is treated using the interventional modalities outlined above (i.e., angioplasty, stenting, atherectomy). All of the comments regarding angioplasty in the setting of the treatment of FP stenoses are applicable in the treatment of FP occlusions. In addition, for long occlusions, it is best to use 150 to 220 mm long balloons (e.g., SAVVY, Cordis), in the interest of time efficiency. Careful attention should be paid to patient discomfort during subintimal angioplasty. Excessive dilation in this circumstance may result in an increased risk of vessel perforation (Fig. 16.8).

Regarding stenting in the treatment of FP occlusions, the authors will typically stent the length of the occlusion, taking care to ensure that the re-entry point is stented if subintimal recanalization has been performed.

Atherectomy should be performed with care in the treatment of FP occlusions. The authors generally favor the concentric Jetstream atherectomy and Laser ablation devices, avoid the Diamondback 360°, and use the Silverhawk catheter with caution in this situation. If a re-entry device has been used to regain entry to the true lumen, atherectomy is generally avoided, reasoning that the need for a re-entry device serves as a marker of deeper subintimal recanalization that may be associated with an increased risk for perforation with atherectomy devices.

OSTIAL SFA DISEASE

Disease at the ostium of the SFA deserves special mention. These lesions are difficult to treat because of the proximity of PFA, and its importance in the arterial supply to the thigh,

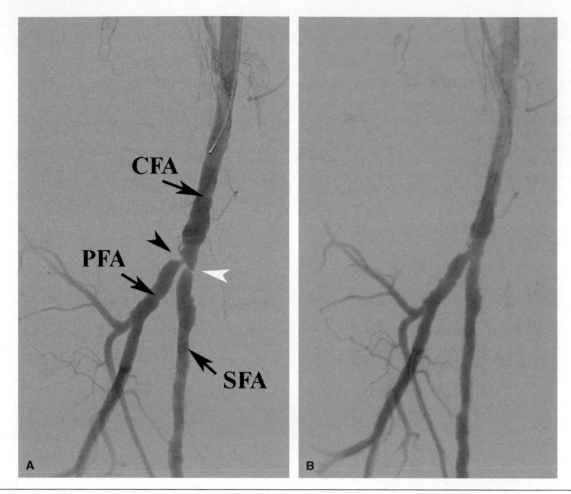

Figure 16.20 • Treatment of ostial superficial femoral artery disease. **A:** Angiogram of the right common femoral artery demonstrating critical ostial disease of the superficial and profunda femoral arteries. **B:** The ostia of both arteries were treated with the Foxhollow atherectomy catheter producing an excellent angiographic result and no compromise of the profunda ostium.

and the arterial supply to the leg and foot via collaterals when the SFA is significantly diseased. The major risk of treatment in this location is plaque shift into the ostium of the PFA that may compromise flow. In assessing the risk of plaque shift, the authors pay particular attention to the caliber of the PFA, the presence of disease at the ostium of the PFA, and the angle between the SFA and the PFA. The combination of a large caliber PFA without disease and at least a 45° between the PFA and SFA is reassuring that any interventional strategy can be applied safely. However, if one or more of these variables is not favorable, the authors have a low threshold for using a debulking strategy with an atherectomy device (Fig. 16.20).

When stenting the ostium of the SFA, most operators advocate extending the stent 1 to 2 mm above the level of the ostium of the SFA (i.e., into the distal CFA) to ensure that the ostium is covered. When deploying long bare-metal self-expanding stents, precise placement at the SFA ostium can be difficult. Where more than one stent is being used to treat the segment of disease in the SFA, one approach to this problem is to choose stent lengths such that the last stent placed is required to treat only a short length of disease at the ostium and proximal SFA (i.e., ~2 to 3 cm). Using a 40 mm length stent to treat the ostium and proximal segment will then be associated

with minimal foreshortening and more accurate placement. The Viabahn covered stent performs very well in this regard as it does not foreshorten making its use at the ostium of the SFA very attractive.

If there is significant plaque shift into the PFA following interventional therapy at the ostium of the SFA, the PFA should be wired, and prolonged low-pressure angioplasty should be performed. An acceptable result is to achieve less than 50% residual stenosis with brisk antegrade flow in the PFA.

POPLITEAL ARTERY DISEASE

The popliteal artery represents the transition between the SFA and tibial circulations. This explains the variation in approach to popliteal artery intervention. For above-knee popliteal artery disease, interventional techniques and tools largely resemble those in the SFA proper. For below-knee popliteal disease, and particularly, when this disease is continuous with tibial arteries, the interventional technique begins to resemble tibial intervention. This latter group can represent some of the more complex interventions performed. Some general principles that the authors use to approach this disease subset are as follows:

1. Stenting should generally be avoided in the popliteal artery due to the exaggerated conformational changes in this vessel with leg motion.
2. Atherectomy of the popliteal artery should be performed with particular care, due to the consequences of perforation in this location (i.e., high likelihood of compartment syndrome). This is particularly true when treating total occlusions, as one cannot be sure of the intraluminal position of the interventional wire along the length of the occlusion.
3. The need for retrograde tibial/pedal access is high when treating occlusions of the distal popliteal artery that extends into the tibial vessels. This needs to be considered carefully when treating patients with claudication, and the risk/benefit ratio of this approach needs to be considered carefully.

FP Artery Intervention—Clinical Efficacy Outcomes

The gold standard for revascularization of the SFA remains surgical bypass, using a venous or prosthetic (e.g., PTFE) graft conduit. For an above-the-knee vein graft using either type of conduit, the primary patency rates at 1 and 4 years are 81% and 70%, respectively (Table 16.2) (18). In analyses of outcomes by individual graft, there does appear to be a benefit in favor of the venous conduit (i.e., 5-year patency of 75% vs. 60%). With below-the-knee grafts, the difference is more dramatic (i.e., 5-year patency of 75% vs. 30%). Based on these data, it is generally recommended to use a venous conduit for both above- and below-the-knee femoropopliteal bypass surgery. However, the use of a venous conduit is complicated by prolonged operative times, an increased risk of wound complications, and the removal of veins that may be subsequently required for other revascularization procedures (e.g., coronary artery bypass surgery). For these reasons, many operators continue to use prosthetic conduits, particularly for above-the-knee bypass surgery, where the potential benefit of the venous conduit on long-term patency is less dramatic.

The patency data for surgical bypass serve as a useful reference for assessing the efficacy of endovascular therapies. However, it should be emphasized that in making the clinical decision to treat by surgical or percutaneous techniques, consideration of these data, together with an assessment of the potential morbidity and mortality from either procedure, should be considered.

ANGIOPLASTY

Angioplasty, alone, is associated with excellent results in patients with focal SFA disease, with patency rates at 1 and 5 years of more than 80% and 70%, respectively (19–21). With the use of hemodynamic assessments of pressure gradients across the lesion to guide optimal angioplasty, these results may be improved upon. However, angioplasty performs poorly for patients with diffuse disease and poor vessel run-off (22). Inclusion of this population of patients in a review by Dorrucci explains the overall 1- and 4-year patency rates for angioplasty of about 58% and 40%, respectively (18). In an analysis of data from published randomized trials, the 12-month primary patency rate for angioplasty of SFA lesions with a mean length of 8.7 cm was 33% (23). These data highlight the unacceptable patency rates associated with angioplasty in more complex FP disease, particularly in patients with claudication, where recurrence of symptoms represents treatment failure.

STENTING

Initial studies using balloon-expandable stents in the SFA demonstrated poor outcomes, with no benefit over angioplasty alone (24,25). These types of stents appear particularly unsuited

TABLE 16.2 Summary of Primary and Secondary Patency Rates Achieved with Various Surgical and Endovascular Interventions for the Treatment of Superficial Femoral Artery Disease

Revascularization Method	Patency Rates (%)									
	6 Months		1 Year		2 Years		3 Years		4 Years	
	1°	2°	1°	2°	1°	2°	1°	2°	1°	2°
Above-knee vein conduit	87	90	81	89	77	86	71	82	70	81
Above-knee prosthetic conduit	85	91	77	86	66	73	59	68	51	61
Covered stents*	62	79	54	75	—	—	—	—	—	—
Hemobahn endoprosthesis	81	89	74	85	73	84	64	80	—	—
Bare-metal stents[†]	81	84	65	75	55	60	55	50	37	52
Nitinol stents	93	96	85	93	—	—	—	—	—	—
Angioplasty	73	80	58	69	51	63	47	53	40	53
Subintimal angioplasty	55	—	46	—	36	—	—	—	—	—

1, primary patency; 2, secondary patency.
*Excluding Hemobahn endoprosthesis.
[†]Balloon-expandable stents.

in the SFA location, where they generate an exaggerated intimal hyperplastic response and are prone to compression from external forces. This led to the use of the stainless-steel self-expanding stents (e.g., Wallstent). Early results with this type of stent were similarly disappointing, suggesting no benefit over angioplasty alone (26–28). In retrospect, studies using these stents have been criticized on the basis of poor interventional technique and suboptimal peri-procedural pharmacotherapy (29). It is unclear if modern techniques and current advances in peri-procedural anticoagulant and antiplatelet regimens would have significantly improve the outcomes achieved in these studies.

Contemporary stenting of the FP artery is achieved using nitinol self-expanding stents, and to a lesser extent, using endovascular stent grafts. The IntraCoil stent is FDA approved for use in the FP artery (30). However, this stent has a number of limitations: it is high profile, the absence of a sheath covering the stent makes it difficult to deliver through calcified lesions (i.e., making predilation mandatory), and precise placement is difficult as a result of the deployment mechanism. For these reasons, the authors do not currently use this stent.

Of the bare-metal self-expanding nitinol stents that are currently used in the FP artery, one has received FDA approval (LifeStent, Bard) for use in the FP artery, and the remainder have received approval for use in the biliary system (Table 16.3). However, in reference to this latter group, a number of ongoing registries are being performed to achieve this approval.

The most reliable data on outcomes with bare-metal nitinol stenting in the FP artery come from the stent arm of

the four randomized controlled trials comparing the performance of contemporary nitinol stents versus angioplasty and one prospective stent registry (6–9) (Table 16.4). These studies differ from observational analyses in that there was rigorous adjudication and core laboratory assessment of outcomes, which help eliminate the clear bias associated with observational studies in this field. Given the hundreds of thousands of these stents that have been implanted worldwide, it is remarkable that the total number of patients receiving stents in these rigorous studies totals only 493. The mean length of disease among this cohort was relatively modest (4.5 to 13.2 cm), and the duration of follow-up is relatively short (12 to 24 months). Primary patency rates at 1 year vary from 65.6% to 81.3%, and the only trial with 2-year data reported primary patency rates at that time point of only 54.3% (31). Although three of the four randomized trials that enrolled patients with longer lesion length did show a benefit of bare-metal nitinol stenting over angioplasty, the patency rates associated with stenting in the FP artery are sobering, and are not near what has been achieved in the coronary circulation. In addition, for younger patients with claudication, it is the anticipated 4- to 5-year patency rates that have greatest clinical relevance. This data is largely unknown.

The Gore Viabahn Endoprosthesis® is the dominant stent graft used in the FP artery, and is composed of a PTFE graft supported by an outer nitinol frame (Chapter 7). This type of stent graft is distinct from older stent grafts that were constructed from vascular grafts and balloon-expandable stents, and were associated with high complication and restenosis rates when used in the SFA location (18). Again, the most reliable data on outcomes with the Viabahn

TABLE 16.3 Self-Expanding Nitinol Stents Used for Superficial Femoral Artery Intervention

Name	Manufacturer	Stent Diameter (mm)	Stent Length (mm)	Sheath Size (Fr.)	Guidewire (inch)
Zilver 518	Cook	6–10	20, 30, 40, 60, 80	5	0.018
Zilver 635	Cook	6–10	20, 30, 40, 60, 80	6	0.035
Sentinol	Boston Scientific	5–8, 10	20, 40, 60, 80	6	0.035
Luminexx	Bard	4–10, 12, 14	20, 30, 40, 50, 60, 80, 100, 120	6	0.035
SMART	Cordis	6–10, 12, 14	20, 40, 60, 80, 100, 150	6, 7	0.035
ABSOLUTE	Abbott Vascular	5–8	20, 30, 40, 60, 80, 100, 120, 150	6	0.035
Protégé EverFlex	ev3	5–9	20, 30, 40, 60, 80, 100, 120, 150	6	0.035
LifeStent	Bard				
• FlexStar	Bard	6–10	20, 30, 40, 60, 80	7	0.035
• FlexStar XL	Bard	6, 7	100, 120, 150, 170	7	0.035
Supera	IDev	4–10	40, 60, 80, 100, 120	7	0.018
Complete	Medtronic	4–10	20–150	6	0.035

TABLE 16.4 Summary of Outcomes Associated with Bare-Metal Nitinol Self-Expanding Stents and Covered Nitinol Stents in the Femoropliteal Artery

Study	N	Stent	Follow-up (months)	Lesion Length (cm)	Cross-over Rate (%)	1° Patency (%)
Bare-metal nitinol stents						
RESILIENT	134	LifeStent	12	7.1	40.3	81.3
Schillinger	51	Absolute	24	13.2	32	54.3
ASTRON	34	Astron	12	9.8	26	65.6
FAST	123	Luminexx	12	4.5	11	68.3
DURABILITY	151	EverFlex	12	9.6	N/A	79.1
Covered nitinol stent (Viabahn)						
McQuade	40	Viabahn	24	25.6	N/A	63
Saxon	97	Viabahn	12	7	N/A	65

stent come from the stent arm of two randomized trials (11,32) (Table 16.4). These two trials enrolled very modest patient numbers (total 137), with limited follow-up (12 to 24 months). However, the lesion length in the Baylor study was 25 cm, which is dramatically longer than any other FP study, and is more reflective of many of the complicated FP anatomies encountered in clinical practice. Patency rates appear to compare favorably with bare-metal nitinol stents, but a head-to-head study is lacking. In the Baylor study, stenting with the Viabahn stent was equivalent with surgical bypass using prosthetic conduit (primary patency at 24 months—63% vs. 64%). The study by Saxon et al. reported a higher patency rate at 12 months in the Viabahn versus the angioplasty group (65% vs. 40%, $p = 0.0003$). Additional data are awaited from the VIBRANT trial, which has been completed, and the VIPER registry that is currently enrolling.

CRYOPLASTY

The PolarCath peripheral balloon catheter system and clinical outcomes associated with its use are reviewed in Chapter 7. In brief, data supporting the use of this system come from single and multicenter registries. In the largest of these registries that enrolled 102 patients with relatively short lesions (mean lesion length 4.7 cm), the patency at 9 months as determined by Duplex ultrasound was 70.1% (33). In a subset of these patients with longer-term follow-up, the clinical patency at 3 years was 75%. A small randomized trial (COBRA) is ongoing that tests the impact of cryoplasty versus routine angioplasty following nitinol stent placement to reduce the rates of in-stent restenosis.

ATHERECTOMY

The data regarding the use atherectomy devices in the FP artery are fully reviewed in Chapter 8. In summary, these data are largely composed of single or multicenter registries of mixed populations of patients (i.e., both claudication and critical limb ischemia), with mixed anatomies including non-FP lesions, without rigorous core-lab or clinical event committee

adjudication of endpoints, and with limited follow-up (typically 12 months). There are no data to demonstrate the superiority of these devices in improving long-term patency over conventional balloon or stent technologies.

BRACHYTHERAPY

Enthusiasm for the use of brachytherapy in FP intervention was founded on the promising results achieved in the coronary circulation for the treatment of in-stent restenosis in the early 2000s. Much of the testing of brachytherapy in the FP artery was as an adjunct to angioplasty. However, the pathologies of in-stent restenosis and restenosis following angioplasty are distinct. Whereas in-stent restenosis is caused entirely by intimal hyperplasia, restenosis following successful angioplasty is secondary to the combination of elastic recoil, constrictive remodeling, and intimal hyperplasia.

Several clinical studies have been performed to evaluate brachytherapy as an adjunct to angioplasty in the prophylaxis of SFA restenosis and the treatment of restenosis following angioplasty. The Vienna-2 Study enrolled 113 patients with claudication or critical leg ischemia, with de novo FP stenosis or occlusion of more than 5 cm in length, and FP restenosis following angioplasty (regardless of length) (34). IR-192 was delivered using a noncentered delivery system with 10-mm safety margins. At 6-months follow-up evaluation, restenosis was observed in 54% of the PTA group and 28% of the PTA and adjunctive brachytherapy group. However, at 5-year follow-up, there was evidence of late catch-up, with equivalent and disappointing restenosis rates in both arms (72.5% in each arm) (35).

Like the Vienna-2 trial, the Peripheral Artery Radiation Investigational Study (PARIS) attempted to investigate the effectiveness of IR-192 using a centered catheter for the prevention of FP restenosis. Patients included in the trial had stenoses between 5 and 15 cm in length or occlusions up to 5 cm. Unfortunately, the randomized trial was terminated early as a result of poor enrollment (data unpublished). An assessment of the randomized cohort enrolled revealed no

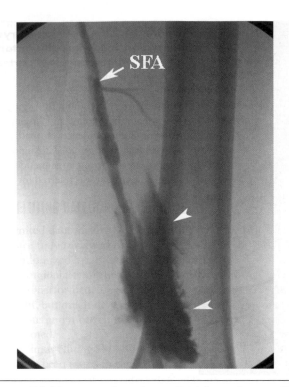

Figure 16.24 • Complicated superficial femoral artery (SFA) perforation. Angiogram of the distal left SFA demonstrating significant perforation and extravasation of contrast into the thigh (indicated by *white arrowheads*). Failure to seal this perforation would place the patient at high risk for a compartment syndrome.

our practice to obtain an ABI at rest and duplex ultrasound of the treated vessel, shortly after endovascular therapy (1 to 4 weeks). These studies serve as a baseline for future comparisons in the event of recurrence of chronic limb ischemia.

In general, patients are routinely seen at 3, 6, 9, and 12 months, and at 6- to 12-month intervals thereafter if patency at 12 months is confirmed. At each time point, the patient is questioned about the presence of recurrent symptoms, and an ABI and duplex ultrasound of the FP artery are performed. Duplex ultrasound is more sensitive than either clinical symptoms or ABI in detecting restenosis. A peak systolic flow velocity greater than 200 cm/sec at the site of the lesion or less than 45 cm/sec distal to the lesion is indicative of a stenosis of more than 50%. Using contemporary techniques and devices for reintervention after the aggressive use of these monitoring strategies may help achieve secondary patency rates of about 90%. However, the recurrence rates following reintervention for restenosis are high (up to 70%), which is unacceptable for most younger patients whose presenting complaint is claudication. If there are repeated recurrences of restenosis, the patient should be considered for an alternative endovascular approach (e.g., covered self-expanding stent), surgical revascularization, or a repeated attempt at aggressive medical therapy that includes exercise. Medical therapy following FP intervention is largely empiric. The authors treat with aspirin and clopidogrel for a minimum of 1 month following intervention. Longer-term dual antiplatelet therapy may be indicated in patients with critical limb ischemia and poor distal run-off. Aggressive secondary risk modification is also indicated in this group at high risk for cardiovascular events.

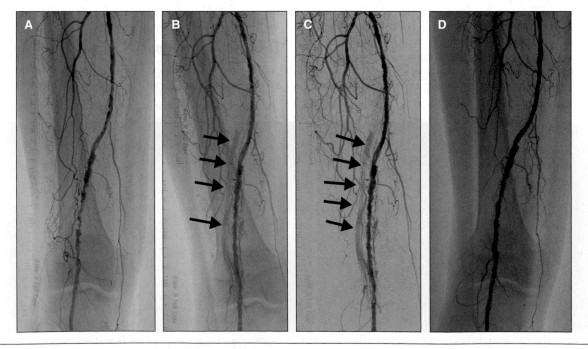

Figure 16.25 • Arteriovenous-fistula formation following femoropopliteal artery intervention. **A:** Baseline angiogram showing severe disease in above-knee popliteal artery. **B,C:** Landscape and subtracted angiogram following atherectomy with Jetstream catheter showing filling of deep vein *(black arrows)* indicating presence of arteriovenous fistula. **D:** Angiogram performed 6 weeks later showing complete resolution of the fistula. The patient was asymptomatic.

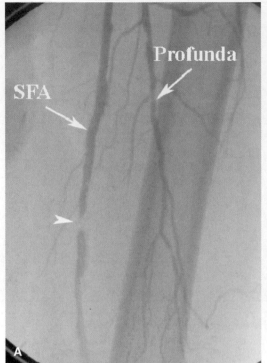

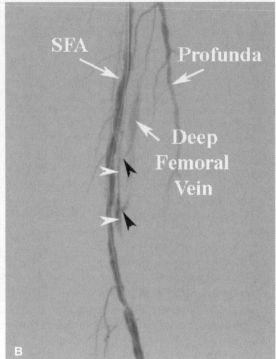

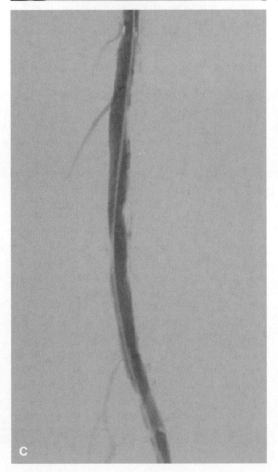

Figure 16.26 • Benign form of superficial femoral artery (SFA) perforation. **A:** Baseline angiogram demonstrating severe stenosis in the left mid-SFA. **B:** Angiogram following angioplasty demonstrating a tear in the wall of the SFA, evidenced by staining of the adventitia *(white arrowheads)*, and flow from the SFA (indicated by *black arrowheads*) into the adjacent deep femoral vein. **C:** Final angiography following deployment of self-expanding stent in the SFA.

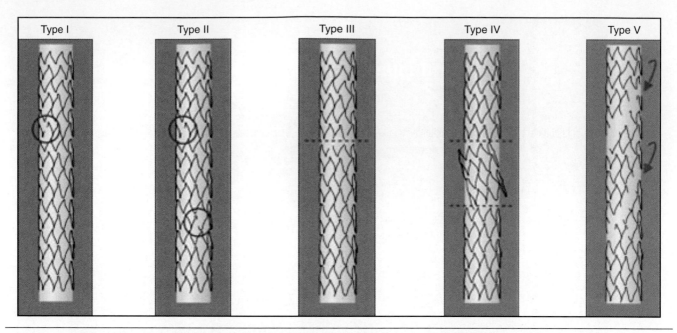

Figure 16.27 • Proposed classification of stent fractures in the femoropopliteal artery. *I*: Single tine fracture. *II*: Multiple tine fractures. *III*: Stent fracture(s) with preserved alignment of the components. *IV*: Stent fracture(s) with malalignment of the components. *V*: Stent fracture(s) in a trans-axial spiral configuration. (Reproduced from Rocha-Singh KJ, Jaff MR, Crabtree TR, et al. Performance goals and endpoint assessments for clinical trials of femoropopliteal bare nitinol stents in patients with symptomatic peripheral arterial disease. *Catheter Cardiovasc Interv.* 2007;69:910–919, with permission of John Wiley & Sons, Inc.)

Figure 16.28 • Stent fracture following femoropopliteal artery stenting. A: Baseline angiogram showing diffuse in-stent restenosis. **B,C:** High magnification unsubtracted images from the proximal and distal stents showing Grade II *(solid arrows)* and Grade III *(dotted arrows)* stent fractures. **D:** Angiography following atherectomy with Jetstream catheter and angioplasty.

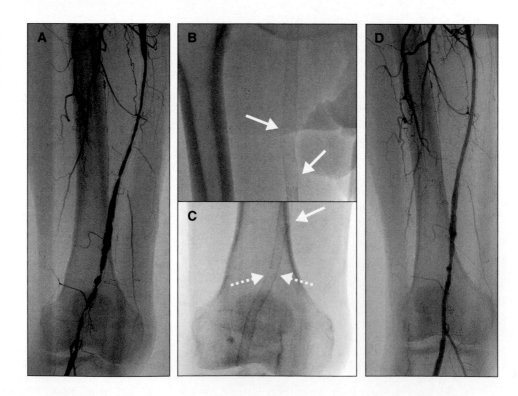

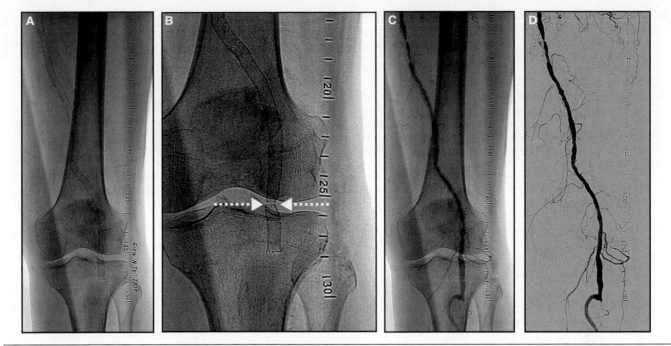

Figure 16.29 • Stent fracture following femoropopliteal artery stenting. **A:** Baseline unsubtracted image. **B:** Magnified view showing Grade III fracture at the level of the knee joint. **C,D:** Unsubtracted and subtracted angiography showing in-stent restenosis that is geographically remote from the site of stent fracture.

References

1. Walsh DB, Powell RJ, Stukel TA, et al. Superficial femoral artery stenoses: characteristics of progressing lesions. *J Vasc Surg.* 1997;25:512–521.

2. Whyman MR, Ruckley CV, Fowkes FG. A prospective study of the natural history of femoropopliteal artery stenosis using duplex ultrasound. *Eur J Vasc Surg.* 1993;7:444–447.

3. Goodney PP, Beck AW, Nagle J, et al. National trends in lower extremity bypass surgery, endovascular interventions, and major amputations. *J Vasc Surg.* 2009;50:54–60.

4. Norgren L, Hiatt WR, Dormandy JA, et al. Inter-society consensus for the management of peripheral arterial disease. *J Vasc Surg.* 2007;45(suppl 1):S5–S67.

5. Feinglass J, McCarthy WJ, Slavensky R, et al. Functional status and walking ability after lower extremity bypass grafting or angioplasty for intermittent claudication: results from a prospective outcomes study. *J Vasc Surg.* 2000;31:93–103.

6. Laird JR, Katzen BT, Scheinert D, et al. Nitinol stent implantation versus balloon angioplasty for lesions in the superficial femoral artery and proximal popliteal artery: twelve-month results from the RESILIENT randomized trial. *Circ Cardiovasc Interv.* 2010;3:267–276.

7. Dick P, Wallner H, Sabeti S, et al. Balloon angioplasty versus stenting with nitinol stents in intermediate length superficial femoral artery lesions. *Catheter Cardiovasc Interv.* 2009;74:1090–1095.

8. Schillinger M, Sabeti S, Loewe C, et al. Balloon angioplasty versus implantation of nitinol stents in the superficial femoral artery. *N Engl J Med.* 2006;354:1879–1888.

9. Krankenberg H, Schlüter M, Steinkamp HJ, et al. Nitinol stent implantation versus percutaneous transluminal angioplasty in superficial femoral artery lesions up to 10 cm in length. *Circulation.* 2007;116:285–292.

10. Mewissen MW, Primary nitinol stenting for femoropopliteal disease. *J Endovasc Ther.* 2009;16(suppl II):1163–1181.

11. Kedora J, Hohmann S, Garrett W, et al. Randomized comparison of percutaneous Viabahn stent grafts vs. prosthetic femoral-popliteal bypass in the treatment of superficial femoral arterial occlusive disease. *J Vasc Surg.* 2007;45:10–16.

12. McQuade K, Gable D, Hohman S, et al. Randomized comparison of ePTFE/nitinol self-expanding stent graft vs. prosthetic femoral-popliteal bypass in the treatment of superficial femoral artery occlusive disease. *J Vasc Surg.* 2009;49:109–115.

13. Saxon RR, Coffman JM, Gooding JM, et al. Long-term results of ePTFE stent-graft versus angioplasty in the femoropopliteal artery: single center experience from a prospective, randomized trial. *J Vasc Interv Radiol.* 2003;14:303–311.

14. Ahmadi R, Schillinger M, Maca T, et al. *Radiology.* 2002;346:345–350.

15. Casserly I. The role of atherectomy in the femoropopliteal artery. *Endovascular Today Suppl.* 2009;(September):3–7.

16. Das T. Crossing peripheral CTOs. *Endovascular Today.* 2006;(March):50–58.

17. Casserly IP, Sachar R, Bajzer C, et al. Utility of IVUS-guided transaccess catheter in the treatment of long chronic total occlusion of the superficial femoral artery. *Catheter Cardiovasc Interv.* 2004;62:237–243.

18. Dorrucci V. Treatment of superficial femoral artery occlusive disease. *J Cardiovasc Surg (Torino).* 2004;45:193–201.

19. Grimm J, Muller-Hulsbeck S, Jahnke T, et al. Randomized study to compare PTA alone versus PTA with Palmaz stent placement for femoropopliteal lesions. *J Vasc Interv Radiol.* 2001;12:935–942.

20. Hunink MG, Wong JB, Donaldson MC, et al. Revascularization for femoropopliteal disease. A decision and cost-effectiveness analysis. *JAMA.* 1995;274:165–171.

21. Johnston KW. Femoral and popliteal arteries: reanalysis of results of balloon angioplasty. *Radiology.* 1992;183:767–771.

22. Capek P, McLean GK, Berkowitz HD. Femoropopliteal angioplasty. Factors influencing long-term success. *Circulation.* 1991;83:I70–I80.

23. Rocha-Singh KJ, Jaff MR, Crabtree TR, et al. Performance goals and endpoint assessments for clinical trials of femoropopliteal bare nitinol stents in patients with symptomatic peripheral arterial disease. *Catheter Cardiovasc Interv.* 2007;69:910–919.

24. Chatelard P, Guibourt C. Long-term results with a Palmaz stent in the femoropopliteal arteries. *J Cardiovasc Surg (Torino)*. 1996;37:67–72.

25. Rosenfield K, Schainfeld R, Pieczek A, et al. Restenosis of endovascular stents from stent compression. *J Am Coll Cardiol*. 1997;29:328–338.

26. Martin EC, Katzen BT, Benenati JF, et al. Multicenter trial of the Wallstent in the iliac and femoral arteries. *J Vasc Interv Radiol*. 1995;6:843–849.

27. Do DD, Triller J, Wolpoth BH, et al. A comparison study of self-expandable stents vs. balloon angioplasty alone in femoropopliteal artery occlusions. *Cardiovasc Intervent Radiol*. 1992;15:306–312.

28. Gray BH, Sullivan TM, Childs MB, et al. High incidence of restenosis/reocclusion of stents in the percutaneous treatment of long-segment superficial femoral artery disease after suboptimal angioplasty. *J Vasc Surg*. 1997;25:74–83.

29. Silver MJ, Ansel GM. Femoropopliteal occlusive disease: diagnosis, indications for treatment, and results of interventional therapy. *Catheter Cardiovasc Interv*. 2002;56:555–561.

30. Ansel GM, Botti CF Jr., George BS, et al. Clinical results for the training-phase roll-in patients in the intracoil femoral-popliteal stent trial. *Catheter Cardiovasc Interv*. 2002;56:443–449.

31. Schillinger M, Sabeti S, Dick P, et al. Sustained benefit at 2 years of primary femoropopliteal stenting compared with balloon angioplasty with optional stenting. *Circulation*. 2007;115:2745–2749.

32. Saxon RR, Dake M, Volgelzang R, et al. Randomized, multicenter study comparing expanded polytetrafluoroethylene-covered endo-prosthesis placement with percutaneous transluminal angioplasty in the treatment of superficial femoral artery occlusive disease. *J Vasc Interv Radiol*. 2008;19:823–832.

33. Laird JR, Biamino G, McNamara T, et al. Cryoplasty for the treatment of femoropopliteal arterial disease: extended follow-up results. *J Endovasc Ther*. 2006;13(suppl II):II52–II59.

34. Minar E, Pokrajac B, Maca T, et al. Endovascular brachytherapy for prophylaxis of restenosis after femoropopliteal angioplasty: results of a prospective randomized study. *Circulation*. 2000;102:2694–2699.

35. Wolfram RM, Budinsky AC, Pokrajac B, et al. Endovascular brachytherapy for prophylaxis of restenosis after femoropopliteal angioplasty: five-year follow-up—prospective randomized study. *Radiology*. 2006;240:878–884.

36. Wolfram RM, Budinsky AC, Pokrajac B, et al. Vascular brachytherapy with ^{192}Ir after femoropopliteal stent implantation in high-risk patients: twelve-month follow-up results from the Vienna-5 trial. *Radiology*. 2005;236:343–351.

37. Rocha-Singh KJ, Scheer K, Rutherford J. Nitinol stent fractures in the superficial femoral artery: incidence and clinical significance. *J Am Coll Cardiol*. 2003;41(suppl 1):79–80.

CHAPTER 17

Infrapopliteal Intervention

Mitchell J. Silver and Gary M. Ansel

The advancing field of percutaneous endovascular therapy has led to a significant increase in options available for the treatment of patients with symptomatic peripheral vascular disease. Previous reticence in applying these techniques to the infrapopliteal arterial bed is slowly giving way, as technological improvements and operator experience have led to predictable and consistently high rates of technical success with low risk of complications.

INDICATIONS FOR INTERVENTION

Critical limb ischemia (CLI), manifest as ischemic rest pain or tissue loss, is the most common clinical indication for infrapopliteal intervention, and presents a significant risk for amputation in that individual (1). In the elderly, who are most at risk, the probability of loss of independence and reduced quality of life from an amputation is significant (2). Currently it appears that whatever treatment successfully prevents major amputation will be cost-effective, with benefit to the individual as well as society (3). In most instances of CLI, the risk–benefit ratio is different from that seen with the claudicant; because of the risk of limb threat in patients with CLI, there is a significantly lower threshold in performing endovascular and surgical procedures of greater complexity (and greater risk). There is also a greater acceptance in performing procedures of more limited durability, since in most circumstances, restenosis following complete wound healing is often clinically silent. The latter observation is based on the fact that the tissue in patients with nonhealing ulcers, or gangrene, requires high levels of oxygen and nutrition for tissue repair. This level of oxygenation is usually only adequately supplied by uninterrupted, straight-line arterial flow by at least one of the tibial vessels (i.e., with an intact pedal arch). However, once wound healing has occurred, the oxygen requirements to maintain tissue integrity are significantly decreased. Thus, if vascular occlusion or restenosis occurs after wound healing, most patients will maintain integrity of the tissue and function satisfactorily. Long-term healing will be particularly successful if patients are instructed in proper foot care, and in the avoidance of foot trauma and infection.

The therapeutic decision process for the treatment of infrapopliteal disease is complex, whether the treatment is medical, surgical, or endovascular. Considerations include such limb variables as the level and degree of tissue destruction, the presence of associated soft tissue or bony infection, and the need for debridement or skin grafting. General patient variables that play a significant role in the decision process include the presence of comorbidities such as cardiopulmonary disease, diabetes and renal insufficiency, the functional and ambulatory status of the patient, and the availability of appropriate vein conduit for surgical revascularization. Anatomic variables such as the distribution, burden, and nature of athereosclerosis in the lower extremities are important in assessing the likely technical success of revascularization. It should be recognized that the primary goal of treatment of significant distal limb ischemia is not necessarily hemodynamic but is that of safe avoidance of amputation and salvage of a functioning limb.

Historically, reconstructive femoral-to-tibial bypass surgery using venous conduit has been successful in preserving limb viability. However, in the absence of adequate venous conduit, results were universally dismal. Recent availability of heparin-bonded bypass conduit appears to be offering some improved results (4). Further larger studies will be required to confirm these initial data. In the interim, there is a general reluctance to use prosthetic grafts to bypass the tibial vessels (5,6). Even when appropriate vein conduit is available, there remain significant issues with distal bypass surgery. Although individual centers may give excellent results, similar results may not be possible in many centers, when audited (7). The problem of postoperative wound infection, necessitating weeks of intensive care, occurs commonly (i.e., 10% to 30%) but is rarely mentioned (8). Interestingly, as seen in distal angioplasty, the patency rates of surgical-bypass grafts may lag behind the limb salvage rates. Similar to restenosis following percutaneous procedures, graft closure after wound healing may not always lead to significant ischemia (9).

The published experience for endovascular intervention of the infrapopliteal arteries began with the advent of balloon angioplasty, but even today, it is still limited. In contrast to early data, current reports have documented endovascular revascularization to be highly efficacious with very low risk (10,11). Widespread application is still debated, primarily on the basis of poor long-term, hemodynamic outcome and lack of comparative trials (12,13). However, the use of endovascular techniques continues to grow rapidly because these procedures are repeatable, may be accomplished quickly, and are safely completed in patients with multiple comorbidities. Whereas restenosis is a major consideration for endovascular procedures performed above the knee (i.e., performed usually for claudication), it should not be a major limiting factor in below-the-knee intervention (i.e., performed usually for limb salvage).

Most of the literature evaluating infrapopliteal endovascular techniques has been reported from studies with

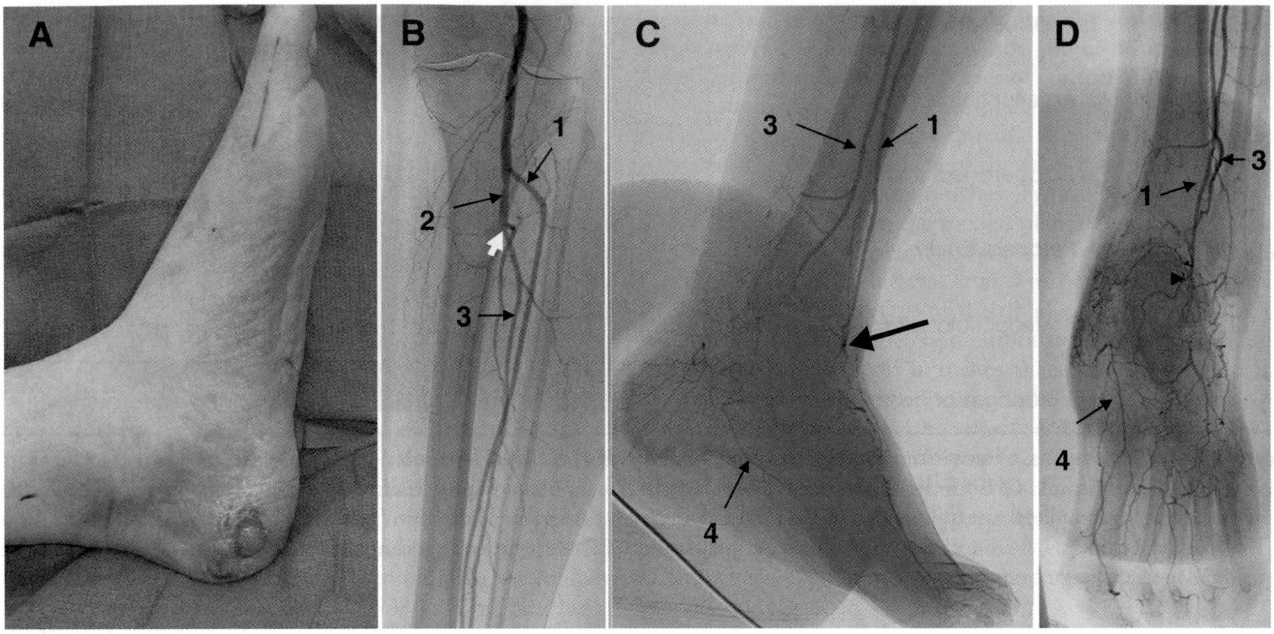

Figure 17.4 • Angiography of the tibial and pedal vessels in a patient with wound on medial aspect of left heel.
A: Appearance of wound on left heel. **B:** Tibial angiography demonstrating occlusion of the posterior tibial artery *(white arrow)*. **C:** Lateral angiogram of the foot demonstrating occlusion of the dorsalis pedis branch *(arrow)* and collateral filling of a plantar branch. **D:** Antero-posterior cranial view of the foot confirming that the plantar branch that fills via collaterals is the medial plantar branch and that the dorsalis pedis branch is occluded *(arrowhead)*.

INTERVENTION

General Strategy

Infrapopliteal intervention is usually reserved for the patient with ischemic rest pain or tissue loss. There are rare patients who have true, lifestyle-limiting, intermittent claudication from isolated infrapopliteal disease. Obtaining a careful history is essential to determine the duration of symptoms, as thrombolytic therapy may be the initial intervention in the patient with an acute change in clinical status. A meticulous physical examination of the area of tissue loss is necessary to elicit any signs of infection or underlying osteomyelitis, either of which may adversely affect the success of any interventional therapy. Nuclear scanning or MRI may be important additional diagnostic modalities to characterize the presence of osteomyelitis.

The initial diagnostic angiogram will typically be obtained from the contralateral, common femoral artery, or brachial artery access, unless the patient has had prior CT or MR angiography. It is important to emphasize that routine invasive angiography remains critical to the accurate assessment of the infrapopliteal anatomy in patients with CLI due to the limitations of currently available noninvasive angiographic techniques. After demonstrating the infrapopliteal anatomy, the decision regarding approach and interventional modality may be made. For proximal, focal, stenotic disease, a contralateral common femoral artery access will usually suffice. For long occlusions and severely calcified or distal disease (i.e., below mid-calf), an antegrade approach is preferable.

In general, to resolve ischemic rest pain or heal an ischemic ulcer, it is necessary to achieve patency to one infrapopliteal vessel to the foot. Since rest pain typically involves the forefoot, the tibial target in this instance should ideally provide the main contribution to the metatarsal arch. In patients with tissue loss, the tibial target should provide flow to the affected area. For wounds that affect the digits (the most common scenario), the tibial target should again supply flow to the metatarsal arch. Less common wound locations such as the heel and malleoli require a careful examination of the arterial anatomy to determine the most appropriate tibial target. These considerations emphasize the need to identify the most appropriate tibial target for revascularization primarily based on the clinical indication, and not on the anticipated complexity of the procedure to open a given tibial vessels. Where two tibial vessels contribute equally to a given area of ischemia, the tibial vessel with the least complex disease can be approached. At times, two vessels may be recanalized without significant additional time, difficulty, or risk to the patient.

Anticoagulation/Antithrombotics

The pattern of infrapopliteal disease (i.e., focal stenotic or diffuse) will dictate the intensity of anticoagulation and antiplatelet therapy. In addition, the clinical presentation (i.e., acute or chronic presentation) will play a role in what pharmacologic adjuncts will be used.

In regard to antiplatelet therapy, the patient should be taking the combination of aspirin and an ADP-receptor inhibitor (e.g., ticlopidine or clopidogrel) prior to coming to the angiographic suite. For patients with diffuse infrapopliteal disease that may be scheduled to undergo rotational atherectomy or excimer laser therapy, intravenous glycoprotein (GP) IIb/IIIa inhibitor use may, theoretically, be useful in preventing platelet aggregation and development of the no-reflow phenomenon. In addition, in the limb salvage situation where there is tissue loss, those patients undergoing stand-alone angioplasty for long-segment disease may also be considered candidates for use of a GP IIb/IIIa inhibitor. However, further study and data are required before routine use can be recommended. As the patient with infrapopliteal disease likely has multivascular bed atherosclerosis, a consideration for chronic combination therapy with aspirin and ADP-receptor inhibitor administration, following infrapopliteal intervention, should be made.

Unfractionated heparin has been used most often as an anticoagulant agent during infrapopliteal intervention. Patients receive 50 to 70 U/kg, intravenously, as a bolus at the start of the procedure, with a goal activated clotting time (ACT) of 250 to 300 seconds. There is limited experience using low-molecular-weight heparin during infrapopliteal intervention, although a comfort level is certainly being established for its application during coronary intervention. The use of low-molecular-weight heparin during peripheral intervention is currently the subject of ongoing clinical trials. In regard to direct thrombin inhibitors for infrapopliteal intervention, the use of bivalirudin was studied as part of the Angiomax Peripheral Procedure Registry of Vascular Events (APPROVE) study (20). The APPROVE study group determined that bivalirudin provided consistent anticoagulation and similar outcomes in all vessel types treated, with low ischemic and bleeding events both in hospital and at 30 days (20).

Guide/Sheath

If intervention is being performed from the contralateral common femoral artery (i.e., crossing over the aortic bifurcation), the crossover sheath, itself, may be used as a guide, especially if treating proximal focal stenotic disease. Flexible 4- to 6-Fr. crossover sheaths (i.e., nonkinking) are now available from a number of vendors. The distal portion of the sheath should be advanced to the distal ipsilateral external iliac artery or mid-common femoral artery. For more complex disease being approached from the contralateral common femoral artery, a long, 4- to 6-Fr. sheath, or a 6-Fr. multipurpose coronary guide catheter telescoped through a standard crossover sheath, may be advanced to the level of the distal SFA or midpopliteal artery. If there is significant SFA disease precluding safe passage of the 6-Fr. multipurpose coronary guide, the SFA disease should be treated first.

If the infrapopliteal intervention is being performed from an antegrade approach, a flexible, hydrophilic, 4- to 6-Fr., 30- to 55-cm sheath, placed to the level of the distal SFA or midpopliteal artery will be sufficient. The antegrade approach is preferred when treating more complex disease such as total occlusions or long, segmental, diffuse disease.

Wires

The interventional treatment of infrapopliteal disease most commonly uses coronary modalities (e.g., balloons, rotational atherectomy, stents, laser) on a 0.014" guidewire platform. The selection of which 0.014" guidewire to use will be driven by the type of disease being treated (i.e., stenotic, occlusive, focal, diffuse). For focal stenotic disease, any commonly used, floppy, 0.014" coronary guidewire may be used (e.g., Asahi Soft—Abbott Vascular, Santa Clara, CA). The guidewire is most easily manipulated if it is supported by an over-the-wire 0.014" coronary balloon catheter (e.g., Maverick—Boston Scientific, Boston, MA), or a 0.014"/0.018" low-profile catheter (e.g., Quickcross catheter—Spectranetics). For total occlusions, the group of 0.014" coronary wires with stiffer tips specifically designed

for crossing occlusions may be used (e.g., Miraclebro, Confianza—Abbott Vascular). Alternatively, a hydrophilic-coated, 0.018" or 0.035" guidewire may be used. The authors have had success using a 0.018" angled hydrophilic wire that has a gold distal marker (manufactured by Terumo) inside of a 0.018" Quickcross support catheter for crossing total occlusions. After successful crossing, the 0.018" angled hydrophilic wire is then exchanged for a supportive, 0.014" coronary-type guidewire (e.g., GrandSlam wire—Abbot Vascular) as a platform to perform the intervention.

When dealing with total occlusions that may not be crossed from the antegrade approach, Dorros and coworkers (21) have described their use of a surgical cut-down procedure on the tibial vessel, to achieve retrograde access in two cases. In similar cases, the authors have successfully entered the distal tibial vessel, using a micropuncture technique for advancement of a 0.018", hydrophilic wire through the occlusion, in a retrograde fashion (22). The wire is then snared at the popliteal artery and externalized through an antegrade femoral sheath. Following removal of the tibial sheath, the endovascular procedure was then completed from the antegrade access (Figs. 17.5 and 17.6).

Angioplasty

Standard 0.014" low-profile balloon catheters, ranging from 1.5 to 4 mm in diameter, may be used in the majority of interventions for focal stenoses, when attempting stand-alone angioplasty for infrapopliteal disease. At experienced centers, the acute technical success of angioplasty in primarily focal infrapopliteal stenoses is excellent, at approximately 98%. The success in treating total occlusions appears to be somewhat less. Clinical results are favorable. When defined by a pain-free extremity and limb salvage, success is reported in up to 84% at 2 to 5 years, in patients treated with angioplasty (23,24).

Traditionally, more diffuse, long-segment, diseased tibial vessels appear to have a lower clinical success rate when treated with stand-alone balloon angioplasty (i.e., 57% at 3 years) (25). Fortunately, there has been a major development and improvement in both angioplasty balloon catheters that are now manufactured for dedicated tibial artery use. The new relevant design characteristics include extremely low-profile tapered 0.014" balloon catheter types, and longer balloon lengths including 120, 150, and 220 mm. While a monorail platform is most efficient, the best pushability and tracking characteristics have been obtained utilizing over-the-wire platforms. Other important technical characteristics applied to these new balloons include low compliance and the ability to sustain medium-high pressure inflations, improving the remodeling of the treated vessel, especially when employing prolonged inflation times.

Utilizing this new generation of long balloons, Graziani et al. (26) have published very impressive clinical outcomes in dialyzed patients with long-segment tibial disease with CLI. Immediate technical success was achieved in 97% of cases, with cumulative limb salvage rates (median follow-up, 22 months) at 12, 24, 36, and 48 months of 96%, 84%, 84%, and 62%, respectively. Limb salvage without any new intervention on the same leg was achieved in 70% of patients, and repeat interventions were performed on 23 (17%) legs.

The authors have experience using coronary cutting balloons for complex, infrapopliteal stenoses, such as lesions at

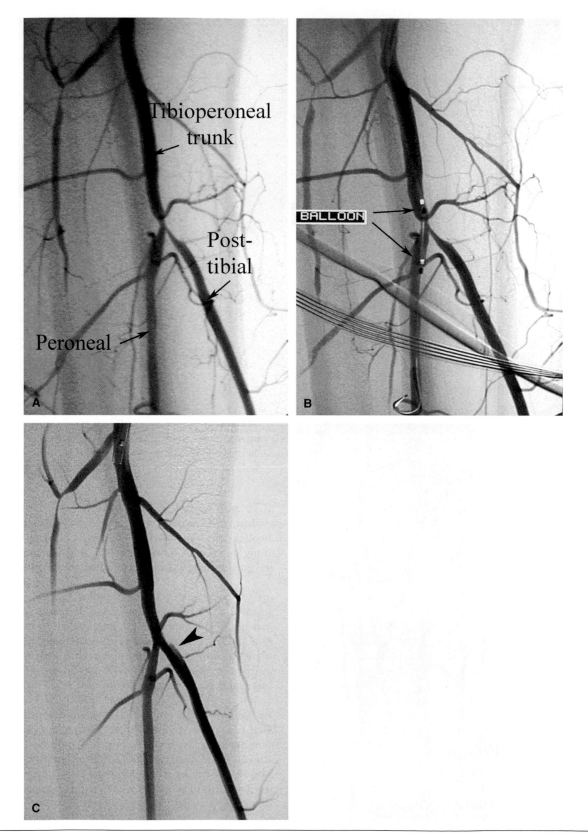

Figure 17.7 • Cutting balloon angioplasty of tibioperoneal bifurcation. A: Preprocedure angiogram of severe stenosis at right tibioperoneal bifurcation, AP projection. B: Cutting balloon dilation of right tibioperoneal bifurcation with cutting balloon into right peroneal artery, AP projection. C: Final angiogram of right tibioperoneal trunk bifurcation after cutting balloon treatment, AP projection. The presence of a non–flow-limiting dissection in the proximal portion of the posterior tibial branch is noted *(arrowhead)*.

restenosis and reocclusion rates are high (33,34). Siablis and colleagues reported a nonrandomized, prospective, single-center study that compared sirolimus-eluting stents (SES) (N = 29) versus BMS (N = 29) used for bailout after infrapopliteal revascularization of patients with CLI. The results at 6 months revealed higher primary patency (92% vs. 68.1%, P < 0.002) and decreased in-stent (4% vs. 55.2%, P < 0.001) and in-segment (32% vs. 66%, P < 0.001) restenosis (35) with SES use.

The Leipzig Cypher below-the-knee registry was a prospective, nonrandomized, single-center registry investigating the long-term clinical outcomes of patients receiving below-the-knee SES intervention for focal symptomatic infrapopliteal disease. All patients had single lesions treatable with a single 33-mm SES with a nominal diameter of 3.5 mm. Both primary and secondary patency rates were acceptable at 6 months (98.2%, 98.2%), 12 months (94.1%, 95.9%), and 24 months (89.2% and 95.9%).

Atherectomy Devices

The presumed benefit of atherectomy is that it debulks/removes obstructing material rather than displacing it, as occurs with angioplasty. These devices are categorized as either excisional (removing and collecting atheromatous material) or ablative (fragmenting the atheroma into small particles).

The Silver Hawk Plaque Excision System (EV3 Endovascular Inc., Plymouth, MN) has been reported to be efficacious in several nonrandomized single-center registries (36–38) for the treatment of patients with CLI. These promising short-term outcomes need to be validated in randomized, controlled trials to ensure data quality regarding long-term outcomes and safety. The Silverhawk ES and DS devices are appropriate for use in most tibial vessels, whereas the Silverhawk SS and SX devices may be used for distal popliteal disease and the proximal segment of larger tibial vessels. Particular care should be exercised in using these devices at angulated segments (e.g., the proximal anterior tibial artery) since wire bias may result in excessive atherectomy at the location where the wire is closest to the vessel wall and increase the risk of complications (i.e., perforation). Severe vessel calcification also significantly limits the ability to successfully use these devices in the tibial vessels.

The use of rotational atherectomy very early after its introduction was associated with poor results. Coronary data have shown improved results when this device is combined with platelet inhibition, using the GP IIb/IIIa inhibitor, abciximab. The authors have since reported its use in 15 consecutive patients with total occlusions, diffuse tibial disease, and limb-threatening ischemia (Fig. 17.8) (39). Only one amputation has occurred at an average of 1-year follow-up evaluation. Using abciximab with rotational atherectomy appeared to prevent significant embolization and poor reflow.

Another ablative atherectomy device has recently entered the clinical arena that utilizes an eccentric, diamond-coated crown to achieve a mechanical sanding process that removes atherosclerotic plaque (Diamondback 360° Orbital Atherectomy System, Cardiovascular Systems, Inc., St. Paul, MN). Orbital atherectomy is performed over a 0.014″ guidewire with a proprietary 0.023″ spring coil tip (Viper wire), in contrast to the

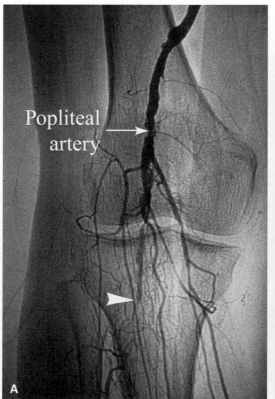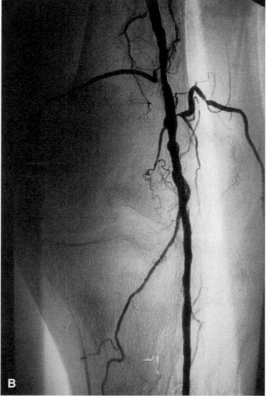

Figure 17.8 • **A:** Angiogram of right distal popliteal and tibioperoneal trunk total occlusion (*arrowhead*), before treatment, AP projection. **B:** Angiogram right popliteal artery postrotational atherectomy, lateral view.

0.009″ wire with rotational atherectomy. Final lumen diameter is dependent on the selected crown size and the rotational speed (80 K to 200 Krpm) during the ablation. As the crown rotates and the orbit increases, centrifugal force presses the crown against the lesion or plaque, ablating a small amount of plaque with each orbit. The authors have found more "stand-alone" results in heavily calcified tibial lesions, rather than "soft" atherosclerotic lesions that may require adjunctive PTA.

Laser Angioplasty

Laser is an attractive option for the treatment of diffuse tibial disease. Typically, the 1.4-mm and 1.7-mm diameter laser catheters are used in tibial vessels, although the 2.0-mm catheter may be used in the proximal segment of good caliber tibial vessels. Adjunctive angioplasty is typically employed following initial treatment with the laser catheter.

Excimer laser recanalization has been studied systematically in a multicenter trial (Laser Angioplasty for Critical Leg Ischemia; LACI 2) (Fig. 17.9) (40). Reports from LACI 2, with a tibial artery intervention strategy that used excimer laser followed by balloon angioplasty, have shown promising results. In LACI 2, 6-month limb salvage was over 90%, with only 16% stent usage in the tibial vessels. Patients in LACI 2 were, by definition, poor surgical candidates.

PROCEDURAL COMPLICATIONS

Vasospasm

The liberal use of intra-arterial nitrates and calcium channel antagonists administered upstream, prior to guidewire passage, may be useful in preventing vasospasm. Certainly, if vasospasm occurs, intra-arterial nitrates or calcium channel antagonists may be successful in treating vasospasm. Doses of 100 to 200 mcg, given intra-arterially (e.g., nitroglycerin, nicardipine, or verapamil), are usually well tolerated. Adenosine is also a consideration for the treatment of vasospasm. Removal of the guidewire from the affected vessel may also be necessary, in refractory cases. A meticulous search for occult dissection also needs to be performed.

No-Reflow

As seen during coronary intervention, "no-reflow" may occur during infrapopliteal intervention, particularly when treating acute limb ischemia. As in the coronary circulation, the cause of no-reflow is often multifactorial, with distal embolization, vasospasm, and skeletal muscle edema as recognized contributors. Occult dissection and thrombosis certainly need to be considered when faced with this issue. A methodic approach to looking for, and treating, the above-mentioned causative mechanisms is required when faced with no-reflow during infrapopliteal intervention. If no underlying cause is identified, no-reflow is typically treated with the administration of vasodilators (e.g., nitroglyerin, adenosine, verapamil, diltiazem). The use of GP IIb/IIIa inhibitors is also employed by some operators.

Thrombosis

Thrombosis that occurs during infrapopliteal intervention may be promptly resolved with catheter-based, mechanical, rheolytic thrombectomy, using the 0.014″ XMI AngioJet catheter Medrad/Possis (Minneapolis, MN). When arterial thrombosis occurs, the operator must be certain the appropriate doses of anticoagulation and antiplatelet therapy have been administered. Occult arterial dissection needs to be ruled out by meticulous angiography. If thrombus persists after catheter-based mechanical thrombectomy, and other causes for thrombosis have been ruled out, thrombolytic therapy should be considered if there are no contraindications.

Perforation

Arterial perforation most commonly occurs when treating long, total occlusions, or when using rotational atherectomy. The majority of perforations that occur during infrapopliteal intervention may be treated with prolonged balloon inflations. Rarely, reversal of anticoagulation and/or platelet administration is necessary. For limb-threatening perforations that may not be controlled with prolonged balloon inflations, deployment of a coronary, covered stent would be an option (e.g., JoStent). This should be an exceedingly rare occurrence.

Flow-Limiting Dissection

The initial approach to managing a flow-limiting dissection that occurs during infrapopliteal intervention would be prolonged balloon inflation. If this approach fails, then bailout stenting is indicated. As described earlier, 0.014″-based coronary stent systems are typically used for this application. If the anatomic location is of concern for a possible crush point (e.g., proximal anterior tibial artery), then a self-expanding stent (e.g., Xpert) would be preferred.

LONG-TERM FOLLOW-UP EVALUATION

One of the limitations in the historic performance of distal limb endovascular techniques is the lack of close follow-up evaluation and noninvasive vascular surveillance. Our surgical colleagues are keenly aware of the need for bypass-graft surveillance (41). It has been the authors' experience that when continued surveillance is completed postendovascular intervention, the limb salvage rates are also improved. Importantly, neither clinical symptoms nor standard ABI measurements are as sensitive as duplex scanning for the detection of recurrent disease or restenosis. A peak systolic velocity greater than 200 cm/sec, or a flow velocity of less than 45 cm/sec distal to the lesion, is quite indicative of a stenosis of 50% or greater. As infrapopliteal intervention is becoming more common place, postprocedure testing should include an ABI evaluation prior to discharge, and then duplex scanning at 3-, 6-, and 12-month intervals. A strict duplex-surveillance program should most certainly lead to higher secondary patency rates than clinical follow-up evaluation, alone.

An often overlooked rule that cannot be overemphasized is that repeat intervention must be completed if there is evidence of recurrent vascular compromise prior to complete wound healing. Infrapopliteal intervention performed by experienced operators will rarely preclude the performance of a subsequent bypass graft, or alter previously planned surgery.

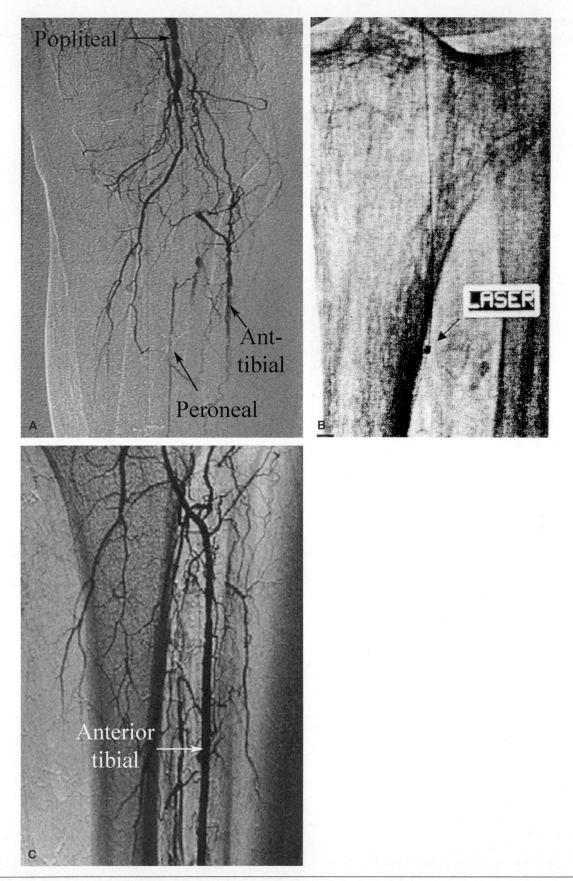

Figure 17.9 • **A:** Preprocedure angiogram of the left lower extremity demonstrating total occlusion of all infrapopliteal vessels, AP projection. **B:** Concentric 2.0 excimer laser of proximal left anterior tibial artery, AP projection. **C:** Final angiogram postlaser treatment demonstrating patent left anterior tibial artery, AP projection.

CONCLUSIONS

The endovascular treatment of infrapopliteal disease continues to improve and allows for successful limb salvage in the majority of patients. The ability of percutaneous procedures to be repeated is often overlooked, and, as discussed, it does *not* appear that long-term patency with endovascular techniques need match surgical results. Maintaining functional limb viability, with the lowest procedural and long-term mortality rates, should be the objective in the care of these patients. When chosen appropriately, both surgical bypass and endovascular therapy may benefit many patients. However, performing procedures that may lead to difficulty in healing or to prolonged hospitalization is not an acceptable outcome.

Treatment should not be entered into lightly or without a clear plan. A team approach, with a close working relationship between the interventionalist and surgeon, allows clear treatment goals and expected treatment outcomes to be determined. Whatever technique is used, the result should create straight-line, distal flow to the foot, preferably leading to distal pulsation. The patient should be followed closely for wound healing, and with noninvasive vascular surveillance to identify restenosis. Regular evaluation should also be continued for associated cardiovascular and cerebrovascular disease. An appropriate exercise program should be instituted, and referral to a smoking cessation program should be offered if required.

References

1. London NJM, Srinavass R, Naylor AR, et al. Changing arteriosclerotic disease patterns and management strategies in lowerlimb threatening ischemia. *Eur J Vasc Surg*. 1994;8:148–155.
2. Houghton AD, Taylor PR, Thurlow S, et al. Success rates for rehabilitation of vascular amputees: implications for preoperative assessment and amputation level. *Br J Surg*. 1992;79:753–755.
3. Cheshire NJW, Wolfe JHN, Noone MA, et al. The economics of femorocrural reconstruction for critical limb ischemia with and without autologous vein. *J Vasc Surg*. 1992;15:167–175.
4. Dorigo W, Di Carlo F, Troisi N, et al. Lower limb revascularization with a new bioactive prosthetic graft: early and late results [abstract]. *Ann Vasc Surg*. 2008;22(1):79–87.
5. Veith FJ, Gupta SK, Ascer E, et al. Six-year prospective multicenter randomized comparison of autologous saphenous vein and expanded polytetrafluoroethylene grafts in infrainguinal arterial reconstructions. *J Vasc Surg*. 1986;3:104–114.
6. Harris PI, How TV, Jones DR. Prospectively randomized clinical trial to compare in situ and reversed saphenous vein grafts for femoropopliteal bypass. *Br J Surg*. 1987;74:252–255.
7. The Iloprost Bypass International Study Group. Effects of perioperative iloprost on patency of femorodistal bypass grafts. *Eur J Vasc Endovasc Surg*. 1996;12:363–371.
8. Schwartz ME, Harrington EB, Schanzer H. Wound complications after in situ bypass. *J Vasc Surg*. 1988;7:802–807.
9. Monteverde-Grether C, Valezy Tello de Meneses M, Nava Lopez G, et al. Percutaneous transluminal ultrasonic angioplasty: preliminary clinical report of ultrasound plaque ablation in totally occluded peripheral arteries. *Arch Invest Med Mexico*. 1991;22:171–179.
10. Brown KT, Moore ED, Getrajdman GI, et al. Infrapopliteal angioplasty: long term follow-up. *J Vasc Interv Radiol*. 1993;4:139–144.
11. Varty K, Bolia A, Naylor AR, et al. Infrapopliteal percutaneous transluminal angioplasty: a safe and successful procedure. *Eur J Vasc Endovasc Surg*. 1995;9:341–345.
12. Fraser SCA, Al-Kutoubi MA, Wolfe JNA. Percutaneous transluminal angioplasty of infrapopliteal vessels: the evidence. *Radiology*. 1996;200:33–36.
13. Ahn SS, Eton D, Moore WS. Endovascular surgery for peripheral arterial occlusive disease. *Ann Surg*. 1992;216:3–16.
14. Ansel G, George BS, Kander NH, et al. Successful limb salvage with superficial femoral artery wall stenting [abstract]. *Circulation*. 1997;96(suppl 8):755.
15. Varty K, Bolosa A, Naylor AR, et al. Infrapopliteal percutaneous angioplasty: a safe and successful procedure. *Eur J Vasc Endovasc Surg*. 1995;9:341–345.
16. Kil S, Jung G. Anatomical variations of the popliteal artery and its tibial branches: analysis in 1242 extremities. *Cardiovasc Interv Radiol*. 2009;32:233–240.
17. Gates J, Hartnell GG. Optimized diagnostic angioplasty in high risk patients with severe peripheral vascular disease. *Radiographics*. 2000;20:121–133.
18. Kreitner KF, Kalden P, Neufang A, et al. Diabetes and peripheral arterial occlusive disease: prospective comparison of contrastenhanced three dimensional MR angiography with conventional digital subtraction angiography. *Am J Roentgenol*. 2000;174:171–179.
19. Oser R, Picus D, Hicks M, et al. Accuracy of DSA in the evaluation of patency of infrapopliteal vessels. *J Vasc Interv Radiol*. 1995;6:589–594.
20. Angiomax Peripheral Procedure Registry of Vascular Events (APPROVE) Study. In hospital and 30-day results. *J Invasive Cardiol*. 2004;16:651–656.
21. Iyer SS, Dorros G, Zaitown R, et al. Retrograde recanalization of an occluded posterior tibial artery by using a posterior tibial cutdown: two case reports. *Catheter Cardiovasc Diagn*. 1990;20:251–253.
22. Botti CF, Ansel GM, Silver MJ, et al. Percutaneous retrograde tibial access in limb salvage. *J Endovasc Ther*. 2003;10:614–618.
23. Bull PG, Mendel H, Hold M, et al. Distal popliteal and tibioperoneal transluminal angioplasty: long-term follow-up. *J Vasc Interv Radiol*. 1992;3:45–53.
24. Wagner HJ, Starch EE, McDermott JC. Infrapopliteal percutaneous transluminal revascularization: results of a prospective study on 148 patients. *J Interv Radiol*. 1993;8:81–90.
25. Matsi PJ, Manninen HI, Suhonen MT, et al. Chronic critical lower-limb ischemia: prospective trial of angioplasty with 1–36 months follow-up. *Radiology*. 1993;188:381–387.
26. Graziani L, Silvestro A, Bertone V, et al. Percutaneous transluminal angioplasty is feasible and effective in patients on chronic dialysis with severe peripheral artery disease. *Nephrol Dial Transplant*. 2007;22:1144–1149.
27. Engelke C, Morgan RA, Belli AM. Cutting balloon percutaneous transluminal angioplasty for salvage of lower limb arterial bypass grafts: feasibility. *Radiology*. 2002;223:106–114.
28. Costa JR, Mintz GS, Carlier SG, et al. Nonrandomized comparison of coronary stenting under intravascular ultrasound guidance of direct stenting without predilation versus conventional predilation with a semi-compliant balloon versus predilation with a new scoring balloon. *Am J Cardiol*. 2007;100:812–817.
29. Ansel GM, Botti C, Silver MJ. Cutting balloon angioplasty of the popliteal and infra-popliteal vessels for symptomatic leg ischemia. *Catheter Cardiovasc Interv*. 2004;61(1):1–4.
30. Laird J, Jaff MR, Biamino G, et al. Cryoplasty for the treatment of femoropopliteal arterial disease. *J Vasc Interv Radiol*. 2005;16:1067–1073.
31. Das T, McNamara T, Gray B, et al. Cryoplasty therapy for limb salvage in patients with critical limb ischemia. *J Endovasc Ther*. 2007;14:753–762.
32. Dorros G, Hull P, Prince C. Successful limb salvage after recanalization of an occluded infrapopliteal artery utilizing a balloon expandable (Palmer–Schatz) stent. *Catheter Cardiovasc Diagn*. 1993;28:83–88.

33. Tsetis D, Belli AM. The role of infrapopliteal angioplasty. *Br J Radiol*. 2004;77:1007–1015.
34. Rastogi S, Stavroploulos SW. Infrapopliteal angioplasty. *Tech Vasc Interv Radiol*. 2004;7:33–39.
35. Siablis D, Kraniotis P, Jarnabatidis D, et al. Sirolimus-eluting versus bare stents for bailout after suboptimal infrapopliteal angioplasty for critical limb ischemia: 6-month angiographic results from a nonrandomized prospective single-center study. *J Endovasc Ther*. 2005;12:685–695.
36. Kandzari D, Keisz R, Allie D, et al. Procedural and clinical outcomes with catheter-based plaque excision in critical limb ischemia. *J Endovasc Ther*. 2006;13:12–22.
37. Zeller T, Rastan A, Schwarzwalder U, et al. Mid-term results after atherectomy-assisted angioplasty of below knee arteries with use of the SilverHawk device. *J Vasc Surg*. 2004;15: 1391–1397.
38. Keeling BW, Shames ML, Stone PA, et al. Plaque excision with the Silverhawk catheter: early results in patients with claudication or critical limb ischemia. *J Vasc Surg*. 2007;45:25–31.
39. George BS, Ansel GM, Noethen AA, et al. Efficacy of rotational atherectomy in the treatment of patients with lower extremity (infra-femoral) ischemia. *Am J Cardiol*. 1997;80(7A):125.
40. LACI 2 Investigators. Laser angioplasty for critical leg ischemia. In: *Report from Circulatory System Devices Advisory Panel of the US Food and Drug Administration (FDA)*. Washington, DC; October 2, 2002.
41. Green RM, McNamara J, Ouriel K, et al. Comparison of infrainguinal graft surveillance techniques. *J Vasc Surg*. 1990;11:207–215.

Endovascular Management of Aneurysmal Disease

CHAPTER 18

Endovascular Management of Abdominal Aortic Aneurysms

Kenjiro Kaneko, Yuji Kanaoka, and Takao Ohki

In the United States, abdominal aortic aneurysm (AAA) is ranked as the 13th leading cause of death and is largely related to the high mortality rate associated with aneurysm rupture (up to 80%). The success rate in treating an intact AAA, however, is over 95%, which underpins the objective of early detection and treatment of AAA before rupture. Until recently the only treatment modality available was open surgical repair, which required general anesthesia and open laparotomy. The first successful surgical repair of an AAA was performed by Dubost et al. in 1952 (1). Since then, significant improvements related to surgical repair of AAAs have been made. Current studies report an impressive surgical mortality rate of 2.1% to 5.8% following open elective repair (2-6). However, it is important to note that there are other risks besides mortality in performing a major laparotomy. These include high rates of major complications including prolonged hospitalization, prolonged recuperation, and sexual dysfunction (7). Moreover, there are patients who are not surgical candidates, owing to comorbid conditions. As a result, there was a significant unmet need for a less invasive approach to treat patients with AAAs. This led to the development of endovascular aneurysmal repair (EVAR), which was first performed and reported by Juan Parodi in the early 1990s. EVAR can accomplish AAA repair without the need for major laparotomy and/or general anesthesia. Since that time, significant improvements in both technique and devices have been made. Currently, five endografts are approved by the Food and Drug Administration (FDA) for EVAR.

This chapter provides a description of the general indications for surgical repair of AAA, the specific indications for EVAR, the various types of endovascular grafts that are currently available for AAA, and the principal techniques used to achieve EVAR.

GENERAL INDICATION FOR AAA THERAPY

At the present time, the same size (i.e., maximal aortic diameter) criteria for open repair should be used for EVAR, as there are no data to justify performing EVAR for smaller aneurysms. In 1966, the first paper discussing the size of AAA as an indication for open repair was published. Measurement on physical examination of more than 6.0 cm was used as a cut-off to proceed with the repair. Since then, extensive studies have been performed to define the standard for management.

There appears to be a consensus opinion, based on estimates of rupture risk with increasing aortic diameter (Table 18.1), that AAA > 5.5 cm should be repaired. Because of this consensus, no randomized controlled trials (RCT) have been performed in this patient cohort.

Although size is a very important factor in predicting AAA rupture risk, there are other factors that appear to play an important role. Each of the following has been found to be an independent risk factor for AAA rupture (3,15,16):

1. chronic obstructive pulmonary disease (COPD);
2. hypertension (HTN);
3. female gender;
4. smoking;
5. symptoms: abdominal or back pain.

Other nonindependent risk factors include:

1. First-degree relatives with AAA (15% to 35% increase rupture risk based on the number of first-degree relatives).
2. The ratio of the AAA diameter to the native aorta diameter.
3. The shape of the aneurysm. Saccular aneurysms have a higher risk than fusiform aneurysm. This is probably related to the significant increase in wall stress with eccentric aneurysms leading to rapid expansion and rupture.
4. The degree of expansion. It continues to be regarded as a significant risk factor for rupture. Aneurysms that enlarge more than 0.6 cm in diameter in 1 year are at a higher risk for rupture, and thus require earlier repair. Smoking, HTN, and mural thrombus are each associated with rapid expansion.

Given the uncertainty regarding the optimal management of patients with aneurysms less than 5.5 cm in diameter, two prospective randomized multicenter studies have been performed in this patient cohort: the United Kingdom Small Aneurysm Trial (UKSAT) (2) and the Aneurysm Detection and Management trial (ADAM trial) (3). Each study prospectively randomized patients ($n = 1090$ and 1136, respectively) with asymptomatic AAAs between 4.0 and 5.5 cm in diameter to undergo early elective open surgery (early surgery group, $n = 563$ and 569, respectively) or surveillance with ultrasonography or computed tomography (CT) scan, every 3 to 6 months (surveillance group, $n = 527$ and 567, respectively). The mean follow-up period for the entire group was 4.6 and 4.9 years in the UKSAT and ADAM trials, respectively. If the diameter of an AAA exceeded 5.5 cm, the AAA expanded by more than 1.0 cm in 1 year, or the patient became symptomatic, surgical repair was recommended. The primary end point was death, and analysis was performed by intention-to-treat.

TABLE 18.1 Estimated Rupture Risk Per Year According to Abdominal Aortic Aneurysm Diameter Alone

Diameter (cm)	Nevitt et al. (8)	Reed et al. (9)	Brown et al. (10)	Scott et al. (11)	Jones et al. (12)	ADAM (13)	Experts Consensus (14)
<4.0	0%	0%	0.3%	0.7%	-	-	0%
4–4.9	0%	1%	1.5%	1.7%	-	-	0.5–5%
5–5.9	5%	11%	6.5%	10%	12%	9.4%	3–15%
6-6.9	—	26%	—	—	14%	10.2%	10–20%
7–8.0	—	—	—	—	—	32%	20–40%
>8.0	—	—	—	—	—	—	30–50%

Both groups had similar cardiovascular risk factors at baseline. At the end of the trial, surgical repair was performed in 90% of the patients in the early surgery groups, and in 60% in the surveillance groups of both studies. Mortality rates did not differ significantly between the two groups at 2, 4, or 6 years. However, the 30-day operative mortality in the early surgery group for the UKSAT was 5.8%, which led to a survival disadvantage early in the trial. In the ADAM trial, the immediate post-operative mortality was significantly lower at 2.7%, but the overall rate of aneurysm-related death in the early surgery group was similar to that in the surveillance group (3.0% vs. 2.6%). Age, sex, or initial aneurysm size did not modify the overall hazard ratio. The conclusion for both studies was that radiographic surveillance with delayed surgery for small AAAs (4.0 to 5.5 cm) is safe, and immediate surgery does not provide a long-term survival advantage.

As a result of these recent findings, the Society for Vascular Surgery Guidelines for the treatment of AAA have been modified. The previous guidelines recommended surgical treatment for an AAA greater than 4.0 cm in diameter. This size threshold has been modified to 5.5 cm (14).

EVAR VERSUS OPEN REPAIR

Short-term Outcome

Intuitively, EVAR seemed to be safer compared with open repair owing to its less invasive nature. However, the EVAR-1 (5) and DREAM trials (4), both of which were randomized trials comparing EVAR and open repair, were pivotal in assessing relative performance of EVAR versus conventional open surgical repair. Both trials randomized patients with AAA that were suitable for both EVAR and open repair. Both trials showed a strikingly similar result, with a one-quarter to one-third reduction in 30-day mortality following EVAR compared with open surgery (EVAR-1: 1.7% vs. 4.8%, DREAM: 1.2% vs. 4.6%, both statistically significant). During the follow-up period, there were many cases of unrelated deaths due to cardiac and pulmonary causes, and death due to cancer. As a result, the overall survival rate was similar in both groups. However, even at 4 years following treatment, the EVAR patients enjoyed a 3% higher freedom from aneurysm-related death, which was unaffected by the aforementioned background noise (i.e., non-aneurysm-related death) (5).

In addition to operative mortality, patients undergoing open repair require several weeks for recovery. Approximately 20%

to 30% of patients suffer from major operative complications including pneumonia, myocardial infarction, intestinal obstruction, bleeding, renal infarction, and peripheral embolism (17,18). Williamson et al. analyzed 139 patients who underwent open repair and found that 36% of the patients were non-ambulatory post-operatively, and 11% required transfer to a nursing home for 4 months or longer post-operatively (18). Furthermore, 80% of patients had post-operative sexual dysfunction.

Based on these favorable results as well as those obtained from observational studies (19), EVAR has become the "default" standard therapy for the treatment of AAA, assuming the anatomy is suitable for EVAR. In fact, it is estimated that more than half of the 60,000 AAA treatments performed per year in the United States are performed with EVAR (17).

Mid-/Long-Term Results

In terms of long-term outcome, open repair has been studied quite extensively owing to its longstanding availability. Although its long-term outcome is very acceptable, it is noteworthy that open repair has not been subjected to the same level of scrutiny that EVAR has been subjected to, and therefore it is highly likely that the late complication rate following open repair is underestimated. For example, in a recent study by Conrad et al., only 57% of the 269 open cases underwent follow-up radiologic studies (i.e., CT or magnetic resonance imaging [MRI]) (20). Keeping this in mind, the reported need for secondary procedures following open repair ranges between 3% and 15%, during 5 to 10 years follow-up (20-22). In order to assure accuracy and minimize the "lost to follow-up" rate, Hallett et al. conducted a survey including only those patients who lived near the hospital (21). This study reported that 9.4% of patients had complications related to open repair or the aortic graft during a mean follow-up period of 5.8 years. Late complications following open repair include graft infection, para-anastomotic aneurysms, aortoenteric fistula, graft thrombosis, ileus, and incisional hernia (20-22). Although the incidence of such complications may not be alarmingly high, once they occur, the operation for treating them is often difficult, and the mortality rate accompanying a secondary operation has been reported to be about 15%.

Durability has been considered the major limitation of EVAR. In fact, high rates of secondary intervention have been reported. However, it is also true that these poor outcomes were mainly based on studies that utilized either homemade or first-generation endografts. Recent studies have shown that the current generation endografts perform better than these early generation devices. As shown in the EVAR-1 and DREAM trials that utilized second-generation endografts, treatment outcomes have improved. Other evidence comes from the FDA-approved Excluder clinical trial (W.L. Gore & Associates, Flagstaff, AZ) that was conducted in the United States. At 5 years follow-up, there were no ruptures in either the open repair group (99 cases) or the EVAR group (235 cases). As for the rate of major adverse events, the EVAR group had a sustained benefit at 5 years compared with the open repair group. In addition, stent migration (clinically relevant), stent fracture, and limb thrombosis were not seen at all.

One unique aspect of late failures following EVAR includes the fact that secondary intervention can almost always be performed with catheter-based techniques and therefore is very safe and minimally invasive (4,5,23).

The operative mortality for open repair is significantly higher if one of the following factors is present (Canadian Aneurysm Study (24), UKSAT (2)):

1. electrocardiographic changes indicating ischemia;
2. congestive heart failure;
3. COPD with forced expiratory volume in 1 minute (% FEV 1.0 L) of less than 70%;
4. elevated serum creatinine greater than 1.8 mg/dL;
5. age older than 75 years.

The 30-day operative mortality may range between 2% and 50%, based on the number of the above factors present. The presence or absence of these risk factors might be helpful in selecting the appropriate treatment modality.

Morbidity rates are significantly lower with EVAR. The relative reduction in complication rates approaches 30% to 70% (14), and this might be attributed to the significant reduction in anesthesia time, blood loss, and fewer cardiac complications. The reduced invasiveness (i.e., avoidance of the laparotomy and exposure of the retroperitoneal cavity) and smaller incisions (usually limited to groin incisions for access) associated with EVAR result in significantly less gastrointestinal complications and less post-operative pain, allowing early ambulation and oral intake. Reducing anesthetic time, incision pain, and early ambulation ultimately reduces post-procedural pulmonary complications. The end result is shorter hospital stays (6,25). The most striking difference between EVAR and open repair is the remarkable difference in recovery time. Up to 30% of patients with open repair did not recover at 34 months postoperatively, and 18% of patients indicated that they would not have open repair again knowing the recovery process. Sexual dysfunction following open repair approaches 60% to 80% in some studies (7). This is significantly less with EVAR because there is no dissection of pelvic nerves. Even in the case of intentional coverage of the internal iliac arteries, the incidence of post-operative sexual dysfunction is less than 1% with EVAR. Early conversion of EVAR to open surgery has significantly decreased from 10% to 2%, as patient selection has improved, devices have become more sophisticated, and surgeons/interventionalists have become more experienced. Reported late conversion rates are now reported at 1% to 2% per year. Typical causes of late conversion include aneurysm enlargement, device migration, structural graft failure, and late rupture of the aneurysm (23,26). Secondary conversion is associated with higher morbidity and mortality rates. All of these factors make open repair ideal for younger patients who are less likely to have high-risk characteristics for open repair. Bush et al. studied patients who underwent EVAR

but were deemed high risk for open repair (27). They found that outcomes after EVAR were excellent and that the procedure is safe even in high-risk patients. Patient choice remains an important factor in selecting the treatment modality (14).

INDICATIONS FOR TREATMENT OF AAA USING EVAR

Since its first introduction in 1991, EVAR has gained significant acceptance (28,29). However, not all patients are anatomically suitable for EVAR. The critical anatomic elements that determine the suitability of a patient for EVAR include (Fig. 18.1):

1. Patent superior mesenteric artery (SMA) or celiac trunk.
2. An infrarenal neck diameter of <32 mm. This is based on the fact that the graft is typically oversized by 10% to 20%, and the largest graft available has a 36-mm diameter (Cook, Zenith; see Table 18.2).

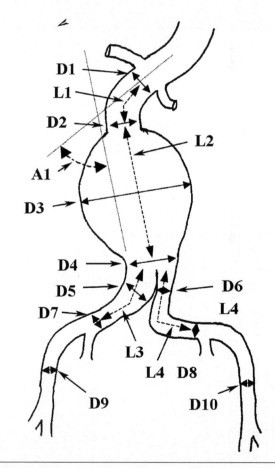

Figure 18.1 • Illustration of diameter, length, and angle measurements made in each patient with an abdominal aortic aneurysm to assess the patient's eligibility for EVAR and also to select the appropriate endograft and the appropriate size of each component of the endograft. These are typically obtained using 3D reconstructed CT scan images. Diameters: D1 and D2, proximal neck of aneurysm; D3, aneurysm; D4, distal neck of aneurysm; D5 and D7, right common iliac artery; D6 and D8, left common iliac artery; D9, right external iliac artery; D10, left external iliac artery. Lengths: L1, length of proximal neck; L2, length of aneurysm; L3, length of right iliac limb; L4, length of left iliac limb; A1, neck angle.

TABLE 18.2 Main Body Grafts

Company	Device(s)	Main Body Length (cm)	Main Body Diameter (mm)	Iliac Leg Length (cm)	Iliac Leg Diameter (mm)	Delivery System Profile OD	Delivery System Profile ID	Fixed Location	Stent Expansion	Stent Material	Graft Material	Markets Available
Cook Medical	Zenith Flex	11.2, 12.5,* 12.6, 14.1, 14.3,* 15.5, 16.1,* 17, 17.9*	22, 24, 26, 28, 30, 32, 36	3.7,‡ 3.9, 5.4,‡ 5.6, 7.1,‡ 7.3, 8.8,‡ 10.5,‡ 10.7,§ 12.2,‡ 12.4,§	8, 10, 12, 14, 16, 18, 20, 22, 24	20, 23, 26 Fr.		Suprarenal	Self-expanding	Stainless steel	Woven polyester	United States, Europe, Asia, Australia, Canada, South America, Middle East, Africa, Japan
Endologix	Powerlink	12, 13.5, 14, 15.5, unibody main size 8, 10	25, 28	4, 5.5	16	21, 22†		Infrarenal	Self-expanding	Cobalt-chromium alloy	High-density ePTFE	United States, Europe, Latin America, Africa, Japan
W.L. Gore & Associates	Excluder AAA Endoprosthesis	12, 13,†,** 14, 15,†,** 16, 17,†,** 18	23, 26, 28.5, 31†	9.5,†,†† 10, 11.5,†† 12, 13.5,†† 14	12, 14.5, 16, 18, 20	18, 20†		Infrarenal	Self-expanding	Nitinol	ePTFE	United States, Canada, Europe, Africa, Asia, Japan, Australia, Latin America, Middle East, South America, India
Medtronic Vascular	AneuRx AAA Advantage	13.5, 16.5	20, 22, 24, 25, 28	8.5, 11.5, 13.5	12, 13, 14, 15, 16, 18, 20 (20, 22, 24 distal flare)	21 Fr.		Infrarenal	Self-expanding	Nitinol	Woven polyester	United States, Latin America, Asia
	Talent Abdominal	14, 15.5, 17	22, 24, 26, 28, 30, 32, 34, 36	7.5, 9, 10.5	8, 10, 12, 14, 16, 18, 20, 22, 24	22, 24 Fr.		Suprarenal				United States, Europe, Middle East, Africa, Asia, Australia, Canada, Latin America, India

*Lengths for 36-mm-diameter grafts only.
†Sizes available outside the United States.
‡Not available in the United States.
§Length for 12- and 14-mm-diameter grafts only.
**Length for 31-mm-diameter graft only.
††Length for 16-, 18-, and 20-mm-diameter grafts only.

3. The length of the proximal neck has to be at least 10 to 15 mm, to allow for a proper seal of the stent graft against the aortic wall.
4. Neck angulation of less than 45 to 60 degrees, since this is associated with a lower incidence of type 1 endoleaks.
5. Calcification and mural thrombus encompassing more than 90 degrees of the circumference of proximal neck is unfavorable (Fig. 18.2).
6. A contour change of the proximal neck of more than 10% is associated with a higher incidence of type 1 endoleaks (i.e., flared neck).
7. The minimal diameter of the external iliac artery should be 6 to 7 mm to allow the passage of the device. The smallest caliber delivery system for the main body of a stent graft in the US market is 18 Fr. (Excluder, W.L. Gore).
8. Distal fixation requires a 10- to 15-mm length of normal vessel in the iliac segment, similar to that required for proximal fixation.
9. The diameter of the common iliac artery (CIA) should be less than 20 mm. If the CIA diameter is greater than 20 mm, an additional cuff is required to extend the stent graft into the external iliac artery following coiling of the internal iliac artery.

These summarize the most common anatomic criteria for a patient to be treated with EVAR. It has been shown that those patients who have unsuitable anatomy do poorly, in both short- and long-term follow-up (30). This is especially true for those who have anatomically unfavorable proximal necks (short, angulated, and wide necks). Thus, we believe that it is of paramount importance to adhere to these anatomic criteria.

PRE-OPERATIVE IMAGING EVALUATION

Computed Tomography

Contrast-enhanced CT is the standard pre-operative imaging modality for EVAR. A high-quality scan can be reconstructed in three dimensions.

The advantages of CT imaging include:

1. The ability to evaluate vessel wall calcification and mural thrombus.
2. Compared with conventional angiography, it is noninvasive, utilizing only a peripheral intravenous (IV) to administer contrast.
3. It enables accurate measurement of all the dimensions needed to perform the EVAR procedure including the diameter, length, and angle of the proximal neck as well as the iliac vessels. If one can utilize the three-dimensional (3D) CT workstation, these measurements will be more precise. A workstation provides a 3D reconstruction of the CT angiogram, and allows one to rotate the images in the sagittal, coronal, and axial axes, and obtain all measurements required for proper graft selection (Fig. 18.3). An additional advantage is that it provides aneurysmal volume measurements, and it shows the precise location and the presence of disease at the orifice of critical branch vessels (i.e., celiac trunk, SMA, inferior mesenteric artery [IMA], renal arteries, and internal iliac arteries).

The disadvantages of CT include:

1. The risk of contrast-induced allergic reaction (1% to 2%).
2. The risk of contrast-induced nephropathy.

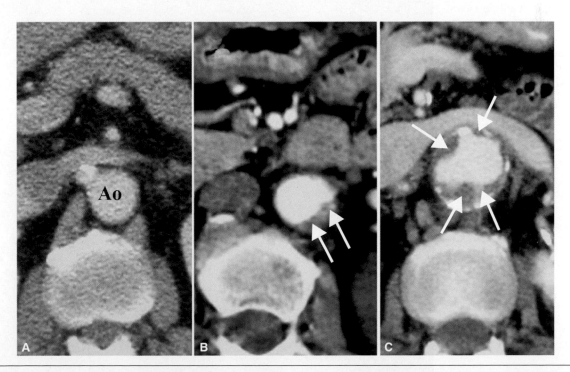

Figure 18.2 • Quality of the proximal neck. **A:** Ideal proximal neck with absence of plaque or mural thrombus (Ao, aorta). **B:** Acceptable neck for EVAR with thrombus *(arrows)* occupying 90 degrees of the aortic circumference. **C:** Illustration of extensive mural thrombus in proximal neck *(arrows)*, which is a contraindication for EVAR.

3. Pitfalls of sizing by CT angiography. A major pitfall of axial imaging using CT is that aortic neck deviation may not be taken into account. As the vessel enlarges, it also elongates, resulting in tortuosity and deviation. This may result in over-estimation of the neck diameter (i.e., when the aortic lumen is oval rather than round) and under-estimation of the neck length. This may be overcome by image processing with curvilinear reformatting, perpendicular to an imaginary line inserted in the center of the vessel lumen. If reformatting is not available, one may estimate the angulation and factor in the extra length. In an effort to guard against an over-estimation of the neck diameter, the minor diameter of the neck should always be used. The authors utilize the Aquarius NetStation (TeraRecon, Inc., Powering Imaging Innovation) to make precise measurements of the length of the neck. This workstation allows simultaneous presentation of 3D volume rendering, multiplanar reconstruction (MPR), maximum intensity projection (MIP), minimum intensity projection (MinIP), RaySum, thick MPR, perspective 3D, and Curved Planar Reformat (CPR) data from the arterial segment of interest. CPR is particularly useful in making measurements of the length of proximal neck, the length from the lower renal artery to the internal iliac artery, and the length of distal neck (Fig. 18.3).

Conventional Angiography

In the vast majority of cases, high-resolution CT scan imaging should be sufficient for thorough evaluation of the anatomy of the AAA, and for accurate graft selection. On rare occasions, pre-operative angiography may be beneficial. However, this can always be performed at the time of EVAR. Pre-operative angiography may be beneficial for beginner interventionists.

The advantages of conventional aortography include better evaluation of aortoiliac occlusive disease and major branch stenosis, including main and accessory renal and mesenteric arteries. However, angiography is not as good as CTA for evaluating vessel calcification, and may not be able to measure the neck diameter accurately, owing to the inability to detect thrombus within the neck.

Magnetic Resonance Angiography

Magnetic resonance angiography (MRA) is an alternative diagnostic modality to CT angiography, with the singular advantage of eliminating the use of ionizing radiation.

The disadvantages of MRA include:

1. MRA is inferior to CT scan in terms of spinal resolution.
2. In 10% to 15% of patients, MRA may not be performed, owing to metal implants that produce artifacts, or patient intolerance due to claustrophobia.

Figure 18.3 • Example of 3D reconstruction of an abdominal aortic aneurysm. **A:** 3D reconstruction image. **B:** Curved Planar Reformat (CPR) presents the abdominal aorta in a straight line, which allows for calculation of the precise length of proximal neck and distal neck. **C:** Axial image. **D:** Multiplanar reconstruction (MPR) image.

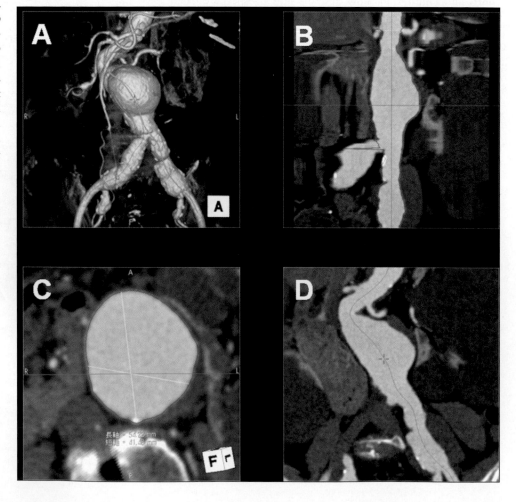

3. MRA is more expensive than CTA.
4. MRA does not demonstrate vessel wall calcification.

Ultrasound

Ultrasound is useful mainly for screening purposes, as it is readily available and is relatively inexpensive. However, it does not provide sufficiently accurate information to allow measurement of critical vessel lengths, diameters, and angulation. It is also highly operator-dependent.

PRE-OPERATIVE CLINIAL EVALUATION

Although EVAR may be performed safely under local or regional anesthesia, one may not be sure that it will be successful. If difficulties are encountered during the course of EVAR, one needs to decide whether to proceed or to discontinue and convert to an open repair. Without knowing the risk of open repair in the individual patient, a sound decision regarding conversion may not be made, and therefore, it is important to perform a thorough pre-operative cardiac and pulmonary evaluation.

Physical Exam

It is important to document the presence or absence of pulsatility in the aneurysm pre-operatively. Once EVAR is performed, an abdominal examination should be performed and compared with the pre-operative exam. This will provide insight into the effectiveness of the aneurysm exclusion. For the same reason, one should document the lower extremity pulse exam prior to any EVAR procedure.

TYPES OF ENDOGRAFTS

The experience with endovascular EVAR had revealed important insights regarding the relationship between endograft design and endograft performance:

1. Small, tapered, and trackable delivery systems ≤20 Fr. in diameter) rarely fail to traverse tortuous iliac arteries.
2. Transmural barbs provide the most secure means of proximal attachment.
3. Modular endografts are more versatile than unibody endografts.
4. Fully stent-supported graft limbs are less prone to thrombosis than unstented graft limbs.
5. Long-trunk/short-limb systems are more stable than short-trunk/long-limb systems.
6. Low-porosity or permeability fabric is associated with lower rates of aneurysm dilatation in the absence of an endoleak.
7. Unpolished (black) nitinol is prone to fracture.

A number of industry-made devices have been approved by the FDA, and have become available in the United States, including the AneuRx (Medtronic, Inc., Santa Rosa, CA), the Zenith (Cook Medical, Bloomington, IN), the Excluder (W.L. Gore & Associates, Flagstaff, AZ), the Powerlink (Endologix, Inc., Irvine, CA), and the Talent (World Medical Corp./ Medtronic, Inc., Minneapolis, MN) stent grafts (Fig. 18.4).

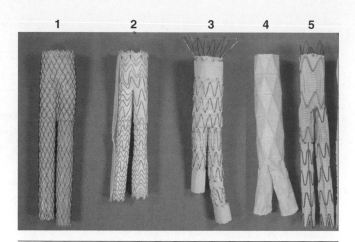

Figure 18.4 • Endovascular grafts (EVGs) approved by the FDA. (1) Medtronic AneuRx, (2) W.L. Gore Excluder, (3) Cook Zenith, (4) Endologix Powerlink, and (5) Medtronic Talent.

DESCRIPTION OF INDIVIDUAL DEVICES APPROVED BY THE FDA FOR EVAR

See Tables 18.2 and 18.3.

AneuRx (Medtronic)

The AneuRx was the first modular device available in the United States. This system has a self-expanding nitinol stent as a fixation device and low-porosity Dacron fabric. It is a modular device composed of a main graft and a separate contralateral limb component (Fig. 18.4). The stent is located on the outside of the graft, which is believed to increase the fixation to the native artery. The chief advantage of this device includes its versatility. The company provides a full line of proximal and distal extension cuffs (12 to 28 mm diameter) that may be used to accommodate a wide range of distal landing zone diameters. Following deployment of the main graft, a contralateral limb is inserted, via the contralateral femoral artery, and deployed. In 2004, an enhanced fabric version of the AneuRx was introduced. Additional improvements included the Xpedient delivery system for accurate and easy deployment, the use of high-density Dacron that eliminates type 4 endoleaks, and availability of larger sizes for treatment of aneurysms with larger diameter proximal and distal landing zones. The outer diameters of the main body and contralateral limb delivery systems are 21 Fr. and 16 Fr., respectively. The AneuRx is suitable for treatment of AAA with proximal aortic neck diameters of 20 to 28 mm, and iliac artery diameters of 12 to 16 mm.

Excluder (W.L. Gore)

The Excluder also employs a nitinol stent as a fixation device and polytetrafluoroethylene (PTFE) fabric. One reason for the difference in sac shrinkage rate following EVAR is the different degree of porosity or permeability of the endograft fabric. The low-permeability Excluder device was introduced in 2004. The additional film layers decreased the overall permeability of the expanded polytetrafluoroethylene (ePTFE) device. It is a modular device, composed of a main graft and a separate contralateral

TABLE 18.3 Ancillary Components

Company	Product	Main Body Extension		Iliac Leg Extension		Aorto-uni-iliac/ Converter		Occulder Diameter (mm)
		Length (cm)	Diameter (mm)	Length (cm)	Diameter (mm)	Length (cm)	Proximal Diameter (mm)	
Cook Medical	Zenith	3.9, 5,* 5.8, 7.3*	22, 24, 26, 28, 30, 32, 36	5.5	8, 10, 12, 14, 16, 18, 20, 22, 24	8, 8.2*	24, 28, 32, 36	14, 16, 20, 24
	Renu	4.3, 5.4, * 6.2, 7.7,* 8.1, 10*		N/A	N/A	9.1, 9.9,* 10.8, 11.3, 11.6,* 12.5, 12.7,* 13.0, 13.3,* 14.4,* 14.7, 16.1*	22, 24, 26, 28, 30, 32, 36	N/A
Endologix	Powerlink	5.5, 7.5, 8, 9.5, 10	25, 28, 34	5.5, 6.5, 8.8	16, 20, 25	N/A	N/A	N/A
Medtronic Vascular	AneuRx AAA Advantage	4	20, 22, 24, 26, 28	5.5, 8.5	12, 13, 14, 15, 16, 18, 20 (20, 22, 24 distal flare)	N/A	N/A	N/A
	Talent Abdominal	2.6, 2.8, 2.9, 3.0	22, 24, 26, 28, 30, 32, 34, 36	7.4, 7.5, 7.9, 8.0, 8.1. 14	8, 10, 12, 14, 16, 18, 20, 22, 24			
W.L. Gore & Associates	GORE Excluder AAA Endoprosthesis	3.3, 4.5†	23, 26, 28.5, 32†	7, 9.5,‡ 11.5,‡ 13.5‡	10, 12, 14.5, 16, 18, 20	N/A	N/A	N/A

*Lengths for 36-mm-diameter grafts only.
†Sizes available outside the United States.
‡Length for 16-, 18-, and 20-mm-diameter grafts only.

limb component (Fig. 18.4). The chief advantage of this device is the small crossing profile, with the main body and contralateral limb being 18 Fr. and 12 Fr., respectively. This has been extremely helpful in treating patients with diseased and/or small caliber iliac vessels. Because the stent graft is flexible, it can be advanced in cases with an extremely tortuous access route and in cases with significant angulation of the aneurysm neck. In addition, the stent is attached to the graft material with thin layers of PTFE rather than sutures, a feature that is thought to result in less endograft failure. The main graft is constrained by an outer wrap, and is deployed by pulling a rip cord that releases the outer wrap. The Excluder does not have an aorto-uni-iliac (AUI) converter (see Fig. 18.12), but two aortic cuffs of the same size are used in the case of a need to convert to an AUI.

Zenith (Cook)

The Zenith is another modular endograft, but unlike the others, it utilizes a stainless steel stent (Fig. 18.4). The Zenith endograft introduced the concept of two docking limb modularity and thus a more user-controlled approach to each attachment site (i.e., aortic, ipsilateral iliac, and contralateral iliac). Also,

it has a large suprarenal stent that is designed to be deployed across the renal artery orifices. In addition, the suprarenal stent has 16 barbs that are believed to decrease the risk of stent migration. Such features may be beneficial in treating patients with shorter necks. In addition, the Zenith has a wide range of iliac diameters allowing treatment of AAAs with large iliac arteries. The US clinical trial has shown an impressive migration (>10 mm) rate of 0% and sac shrinkage/stabilization rate of 98% at 2 years. Fenestrated and branched endografts that can treat pararenal aneurysms are in the pipeline.

The FDA approved Cook's next-generation Zenith Flex® AAA Endovascular Graft in 2004. This system is designed specifically to provide increased flexibility and improved conformability in the aorta and iliac artery.

Powerlink (Endologix)

A more recent introduction to the US EVAR portfolio was the Endologix Powerlink graft, approved for clinical use in the United States in 2004. This graft introduced a variety of unique aspects to EVAR technology. The Powerlink is a unibody bifurcated self-expanding endograft that avoided the complications related to modular limb dysjunction. The endoskeleton is a continuous cobalt-chromium wire woven into a double spine without structures or welds. The endoskeleton is covered with graft material made of ePTFE (Fig. 18.4). Like all endografts, it has a fully stented design, but the stent is on the inside of the graft material and only sewn to the graft at the top and bottom, allowing the graft material to "float away" from the stent in the aneurysmal segments of the anatomy and prevent stent-on-graft erosion. It does not incorporate any hook or barb fixation and migration was a risk in its early use. As experience with the graft progressed, the technique of anatomic fixation was used to overcome this limitation. This technique involves the deployment of the bifurcation of the main body of the endograft onto the bifurcation of the native aorta such that the graft is sitting on the aortic bifurcation. Another advantage of this device is the requirement for only one surgically exposed femoral artery since the contralateral limb can be deployed percutaneously. This feature may reduce the morbidity of an additional groin wound.

Talent (Medtronic)

The FDA approved the Medtronic's Talent™ abdominal stent graft for repairing aortic aneurysms in 2008. This system is made of multiple self-expandable nitinol stents attached with sutures to the inside of a thin Dacron graft (Fig. 18.4). It uses suprarenal bare stents for fixation but has no hooks or barbs. The nitinol stents in the iliac limbs are placed on the outside of the graft. It accommodates 22- to 32-mm diameter aortic necks and 8- to 20-mm diameter iliac arteries. It is delivered via a 20 to 24 Fr. outer diameter main body sheath and an 18 Fr. outer diameter iliac limb sheath. An advantage of this system is its ability to treat AAAs with larger aortic necks.

It is important to become fully acquainted with the respective features as well as the disadvantages of endografts. Some other endografts are available in the European Union (EU), and some trials with new endografts are in progress including the following:

Anaconda (Vascutek Ltd., a Terumo company, Renfrewshire, Scotland);

Aorfix (Lombard Medical, Oxfordshire, England);

Aptus Endovascular AAA Repair System (Aptus Endosystems, Sunnyvale, CA);

Endurant (Medtronic);

Nellix Fillable Sac Anchoring Prosthesis (Nellix Endovascular, Palo Alto, CA);

TriVascular2 (Santa Rosa, CA).

REQUIRED EQUIPMENT FOR EVAR

The vast majority of endograft procedures are currently performed in an operating room (OR) using a portable C-arm digital fluoroscope or fixed type fluoroscope with subtraction capabilities. The rationale for performing the procedure in the OR includes:

1. the need to be able to convert rapidly to an open major surgical procedure when necessary, without any delay;
2. a mandatory sterile environment, as all the devices currently require surgical exposure of the femoral artery, and the risk of graft infection must be minimized;

3. the ability to perform a simultaneous open procedure, such as creation of a conduit for iliac access, or a femoral-femoral bypass in conjunction with insertion of an endovascular graft.

However, with improved endografts accompanied by increased experience, the need for urgent surgical bailout maneuvers has become insignificant, and therefore performing EVAR in the cardiac catheterization laboratory, or an angiography suite with peripheral capabilities and appropriate sterile environment, is a reasonable alternative.

The Basic Setup of the Operation Room

Owing to the improvement in devices and increased experience, acute conversion to open repair is becoming less frequent. However, it is still advisable to sterilize the patient from the nipple down to the upper thigh so that one can perform a laparotomy without delay, if needed. The operator and first assistant usually stand on the right side of the patient, and the monitor displaying the fluoroscopic image is placed so that it faces the operator. The operating table must be radiolucent, and have the ability to be controlled by the interventionist/surgeon. An extension table is attached caudal to the operating table to provide support for the lengthy guidewires and catheters. This extension table may have wheels so that it can simultaneously move with the operating table. Alternatively, a Mayo stand placed at the caudal end of the OR table may suffice.

INTERVENTIONAL TECHNIQUE

Techniques to Obtain Vascular Access

All currently available devices typically require surgical exposure and an arteriotomy, owing to the large profiles of the introducer systems. The oblique incisions are placed higher (i.e., closer to the inguinal ligament) than for a standard femoral-popliteal bypass, and retraction or partial division of the inguinal ligament may be necessary in order to dissect the external iliac artery. This technique is helpful in straightening a tortuous external iliac artery, which is not an uncommon finding in complex AAA cases. In addition, it allows access to a larger section of the iliac artery.

Following arterial exposure, vessel loops are placed around the artery proximal and distal to the puncture site, and around adjacent branches. It is not necessary to dissect the origin of the deep femoral artery. An 18-gauge needle is used to puncture the artery, and a 0.035" guidewire is inserted through the needle. The needle is then removed and an introducer sheath (7 to 9 Fr., 10 to 25 cm long) is inserted over the guidewire. The same steps are repeated in the contralateral femoral artery.

Alternatively, one may perform EVAR percutaneously (31). Although no closure device is designed for closure of puncture sites as large as those of the EVAR delivery systems, by deploying the suture-mediated closure device prior to introduction of the endograft, it may be performed with a reasonable success rate. This technique has been performed using the Prostar XL device, and has been termed the "preclose" technique. Not every patient is a candidate for this percutaneous approach. Patients with small diseased femoral arteries, preexisting femoral artery plaque and calcification, and femoral aneurysms should undergo open access. The advantage of a percutaneous approach is that one can perform EVAR with minimal or no anticoagulation, in addition to the obvious advantage of avoiding a surgical incision.

Aortogram

A marker pigtail catheter is inserted into the abdominal aorta and placed just above the level of the renal arteries. If the catheter is placed proximal to the SMA, the SMA may obscure the right renal artery orifice and the proximal neck. This pigtail catheter should be introduced from the common femoral artery that is contralateral to the side for which the main endograft deployment is planned. One should use a contrast injector that delivers 15 to 20 mL of contrast at a rate of 15 mL/sec. If preoperative angiography has not been obtained, the proximal and distal neck diameter, as well as the length of the required endograft, should be confirmed. As the internal iliac artery arises off the CIA in a posterior-medial direction, a contralateral oblique projection may be used to best visualize the orifice of the internal iliac artery. Alternatively, the authors use intravascular ultrasound (IVUS) to size the proximal/distal diameters and length, as well as checking for other anatomic considerations (e.g., vessel calcification, presence of mural thrombus, and dissection).

Coil Embolization of the Internal Iliac Artery

If the common iliac arteries are aneurysmal and lack an adequate landing zone, one may decide to extend the limb of the graft into the external iliac artery. It is generally believed that bilateral internal iliac artery occlusion carries a risk of colonic

or pelvic ischemia. However, if this may not be avoided, it may be performed with a relatively low complication rate, accepting that buttock claudication will occur in up to 30% to 40% of patients. Coil embolization can be performed at the time of EVAR or it may be performed in a staged manner prior to the EVAR procedure. In order to preserve as many collateral vessels as possible, the embolization coils are placed as close to the ostium of the internal iliac artery as possible (Fig. 18.5).

If the external iliac artery is tortuous, selective cannulation of the internal iliac artery from the ipsilateral approach may be difficult. In such cases, a contralateral approach may be preferred (Fig. 18.5). Achieving immediate and complete cessation of antegrade flow is not mandatory, as antegrade flow will be obstructed by placement of the endograft limb.

Determining the Femoral Access Site for Endograft Introduction

Once the decision to proceed with EVAR is made, a super-stiff wire (i.e., Amplatz Super Stiff wire, Lunderquist wire) is introduced from the side where the endograft is to be deployed. This is performed to straighten any tortuosity in the access vessel(s) and to improve the tracking capability of the endograft. The tip of the wire should be carefully placed, under fluoroscopic guidance, across the arch into the ascending aorta. With the wire in this position, the location of the caudal end of the wire should be marked on the operating table, for future reference. In choosing the femoral access site for insertion of the main body of the graft, several factors should be considered. These include the size, tortuosity, and degree of calcification of the iliac artery. Using the larger, less tortuous, and less calcified

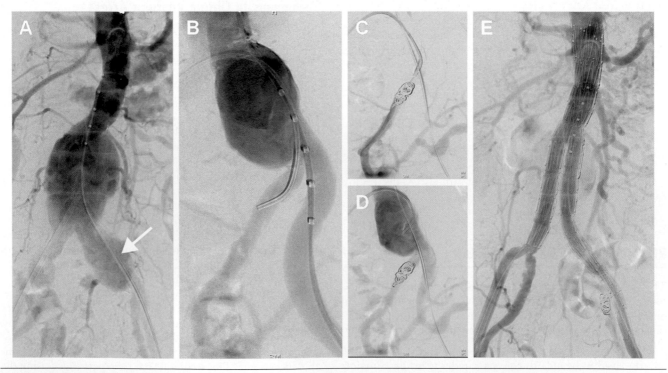

Figure 18.5 • Coil embolization of a left internal iliac artery. **A:** Initial angiogram shows abdominal aortic aneurysm and left common iliac artery aneurysm *(arrow)*. **B:** Selective catheterization of the left common iliac artery is performed via the contralateral approach, using a KMP catheter. **C,D:** Coils were placed at the orifice of the outflow vessel to preserve collateral circulation between distal branch vessels and reduce the risk of buttock claudication. **E:** Completion angiogram.

iliac artery is obviously better. If both iliac arteries have similar characteristics, introduction through the right femoral artery is more convenient.

Introduction of the Endograft

Systemic heparin is administered (usual dose 100 U/kg) prior to insertion of the endograft (Fig. 18.6). The target activated clotting time (ACT) is 250 to 300 seconds. The femoral artery designated for introduction of the main body of the graft is then clamped proximal and distal to the sheath insertion site, and the short sheath is removed. A horizontal arteriotomy is then created in the femoral artery with a scalpel in preparation for insertion of the large sheath containing the main body of the graft.

During introduction of this sheath, difficulties may be encountered for several reasons. First, the iliac artery may be diseased or too small. In such case, balloon angioplasty of the lesion may be helpful. Stenting should be avoided, as insertion of the endograft may dislodge the stent. In addition, the stent may damage the delivery system.

If the difficulty is related to tortuosity, one should use the push-and-pull technique. This is done by simultaneously pulling on the super-stiff wire while introducing the endograft. Having sufficient wire purchase, based on the location of the wire tip in the ascending thoracic aorta, should help the operator perform this maneuver. Alternatively, one may stabilize the tortuous vessel by applying external pressure onto the access vessel of the aneurysm (Fig. 18.7).

If such maneuvers are ineffective, a pull-through method may be effective. After placing a 4 Fr. short sheath in the right brachial artery, the Radifocus guidewire is inserted into the descending thoracic aorta. A snare is then inserted from the femoral artery in order to capture the Radifocus guidewire. The snare is then used to externalize the Radifocus wire out of the femoral artery. By tugging on both ends of the guidewire, the deliverability of the endograft over the wire is increased dramatically (Fig. 18.8).

Finally, a limited retroperitoneal exposure of the CIA may be made to bypass the diseased external iliac artery (Fig. 18.9). A temporary conduit may be made by anastomosing a vascular graft to the CIA, or an arteriotomy may be made in the iliac artery to allow direct insertion of the graft. If persistent difficulties are encountered, and the patient is a reasonable candidate for open surgery, one should also consider the option of performing a standard open repair.

Deployment Of The Endograft

Once the introducer sheath is advanced to the proximal neck of the AAA, an angiogram is performed via the pigtail catheter inserted from the contralateral side, to identify the location of the lowest renal artery. It is important to magnify the image and also to place the renal artery in the center of the image field, to minimize parallax. Also, if there is any anterior-posterior angulation to the proximal neck, the image intensifier should be positioned appropriately (i.e., perpendicular to the neck) (Fig. 18.10). In addition, one should position the image intensifier in the appropriate oblique view to visualize the origin of the renal artery accurately (left anterior oblique [LAO] or right anterior oblique [RAO]). The position of the sheath containing the stent graft is adjusted, based on this angiogram. Each endograft has a unique deployment mechanism, and one should refer to the manufacturers instructions for use for specific details.

Deployment of the Contralateral Limb

For modular endografts, it is necessary to deploy a separate contralateral iliac graft limb. A 7 Fr. sheath should be introduced into the aneurysm sac. This serves to straighten the iliac artery, which allows for improved control of the directional catheter that is used to cannulate the contralateral gate of the main body of the graft (Fig. 18.6B). In general, a single curve catheter, such as the RIM, Vertebral, or Bernstein, is sufficient. An angled

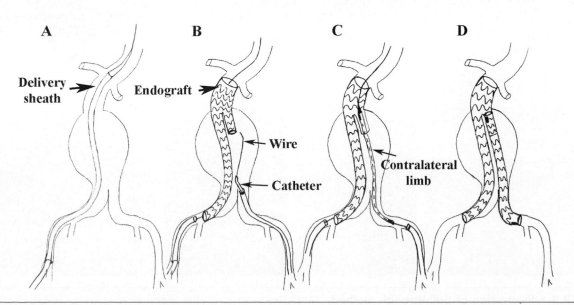

Figure 18.6 • Deployment of the endograft. **A:** Endograft delivery sheath is introduced from the femoral artery. **B:** After confirming that the endograft is in the correct direction (i.e., short limb facing the contralateral iliac) and confirming the location of the lowest renal artery, the endograft is deployed. **C:** Short limb is cannulated from the contralateral side. **D:** Deployment of the contralateral limb completes the procedure.

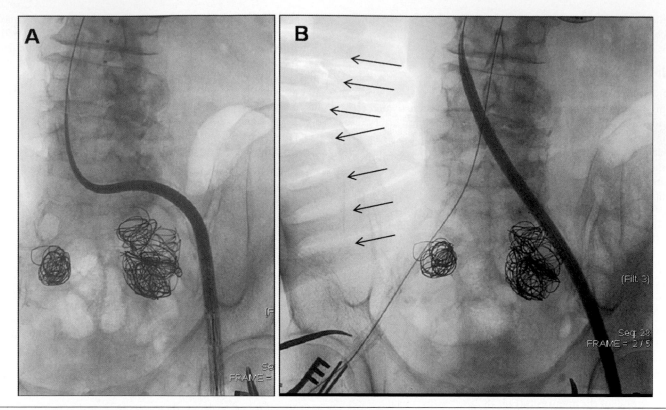

Figure 18.7 • External compression to facilitate stent graft delivery. **A:** Fluoroscopic image shows difficulty introducing the endograft delivery system through the left iliac artery due to vessel tortuosity. **B:** External compression applied on the abdominal wall prevents kinking of the delivery system and facilitates introduction. Note hands *(arrows)* compressing the AAA sac and the iliac artery.

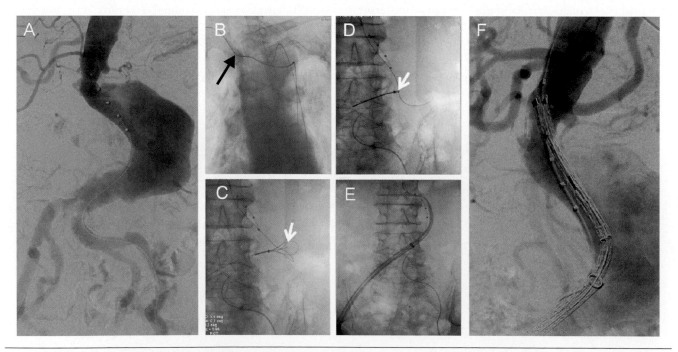

Figure 18.8 • Illustration of pull-through method. **A:** Owing to tortuosity, it was difficult to insert the endograft safely. **B–D:** The Radifocus guidewire *(black arrow)* was inserted from the right brachial artery and grasped by the snare *(white arrow)*, inserted from the ipsilateral femoral artery, and externalized. This "pull-through" method is helpful to facilitate safe introduction of the endograft. **E,F:** By tugging on to both ends of the guidewire, both trackability and pushability of the endograft increase such that the endograft could be delivered successfully.

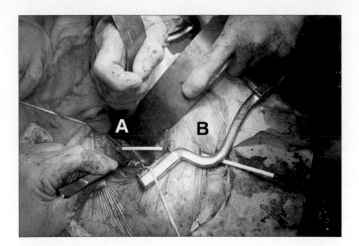

Figure 18.9 • Open iliac access in patient with difficult femoral access. Retroperitoneal exposure of the common iliac artery was achieved and the endograft sheath was inserted directly into the common iliac artery **(A)**. A counterincision made in the abdominal wall avoids kinking of the endograft during introduction **(B)**.

guidewire is used in conjunction with the directional catheter to facilitate this maneuver. In order to increase the chance of contralateral gate cannulation, the directional catheter is placed close to the iliac orifice and away from the short limb of the main body of the graft.

By changing the direction and the position of the catheter, as well as by torquing the guidewire, cannulation of the contra lateral gate may be performed in most cases. However, in some cases, this approach may be difficult and time consuming. As it is easy to lose track of time during the procedure, and as overheating of the portable C-arm fluoroscope may be encountered, it is a good practice to time this step. An alternative approach should be attempted if this step takes longer than 10 minutes. Alternative approaches include the contralateral up-and-over technique and the brachial approach. With the contralateral approach, a curved catheter, such as the SH or RIM catheter, is placed at the flow divider of the endograft and a glidewire is introduced into the sac, where the wire can be snared and externalized from the contralateral femoral access. If it is possible to guide this wire into the contralateral iliac artery, it may be easier to snare the wire in the iliac artery, as opposed to attempting to do so within the sac. In some instances,

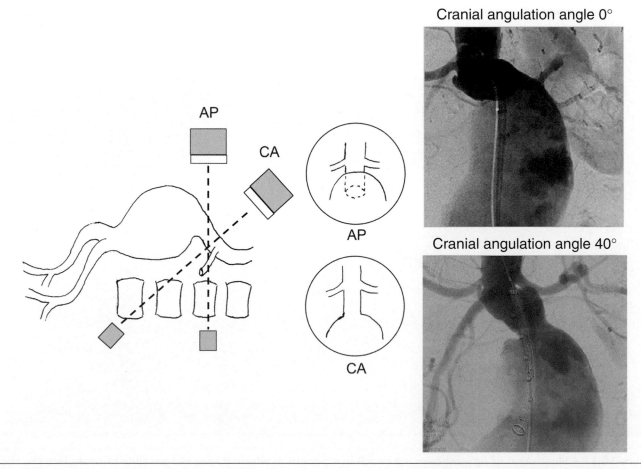

Figure 18.10 • Illustration of appropriate positioning of the image intensifier in a patient with severe anterior–posterior angulation of the aneurysm neck. If the image intensifier is positioned incorrectly (i.e., straight anteroposterior [AP]), one may not appreciate the true length of the neck. Appropriate cranial angulation (CA) provides optimal visualization of the neck without foreshortening.

it is also possible to guide the wire into the contralateral sheath (Fig. 18.11). If one decides to snare the wire inside the sac, the Microvena gooseneck snare (ev3, Plymouth, MN) or the En-snare (MD Tech, CA) is useful.

Once cannulation has been accomplished, it is important to confirm that the guidewire is located within the endograft, and not outside (i.e., in between the proximal stent and the aortic wall). Also, one needs to confirm that the wire has not traversed between the stent and the graft material. A pigtail-type catheter is introduced over the guidewire, and a "spinning test" is then performed within the proximal stent. If the catheter spins freely without resistance, one can be sure that the catheter is within the endograft.

The next step is to deploy the contralateral limb. A final confirmation of the length as well as diameter should be made with an angiogram. The marker pigtail may be used to measure the distance between the short limb of the main body of the graft and the origin of the internal iliac artery. When obtaining this angiogram, it is important to obtain a contralateral oblique view, to visualize the orifice of the internal iliac artery. Also, as it is difficult to obtain another angiogram once the delivery system of the limb is inserted, one should obtain this angiogram with both the short stump and the internal iliac artery within the same field of view.

By doing so, and by marking the two target sites on the fluoroscopic screen, or using the roadmap function, one may deliver and deploy the contralateral limb at the desired position without the need to move the table or the image intensifier. In some instances, it may be impossible to cannulate the short limb and deploy the contralateral limb. This may be encountered when the orifice of the short limb is obstructed, the contralateral iliac artery is occluded, or the distal aorta is too small to accommodate two endograft legs. In such case, use of an AUI converter, followed by creation of a femoral-femoral bypass and occlusion of the contralateral CIA, should be performed (Fig. 18.12).

In cases with a large distal landing zone, one may use the "bell bottom" technique. This is done by deploying an oversized proximal extension cuff at the distal attachment site. In doing so, one needs to terminate the first limb 3 to 4 cm above the landing zone, because the second oversized stent needs some room for it to flare out (Fig. 18.13).

Touch-up Ballooning of the Endograft

Although all the stents are self-expanding, "touch-up" balloon angioplasty should be performed. This maneuver is performed at both the proximal and the distal attachment

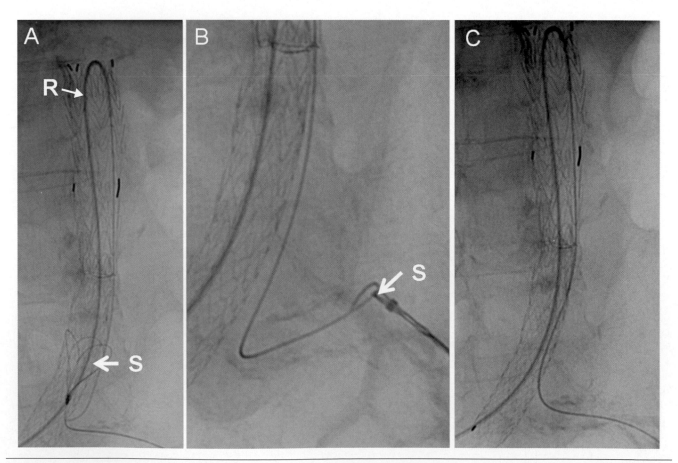

Figure 18.11 • Illustration of up-and-over approach in a patient in whom it was not possible to cannulate the short limb of the main body of the graft from the contralateral femoral approach. **A:** The guidewire is introduced into the contralateral gate from the ipsilateral side with the RIM catheter *(R)*. **B,C:** The snare *(S)* is advanced through the contralateral access and ensnares the guidewire within the sac. The guidewire is then externalized through the contralateral sheath.

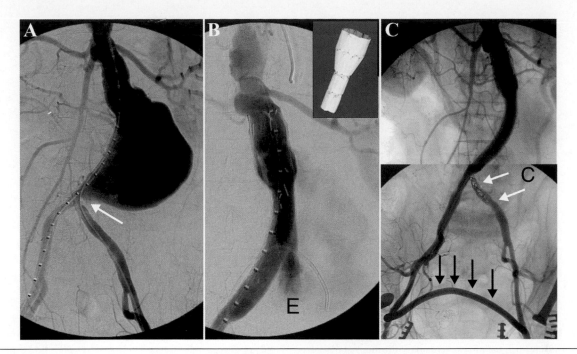

Figure 18.12 • Example of use of aorto-uni-iliac (AUI) converter in a patient in whom it was impossible to access the contralateral limb. **A:** Pre-operative angiogram shows a large abdominal aortic aneurysm with a tight aortic bifurcation *(arrow).* **B:** Contralateral limb cannulation was not possible, due to a lack of space at the aortic bifurcation. Angiography shows an endoleak *(E)* through the short limb. **C:** An AUI converter was placed within the endograft (see figure inset). A femoral–femoral bypass *(black arrows)* was performed and coil embolization *(C)* of the common iliac artery completed the procedure.

sites. Also, any junction of the modular components should be touched up. It is important to use a compliant balloon and to avoid high-pressure dilatation that may damage the endograft and artery. In addition, it is important to introduce the touch-up balloon over a super-stiff wire, and to keep the balloon catheter stationary during inflation. This is performed to prevent downward movement of the balloon as it inflates. This may potentially dislodge the previously deployed endograft distally.

Completion Angiogram

A completion angiogram should be obtained with a power injector. It is important to visualize the late phase, as well as the early phase, in order to detect subtle endoleaks such as small type 1 or 3 endoleaks, or type 2 and 4 endoleaks (Fig. 18.14). The authors perform IVUS within the body of the endograft after the completion angiogram to help detect a wrinkle or a kink of the endograft, which cannot generally be seen with routine angiography. Dissection of the iliac artery is also best detected by IVUS. If a wrinkle or kink in the endograft is detected, further touch-up balloon angioplasty may be effective, while an iliac dissection may require placement of an iliac stent. All the sheaths and wires are removed and the femoral arteriotomy or puncture area is closed with running sutures. In cases with small or diseased femoral arteries, a patch closure of the arteriotomy may be performed.

TROUBLESHOOTING

Diagnosis and Management of Endoleaks

Endoleaks have been classified into five different types (32). The types of endoleaks and their managements are detailed below and in Figures 18.15 and 18.16.

TYPE 1 ENDOLEAK

Type 1 endoleaks arise from the proximal and/or distal attachment sites. Causes of type 1 endoleaks include: (1) undersizing the stent, (2) poor sealing, (3) neck dilatation, (4) stent fracture or separation, and (5) poor patient selection (i.e., those with short, angulated, or irregular aneurysmal necks). If there is a type 1 endoleak, it is generally agreed that the aneurysm is untreated and immediate treatment is required. However, there is one exception. If the endoleak channel is small in diameter and length, one can expect a significant pressure reduction after it thromboses and, therefore, it is reasonable to leave it untreated if it is difficult to treat. If the type 1 endoleak arises from too low a deployment of the graft, deployment of an additional proximal cuff may be attempted. In doing so, one needs to know the length of the graft body (Fig. 18.17; Table 18.2) as well as the length of the cuff, since the distal end of the cuff needs to be placed above the flow divider in the main body of the graft. During this step, it is useful to place a curved catheter on the flow divider to denote its location and to avoid deploying the distal end of the cuff into the ipsilateral limb (Fig. 18.18).

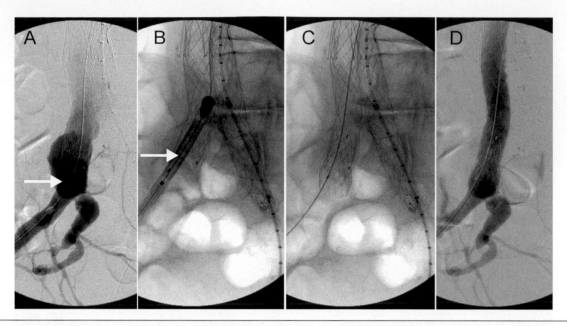

Figure 18.13 • "Bell bottom" technique to facilitate treatment of large iliac artery. **A:** A short main endograft was chosen so that the distal end will terminate 3 cm above the internal iliac artery. Note presence of a distal type 1 endoleak *(arrow)*. **B,C:** Appropriately sized proximal extension cuff *(arrow)* is deployed above the internal iliac artery. **D:** Completion angiogram shows satisfactory result.

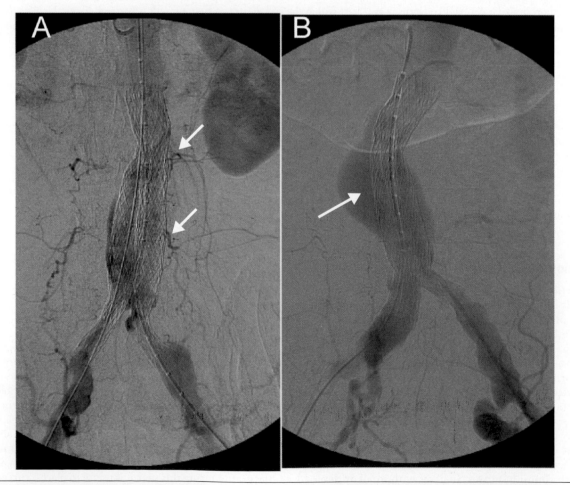

Figure 18.14 • Delayed phase angiogram at completion of procedure may reveal various types of endoleaks. **A:** Type 2 endoleak (note presence of lumbar branches - arrows). **B:** Type 4 endoleak with persistent filling of aneurysmal sac *(arrow)*.

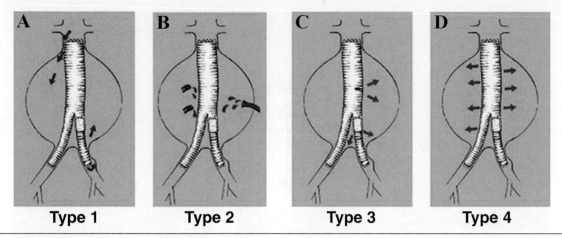

Figure 18.15 • Schematic illustration of various types of endoleaks. **A:** Type 1 endoleak (i.e., peri-prosthetic) occurs at the proximal or distal attachment zones. **B:** Type 2 endoleak is caused by retrograde flow from patent lumbar, inferior mesenteric, or internal iliac arteries. **C:** Type 3 endoleak arises from a defect in the graft fabric, inadequate seal, or disconnection of modular graft components. **D:** Type 4 endoleak is the result of graft fabric porosity, often resulting in a generalized mild blush of contrast within the aneurysm sac. (Reprinted from White GH, May J, Waugh RC, et al. Type III and type IV endoleak: toward a complete definition of blood flow in the sac after endoluminal AAA repair. *J Endovasc Surg.* 1998:5:305–309, with permission from Allen Press Publishing Services.)

If the type 1 endoleak is due to poor apposition of the stent, caused by an angulated or irregular aneurysmal neck, performing additional touch-up balloon angioplasty may be attempted. If this is unsuccessful, deployment of a balloon-expandable stent is usually required. The authors prefer to use the extra-large Palmaz stent (Cordis) deployed with a Maxi LD balloon (Cordis) or a Braun balloon. When doing so, it is important to avoid dilatation of the iliac limb with the shoulder of the large balloon (Fig. 18.19). As deployment of an extra-large stent in a large caliber aorta may be difficult, it is highly recommended to test it outside the patient's body and to learn how the stent expands before insertion (Figs. 18.20 and 18.21).

Distal type 1 endoleaks may be treated in the same manner as the proximal type 1 endoleaks (i.e., with an appropriately sized stent or a cuff).

TYPE 2 ENDOLEAK

Type 2 endoleaks result from retrograde filling of the aneurysmal sac via a lumbar or internal iliac artery, and are more benign compared with type 1 or 3 endoleaks (33). Consequently, the indication for treatment is controversial. However, many agree that those that result in enlargement of the aneurysmal sac should be treated. Treatment options include transarterial embolization, translumbar embolization, and surgical ligation via a laparoscopic or open surgical approach. Owing to its high success rate and minimally invasive nature, the authors prefer the translumbar approach.

The translumbar approach is performed by placing the patient in a prone position. Using fluoroscopic guidance, the location of various bony landmarks, such as the lumbar spine, iliac crest, and the endograft, is outlined on the patient's skin. The location of the endoleak nidus, relative to these bony landmarks, should also be outlined (Fig. 18.22).

An ATLA needle (Boston Scientific Corp.) is used for percutaneous access to the sac. The puncture site should be four-finger breadths lateral to the midline, and the needle should be pointed medially toward the aneurysm sac. If the endoleak nidus cannot be accessed with this needle, then a sheath should

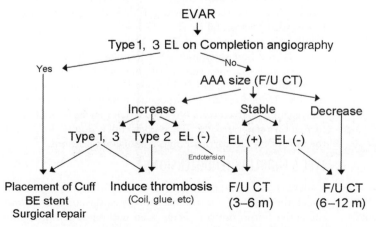

Treatment Strategy for Endoleaks

Figure 18.16 • Summary of treatment strategy for various endoleaks. BE, balloon-expandable stent; EL, endoleak.

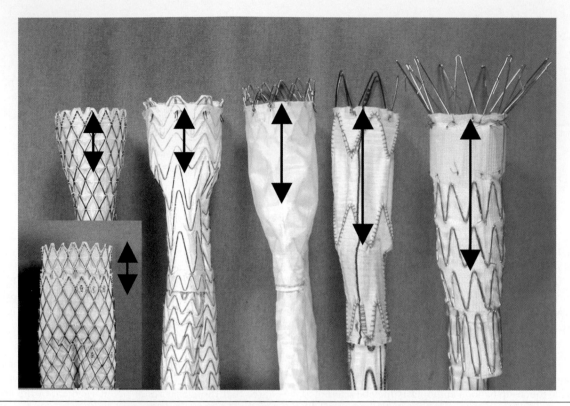

Figure 18.17 • Pitfalls in the deployment of a proximal cuff. Each endograft is available in various body lengths (i.e., length above the flow divider). The body length and the length of the proximal cuff used should be kept in mind when deploying a proximal cuff in order to avoid deploying the distal end of the cuff within the iliac limb and to avoid covering the renal arteries. Inset shows the protrusion of the AneuRx extension cuff from the AneuRx endograft as the cuff is longer than the body of the endograft.

be placed inside the aneurysmal sac and an appropriate directional catheter can then be used. Once the catheter is placed inside the endoleak nidus, an adequate number of coils are deployed to interrupt the communication between the inflow and outflow vessels (Fig. 18.23). It is not necessary to selectively embolize each feeding vessel.

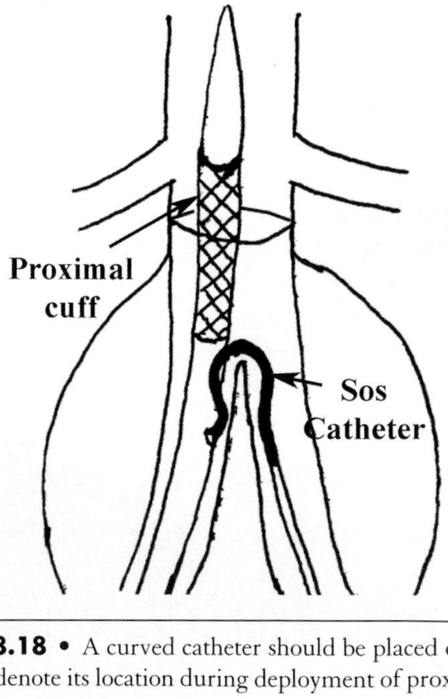

TYPE 3 ENDOLEAK

Type 3 endoleaks result from limb separation or fabric wear. Depending on the location of the endoleak, deployment of an additional cuff may be effective. If the leak is located close to the flow divider, this may be difficult, and either surgical conversion or endovascular conversion to an AUI configuration may be required.

TYPE 4 ENDOLEAK

This type of endoleak is due to the porosity of the fabric material and can be seen following EVAR using grafts with a thin-walled Dacron fabric (Fig. 18.15). The treatment of type 4 endoleaks is controversial. Many believe that the aneurysmal sac will thrombose spontaneously without any clinical sequelae. If one decides to treat a type 4 leak, one of the options includes the addition of cuff(s) inside the graft. If the endoleak is close to the flow divider, it may be impossible to seal it. In this circumstance and if open conversion is needed, it may be better to perform it on a separate occasion, as open conversion performed at the time of EVAR carries a high risk of complications.

TYPE 5 ENDOLEAK (ENDOTENSION)

Endotension (i.e., type 5 endoleak) refers to the circumstance in which the intra-sac (i.e., the space between the aortic graft and the native aorta) pressure is elevated without a demonstrable

Figure 18.18 • A curved catheter should be placed on the flow divider to denote its location during deployment of proximal cuff.

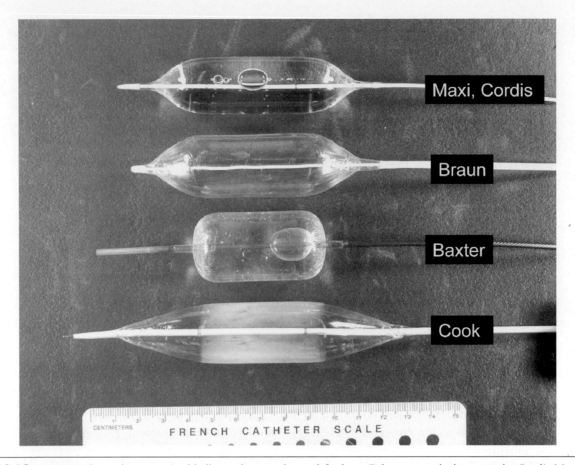

Figure 18.19 • Various large diameter-sized balloons that may be used for large Palmaz stent deployment: the Cordis Maxi LD, the Braun valvuloplasty balloon, the Edwards balloon, and Cook balloon. Note the difference in the length of the shoulders.

endoleak, as seen on a delayed-contrast CT scan. The exact etiology as well as the natural history of endotension is unknown and therefore an appropriate treatment strategy has not been established. The possible causes of endotension include missed endoleak, thrombosed endoleak, hygroma, infection, fluid accumulation caused by hyperosmolarity, and transgraft flow (Fig. 18.24).

Iliac Artery Injury

Dissection and perforation of the access vessel is becoming increasingly less frequent, as a result of the development of lower profile, more flexible devices. The treatment is rather straightforward once the diagnosis is made, but one can easily overlook this complication. When obtaining the completion angiogram,

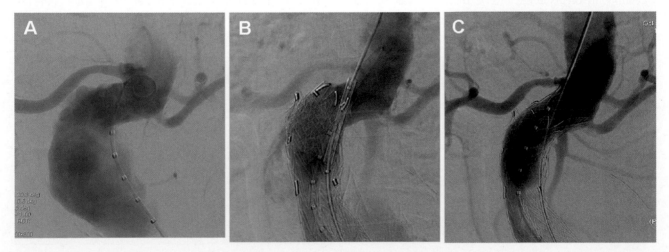

Figure 18.20 • Treatment of type 1 endoleak caused by severe angulation of aneurysm neck. A: Pre-operative angiogram shows severe angulation of the proximal neck of the aneurysm. B: The severe neck angulation resulted in misalignment of the stent and a type 1 endoleak that persisted despite touch-up balloon angioplasty and placement of an additional aortic cuff. C: A large Palmaz stent was deployed within the proximal stent and completion angiography showed a satisfactory result.

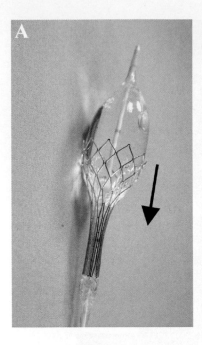
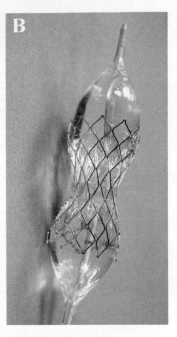

Figure 18.21 • Deployment of a large balloon-expandable (Palmaz) stent and importance of appropriate mounting. **A:** If the stent is not mounted properly in the center of the balloon, the stent may migrate proximally or distally during inflation of the balloon. **B:** Appropriate stent deployment.

the femoral vessels are usually clamped and, therefore, visualization of the external iliac artery is difficult. Prior to removing the guidewires from the access vessels, placement of a 5 to 7 Fr. sheath into the external iliac artery is recommended, to perform a retrograde injection. If a dissection is detected, placement of an appropriate self-expanding stent may readily treat this condition, so long as the wire is still in place. For iliac artery perforation, deployment of a covered stent is indicated. Temporarily occluding the perforation site with an appropriately sized balloon is essential, while one prepares the covered stent. Either the Viabahn or Wallgraft is preferred, due to its ease of use, flexibility, and the availability of appropriate sizes (Fig. 18.25).

Embolization

Embolization may take place at any step of the procedure. It most commonly occurs in the lower extremity vessels, but may also be seen in the visceral, renal, and internal iliac arteries. As the

treatment of embolization is generally difficult, prevention is of paramount importance. Gentle manipulation of endovascular devices during the procedure, as well as avoiding cases with mural thrombus within the proximal neck or distal thoracic aorta, is advised (Fig. 18.2). Comparing the post-operative status with the pre-operative status of the lower extremity pulses is important in the detection of lower extremity embolization. If lower extremity embolization is suspected, one should proceed with lower extremity angiography and perform any treatment required at the time of EVAR, and before the patient leaves the OR.

Kinking of Endograft Limbs

Kinking may occur as a result of pre-existing iliac artery tortuosity or stenosis. It also may be caused by the presence of a small distal aorta. In such cases, deployment of a self-expanding or balloon-expandable stent is indicated. If the kink is the result of a small distal aorta, a kissing balloon angioplasty should be

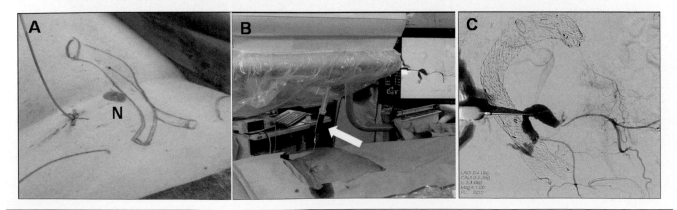

Figure 18.22 • Translumbar angiogram and embolization for treatment of a type 2 endoleak. **A:** The bony landmarks as well as the location of the endoleak nidus *(N)* are depicted on the patient's skin to facilitate needle access of the aneurysm sac and the endoleak nidus. **B:** The needle *(arrow)* is placed inside the aneurysmal sac under fluoroscopic guidance. **C:** Translumbar angiogram of the endoleak nidus shows multiple inflow and outflow vessels.

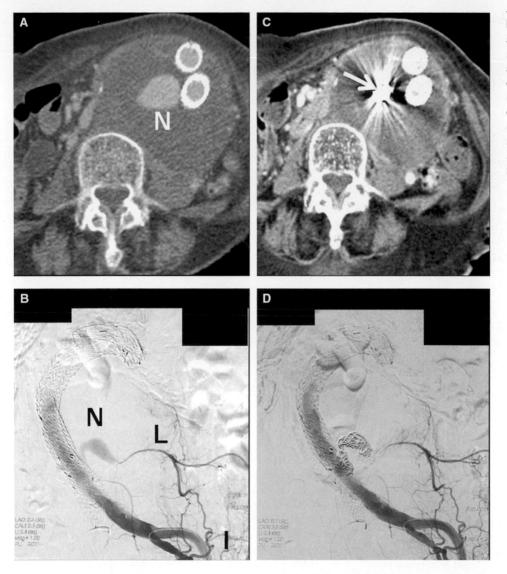

Figure 18.23 • **A:** CT scan shows a type 2 endoleak. A well-defined nidus *(N)* is seen. **B:** Pre-operative angiogram demonstrated a type 2 endoleak arising from internal iliac *(I)* and lumbar *(L)* arteries. **C:** Post-operative CT angiogram. Coils *(arrow)* are visualized within the nidus. **D:** Completion angiogram. Embolization resulted in stagnant flow within the sac.

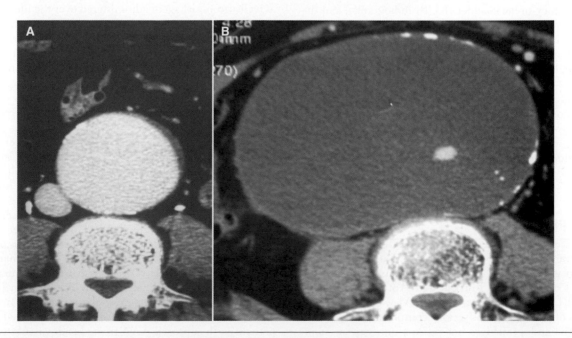

Figure 18.24 • A,B: An example of an endotension (i.e., type 5 endoleak). The aneurysm diameter measured 5.5 cm pre-operatively. Three years later, the aneurysm has grown to 16 cm, without a demonstrable endoleak.

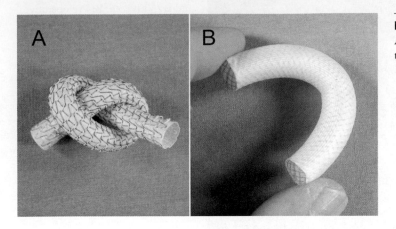

Figure 18.25 • Examples of covered stents.
A: Viabahn endoprosthesis (W.L. Gore). **B:** Wallgraft (Boston Scientific Corp.).

performed within the graft. In some cases, making the diagnosis of a kinked endograft may be difficult, as the angiogram only provides a single-plane image. In such cases, the use of IVUS is extremely helpful. Alternatively, one may perform a pull-back pressure gradient study, after the femoral artery is closed and outflow is re-established.

LATE FAILURES

EVAR may fail in a number of ways, and success in the acute condition does not always guarantee long-term treatment success (7). For this reason, the use of EVAR in low-risk patients who are good candidates for open surgery has been controversial. Owing to the frequent need for secondary procedures, and the continued risk of rupture, lifelong surveillance of these patients has been recommended. In addition to periodic physical examination, various imaging modalities have been used, including CT with intravenous contrast enhancement, MRA or MRI, kidney-ureter-bladder (KUB) radiography, and duplex ultrasonography. If failure is detected, an angiogram may be indicated.

Although late endograft failure and endoleaks have been thought to be the Achilles heel of EVAR, it is noteworthy that most failures following EVAR may be managed endovascularly, and should not always be considered clinical failures. For example, Arko et al. showed that the overall aneurysm-related death was seven times higher following open surgery, compared with EVAR (34). This is related to the reduced peri-operative mortality as well as the fact that secondary procedures following EVAR are relatively benign.

FUTURE PERSPECTIVES

It has become clear from past experience that proximal stent migration is one of the most serious forms of device failure that is often difficult to treat. The Aptus EndoStapling endograft (Aptus Inc., Santa Rosa, CA) was developed in the hopes of preventing this serious complication. The main body of the endograft does not possess unnecessary stents and the fixation of the endograft almost completely relies

on the endostapling device that sutures the endograft to all three layers of the aorta, mimicking surgical suturing of an aortic graft. Miniaturization of the delivery system is also making progress. Cordis (Johnson and Johnson, New Brunswick, NJ) is developing an endograft that can be delivered via a 13 Fr. sheath (outer diameter). This endograft can potentially be delivered completely percutaneously and avoid the need for a surgical cut down. In addition, complications such as dissection or rupture of the iliac artery will definitely decrease as the size of delivery systems gets smaller.

As mentioned earlier, there are several anatomic restrictions in performing EVAR. A short proximal neck is the most common reason to be rejected for EVAR. Fenestrated or branched endografts (Cook) have been developed to tackle those with short or absent proximal necks (i.e., pararenal AAA or thoracoabdominal aneurysms).

One disadvantage of EVAR includes the fact that the patient must be subjected to lifelong radiologic imaging surveillance. The adverse effect of the cumulative dose of radiation as well as contrast agent administered over the life of a patient cannot be underestimated. In order to overcome this problem, a wireless pressure sensor was developed (35). This sensor can be inserted inside the sac but outside the endograft at the time of the endograft procedure. It is hoped that by monitoring the sac pressure, one can reduce the number of imaging studies and detect fatal device failures sooner by being able to measure the intrasac pressure more often than the typical frequency of CT scans.

Despite the significant progress that has been made in transportation, anesthesia, and post-operative care of patients with ruptured AAA, surgical mortality rates still remain high (40% to 50%) and have largely been unchanged over the last four decades. Thus, there remains plenty of room for improvement. Applying EVAR in this setting is an obvious thought, but in reality there are a number of technical as well as logistical problems. In order to overcome these problems, the authors have developed a system that features the following features: (1) permissive hypotension, (2) use of a thoracic occlusion balloon, and (3) use of an endograft that is of one size and fits most anatomies (36). In our limited experience, the mortality rate in an unselected group of patients with ruptured AAA treated endovascularly was 8% and appears to hold great promise.

References

1. Dubost D, Allary M, Oeconomos NA. Resection of an aneurysm of the abdominal aorta: reestablishment of the continuity by a preserved human arterial graft, with result after five months. *AMA Arch Surg.* 1952;64:405–408.
2. The UK Small Aneurysm Trial Participants. Mortality results for randomised controlled trial of early elective surgery or ultrasonographic surveillance for small abdominal aortic aneurysms. *Lancet.* 1998;352:1649–1655.
3. Lederle FA, Wilson SE, Johnson GR, et al. Immediate repair compared with surveillance of small abdominal aortic aneurysms. *N Engl J Med.* 2002;346:1437–1444.
4. Dutch Randomized Endovascular Aneurysm Management (DREAM) Trial Group. Two-year outcomes after conventional or endovascular repair of abdominal aortic aneurysms. *N Engl J Med.* 2005;352:2398–2405.
5. EVAR Trial Participants. Endovascular aneurysm repair versus open repair in patients with abdominal aortic aneurysm (EVAR trial 1): randomised controlled trial. *Lancet.* 2005;365: 2179–2186.
6. Veterans Affairs Cooperative Study Group. Outcomes following endovascular vs. open repair of abdominal aortic aneurysm: a randomized trial. *JAMA.* 2009;302:1535–1542.
7. Lederle FA, Johnson GR, Wilson SE, et al. Aneurysm Detection and Management Veterans Affairs Cooperative Study. Quality of life, impotence, and activity level in a randomized trial of immediate repair versus surveillance of small abdominal aortic aneurysm. *J Vasc Surg.* 2003;38:745–752.
8. Nevitt MP, Ballard DJ, Hallett JW Jr. Prognosis of abdominal aortic aneurysms. A population-based study. *N Engl J Med.* 1989;321:1009–1014.
9. Reed WW, Hallett JW Jr, Damiano MA, et al. Learning from the last ultrasound. A population-based study of patients with abdominal aortic aneurysm. *Arch Intern Med.* 1997;157:2064–2068.
10. Scott RA, Tisi PV, Ashton HA, et al. Abdominal aortic aneurysm rupture rates: A 7-year follow-up of the entire abdominal aortic aneurysm population detected by screening. *J Vasc Surg.* 1998;28:124–128.
11. Jones A, Cahill D, Gardham R. Outcome in patients with a large abdominal aortic aneurysm considered unfit for surgery. *Br J Surg.* 1998;85:1382–1384.
12. Lederle FA, Johnson GR, Wilson SE, et al. Rupture rate of large abdominal aortic aneurysms in patients refusing or unfit for elective repair. *JAMA.* 2002;287:2968–2972.
13. Brewster DC, Cronenwett JL, Hallett JW Jr, et al. Guidelines for the treatment of abdominal aortic aneurysms. Report of a subcommittee of the Joint Council of the American Association for Vascular Surgery and Society for Vascular Surgery. *J Vasc Surg.* 2003;37:1106–1117.
14. Sterpetti AV, Cavallaro A, Cavallari N, et al. Factors influencing the rupture of abdominal aortic aneurysms. *Surg Gynecol Obstet.* 1991;173:175–178.
15. Lederle FA, Larson JC, Margolis KL, et al. Abdominal aortic aneurysm events in the women's health initiative: cohort study. *BMJ.* 2008;337:a1724.
16. McPhee JT, Hill JS, Eslami MH. The impact of gender on presentation, therapy, and mortality of abdominal aortic aneurysm in the United States, 2001-2004. *J Vasc Surg.* 2007;45: 891–899.
17. Williamson WK, Taylor LM Jr, Porter JM, et al. Functional outcome after open repair of abdominal aortic aneurysm. *J Vasc Surg.* 2001;33:913–920.
18. Schermerhorn ML, O'Malley AJ, Jhaveri A, et al. Endovascular vs. open repair of abdominal aortic aneurysms in the Medicare population. *N Engl J Med.* 2008;358:464–474.
19. Conrad MF, Crawford RS, Pedraza JD, et al. Long-term durability of open abdominal aortic aneurysm repair. *J Vasc Surg.* 2007;46:669–675.
20. Hallett JW Jr, Marshall DM, Petterson TM, et al. Graft-related complications after abdominal aortic aneurysm repair: reassurance from a 36-year population-based experience. *J Vasc Surg.* 1997;25:277–284 [discussion 285–286].
21. Adam DJ, Fitridge RA, Raptis S. Late reintervention for aortic graft-related events and new aortoiliac disease after open abdominal aortic aneurysm repair in an Australian population. *J Vasc Surg.* 2006;43:701–705 [discussion 705–706].
22. Ohki T, Veith FJ, Shaw P, et al. Increasing incidence of midterm and long-term complications after endovascular graft repair of abdominal aortic aneurysms: a note of caution based on a 9-year experience. *Ann Surg.* 2001;234:323–334 [discussion 334–335].
23. Johnston KW. Multicenter prospective study of nonruptured abdominal aortic aneurysm. Part II. Variables predicting morbidity and mortality. *J Vasc Surg.* 1989;9:437–447.
24. May J, White GH, Yu W, et al. Concurrent comparison of endoluminal versus open repair in the treatment of abdominal aortic aneurysms: analysis of 303 patients by life table method. *J Vasc Surg.* 1998;27:213–220 [discussion 220–221].
25. Harris PL, Vallabhaneni SR, Desgranges P, et al. Incidence and risk factors of late rupture, conversion, and death after endovascular repair of infrarenal aortic aneurysms: the EUROSTAR experience. European Collaborators on Stent/graft techniques for aortic aneurysm repair. *J Vasc Surg.* 2000;32:739–749.
26. Bush RL, Johnson ML, Hedayati N, et al. Performance of endovascular aortic aneurysm repair in high-risk patients: results from the Veterans Affairs National Surgical Quality Improvement Program. *J Vasc Surg.* 2007;45:227–233 [discussion 233–235].
27. Chaikof EL, Blankensteijn JD, Harris PL, et al. Reporting standards for endovascular aortic aneurysm repair. *J Vasc Surg.* 2002;35:1048–1060.
28. Ahn SS, Rutherford RB, Johnston KW, et al. Reporting standards for infrarenal endovascular abdominal aortic aneurysm repair. Ad Hoc Committee for Standardized Reporting Practices in Vascular Surgery of The Society for Vascular Surgery/International Society for Cardiovascular Surgery. *J Vasc Surg.* 1997;25:405–410.
29. Stanley BM, Semmens JB, Mai Q, et al. Evaluation of patient selection guidelines for endoluminal AAA repair with the Zenith stent-graft: the Australasian experience. *J Endovasc Ther.* 2001;8:457–464.
30. Howell M, Villareal R, Krajcer Z. Percutaneous access and closure of femoral artery access sites associated with endoluminal repair of abdominal aortic aneurysms. *J Endovasc Ther.* 2001;8:68–74.
31. White GH, May J, Waugh RC, et al. Type III and type IV endoleak: toward a complete definition of blood flow in the sac after endoluminal AAA repair. *J Endovasc Surg.* 1998;5:305–309.
32. van Marrewijk CJ, Fransen G, Laheij RJ, et al. Is a type II endoleak after EVAR a harbinger of risk? Causes and outcome of open conversion and aneurysm rupture during follow-up. *Eur J Vasc Endovasc Surg.* 2004;27:128–137.
33. Arko FR, Lee WA, Hill BB, et al. Aneurysm-related death: primary endpoint analysis for comparison of open and endovascular repair. *J Vasc Surg.* 2002;36:297–304.
34. Ohki T, Ouriel K, Silveira PG, et al. Initial results of wireless pressure sensing for endovascular aneurysm repair: the APEX Trial—Acute Pressure Measurement to Confirm Aneurysm Sac EXclusion. *J Vasc Surg.* 2007;45:236–242.
35. Ohki T, Veith FJ. Endovascular grafts and other image-guided catheter-based adjuncts to improve the treatment of ruptured aortoiliac aneurysms. *Ann Surg.* 2000;232:466–479.

CHAPTER 19

Endovascular Treatment of Thoracic Aortic Aneurysms

Karthikeshwar Kasirajan

For patients with descending thoracic aortic aneurysms (TAA), thoracic endografts have demonstrated a dramatic improvement in patient outcome compared with open surgical repair. Dreaded complications, such as paraplegia, have a significantly lower incidence in patients treated with endografts compared with reports from open aneurysm repair (3% vs. 15%), and procedural mortality is also significantly reduced (1,2). However, a new set of complications, largely related to arterial access issues, has been noted that are specific to the use of these endografts. Many of these complications can easily be avoided by careful patient selection, preprocedural planning, and attention to details during the procedure.

There are currently three thoracic endografts approved for use in the United States. Each device has certain unique features, specifically related to the deployment technique. Many physicians view the descending thoracic aorta as a simple, straight tube, and thus surmise that the endovascular treatment of TAA using endografts is technically less challenging than that of infrarenal abdominal aortic aneurysms (AAA). However, the thoracic aorta presents unique challenges that have resulted in a significant time lag between the availability of AAA endografts and FDA-approved thoracic endografts. This chapter summarizes the general principles for performing endovascular repair of TAA, highlighting tips to avoid common pitfalls. Technical steps specific to each unique device are not discussed in detail.

ARTERIAL ACCESS

Arterial access continues to represent a major challenge for endovascular repair of TAA. This is largely based on the requirement for large diameter access sheaths to deliver large diameter devices (Fig. 19.1). The single most frequently encountered complication in thoracic stent graft trials involves the arterial access and conduit iliac vessels. Vascular trauma or thrombosis of the iliac vessels was noted in 14% of patients in the thoracic aortic graft (TAG) phase II muticenter trial, and in 6% of patients in the phase III study (1). Access complications are most commonly encountered when using a 24-Fr. sheath in patients with borderline iliac diameters. Smaller iliac diameters combined with calcification and tortuosity further increase the risk of iliac dissection or rupture. Preoperative planning should involve computed tomography (CT) scans that image caudally to the level of the common femoral artery. Both contrast and noncontrast CT scans need to be evaluated to measure the smallest common femoral and iliac artery diameter and the extent of calcification (Fig. 19.2). Tortuosity is best evaluated with 3D reconstruction of CT data or

conventional angiography (Fig. 19.3). The author typically performs conventional diagnostic angiography with a marker pigtail catheter to supplement CT data.

It is important to watch the sheath move into the aorta at all times under fluoroscopy. The sheath is ideally best introduced over a stiff wire (e.g., Lunderquist or Meier). Additionally, it is important to remember that the vast majority of iliac injuries are noticed during sheath withdrawal. Hence, if excessive force is required to introduce a sheath, an iliac tear may be encountered during sheath withdrawal (Fig. 19.4). If the sheath is not easily withdrawn, it may be advisable to plan for an iliac exposure with the sheath in place or to have an adequate diameter contralateral femoral sheath (12 Fr.) and an aortic occlusion balloon (e.g., Reliant or Coda) readily available to allow for control of aortic inflow, if required. It is also important not to lose wire access as temporary tamponade of iliac injuries may sometimes be achieved by reintroducing the sheath and dilator until a definitive repair is undertaken.

Occasionally, during sheath withdrawal, an intimal flap may be noted to be adherent to the sheath. In these cases, after closure of the femoral arteriotomy, a completion pelvic angiogram using contralateral femoral or brachial access may help in the early identification of an iliac pseudoaneurysm that may result in a delayed rupture (Fig. 19.5). In the event that two or more thoracic endograft devices are required, a long introducer sheath is advisable as this prevents repeated trauma to the iliac/femoral artery during introduction of each subsequent device.

USE OF CONDUIT

As a rule, when in doubt, it is advisable to obtain arterial access through a conduit. Overall, 15% of patients in the TAG (99-01) clinical trial had a conduit to the aortoiliac segment to facilitate access. Iliac conduits are best performed through a left flank incision. The author prefers to use a left common iliac artery conduit, as the left iliac vein is less prone to injury in this location. A 10-mm Dacron graft is sewn in an end-to-side fashion (Fig. 19.6A) and brought out through a stab wound in the lower part of the abdomen (Fig. 19.6B). This allows for a straight and easy access as opposed to introducing the device directly into the common iliac artery. Clamping the distal end of conduit (Fig. 19.6B), and accessing it as though it were an artery, allows for better control of blood loss. This technique allows the physician to make an incision into the conduit only as big as the required sheath. Use of vessel loops, and/or umbilical tapes, around the conduit can also help decrease blood

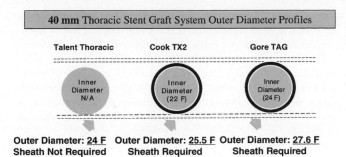

Figure 19.1 • Large diameter introducer sheaths required for the thoracic stent grafts.

loss when the sheath is in place. At the completion of the procedure, the author usually converts the conduit to an iliofemoral bypass. This allows for a ready access site in the event of a need for a delayed intervention in the future.

Occasionally, the common iliac artery is of inadequate caliber and a direct aortic conduit is required (Fig. 19.7). In the author's experience, this is usually only required at the time of visceral debranching procedures or in young trauma patients with traumatic thoracic aortic pseudoaneurysms with small iliac vessels.

DEVICE INTRODUCTION AND PLACEMENT

Regardless of the location of the TAA, it is routine practice to place a stiff wire with the distal tip against the aortic valve to facilitate device delivery. Once guidewire placement has been confirmed on fluoroscopy, the operating room (OR) table is locked in position with the location of the back end of the access wire marked on

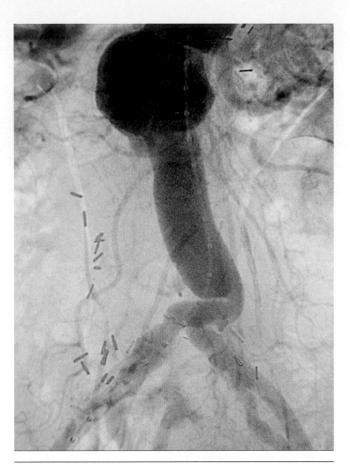

Figure 19.3 • Diagnostic angiogram of abdominal aorta and iliac vessels demonstrates significant iliac limb tortuosity.

the table. Thoracic endografts are available in 20-cm lengths and, depending on the size of the field of view of the imaging system, cannot always be captured within a single fluoroscopic image. For example, if the distal end of a 20-cm graft needs to be deployed immediately proximal to the celiac axis, the proximal end of the graft may not be visualized during this maneuver. Hence, a fixed

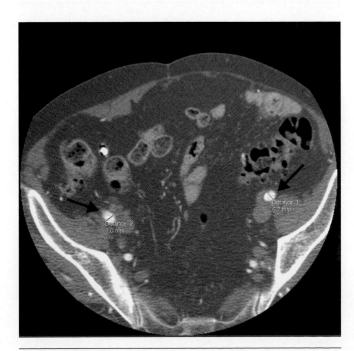

Figure 19.2 • Measurement of external iliac artery diameter from a CT scan.

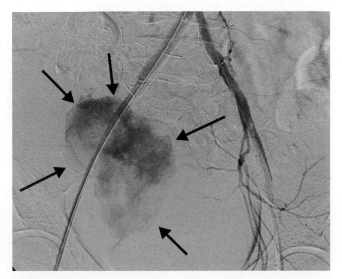

Figure 19.4 • Right external iliac artery rupture noticed after sheath withdrawal.

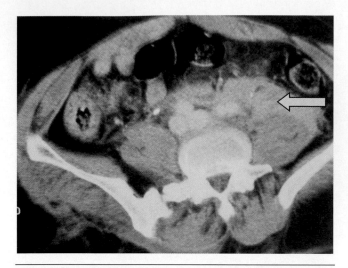

Figure 19.5 • Delayed retroperitoneal hematoma *(arrow)* that developed following a missed iliac artery pseudoaneurysm.

wire position avoids a proximal "unseen" complication that may result from inadvertent distal migration of the guidewire. Loss of wire from the proximal end of the graft may result in the graft folding within the aneurysm and subsequent inability to achieve wire access beyond the graft. Figure 19.8 demonstrates the first portion of a thoracic endograft that has been deployed; it is obvious that loss of guidewire access at this point would result in the proximal end of the stent graft folding within the aneurysm. It is also important to fluoroscopically visualize the leading point of the graft at all times. At no point is it recommended that grafts be moved without visualizing the leading edge.

DIFFICULTY WITH DEVICE TRACKING

Occasionally, the descending thoracic aorta has acute angulation that prevents the device from easily tracking to the desired location (Fig. 19.9). Various maneuvers may help overcome this problem. First, the use of a stiffer wire (e.g., Lunderquist) and placing the wire in as proximal a location (i.e., aortic root) as possible will provide more support. If this does not help, the use of a stiff "buddy-wire" from the contralateral femoral access may help straighten the descending thoracic aorta. Lastly, if these maneuvers are unsuccessful, the use of a "brachiofemoral" wire may prevent buckling of the wire in the descending thoracic aorta ("body-floss" technique). The author's preference is to place a sheath in the left artery using a percutaneous technique with a micropuncture kit. Although right brachial access may be more convenient for the operator, as it is on the same side as the operator, the guidewire is positioned across origin of the right common carotid artery, potentially increasing the risk of an anterior hemispheric event. Thereafter, the author's practice is to snare the wire introduced through the brachial access in the descending thoracic aorta rather than the ascending thoracic aorta, in an attempt to minimize the risk of a cerebrovascular event. In patients with more complicated aortic arch anatomies, a Sos or Cobra 2 catheter may be required to help navigate the wire from the subclavian to the descending thoracic aorta. Once the wire is snared and externalized through the femoral/iliac access, a long 6-Fr. Pinnacle destination sheath is placed across the subclavian–aortic junction from the left brachial location. The externalized glidewire is then exchanged for a Lunderquist wire introduced from the femoral/iliac access over a brachiofemoral exchange catheter. Placement of the Pinnacle sheath across the subclavian–aortic junction minimizes the risk of a possible dissection or tear in the subclavian–aortic junction during these maneuvers. This technique has frequently allowed the device to track across a tortuous descending thoracic aorta by preventing the wire from buckling. If the plan is to cover the left subclavian artery, right brachial access is employed. Occasionally, selective cannulation of the left subclavian artery from the femoral/iliac access and delivery of a stiff guidewire into the left brachial artery has provided enough support to help track a device across a tortuous descending thoracic aorta.

GRAFT DEPLOYMENT

Once the graft(s) of appropriate diameter and length are chosen, the proximal and distal landing zones need to be appropriately imaged to avoid maldeployment. Aggressive oversizing/undersizing can result in fracture, endoleak, infolding, or

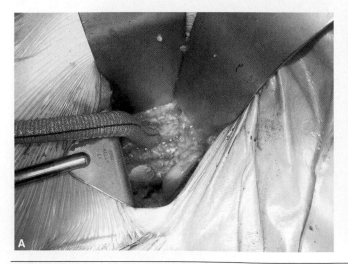

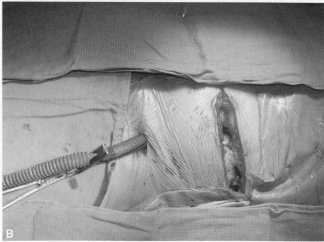

Figure 19.6 • **A:** A 10-mm Dacron graft conduit from the left common iliac artery. **B:** Conduit is tunneled through a stab wound in the lower abdomen to permit a straight access to the iliac artery.

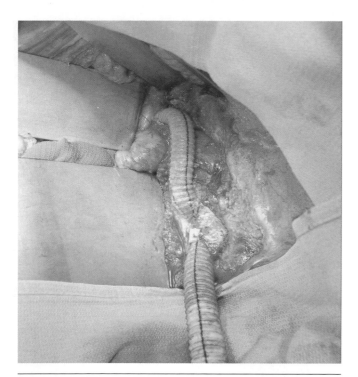

Figure 19.7 • Direct aortic conduit in a patient who had a combined aorto-superior mesenteric artery bypass to increase his distal seal zone.

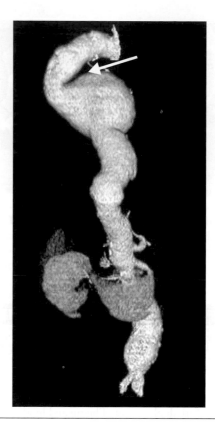

Figure 19.9 • Example of severe aortic angulation seen in a patient with a thoracic aortic aneurysm.

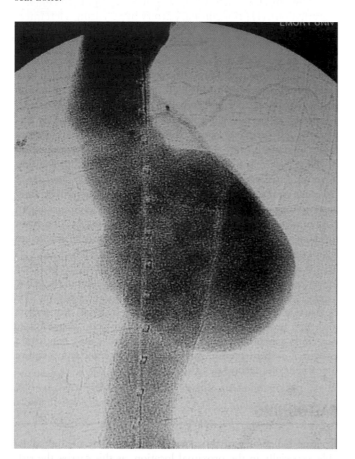

Figure 19.8 • Migration of graft into the aneurysm is prevented by maintaining guidewire access until the second graft can be deployed.

compression of the device (3). It is recommended to closely follow the manufacturers' guidelines (~7% to 18% oversizing).

Multiple devices may be required in the following situations: (1) total length to be treated is longer than the device length available; (2) proximal and distal neck diameters are different and do not fit in the size range of one device; (3) if an endoleak is visible and needs to be treated. If the treatment length is less than 10 cm, proximal and distal neck diameters must be appropriate for a single device, as the shortest device length is 10 cm. It is best to avoid overlapping devices of similar sizes. The author has found this practice to be associated with late device migration and development of type III endoleaks. When using multiple devices (Fig. 19.10), the smaller device is generally deployed first followed by deployment of the larger diameter device into smaller diameter device. Typically, the author upsizes the larger device by 1 or 2 diameter sizes, and uses a minimum of 5-cm overlap between devices, if possible (Fig. 19.10C). If three devices are required, the proximal and distal devices are first deployed and then ballooned, followed by bridging of the gap between these devices with a larger diameter device (Fig. 19.11A–D).

The proximal and distal landing zone lengths need to be at least 2 cm to allow an adequate seal and prevent device migration. In the proximal location, due to the curvature of the aortic arch, this length is best measured along the lesser curvature. Lengths taken along the greater curvature may be inadequate to achieve an adequate proximal seal.

The device is advanced past the target location and brought back to the target landing zone to relieve any stored forward

CHAPTER 20

Endovascular Management of Visceral Artery Aneurysms

Jayer Chung and Ross Milner

VISCERAL ANEURYSMS AND PSEUDOANEURYSMS

Visceral artery aneurysms and pseudoaneurysms are defined as localized arterial dilatations ≥1.5 times the expected diameter of the normal artery. These aneurysms include dilations found in the splenic, celiac, hepatic, superior mesenteric, inferior mesenteric, and renal arteries. Although the true prevalence is not known, autopsy reports suggest that visceral artery aneurysms and pseudoaneurysms have a prevalence ranging from 0.1% to 2% (1). The increasing use of ultrasound and computed tomography has concomitantly increased the incidence of the incidental finding of visceral artery aneurysms. In addition, increased instrumentation of the pancreaticobiliary tract and nonoperative hepatic trauma management has also increased the incidence and detection of visceral pseudoaneurysms (2). Although rare, rupture of these aneurysms and pseudoaneurysms result in mortality rates ranging from 21% to 100% (1).

Historically, management of visceral artery aneurysms consisted of either serial observation, open surgical ligation, or aneurysmectomy (3). However, since the initial reported cases of endovascular repair, endovascular techniques have emerged as a safe and efficacious alternative treatment to open surgical repair. This improved efficacy and decreased morbidity have resulted in preferential utilization of endovascular methods to manage visceral arteries aneurysms and pseudoaneurysms (4) by many vascular surgery and interventional groups. Because the natural history of the visceral aneurysms and pseudoaneurysms is unclear, endovascular repair is particularly attractive in that they allow physicians to avoid the morbidity associated with a laparotomy. Endovascular techniques are continually evolving, but the present mainstays at the time of publication include the instillation of liquid embolization, coil embolization, and, more recently, stent graft exclusion with both balloon-expandable and self-expanding covered stent technology (1–6).

This chapter will summarize the techniques and materials available to interventionalists to exclude visceral aneurysms and pseudoaneurysms. Special emphasis will be placed upon the techniques utilized by our vascular surgery group. Moreover, the chapter will discuss patient selection, periprocedural management and outcomes of the patients, as well as a discussion of intra- and postprocedural complications. The focus of this chapter will be upon splenic and renal artery aneurysms, with brief mention of hepatic and superior mesenteric artery aneurysms and pseudoaneurysms.

ANATOMIC CONSIDERATIONS

The branches of the abdominal aorta are among the most variable in the human body, with some authors stating that less than 25% of the splanchnic vessels studied follow the "classic" course (7). The renal vessels are more consistent, though there are several variations that are important to recognize. Although multidetector computed tomography (CT) with three-dimensional reconstructions will help identify most anomalous anatomy, knowledge of the common variations is vital to accurately localizing and approaching target vessels, and avoiding technical misadventure.

The celiac trunk is present in approximately 99% of patients (7,8). The "classic" description of the left gastric, splenic, and proper hepatic arteries arising from a common trunk is found in 60% to 89% based on cadaveric dissections and review of CT angiographic data (8). The most common variant is the "gastrosplenic" trunk, which occurs in 5% to 8% of patients and is composed of a common trunk for the left gastric and splenic arteries, and a separate hepatic artery that arises independently from the aorta. Other uncommon variants include the hepatosplenic and hepatogastric trunks. Most rarely, the superior mesenteric artery will arise from the celiac trunk (7,8). An important landmark for the origin of the celiac trunk is the top of the L1 vertebral body (7).

The normal hepatic arterial anatomy is present in 70% to 80% of the time (7,9). The most frequent anomaly encountered in the hepatic arterial tree is an aberrant right hepatic artery, arising from the superior mesenteric artery in 12% to 20% of individuals. The aberrant left hepatic artery arising from the left gastric artery is the next most common variant, occurring in approximately 3% of individuals. With respect to the origin of the common hepatic artery, there are two anomalies that the interventionalist should be aware of: (1) an absent common hepatic artery, occurring in approximately 12% of individuals and (2) an anomalous common hepatic artery, arising as a branch of the superior mesenteric artery, occurring in approximately 4% of individuals (7,9).

The splenic artery usually arises from the celiac axis just distal to the origin of the left gastric artery and follows a serpiginous, retroperitoneal path along the dorsal border of the pancreas (1,7,8). Along the way, the splenic artery will provide the dorsal pancreatic branch and several smaller pancreatic branches, before dividing into four to five branches at the splenic hilum. After providing the splenic hilar branches, the splenic artery will then give off the short gastric arteries within the gastrosplenic ligament. The terminal branch of the splenic artery becomes the left gastroepiploic artery, within the gastrocolic ligament (1,7).

The last major splanchnic vessel to be discussed is the superior mesenteric artery. The superior mesenteric artery most frequently arises from the aorta at the level of the bottom of the L1 vertebra (7). Variations in this vessel mostly occur in the colic branches, in the form of either absent colic branches, or accessory colic branches. Otherwise, anomalous origin of the right hepatic artery or the common hepatic artery from the superior mesenteric artery also frequently occurs (7–9).

The renal arteries typically arise within 2 cm of the L1–L2 disc space, with the origin of the right renal artery being typically higher than the left. In three quarters of cases, there is a single hilar vessel supplying each kidney (7,10). Supernumerary arteries are classified as either hilar or polar accessory vessels, with a combined frequency of 24% (10). Bilateral supernumerary renal vessels occur in 5% of individuals. Prehilar branching of the renal artery is frequent, occurring in 8-13% of individuals (7,10).

EPIDEMIOLOGY, CLINICAL PRESENTATIONS, AND INDICATIONS FOR INTERVENTION

Splenic Artery Aneurysms

Splenic artery aneurysms have the highest prevalence among visceral artery aneurysms, comprising 60% to 75% of all visceral artery aneurysms (1–3,11). The majority (>70%) of splenic artery aneurysms are true aneurysms. Most patients (up to 80%) are female and present in their early sixties (1,11). Presentation with rupture occurs infrequently (<5%), with over 90% of patients presenting with the splenic artery aneurysm as an asymptomatic finding on plain radiograph, CT, or arteriogram (1–3,11). Patients with splenic artery aneurysms are more frequently multiparous (1,11), hypertensive, and obese (11). Other frequent comorbidities include coronary artery disease, hypercholesterolemia, peptic ulcer disease, and cirrhosis. Multiple visceral artery aneurysms can occur in up to one third of patients (1). The most frequent location of visceral aneurysms associated with splenic artery aneurysms include the renal artery (7.4%) and extrahepatic hepatic

artery (2.3%) (11). Although arteriography remains the gold standard for diagnosis, CT angiography has evolved sufficiently to allow the diagnosis to be made by CT angiogram alone, with arteriography reserved for patients undergoing a planned repair of the aneurysm (1).

The largest series of splenic artery aneurysms was published by Abbas et al. (11) who reported a retrospective single-center experience of 217 consecutive splenic artery aneurysms over 18 years. The vast majority (95%) of splenic artery aneurysms were solitary. Ruptured splenic artery aneurysms were larger, particularly in males, with a mean diameter at rupture of 3.1 cm, versus 2.2 cm for nonruptured. The mean aneurysm diameter at the time of repair for elective aneurysms was 2.7 cm. Mean aneurysm growth rate was 0.06 cm/year. Mortality for a ruptured aneurysm was 20% in their series, whereas the mortality after an electively repaired splenic artery aneurysm was 5.1%. Among pregnant patients, the rates of maternal mortality (>20%) and fetal mortality (>90%) were extraordinarily high in those with rupture. Because of the high mortality associated with rupture, intervention is recommended for all patients presenting with symptomatic aneurysms, those women with aneurysms discovered during pregnancy or of childbearing age, and those discovered incidentally in a patient undergoing evaluation for liver transplantation (1,11). Abbas et al. (11) recommend treatment for splenic artery aneurysms greater than 2 cm in patients who are "reasonable" operative candidates with a ≥2 year life expectancy.

Operative options include ligation (open or laparoscopic) or resection and reanastamosis (Figs. 20.1 and 20.2). Both operative techniques may or may not include a splenectomy or distal pancreatectomy (1,11). Endovascular options include embolization (glue or coil) and/or exclusion using a covered stent (1–4,11). Although there are some that preferentially utilize endovascular methods of repair (3,4), open surgical repair is still the gold standard, with endovascular options being reserved for high-risk surgical patients (11). Moreover, some series report a high incidence of splenic and pancreatic tail infarcts with embolization of distal splenic artery aneurysms at the hilum and recommend open surgical repair for these patients (3).

Pregnancy is not a contraindication to endovascular repair; however, the risks of catheter-based intervention

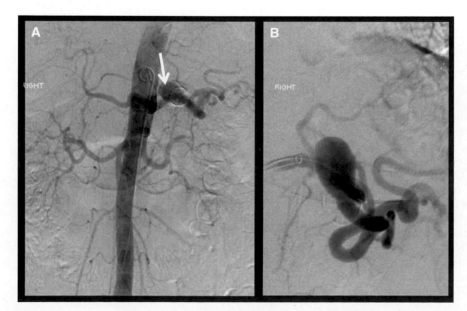

Figure 20.1 • Abdominal aortogram and selective splenic arteriography for treatment planning. **A** reveals a splenic artery aneurysm as demonstrated on AP abdominal aortic imaging. The white arrow is directed toward the calcified appearing aneurysm. **B** is a selective arteriogram of the splenic artery demonstrating the significant tortuosity that can make endovascular therapy challenging in this location.

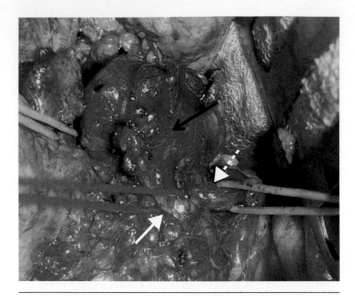

Figure 20.2 • Intraoperative photograph prior to resection of a splenic artery aneurysm and an end-to-end arterial anastomosis to preserve splenic artery flow. The vessel loop has been placed on the proximal artery *(solid white arrow)*. An additional vessel loop has been placed on the vessel distal to the aneurysm and proximal to the hilum of the spleen *(interrupted white arrow)*. The *black arrow* shows the saccular-like aneurysm prior to resection.

during pregnancy (i.e., radiation and iodinated contrast) must be weighed against the risk of conservative management. The maximum allowed fetal dose of radiation is 5 rad, with the most critical time being between 10 and 17 weeks of gestation, where central nervous system development is most prolific (12). During pregnancy, iodinated contrast does not show any adverse teratogenic effects, though there is the potential to suppress neonatal thyroid function. Therefore, it is recommended that thyroid function be evaluated during the first week of life (13). If a pregnant patient presents with a ruptured splenic artery aneurysm, however, celiotomy (incision into the abdominal cavity) is recommended so that an emergent caesarean section can be attempted (11).

Renal Artery Aneurysms

Renal artery aneurysms are also rare, occurring in approximately 0.09% of the population (14). Most patients are multiparous women in their early fifties (14), though patients presenting for repair are typically a decade older (15). Frequent comorbid conditions include fibromuscular dysplasia, atherosclerotic disease, chronic obstructive pulmonary disease, tobacco abuse, and synchronous aneurysms (14,15).

The largest report of renal artery aneurysms was a single-center, retrospective series of 168 patients (252 aneurysms) by Henke et al. (14). Multiple aneurysms were present in 53 patients and 32 had bilateral renal aneurysms. Mean aneurysm size was 1.5 cm, with almost 80% being saccular. The most common site for an aneurysm was the renal artery bifurcation, with the least frequent site being the proximal renal artery.

The natural history of untreated renal artery aneurysms is ill defined, but sequelae include rupture, renovascular hypertension, and renal infarcts resulting in pain, hematuria,

and renal failure (14). The criteria for intervention also lack precise definition. Generally accepted criteria for repair include size ≥ 2.0 cm, renovascular hypertension, dissection, symptoms (pain or hematuria), and the finding of a renal aneurysm in a woman of childbearing age (14,15).

The gold standard of repair includes open operative management strategies such as aneurysmectomy with arterial reconstruction (bypass graft or reimplantation) or nephrectomy (14). Endovascular methods include embolization (liquid and/or coils) with or without exclusion with a stent graft (5,6,15). Endovascular therapies are technically more difficult, as the embolization of a small renal branch or accessory renal artery may have a significant impact on renal function. Moreover, the renal artery is prone to dissection, making endovascular approaches more challenging and risky (14). While endovascular methods of repair are becoming more frequent with evolving technology and operator expertise, care must still be individualized to the patients' anatomy and comorbidities (15).

Hepatic Artery Aneurysms

Hepatic artery aneurysms account for 10% to 20% of visceral artery aneurysms (1–4,16). Approximately 50% of the aneurysms are pseudoaneurysms, with most of the true aneurysms occurring in the extrahepatic hepatic arteries (1). In contradistinction to splenic and renal artery aneurysms, many of these are symptomatic at presentation, especially pseudoaneurysms (2). Over 20% present with either hemoperitoneum or hemobilia (1). Risk factors for rupture are poorly elucidated, but include a diameter ≥ 2 cm, the presence of symptoms (pain, hemobilia), a history of synchronous aneurysms, and aneurysms resulting from a nonatherosclerotic etiology (1–4).

The mainstay of operative management is ligation with arterial reconstruction (1–4,16). Endovascular approaches include embolization (liquid or coil) of the aneurysm, or stent graft exclusion of the aneurysm. Some patients may be managed with a combination of techniques, such as endovascular embolization of the proper hepatic followed by open splenohepatic bypass with saphenous vein. Typically, endovascular techniques are reserved for high-risk surgical patients, with open surgery still being the gold standard (1).

ENDOVASCULAR PROCEDURAL TECHNIQUES

Although open surgery remains the gold standard for the treatment of visceral artery aneurysms, endovascular techniques have been rapidly emerging as a viable alternative, particularly in high-risk populations. This section will delineate several of the interventional techniques utilized to manage splanchnic and renal artery aneurysms. For all planned interventions, the authors recommend assessing the patient's surgical risk, as intraprocedural complications may necessitate expeditious conversion to an open surgical procedure.

Periprocedural Pharmacology

Typically, patients are not placed on antiplatelet agents preoperatively, unless otherwise indicated for preexisting atherosclerotic disease. Patients are placed upon either aspirin or clopidogrel postoperatively if a stent is utilized to exclude an aneurysm, but not both. The patient is typically given a bolus of unfractionated heparin of 70 to 100 U/kg IV after the long destination sheath has been placed, with additional boluses to maintain an ACT of 250 to 300 seconds. We usually allow the heparin to dissipate without reversal at the end of the procedure with protamine. The authors do not utilize low-molecular-weight heparins during interventional procedures. Direct thrombin inhibitors can be used if the patient has a history of heparin-induced thrombocytopenia. General anesthesia is almost never utilized during these procedures.

Access and Sheath Placement

Virtually all patients are accessed via the right common femoral artery, using the 21-guage micropuncture kit followed by placement of a 5-Fr. sheath. This is followed by the placement of a soft-tipped wire and a flush catheter to the level of the L1 vertebral body to perform an aortogram. The initial aortogram serves to isolate the precise location of the orifice of the desired vessel, as well as to delineate any anatomic variants, and the degree of concomitant atherosclerotic disease that may be present. After the orifice location is isolated, typically the 5-Fr. sheath is exchanged for a 6-Fr. 45-cm angled Pinnacle destination sheath (Terumo Medical Corporation, Somerset, NJ). This sheath is placed to provide (1) a rigid support for the catheters and wires and (2) a large enough inner diameter to allow delivery of a stent, if necessary. For all of the visceral artery branches, a reverse-curve catheter is utilized to select the desired artery. Using a glidewire (Terumo Medical Corporation, Somerset, NJ), the target vessel is selected and a catheter is placed.

Alternatively, if the common femoral arteries cannot be accessed, then the left brachial artery is accessed in a similar fashion as mentioned above. A left brachial cut-down can be useful if a sheath larger than 6-Fr. needs to be placed in the brachial artery, to allow for appropriate closure of the arteriotomy at the end of the procedure. Proximal and distal control can be obtained by encircling the brachial artery with vessel loops. These also help to elevate the artery slightly for better visualization. The puncture site can be later closed with 6.0 or 7.0 Prolene suture.

Embolization

Saccular aneurysms and pseudoaneurysms can be treated similarly with liquid or coil embolization. Ideally, embolization is utilized for lesions with narrow necks (≤4 mm, or with a dome-neck ratio of 2:1). The narrow neck prevents migration of the glue into the parent vessel. After the target vessel is selectively catheterized with the guide catheter, the glidewire is exchanged and we typically place a microcatheter, such as a Tracker-18 (Boston Scientific, Natik, MA) in a coaxial fashion. Typically, the microcatheter is placed in the most dependent portion of the aneurysm. After withdrawing the wire and while slowly withdrawing the microcatheter, glue is instilled into the aneurysm until all blood flow within the aneurysm ceases.

We most commonly utilize *N*-butyl cyanoacrylate (NBCA) (Histacryl, B Braun, Germany), which polymerizes on contact with water, forming a plug in the shape of the vessel in which it is injected, thereby obliterating the aneurysm sac. NBCA is mixed with oil dye Lipiodol (Guerbet,

France), which increases the viscosity of the mixture, and permits the mixture to become radio-opaque. Lipiodol is completely inert with respect to NBCA. We usually use a 3:1 mixture of Lipiodol to NBCA, though this can be altered to modify the viscosity and polymerization time to the clinical situation. Tantalum powder is added so that the mixture can be visualized.

Another liquid embolic agent used by the authors is Onyx (ev3, Irvine, CA), which is ethylene vinyl alcohol (EVOH) dissolved in dimethyl sulfoxide (DMSO). Onyx is available with varying concentrations of EVOH. Lower percentages of EVOH result in lower viscosities of the mixture, allowing it to travel further from the injection site prior to polymerization. Onyx also polymerizes on contact with water. Similar to NBCA, it also forms a cast of the aneurysm it is injected into, thereby preventing blood from entering the sac. It is important to utilize a DMSO-compatible catheter when using Onyx, to prevent polymerization within the catheter itself. Roadmapping is frequently utilized to improve the accuracy of both NBCA and Onyx placement.

Coil embolization can also be performed via selective microcatheters. Similar to the liquid agents, saccular aneurysms with narrow necks are well suited to coil embolization. There are a variety of coils available, with various methods of deployment (detachable, injectable). All of the coil types appear to have similar efficacy. The coils are thrombogenic and are deployed sequentially until the entire aneurysm sac is filled with coils and thrombus or until the aneurysm is completely excluded. Frequently, the authors will utilize a combination of both coils and liquid embolization to effect aneurysm exclusion, particularly for larger visceral aneurysms.

With embolization maneuvers, encroachment of the parent vessel lumen is a risk. A wire is placed distally in the parent vessel beyond the aneurysm, followed by balloon angioplasty, to shape the NBCA or the Onyx away from the parent vessel lumen. Angioplasty can also be helpful in tightly packing coils into the sac, preventing them from protruding into the parent vessel. Stent-grafting or bare metal stents are not required, though they can be helpful if angioplasty alone fails to maintain patency of the parent vessel.

Occlusion of the parent vessel and distal embolization of liquid embolic materials is a known risk. The risk of embolization can be minimized by placing coils distal to where the liquid embolic agents are injected. If embolization or occlusion does occur, the treatment depends upon the severity of end-organ damage. For the splenic artery, expectant management is usually successful in the author's experience. For the renal and hepatic arteries, however, occlusion and distal embolization requires more urgent open surgical revascularization. Open embolectomy alone is typically not effective, nor is intra-arterial thrombolytic therapy. Attempts at angioplasty to recanalize an occluded vessel are seldom successful.

Stent Graft Exclusion

In spite of the development of lower-profile, more flexible devices, stent graft exclusion of visceral artery aneurysms has been infrequently documented in the literature (1–4,6). There are multiple anatomic variables that explain the difficulty of applying this technology in the treatment of visceral aneurysms including: (1) The tortuosity and small diameter of the vessels, particularly the splenic artery, prevent navigation of the device to the desired location. (2) Insufficient landing zones, which increases the risk of covering a vital branch of the parent vessel. In addition, the absence of an appropriate proximal and distal landing zone increases the risk of a persistent type I endoleak following stent deployment and of stent migration. (3) Inability to prevent side branches from filling the sac with a stent graft alone. Limited success has been noted, however, especially with fusiform aneurysms and saccular aneurysms with wide necks, with landing zones of 15 mm on either side of the aneurysm (6).

After obtaining access and selecting the target vessel as described earlier, the authors typically use a glidewire (Terumo Medical Corporation, Somerset, NJ) to cross the vessel where the neck of the aneurysm is located. After wire purchase is gained, a guide catheter is placed across the neck of the aneurysm. Roadmapping is usually used to mark the location of the desired landing zones and make a size determination of the stent required. If no other embolization of the aneurysm is to be performed, a PolyTetraFluoroEthylene (PTFE)-covered stent is required to exclude arterial flow from the sac. The author's greatest experience has been with the Viabahn stent graft (W.L. Gore & Associates Inc., Flagstaff, AZ). After stent placement, balloon angioplasty is performed to ensure optimal apposition of the stent graft on the vessel wall. Balloon-expandable technology (i.e., iCast by Atrium, Hudson, NH or GraftMaster, Abbott Vascular, Santa Clara, CA) can also be utilized and usually requires a smaller delivery sheath that varies according to the size of stent selected (Fig. 20.3).

Endoleaks can occur at the fixation sites (i.e., Type I endoleak). If a sufficient landing zone exists, another slightly larger stent can be placed to enhance fixation and seal. Persistent flow within the aneurysm sac, or a "type II" endoleak, is usually managed expectantly, with serial imaging to assess aneurysm size and flow. If endoleaks at the fixation sites cannot be treated appropriately, or the aneurysm continues to be pressurized, open repair may be required.

Vessel rupture can occur when the stent is not sized appropriately, or if the angioplasty is too vigorous. Treatment of vessel rupture entails passage of a balloon catheter, with inflation in the area of stent placement or suspected rupture. This is followed by placement of a covered stent in the area of rupture. If this cannot be achieved, open surgical repair will be required.

Combination Therapy

Embolization in conjunction with stent graft placement is often required to optimize exclusion of aneurysms while maintaining flow within the main vessel. This technique is particularly useful for aneurysms with wide necks. Liquid embolic agents can be used to augment sac thrombosis and occlude any side branches after a coil has been placed. Typically, the authors will place an appropriately sized bare nitinol stent. A microwire and microcatheter will be then placed through the interstices of the stent to permit delivery of coils and liquid embolic agents. Alternatively, a microcatheter can be placed in the aneurysm prior to covered stent graft placement. After the stent has been placed, the microcatheter can then be used to place liquid embolic agents or coils in the sac. Bilateral femoral punctures are required for the latter technique.

CLINICAL OUTCOMES

Early reports of technical success of endovascular repair of visceral aneurysms were discouraging, with technical success rates of ~ 80% (4); however, more recent reports document initial technical success rates of approximately 98% (2,3). Improved experience and improved liquid embolic agents (NBCA or Onyx instead of thrombin-soaked gelfoam) appear to have contributed to the improved rates of initial aneurysm exclusion. Few intraprocedural complications have occurred (3).

Thirty-day complication rates are infrequent with endovascular repair, but are much higher in patients presenting with symptomatic aneurysms. Overall 30-day mortality ranges from 0% to 8.3% (2–4); however, for symptomatic visceral artery aneurysms, the 30-day mortality rate can be as high as 20% (2,11).

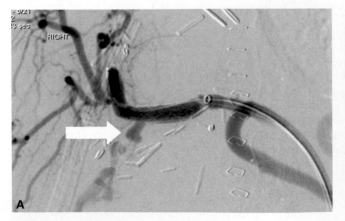
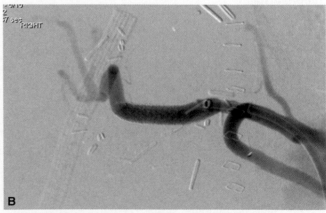

Figure 20.3 • Selective hepatic arteriography as part of the treatment of a hepatic artery pseudoaneurysm. A shows extravasation of contrast at the junction of the proper hepatic, common hepatic, and gastroduodenal arteries. A covered stent graft is in place but has not achieved complete exclusion of the pseudoaneurysm. B shows the pseudoaneurysm to be excluded by the placement of an additional stent graft as well as treatment of the covered balloon-expandable stents with an angioplasty balloon.

End-organ ischemia is infrequently noted in the splenic bed, but is seen particularly in patients treated for distal splenic artery aneurysms. These result mostly in symptomatic splenic infarcts, and occasionally in acute pancreatitis (2–4). Hepatic and mesenteric ischemic complications are rare.

Mid-term clinical outcomes support the opinion that endovascular exclusion of visceral artery aneurysms is a reasonably durable therapy, with only 6% to 12% of aneurysms recanalizing after 6 to 8 months (2–4). Aneurysms that recanalize are often amenable to further attempts at combination therapy, as described earlier (2). Some series suggest there is a slightly higher mortality in the endovascular arm, though there is also a trend toward an increased prevalence of medical comorbidities in patients in the endovascular arms of such studies. There was no statistically significant difference noted in mortality in observational analyses comparing endovascular and open therapies (2–4). Insufficient data exist for outcomes of endovascular aneurysm exclusion beyond 1 year (2–4). Because of the lack of long-term data, but the known risk of aneurysm recanalization, lifelong follow-up imaging is required. Liquid embolic agents, coils, and stents are all radio-opaque resulting in significant artifact on CT scans; therefore, the authors recommend using either ultrasound or magnetic resonance angiography to follow these patients. Typically, patients are followed at 1-, 6-, and 12-month intervals postprocedurally, with yearly studies subsequently.

CONCLUSIONS

Visceral artery aneurysms are rare, though rupture is highly lethal. While open repair remains the gold standard for repair, endovascular exclusions are becoming more rapidly accepted, especially in high-surgical risk populations. Angiography is still recommended to accurately delineate the visceral vascular anatomy. With the rapid evolution in technique, operator experience, and interventional tools (e.g., embolic agents, coils, and stents), making comparisons between endovascular and surgical outcomes is difficult. Early results are encouraging, however, with initial technical success >95%. Follow-up with radiologic imaging is required; however, there is a poorly defined late failure rate.

References

1. Pasha SF, Gloviczki P, Stanson AW, et al. Splanchnic artery aneurysms. *Mayo Clin Proc.* 2007;82:472–479.
2. Tulsyan N, Kashyap VS, Greenberg RK, et al. The endovascular management of visceral artery aneurysms and pseudoaneurysms. *J Vasc Surg.* 2007;45:276–283.
3. Saltzberg SS, Maldonado TS, Lamparello PJ, et al. Is endovascular therapy the preferred treatment for all visceral artery aneurysms? *Ann Vasc Surg.* 2005;19:507–515.
4. Salam TA, Lumsden AB, Martin LG, et al. Nonoperative management of visceral aneurysms and pseudoaneurysms. *Am J Surg.* 1992;164:215–219.
5. Vallina-Victorero Vazquez MJ, Vaquero Lorenzo F, Salgado AA, et al. Endovascular treatment of splenic and renal aneurysms. *Ann Vasc Surg.* 2009;23:258.e13–258.e17.
6. Abath C, Andrade G, Cavalcanti D, et al. Complex renal artery aneurysms: liquids or coils? *Tech Vasc Interventional Rad.* 2007;10:299–307.
7. Valentine RJ, Wind GG, eds. *Anatomic Exposures in Vascular Surgery.* 2nd ed. Philadelphia, PA: Lippincott Williams & Wilkins; 2003.
8. Iezzi R, Cotroneo AR, Giancristofaro D, et al. Multidetector-row CT angiographic imaging of the celiac trunk: anatomy and normal variants. *Surg Radiol Anat.* 2008;30:303–310.
9. Koops A, Wojciechowski B, Broering DC, et al. Anatomic variations of the hepatic arteries in 604 selective celiac and superior mesenteric angiographies. *Surg Radiol Anat.* 2004;26:239–244.
10. Ozkan U, O_uzkurt L, Tercan F, et al. Renal artery origins and variations: angiographic evaluation of 855 consecutive patients. *Diagn Interv Radiol.* 2006;12:183–186.
11. Abbas MA, Stone WM, Fowl RJ, et al. Splenic artery aneurysms: two decades experience at Mayo Clinic. *Ann Vasc Surg.* 2002;16:442–449.
12. Toppenberg KS, Hill DA, Miller DP. Safety of radiographic imaging during pregnancy. *Am Fam Physician.* 1999;59:1813–1818, 1820.
13. Atwell TD, Lteif AN, Brown DL, et al. Neonatal thyroid function after administration of IV iodinated contrast agent to 21 pregnant patients. *AJR Am J Roentgenol.* 2008;191:268–271.
14. Henke PK, Cardneau JD, Welling TH III, et al. Renal artery aneurysms: a 35-year clinical experience with 252 aneurysms in 168 patients. *Ann Surg.* 2001;234:454–463.
15. Hislop SJ, Patel SA, Abt PL, et al. Therapy of renal artery aneurysms in New York state: outcomes of patients undergoing open and endovascular repair. *Ann Vasc Surg.* 2009;23:194–200.
16. Pulli R, Dorigo W, Troisi N, et al. Surgical treatment of visceral artery aneurysms: a 25-year experience. *J Vasc Surg.* 2008;48:334–342.

CHAPTER 21

Endovascular Management of Extra-Aortic Arterial Aneurysms

Albert W. Chan and Christopher J. White

An aneurysm has been traditionally defined as a localized dilation of an arterial segment by more than 50% of the reference diameter (1). Although more than 95% of the arterial aneurysms are located in the aorta, they may develop in any artery of the body. A true aneurysm is one that involves dilation of all three layers (i.e., adventitia, media, and intima) of the arterial wall, characterized pathologically by extensive atrophy of the media. In contrast, a false aneurysm, or pseudoaneurysm, is the result of the disruption of at least one of the three layers of the vessel wall, and blood is contained within the adventitia or by the surrounding tissue. While pseudoaneurysms are mainly caused by trauma, a myriad of etiologies are related to the formation of true aneurysms (Table 21.1).

With the refinement of endovascular technologies, many aneurysms may be managed by an endovascular approach, rather than by surgery. Endovascular therapy has the advantage of lowering morbidity (e.g., perioperative myocardial infarction, infection, prolonged recovery) by obviating the need for general anesthesia, avoiding blood loss, and by reducing in-hospital recuperation time, when compared to surgical treatment. This chapter reviews the contemporary endovascular management of the aneurysms in the extra-aortic vessels.

INDICATIONS FOR REPAIR

In general, the indications for aneurysm repair include (1) symptom(s) caused by the aneurysm (e.g., thromboembolism, compression on surrounding tissues and organs); (2) prevention of impending rupture; and (3) evidence of aneurysm expansion detected by serial imaging studies.

It is important to realize that angiography only provides a lumenogram of an artery, and the actual size of the aneurysm may be underestimated in the presence of a layered, intramural thrombus. Imaging modalities such as ultrasound, computed tomography (CT), or magnetic resonance imaging (MRI) should be performed in order to identify the vessel wall and to provide the actual measurement of the size of an aneurysm.

STRATEGIES OF ENDOVASCULAR TREATMENT OF ANEURYSMS

Many factors should be taken into consideration when determining the appropriate management strategy for an aneurysm. These include the patient's clinical presentation, comorbidities, the location, size, and morphology (saccular or fusiform) of the aneurysm, and the anatomy of the vascular bed involved. The aim of the treatment is to exclude the aneurysmal sac, while maintaining the long-term patency of the parent vessel.

Endovascular strategies for aneurysm repair may be classified into two categories, namely *stent graft* placement (Table 21.2 and Figs. 21.1 and 21.2) and *embolization* (Table 21.3).

Stent grafts exclude the aneurysm and maintain long-term patency of the main vessel. Both self-expanding and balloon-expandable stent grafts are available. For a fusiform aneurysm, the presence of a proximal and distal neck is necessary for successful endovascular repair. The choice of stent graft largely depends on the location of the aneurysm, and the size of the parent vessel. For a large vessel subject to compression or flexion, a self-expanding Wallgraft (Fig. 21.2A) or Viabahn may be used, with a large delivery sheath (Table 21.2).

The Wallgraft endoprosthesis is composed of a stainless steel, monofilament wire, covered by polyethylene (PET) graft material. The Viabahn endoprosthesis is made up of polytetrafluoroethylene (PTFE) lining, with an external nitinol skeleton extending along its entire length. Since a self-expanding stent graft may resist deformation, it is ideally suited for the treatment of aneurysms located in vascular regions that are subject to compression or flexion, such as those in the common carotid artery, proximal internal carotid artery, axillary artery, femoral artery, and popliteal artery (Figs. 21.3 and 21.4). The size of a self-expanding stent graft should be 0.5 to 1.0 mm larger than the estimated reference diameter of the target vessel, in order to minimize shortening of the stent graft, and to ensure adequate apposition of the stent with the vessel wall.

TABLE 21.1 Etiology of Aneurysms

Atherosclerosis/degenerative
Trauma
Vasculitis
Infection
Fibromuscular dysplasia
Chronic dissection
Connective tissue disorders

TABLE 21.2 Various Intraluminal Stent Grafts Available for the Treatment of Extra-Aortic Aneurysms

Type	Delivery System	Guidewire (in.)	Diameter (mm)	Length (mm)
Wallgraft[†]	9- to 12-Fr. sheath	0.035	6.0–14.0	20–70
Viabahn[‡]	7- to 12-Fr. sheath	0.035	5.0–13.0	2.5, 5, 10, 15
Jostent[§]	6-Fr. guide	0.014	3.0–5.0	9, 12, 16, 19, 26
ICAST[**]	6- 7 Fr. sheath	0.035	5.0–10	16, 22, 38, 59

[†]Boston Scientific/Meditech, Natick, MA.
[‡]W.L. Gore, Flagstaff, AZ.
[§]Abbott Vascular Devices, Redwood City, CA.
[**]Atrium, Hudson, NH.

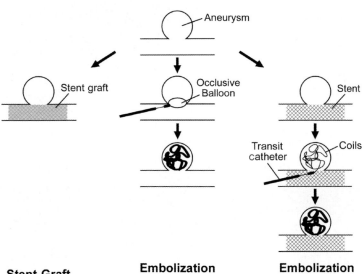

Stent Graft

Embolization without stent

Embolization with stent

A

Figure 21.1 • Schematic diagrams depicting the strategies of endovascular repair of **(A)** a saccular aneurysm and **(B)** a fusiform aneurysm. In **(A)**, the aneurysm may be isolated by a stent graft within the parent artery, treated with embolization coil(s) alone, or bare metal stent placement in the parent vessel and embolization of the aneurysm. In **(B)**, the aneurysm may be treated with a stent graft or a bare metal stent combined with embolization coil(s) within the peri-graft space to induce thrombosis.

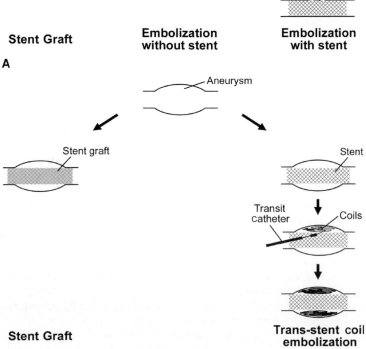

Stent Graft

Trans-stent coil embolization

B

Figure 21.2 • **A:** Wallgraft™. **B:** Jostent™ covered stent.

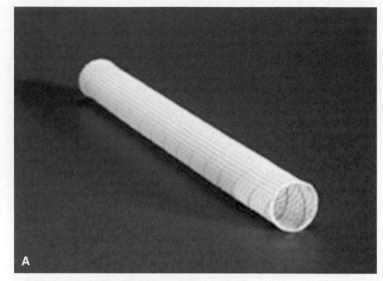

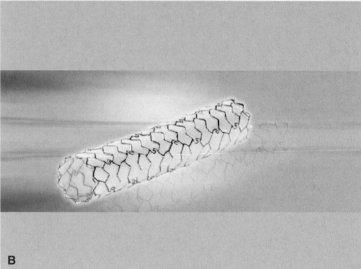

For vessels with smaller diameters (up to 5.0 mm), a balloon-expandable, covered stent (e.g., Jostent) may be used with the advantage of precise stent placement, and immediate exclusion of the aneurysm (Figs. 21.2B and 21.5). The Jostent is constructed by sandwiching an ultrathin layer of PTFE graft material between two stents that are welded at the ends. Recently, pre-mounted Jostents have become available. The diameter of these stents is chosen to match the reference diameter of the target vessel. Occasionally, operators may find it useful to perform intravascular ultrasonography, to determine the reference vessel diameter. High-pressure inflation (12 to 18 atm) should be used to ensure full expansion and apposition of the stent. For aneurysms in larger vessels (i.e., >75 mm) that are not subject to compression or flexion, the iCAST covered balloon-expandable stent offers an important low-profile alternative to self-expanding covered stents.

Before discussing embolization strategies for the treatment of aneurysms, it is worth providing a brief outline of the coils that have been developed for vascular occlusion. Most coils are composed of stainless steel or platinum, with attached Dacron strands to enhance thrombogenicity. The coils are delivered from within a hollow, linear, metal tube (called the loading canula/cartridge) and when released, assume a variety of shapes: straight, curved, helical, or tapered helical (e.g., tornado). Coils are also defined by the diameter of the metal coil (e.g., 0.018″ to 0.052″), the diameter assumed by the unconstrained coil (e.g., 2 to 10 mm), and the linear length of the coil when constrained in its linear form by the loading canula (e.g., 2 to 10 cm).

In general, delivery of the coil is achieved by putting the metal loading canula into the hub of the delivery catheter whose tip has been positioned at the desired location for coil delivery. The coil is then extruded from the loading canula

TABLE 21.3 Embolization Coils and Delivery Catheters That May Be Used for Transcatheter Embolization of an Aneurysm

Coils	Delivery Catheters
Flipper® detachable embolization coil*	Tapered angiographic catheters
Hilal® embolization microcoil*	Tracker® coaxial infusion catheter
Tornado® embolization microcoil*	MicroFerret® infusion catheter
Microplex®ᵠ	Heishima® Microcatheter
Hydrocoil®ᵠ	
GDC® detachable coilᶲ	

*Cook Inc., Bloomington, IN.
ᵠMicroVention, Aliso Viejo, CA.
ᶲBoston Scientific Inc., Natick, MA.
GDC, Guglielmi Detachable Coil.

into the delivery catheter by pushing a wire guide into the proximal end of the loading canula. Continued advancement of the wire results in extrusion of the coil from the distal end of the delivery catheter.

For each coil, the manufacturer provides the recommended minimum and maximum internal diameter of the delivery catheter. Strict adherence to these recommendations is advised. A variety of delivery catheters are available (Table 21.3). The use of polyurethane catheters is discouraged because of the risk of the coil becoming lodged in the catheter. For each coil, the manufacturer will also recommend the appropriate diameter of the wire guide. This will vary from 0.018″ to 0.035″. While certain guidewires are available for use with specific delivery catheters (e.g., Tracker), the stiff end of any appropriately sized wire may be used. Attention to coil sizing during treatment of aneurysms is important. If a coil is too small, there is an increased risk of embolization. Alternatively, using too large a coil will result in the coil remaining elongated, and decrease the likelihood of occlusion of the aneurysmal sac. In addition, the proximal end of the coil may protrude through the neck of the aneurysm, or the interstices of a stent, and provide a nidus for thrombus formation.

Saccular aneurysms may be effectively treated using coil embolization, with or without stent placement in the main vessel. When embolization coils are used, placing a stent within the parent vessel may prevent coil herniation and hence promote thrombogenesis within the aneurysm (Figs. 21.1A,B). For a narrow neck, saccular aneurysm, an occlusion balloon catheter (e.g., Fogarty balloon catheter) may be first advanced into the aneurysm over a directionally controlled guidewire (Fig. 21.1A). With the balloon inflated, the catheter is then pulled back snugly to the neck, to prevent coil embolization. Alternatively, coil embolization may be performed via a microcatheter (e.g., Transit catheter) within the aneurysm (Figs. 21.1A and 21.6).

For fusiform aneurysms, a bare metal, self-expanding stent may be deployed across the lesion (Fig. 21.1B). A Transit catheter may then be placed within the aneurysm, through the stent struts, over a 0.014″ guidewire. The guidewire is then removed, and coils may be deployed into the aneurysmal cavity by pushing with the stiff end of a 0.018″ wire through the Transit catheter. The number of coils needed is determined by the size of the cavity. Attention needs to be paid to avoid disengaging the Transit catheter out of the aneurysm while deploying the coils. The diameter of the coil should be about 1 mm larger than that of the target vessel.

Endoleaks (Table 21.4) occur as a result of failure of a graft to seal an aneurysm completely and are typically classified into four types (see Chapter 18, p 295–299 for full details).

Persistence of an endoleak may result in continuous aneurysmal expansion and rupture. Patients should be followed up with ultrasound, CT angiography, or invasive angiography, to detect the presence of any endoleak after endovascular repair of an aneurysm. The specific therapy for an endoleak will depend on the particular mechanism of the endoleak. (Fig. 21.4).

SPECIFIC CONSIDERATIONS BASED ON ANEURYSM LOCATION

Extracranial Carotid Artery

Aneurysms located in the common carotid artery are usually caused by atherosclerosis, trauma, or post-infectious changes, whereas those in the carotid bulb are most commonly seen after surgical endarterectomy. Carotid aneurysms related to fibromuscular dysplasia (FMD) are usually located in the distal internal carotid artery. The presence of carotid FMD should prompt a search for FMD in other arterial territories, particularly within the vertebral, renal, and intracranial arteries (2). Spontaneous dissections are frequently associated with FMD (Fig. 21.5).

Extracranial carotid aneurysms may be asymptomatic and may only be detectable by palpation underneath the angle of the jaw on physical examination. Occasionally, the lesions may be associated with cervical pain, transient ischemic attacks, or stroke resulting from embolization. Patients may provide a history of invasive tests or cervical manipulation (e.g., insertion of internal jugular venous catheter). Although ultrasonography, CT angiography, or magnetic resonance angiography usually is the initial imaging modality, contrast angiography is often required both for confirmation of the diagnosis and guidance of management. Knowledge of the intracranial vascular anatomy and any associated cerebrovascular obstructive disease or dissection is necessary in order to select the appropriate management strategy.

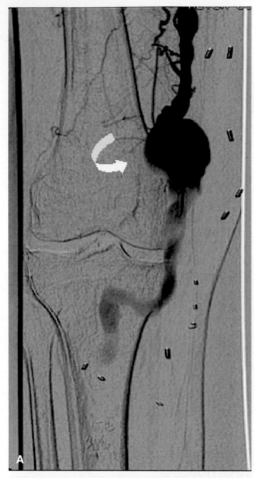

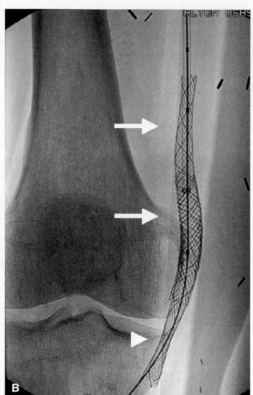

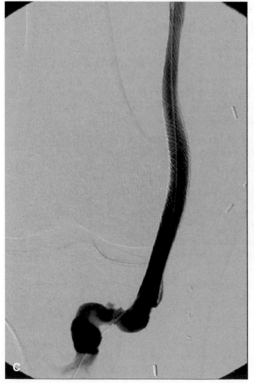

Figure 21.3 • Endovascular treatment of popliteal artery aneurysm.
This patient had a history of coronary artery bypass surgery, ischemic cardiomyopathy, and infrarenal abdominal aortic aneurysm repair with an endovascular graft. Endovascular exclusion of the popliteal artery aneurysm *(curved arrow)* was performed because of multiple embolic events to the foot **(A).** Antegrade arterial access with a 12-Fr. sheath was established in the right common femoral artery. Over a stiff-angled glidewire, two 10-mm-diameter × 70-mm-long Wallgraft stents *(arrows)* were placed sequentially across the popliteal artery aneurysm. Post-dilation with 10-mm-diameter × 40-mm-long balloon catheter was performed. A residual leak was demonstrated on repeat angiography and this necessitated placement of a 12-mm-diameter × 50-mm-long Wallgraft *(arrowhead)* distally followed by post-dilation with a 12-mm-diameter × 40-mm-long balloon catheter **(B).** Final angiogram revealed adequate exclusion of the aneurysm **(C).** Aspirin, clopidogrel, and warfarin were provided after the procedure.

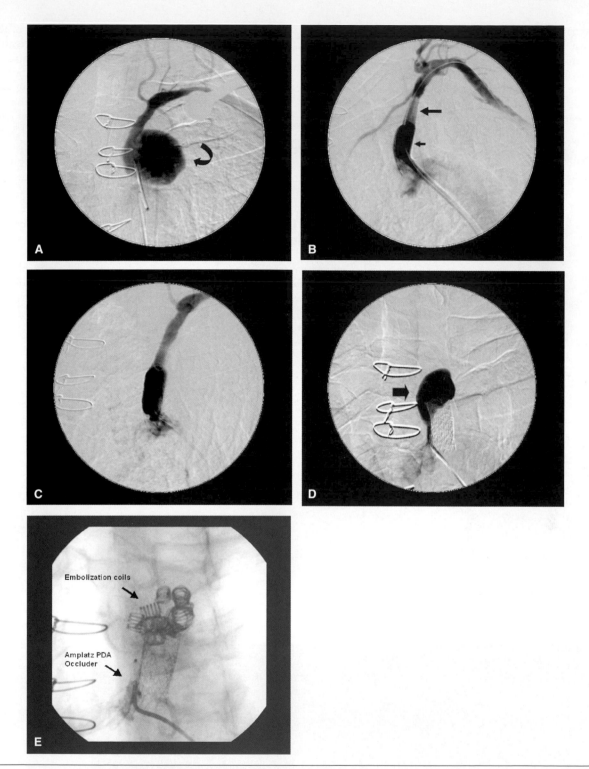

Figure 21.4 • Endovascular repair of left subclavian artery pseudoaneurysm. This 79-year-old man complained of left upper extremity numbness following coronary bypass surgery (involving the use of a left internal mammary artery conduit). He had a history of hypertension and surgical repair of an abdominal aortic aneurysm 20 years previously. A large pseudoaneurysm *(curved arrow)* was demonstrated in the proximal left subclavian artery **(A)**. Via a 12-Fr. sheath inserted through the right common femoral artery, an 11-mm-diameter × 50-mm-long Viabahn endoprosthesis *(large arrow)* was advanced over a 0.018″ Roadrunner wire and was deployed across the aneurysm. Post-dilation was performed with a 12-mm-diameter × 40-mm-long balloon catheter. A 12-mm-diameter × 26-mm-long Intrastent® *(small arrow)* was deployed within the inflow of the covered stent in a bid to seal off the residual leak **(B)**. A year later, repeat angiography revealed a patent subclavian artery and persistence of a large perigraft aneurysmal sac **(C,D,** *block arrow)*. Via a 4-Fr. multipurpose catheter, a total of three Flipper® detachable embolization coils (0.035″ × 5 cm × 8 mm, two 0.035″ × 12 cm × 8 mm), two Hilal® embolization coils (0.038″ × 8 cm × 5 mm), and eight embolization coils (0.038″ × 8 cm × 5 mm) were deployed. An Amplatz PDA® occluder (8 mm × 6 mm) was deployed via a 7-Fr. Shuttle sheath in order to seal the entrance of the aneurysm **(E)**.

The natural history of an untreated carotid aneurysm is not known. In the past, surgical repair was recommended because cerebral ischemia was common, and most patients remained asymptomatic after surgery (3–5). Endovascular repair has become a more attractive approach because it eliminates the use of general anesthesia and the potential complications related to surgery (e.g., cranial nerve palsy or stroke). Percutaneous treatment is the therapy of choice for patients with appropriate anatomic features.

The technique of carotid angiography and choice of guide catheters has been described in Chapter 10. During angiography, it is critical to identify the location of the neck of the aneurysm, in order to ensure successful treatment of the aneurysm. For aneurysms (saccular or fusiform) and pseudoaneurysms located in the common carotid artery or at the carotid bifurcation, coil embolization or stent graft placement has been performed successfully (6–9). The balloon-expandable covered stent, Jostent, has been used for treatment of distal internal carotid artery aneurysms (Fig. 21.5) (10). All patients should undergo ultrasound and Doppler study prior to discharge, and again in 1 month, 6 months, 1 year, and annually thereafter.

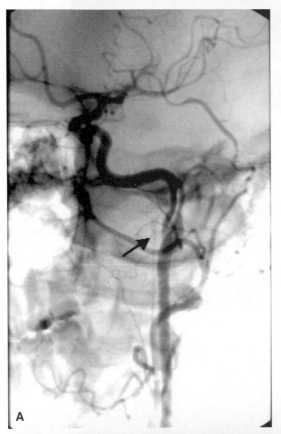

Figure 21.5 • Endovascular treatment of internal carotid artery aneurysm. This 41-year-old woman complained of left-sided tinnitus and right-sided hemiparesthesia. **A:** Angiogram revealed an aneurysm in the distal left internal carotid artery associated with a dissection. Fibromuscular dysplasia (FMD) was evident in the vertebral artery as well as the renal arteries. A 0.014″ BMW wire was placed across the aneurysmal segment (arrow). **B:** Intracarotid ultrasound across the lesion demonstrated simultaneous filling of both chambers with agitated saline contrast ("*" denotes the false lumen).

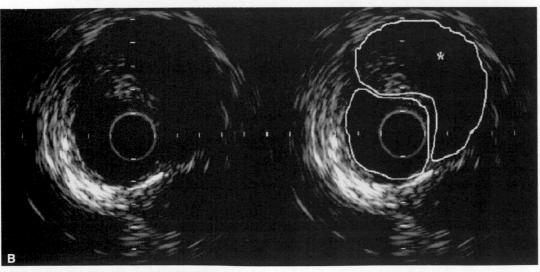

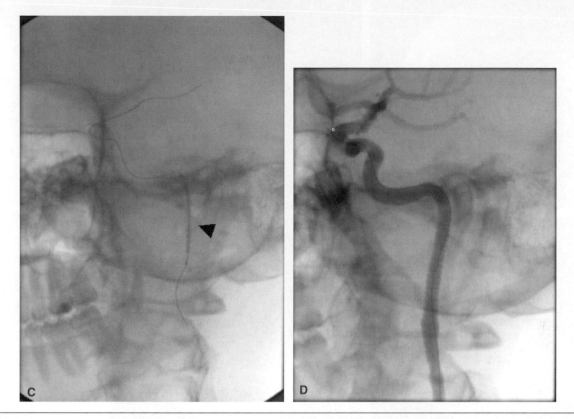

Figure 21.5 • *(Continued)* **C:** The Jostent *(arrowhead)* was placed across the distal part of the aneurysm over a Synchro® Neuro guidewire. **D:** Sequential placement of two Jostent covered stents resulting in complete coverage of the aneurysm and dissection. Symptoms were resolved post-procedure, and the patient was started on daily aspirin and clopidogrel. Ultrasound revealed a patent vessel in 1 year. (Reprint from Chan AW, Yadav J, Kreiger D, et al. Endovascular repair of carotid artery aneurysm with Jostent™ covered stent: initial experience and one-year result. *Cathet Cardiovasc Intervent.* 2004;63(1):15–20. with permission from John Wiley and Sons.)

Vertebral Artery

Extracranial vertebral artery aneurysms are exceedingly rare, and the majority of them are related to trauma. FMD of the vertebral artery can result in a spontaneous dissection and/or pseudoaneurysm formation. Symptoms may range from cervical or occipital pain, to vertebrobasilar insufficiency (e.g., nausea, vertigo, diplopia, hemiplegia, hemiparesis). Coil embolization or stent graft placement may be considered for symptomatic patients. A stent graft is contraindicated if a major side branch (e.g., posterior inferior cerebellar artery) is involved by the aneurysm.

Renal Artery

Renal artery aneurysms (RAA) are reported in 0.1% to 1.0% of all patients undergoing renal angiography (11,12). Bilateral RAA may occur in about 15% of these patients (11,13). They are usually discovered as an incidental finding during imaging studies, but occasionally they may present with rupture (13). RAA may result in secondary hypertension, by causing ischemia stemming from compression of the artery, altering antegrade blood flow, or causing renal infarction arising from embolization of mural thrombus. Pregnancy poses a particular risk for rupture (14). The indications for RAA repair include the presence of symptoms, demonstration of progressive

enlargement, expectation of pregnancy, intractable hypertension, and renal infarction (15). Whether or not the size of the aneurysm should be a factor in determining treatment remains debatable. In the surgical literature, a minimum size of 2 cm in the diameter of an aneurysm has been required by some centers for surgical repair (15–19), whereas others reported that rupture may still occur even when the aneurysm was smaller than 2 cm (20).

Surgical ligation and renal artery reconstruction have been the standard treatment for RAA, but percutaneous treatment has become available in the past several years. Aneurysms in the main renal artery may be treated with coil embolization or implantation of a stent graft (21). Those located in the distal renal arteries may be treated with coil embolization, using microembolization coils (Table 21.3), resulting in small, segmental, renal infarction and elimination of the aneurysm. This may be achieved by advancing a Transit catheter to the target renal artery over a 0.014″ floppy coronary guidewire, and one or more microembolization coils may be used to occlude the artery that feeds the aneurysm.

FMD in the renal artery is usually associated with fusiform aneurysms (22). The classic angiographic appearance of a "string of beads," represents a series of stenoses with intervening areas of dilation, and are typically located proximal to the first branch of the main renal artery (Fig. 21.6E).

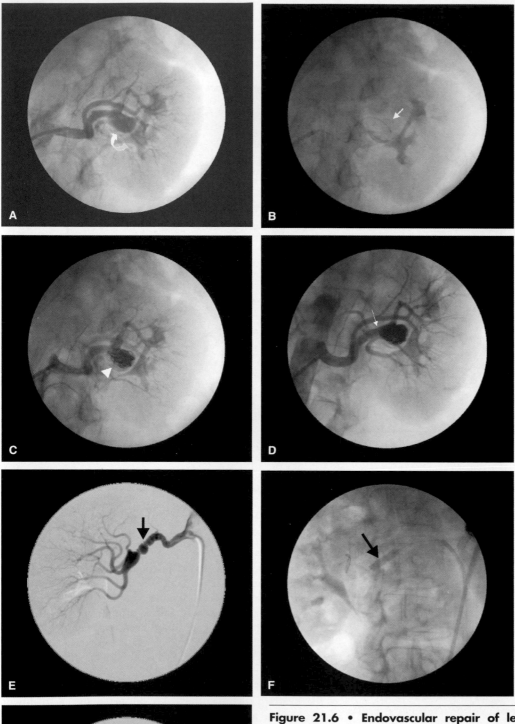

Figure 21.6 • Endovascular repair of left renal artery aneurysm and right renal artery stenosis. **A:** A 67-year-old woman with a long-standing history of refractory hypertension was referred for back pain and investigation revealed a large left renal artery saccular aneurysm *(curved arrow)* associated with bilateral fibromuscular dysplasia. **B:** Through a 6-Fr. Hockey Stick Pinnacle sheath and over a Choice PT wire, a 4-Fr. Transit catheter *(white arrow)* was advanced into the aneurysmal sac. Unfractionated heparin was given for anticoagulation. **C:** Four Hydrocoils (i.e., 20 mm × 20 mm, 14 mm × 20 mm, 14 mm × 15 mm, 12 mm × 20 mm) and two Microplex detachable coils (i.e., 18 mm × 43 mm, 12 mm × 27 mm) were inserted into the aneurysm *(arrowhead)*. **D:** A 5-mm-diameter × 31-mm-long Magic Wallstent *(white arrow)* was placed within the dysplastic main renal artery and covered the entry of the aneurysm. **E:** Fusiform aneurysms within right renal artery with angiographic appearance consistent with fibromuscular dysplasia. **F:** Balloon angioplasty with balloon catheter *(arrow)* that matched the reference diameter of the vessel. **G:** Angiographic appearance following angioplasty showing little change from baseline, which is typical in patients with FMD.

TABLE 21.4 Classification of Endoleaks

Types	Description
I	Inadequate seal at the proximal or distal landing zones
II	Retrograde filling of the aneurysmal sac through a side branch
III	Leak as a result of defect in graft fabric or separation of overlapping stents
IV	Contrast blush through the stent graft as a result of graft porosity

Duplex ultrasound, CT angiography, and MRI are the non-invasive modalities that may be used to detect this pathology (Fig. 21.7). Blood pressure usually responds to angioplasty, alone, in FMD (23), and placement of a bare metal stent is indicated only for failed angioplasty. Long-term patency of a balloon-expandable covered stent has been reported in the treatment of FMD-related RAA (24).

Iliofemoral Artery

The prevalence of an iliac artery aneurysm (IAA) ranges from 0.01% to 0.03% of the US population, many of which are in

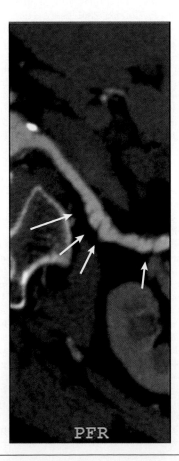

Figure 21.7 • Computed tomography angiogram of FMD (arrows) within a renal artery.

continuity with infrarenal aortic aneurysms (25–27). Most IAAs are caused by atherosclerosis. These aneurysms may be detected incidentally, during physical examination, or during investigation for obstructive arterial disease in the extremities. They may also be diagnosed as a result of complaints related to ureteral obstruction, hydronephrosis, or rupture (28,29). IAAs appear more likely to be underdiagnosed, relative to abdominal aortic aneurysms, but the mortality rate (i.e., 50%) associated with IAA rupture is comparable to that of aortic aneurysm rupture (27,29). Therefore, early recognition and prompt treatment of IAAs, to prevent rupture, are important.

A longitudinal study reported by the Veterans Administration Medical Center suggested that the expansion rate of IAA of less than 3.0 cm in diameter was about 0.11 ± 0.02 cm/year; this became significantly greater when the size of IAA was 3.0 to 5.0 cm (i.e., 0.26 ± 0.10 cm/year) (30). In addition, all patients suffering from IAA rupture in that series had a diameter more than 4.0 cm. Hence, in addition to symptoms and evidence of aneurysm enlargement, an aneurysm larger than 3.0 cm is an indication for repair (25,26,29–31). The success rate for endo-vascular therapy of anatomically suitable IAA is nearly 100% (32–35). The primary patency rates of the stent grafts are 88% to 92%, in 3 years (33,34). There is no evidence of aneurysm expansion after successful exclusion. Successful placement of a stent graft relies on the presence of a suitable, proximal, and distal anchor zone. For isolated IAA repair, Wallgraft placement has been successful (36,37). When the proximal neck is absent, or an infrarenal aortic aneurysm coexists, an aortic bi-furcated stent graft (e.g., AneuRx; Vanguard; Excluder) with an iliac extender cuff is required (38–40).

Fahrni et al. described five morphologies of iliac aneurysms that may be treated successfully with a stent graft, combined with coil embolization of the internal iliac artery (Fig. 21.8) (32). When a stent graft is required for treating a common, or external IAA, coil embolization of the internal iliac artery is important, to prevent retrograde filling of the aneurysmal sac and late rupture.

Isolated femoral artery aneurysms are mostly of the fusi-form type and are related to degenerative changes secondary to atherosclerosis. Saccular aneurysms at this location are typically pseudoaneurysms related to iatrogenic trauma (e.g., after catheterization).

Popliteal Artery

Popliteal artery aneurysms are the most common, extra-aortic arterial aneurysm, and account for 70% of all extra-aortic aneurysms (41). They have been documented in 1 of every 8 to 15 patients with abdominal aortic aneurysms, with a male pre-dominance (i.e., greater than 95%) (41,42). Under-reporting, owing to the absence of symptoms, implies that this disease is more prevalent than the reported data suggest. Pooling the results from 29 published reports that included a total of 1673 patients with popliteal aneurysms, Dawson and coworkers reported that ischemic events during follow-up evaluation occurred at a mean rate of 36% (43).

Symptoms are manifested as "blue toes" or "trash-foot," and mortality or amputation rates with these conditions may be as high as 20% (44). Repair of the popliteal artery aneurysm has been recommended not only for the symptomatic patients but also for asymptomatic patients with aneurysm sizes greater than 2.0 cm (45). Conservative follow-up evaluation of an aneurysm

Figure 21.8 • Various endovascular treatment options for solitary common and internal iliac artery aneurysms. **A:** Type 1a: Common iliac artery aneurysm with a proximal neck; coil embolization of the internal iliac artery is needed to avoid retrograde feeding of the aneurysmal sac via pelvic collaterals into the internal iliac artery. **B:** Type 1b: Common iliac artery aneurysm without a proximal neck; this necessitates stent graft placement in the aortic bifurcation. **C:** Internal iliac artery aneurysm may be treated with distal coil embolization combined with either proximal stent graft coverage (type 2a) or coil embolization (type 2b). Coil embolization alone may be used for those without a proximal neck (type 2c). (Adapted from Fahrni M, Lachat MM, Wildermuth S, et al. Endovascular therapeutic options for isolated iliac aneurysms with a working classification. *Cardiovasc Intervent Radiol*. 2003;26:443–447.)

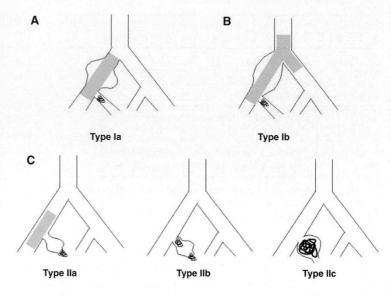

Type Ia Type Ib

Type IIa Type IIb Type IIc

of up to 2.0 cm appears to be safe (41,46). Thrombolysis may be used for acute or recent thrombotic occlusion (47,48). Failed thrombolysis may indicate poor runoff, and may predict poor, long-term outcome, with revascularization (49). Several centers have suggested that placement of a self-expanding stent graft is reasonable, with primary and secondary patency rates, at 18 months, of between 47% to 74% and 67% to 92%, respectively (Fig. 21.3) (50,51). These results are comparable to the surgical results (i.e., 2-year graft patency rate is about 75% to 80%) (43,52). Adequate outflow (i.e., at least two vessels run off) is beneficial in maintaining long-term patency of the stent graft (53).

Axillosubclavian Artery

Aneurysms in the axillosubclavian artery are extremely rare, and the majority of these are, in fact, pseudoaneurysms secondary to trauma (Fig. 21.4). As a result, the experience with endovascular repair of these aneurysms is in case report form only. Overall, these reports suggest that endovascular repair is feasible and may be an alternative to surgical treatment. An aneurysm associated with thoracic-outlet syndrome probably should be treated surgically, rather than with stents (54).

References

1. Johnston KW, Rutherford RB, Tilson MD, et al. Suggested standards for reporting on arterial aneurysms. Subcommittee on Reporting Standards for Arterial Aneurysms, Ad Hoc Committee on Reporting Standards, Society for Vascular Surgery and North American Chapter, International Society for Cardiovascular Surgery. *J Vasc Surg*. 1991;13:452–458.
2. Cloft HJ, Kallmes DF, Kallmes MH, et al. Prevalence of cerebral aneurysms in patients with fibromuscular dysplasia: a reassessment. *J Neurosurg*. 1998;88:436–440.
3. Moreau P, Albat B, Thevenet A. Surgical treatment of extracranial internal carotid artery aneurysm. *Ann Vasc Surg*. 1994;8:409–416.
4. Pulli R, Gatti M, Credi G, et al. Extracranial carotid artery aneurysms. *J Cardiovasc Surg (Torino)*. 1997;38:339–346.
5. Sahlman A, Salo J, Kostiainen S, et al. Extracranial carotid artery aneurysms. *Vasa*. 1991;20:369–373.
6. Assali AR, Sdringola S, Moustapha A, et al. Endovascular repair of traumatic pseudoaneurysm by uncovered self-expandable stenting with or without transstent coiling of the aneurysm cavity. *Catheter Cardiovasc Interv*. 2001;53:253–258.
7. Bush RL, Lin PH, Dodson TF, et al. Endoluminal stent placement and coil embolization for the management of carotid artery pseudoaneurysms. *J Endovasc Ther*. 2001;8:53–61.
8. Redekop G, Marotta T, Weill A. Treatment of traumatic aneurysms and arteriovenous fistulas of the skull base by using endovascular stents. *J Neurosurg*. 2001;95:412–419.
9. Mukherjee D, Roffi M, Yadav JS. Endovascular treatment of carotid artery aneurysms with stent grafts. *J Invasive Cardiol*. 2002;14:269–272.
10. Chan AW, Yadav J, Kreiger D, et al. Endovascular repair of carotid artery aneurysm with Jostent™ covered stent: initial experience and one-year result. *Catheter Cardiovasc Interv*. 2004;63(1):15–20.
11. Tham G, Ekelund L, Herrlin K, et al. Renal artery aneurysms. Natural history and prognosis. *Ann Surg*. 1983;197:348–352.
12. Stanley JC, Rhodes EL, Gewertz BL, et al. Renal artery aneurysms. Significance of macroaneurysms exclusive of dissections and fibrodysplastic mural dilations. *Arch Surg*. 1975;110:1327–1333.
13. Henke PK, Cardneau JD, Welling TH III, et al. Renal artery aneurysms: a 35-year clinical experience with 252 aneurysms in 168 patients. *Ann Surg*. 2001;234:454–462.
14. Cohen JR, Shamash FS. Ruptured renal artery aneurysms during pregnancy. *J Vasc Surg*. 1987;6:51–59.
15. Martin RS III, Meacham PW, Ditesheim JA, et al. Renal artery aneurysm: selective treatment for hypertension and prevention of rupture. *J Vasc Surg*. 1989;9:26–34.
16. Dzsinich C, Gloviczki P, McKusick MA, et al. Surgical management of renal artery aneurysm. *Cardiovasc Surg*. 1993;1:243–247.
17. Soussou ID, Starr DS, Lawrie GM, et al. Renal artery aneurysm. Long-term relief of renovascular hypertension by in situ operative correction. *Arch Surg*. 1979;114:1410–1415.
18. Hageman JH, Smith RF, Szilagyi E, et al. Aneurysms of the renal artery: problems of prognosis and surgical management. *Surgery*. 1978;84:563–572.
19. Bastounis E, Pikoulis E, Georgopoulos S, et al. Surgery for renal artery aneurysms: a combined series of two large centers. *Eur Urol*. 1998;33:22–27.
20. Reiher L, Grabitz K, Sandmann W. Reconstruction for renal artery aneurysm and its effect on hypertension. *Eur J Vasc Endovasc Surg*. 2000;20:454–456.
21. Schneidereit NP, Lee S, Morris DC. Endovascular repair of a ruptured renal artery aneurysm. *J Endovasc Ther*. 2003;10:71–74.

22. Alimi Y, Mercier C, Pellissier JF, et al. Fibromuscular disease of the renal artery: a new histopathologic classification. *Ann Vasc Surg*. 1992;6:220–224.

23. Sos TA, Pickering TG, Sniderman K, et al. Percutaneous transluminal renal angioplasty in renovascular hypertension due to atheroma or fibromuscular dysplasia. *N Engl J Med*. 1983;309:274–279.

24. Bisschops RH, Popma JJ, Meyerovitz MF. Treatment of fibromuscular dysplasia and renal artery aneurysm with use of a stent-graft. *J Vasc Interv Radiol*. 2001;12:757–760.

25. Lawrence PF, Lorenzo-Rivero S, Lyon JL. The incidence of iliac, femoral, and popliteal artery aneurysms in hospitalized patients. *J Vasc Surg*. 1995;22:409–415; discussion 415–416.

26. Brunkwall J, Hauksson H, Bengtsson H, et al. Solitary aneurysms of the iliac arterial system: an estimate of their frequency of occurrence. *J Vasc Surg*. 1989;10:381–384.

27. Vammen S, Lindholt J, Henneberg EW, et al. A comparative study of iliac and abdominal aortic aneurysms. *Int Angiol*. 2000;19:152–157.

28. Unno N, Kaneko H, Uchiyama T, et al. The fate of small aneurysms of the internal iliac artery following proximal ligation in abdominal aortic aneurysm repair. *Surg Today*. 2000;30:791–794.

29. Minato N, Itoh T, Natsuaki M, et al. Isolated iliac artery aneurysm and its management. *Cardiovasc Surg*. 1994;2:489–494.

30. Santilli SM, Wernsing SE, Lee ES. Expansion rates and outcomes for iliac artery aneurysms. *J Vasc Surg*. 2000;31:114–121.

31. Kasirajan V, Hertzer NR, Beven EG, et al. Management of isolated common iliac artery aneurysms. *Cardiovasc Surg*. 1998;6:171–177.

32. Fahrni M, Lachat MM, Wildermuth S, et al. Endovascular therapeutic options for isolated iliac aneurysms with a working classification. *Cardiovasc Intervent Radiol*. 2003;26:443–447.

33. Henry M, Amor M, Henry I, et al. Percutaneous endovascular treatment of peripheral aneurysms. *J Cardiovasc Surg (Torino)*. 2000;41:871–883.

34. Scheinert D, Schroder M, Steinkamp H, et al. Treatment of iliac artery aneurysms by percutaneous implantation of stent grafts. *Circulation*. 2000;102:III253–III258.

35. Henry M, Amor M, Cragg A, et al. Occlusive and aneurysmal peripheral arterial disease: assessment of a stent-graft system. *Radiology*. 1996;201:717–724.

36. Curti T, Stella A, Rossi C, et al. Endovascular repair as first-choice treatment for anastomotic and true iliac aneurysms. *J Endovasc Ther*. 2001;8:139–143.

37. Kumins NH, Owens EL, Oglevie SB, et al. Early experience using the Wallgraft in the management of distal microembolism from common iliac artery pathology. *Ann Vasc Surg*. 2002;16:181–186.

38. Zarins CK, White RA, Moll FL, et al. The AneuRx stent graft: four-year results and worldwide experience 2000. *J Vasc Surg*. 2001;33:S135–S145.

39. Zarins CK, White RA, Schwarten D, et al. AneuRx stent graft versus open surgical repair of abdominal aortic aneurysms: multicenter prospective clinical trial. *J Vasc Surg*. 1999;29:292–305; discussion 306–308.

40. Kibbe MR, Matsumura JS. The Gore Excluder US multicenter trial: analysis of adverse events at 2 years. *Semin Vasc Surg*. 2003;16:144–150.

41. Duffy ST, Colgan MP, Sultan S, et al. Popliteal aneurysms: a 10-year experience. *Eur J Vasc Endovasc Surg*. 1998;16:218–222.

42. Diwan A, Sarkar R, Stanley JC, et al. Incidence of femoral and popliteal artery aneurysms in patients with abdominal aortic aneurysms. *J Vasc Surg*. 2000;31:863–869.

43. Dawson I, Sie RB, van Bockel JH. Atherosclerotic popliteal aneurysm. *Br J Surg*. 1997;84:293–299.

44. Wingo JP, Nix ML, Greenfield LJ, et al. The blue toe syndrome: hemodynamics and therapeutic correlates of outcome. *J Vasc Surg*. 1986;3:475–480.

45. Szilagyi DE, Schwartz RL, Reddy DJ. Popliteal arterial aneurysms. Their natural history and management. *Arch Surg*. 1981;116:724–728.

46. Galland RB, Magee TR. Management of popliteal aneurysm. *Br J Surg*. 2002;89:1382–1385.

47. Dorigo W, Pulli R, Turini F, et al. Acute leg ischaemia from thrombosed popliteal artery aneurysms: role of preoperative thrombolysis. *Eur J Vasc Endovasc Surg*. 2002;23:251–254.

48. Varga ZA, Locke-Edmunds JC, Baird RN. A multicenter study of popliteal aneurysms. Joint Vascular Research Group. *J Vasc Surg*. 1994;20:171–177.

49. Marty B, Wicky S, Ris HB, et al. Success of thrombolysis as a predictor of outcome in acute thrombosis of popliteal aneurysms. *J Vasc Surg*. 2002;35:487–493.

50. Tielliu IF, Verhoeven EL, Prins TR, et al. Treatment of popliteal artery aneurysms with the Hemobahn stent-graft. *J Endovasc Ther*. 2003;10:111–116.

51. Gerasimidis T, Sfyroeras G, Papazoglou K, et al. Endovascular treatment of popliteal artery aneurysms. *Eur J Vasc Endovasc Surg*. 2003;26:506–511.

52. Sarcina A, Bellosta R, Luzzani L, et al. Surgical treatment of popliteal artery aneurysm. A 20 year experience. *J Cardiovasc Surg*. 1997;38:347–354.

53. Lagana D, Mangini M, Marras M, et al. Percutaneous treatment of femoral-popliteal aneurysms with covered stents. *Radiol Med*. 2002;104:322–331.

54. Phipp LH, Scott DJ, Kessel D, et al. Subclavian stents and stent-grafts: cause for concern? *J Endovasc Surg*. 1999;6:223–226.

Miscellaneous

CHAPTER 22

Renal Artery Intervention

Joel P. Reginelli and Christopher J. Cooper

INDICATIONS AND PIVOTAL TRIALS

Natural History of Renal Artery Stenosis

The prevalence of renal artery stenosis (RAS) in patients with hypertension (HTN) has been estimated at 1% to 5%; however, angiographic studies suggest this may be an underestimate (1). Among patients with documented atherosclerotic disease in other peripheral vascular beds, the prevalence of RAS may be as high as 30% to 40% (2).

Fibromuscular dysplasia (FMD) and atherosclerosis are the two primary pathologic etiologies of RAS. FMD accounts for about 10% of all RAS cases, typically occurs in younger (i.e., less than 50 years) women, and has the classic "beads on a string" appearance at angiography (Fig. 22.1). A young woman with new-onset HTN that is accelerating or refractory to antihypertensive therapies suggests the diagnosis of FMD.

Atherosclerosis is responsible for approximately 90% of all RAS cases and generally occurs in an older population (i.e., greater than 50 years) with vascular risk factors. There is no gender preference observed in atherosclerotic RAS, and these patients may present in a myriad of ways: refractory or accelerating HTN, worsening renal function, angiotensin-converting enzyme (ACE) inhibitor-induced renal failure, flash pulmonary edema, or as an incidental finding during other testing.

The natural history of RAS depends largely upon the underlying etiology. FMD may involve the intimal, medial, or adventitial layer of the vessel, but medial FMD accounts for the overwhelming majority of cases (i.e., about 90%) (3). Progressive narrowing occurs in one third of patients with medial FMD; however, progression to complete occlusion is an extremely rare event. In contrast, atherosclerotic RAS is a progressive disease that may culminate in occlusion of the vessel. In one series, patients with RAS of less than 60% severity had a rate of progression to significant disease (i.e., greater than 60% severity) of approximately 20% per year. Among patients with vessels who had an initial stenosis of greater than 60% severity, there was progression to complete occlusion in 5% of patients at 1 year and 11% at 2 years; however, some investigators have been unable to demonstrate a relationship between stenosis severity and renal function (4–6). While one might conclude from this that stenoses do not cause renal dysfunction, such a conclusion would be unfounded. Fundamentally, the kidney requires blood flow to function. Thus, it is absolutely clear that severe stenoses and occlusions yield a nonfunctioning kidney.

Why then is there difficulty relating stenosis severity to function? Clearly, there are factors beyond the degree of stenosis that influence function. Some are intrinsic to RAS, including the duration of the insult, atheroemboli, hypertensive nephrosclerosis of the contralateral kidney, activation of the renin–angiotensin system, and finally the characteristics and effects of the stenosis (including lesion length, minimal lumen diameter, etc.) on renal blood flow and intrarenal pressure. Additionally, other factors, such as essential HTN, diabetes, concomitant medications, generalized atherosclerosis progression, and aging, play roles in determining overall renal function.

Renal Artery Revascularization

An early, nonrandomized comparison suggested a benefit of surgical revascularization of severely narrowed renal arteries; however, surgery has been associated with significant perioperative complications and mortality (7). Most patients with RAS have lesions in other vascular beds, making them high-risk operative candidates; therefore, percutaneous transluminal renal angioplasty (PTRA) became an attractive alternative. Notably, the results of PTRA and surgery appear equivalent, when compared directly (8). PTRA was associated with improved blood pressure (BP) control and a decrease in need for antihypertensive medications in retrospective studies; however, PTRA is associated with a high restenosis rate for atherosclerotic lesions involving the ostium, which is the location of 80% to 85% of all atherosclerotic RAS lesions. With the advent of stents, the problems associated with angioplasty may be circumvented.

Rees et al. reported 96% technical success rate with Palmaz® stents in ostial lesions (9), and perhaps more importantly, stents appear to be superior to PTRA, when compared directly (10). For these reasons, stents have become the dominant mode of revascularization for ostial-atherosclerotic lesions of the renal artery.

DATA SUPPORTING PERCUTANEOUS RENAL ARTERY REVASCULARIZATION

The primary goals of treatment in RAS are to improve the management of refractory HTN and to preserve or improve renal function (Table 22.1).

While there is general agreement that PTRA/stent procedures offer benefits for patients with the aforementioned conditions, who are found to have bilateral renal artery stenoses, the indications for PTRA/stent procedures in similar patients with unilateral disease are more contentious.

In three randomized trials that compared balloon angioplasty to medical therapy for the treatment of HTN in patients with RAS, there was no difference in BP control or serum creatinine among the two treatment groups; however, the need for fewer antihypertensive medications in patients

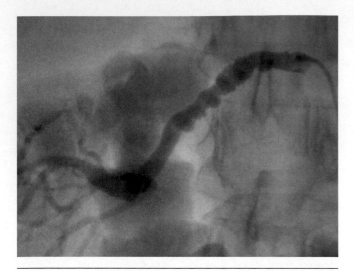

Figure 22.1 • Right renal artery angiogram in a 40-year-old female demonstrating "beaded" appearance of vessel lumen, consistent with a diagnosis of fibromuscular dysplasia.

treated with angioplasty was a consistent finding in each of the studies (11–13). These trials were limited by the high rate of crossover in the treatment arms (i.e., from medical arm to angioplasty arm)—the small number of patients enrolled, the treatment of patients with stenoses that may not have been physiologically significant, and the use of angioplasty without stenting. The recently published Angioplasty and Stenting for Renal Artery Lesions (ASTRAL) trial represents the

TABLE 22.1	Indications for Percutaneous Revascularization for Renal Artery Stenosis
Indication	
Medically refractory hypertension Requiring ≥ 3 antihypertensive medications at maximal doses	
Significant hypertension in the setting of fibromuscular dysplasia	
Acute renal failure after the initiation of angiotensin-converting enzyme (ACE) inhibitors	
Recurrent flash pulmonary edema in setting of uncontrolled hypertension	
Severe renal artery stenosis in a solitary kidney	
Severe bilateral renal artery stenoses	
Severe unilateral renal artery stenosis with Evidence of decreased filtration in the affected kidney Hyperfiltration in the contralateral kidney (i.e., lateralization)	
Subacute renal failure (<6 months), Particularly if creatinine < 3.0 and kidney size ≥ 9 cm in length	

first randomized controlled trial (RCT) that compared contemporary renal artery revascularization using stents plus optimal medical therapy versus optimal medical therapy alone (14). In this trial, 806 patients diagnosed with RAS in which the physician was unclear of the clinical benefit of renal artery revascularization were enrolled. The primary end point of the study was the change in renal function over time, measured as the slope of the reciprocal of serum creatinine. There was no significant difference in the two treatment groups. Likewise, there were no differences noted in the two treatment groups with regard to the prespecified secondary end points that included BP control, time to first renal event, time to first major cardiovascular event, and mortality. This trial has been heavily criticized by proponents of renal artery revascularization (15). The major criticisms include the decision to enroll patients with an uncertain clinical indication for renal revascularization, which clearly makes it difficult to demonstrate a clinical benefit. The choice of the rate of decline in renal function as the primary end point is also problematic, given that 25% of patients in the study had normal renal function and an additional 15% had near-normal renal function. A significant proportion of patients in the study did not appear to have a physiologically significant stenosis, with 40% of patients being documented to have ≤70% stenosis of the renal artery. With the absence of any core lab for the study, it would appear likely that this represents an underestimate. Finally, the quality of the interventional operators in this study is questionable, given the high rate of major adverse events (9%) when compared with other contemporary renal artery stent studies (~2%). For this reason, it seems fair to conclude that the major finding of the ASTRAL trial is that routine renal artery revascularization is not indicated in patients without a clear clinical indication. The ongoing Cardiovascular Outcomes in Renal Atherosclerotic Lesions (CORAL) trial does address some of the shortcomings of the ASTRAL trial and will be pivotal in determining the future role of renal artery revascularization.

PATIENT SELECTION

In the absence of clear data from RCTs guiding treatment decisions in patients with RAS, the interventionist must determine the appropriateness of renal artery revascularization for each individual patient who presents for evaluation. In essence, one must ask two fundamental questions: (1) Is the patient's clinical condition being caused by RAS? and (2) having fulfilled that condition, does the patient have a reasonable chance of clinical benefit from revascularization? It is important to emphasize that a patient's clinical condition may be caused by RAS, but he or she may not benefit from revascularization. For example, a patient may have a critical stenosis of a renal artery that results in profound ischemic changes in the affected kidney resulting in atrophy of the kidney. If the indication for revascularization is restoration of renal function, then revascularization of an atrophic kidney is unlikely to provide the patient with any clinical benefit and the patient should be managed medically.

In attempting to answer these two critical questions, the synthesis of data from a number of sources is required including clinical history and exam, serum Cr (including the trajectory of the serum Cr over time), urinary protein, and imaging data. The presence of a clear clinical indication is important. If a young woman is diagnosed with RAS due to FMD, then the clinical indication driving the need for intervention will be the presence of HTN. Likewise, in patients with RAS due to atherosclerotic disease, the following clinical indications should be present before considering renal artery revascularization: refractory HTN, ACE inhibitor–induced renal failure, recurrent flash pulmonary edema in the setting of HTN, unexplained hypokalemia, subacute (i.e., 6 months) onset of renal insufficiency, or an incidental finding of decreased kidney size on imaging studies obtained for other reasons (16).

The serum Cr is an important variable that should be examined in patients with atherosclerotic RAS. As mentioned previously, the patients who typically stand to benefit from renal artery revascularization in terms of improvements or stabilization of renal function include those with a recent deterioration in renal function. The more acute this deterioration (assuming the absence of other etiologies), the more likely the patient will recover renal function following revascularization. A patient who presents with significant fluctuation in renal function over a long period of time is unlikely to benefit, as the underlying etiology of the fluctuation in renal function is unlikely to be due to RAS. The limitations of serum Cr as a marker of renal function should be accepted, however, particularly in patients with unilateral RAS. In such cases, as disease progresses in one kidney, there is often lateralization or hyperfiltration of the unaffected kidney, which maintains the serum creatinine within a relatively normal range despite significant renal impairment in the affected kidney.

Urinary protein measurements are a crude method of assessing the parenchymal function of the kidney(s). Urinary protein measurements > 1 g/24 hr suggest significant parenchymal disease and make it less likely that revascularization of the main renal artery will result in a significant clinical benefit.

Imaging data may be derived from purely anatomic studies (i.e., CT and MR angiography) or from ultrasound that provides both anatomic and important functional data. Anatomic assessments of the severity of RAS are important, as most physiologically significant stenoses will be in the severe to critical range, and as a result are more likely to have a clinical response to revascularization. The vertical kidney size provided by these modalities is also an important variable as it serves as a crude assessment of the health of the kidney parenchyma. Most experts would agree that a kidney size < 8 cm suggests severe parenchymal disease with minimal effective residual renal function and should raise the threshold for revascularization.

Much has been written regarding the value of the resistive index (RI) measurements from the renal parenchyma in determining the clinical response to renal revascularization. The RI is calculated as 1 − EDV/PSV (EDV, end-diastolic velocity, and PSV, peak systolic velocity) from Doppler waveforms sampled from the superior, mid, and inferior segments of both kidneys. A high RI (i.e., >0.8) has been regarded as an indication of severe parenchymal disease and as a marker of a lack of clinical response to revascularization. However, this measurement needs to be examined critically, as it can be influenced by a variety of factors. For example, the presence of a severe main RAS will result in a parvus tardus waveform (i.e., reduction in the PSV measurement), thus resulting in a reduction in the RI measurement. Thus, a patient with concomitant severe parenchymal disease and severe main RAS could have a normal RI measurement based on the balance of these two influences on the RI. Additional variables that can influence the RI measurement include the presence of valvular heart disease (e.g., aortic stenosis—decrease, aortic regurgitation—increase, and stiff calcified aorta—increase). Unfortunately, the RI is poorly understood by many interventionalists and general medicine physicians. It should be viewed in the context of the entire body of information gathered from the patient and its limitations should be clearly understood.

A typical screening and treatment algorithm for RAS is outlined in Figure 22.2.

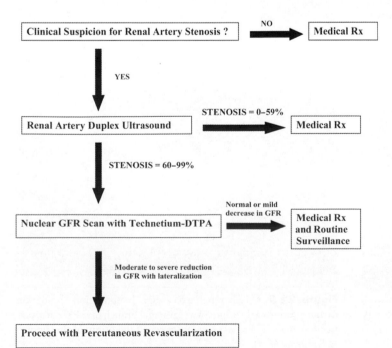

Figure 22.2 • Algorithm for diagnosis and management of patients with suspected renal artery stenosis.

ANATOMY

Paired renal arteries arise from the lateral aspect of the abdominal aorta at the level of the first and second lumbar vertebrae, just inferior to the anterior origin of the superior mesenteric artery. The origin of the right renal artery is often slightly higher than that of the left renal artery. The main renal artery remains intact for a variable length, prior to subdividing into segmental arteries. These segmental arteries further subdivide into interlobar arteries that subsequently divide into the arcuate and interlobular arteries. The arcuate and interlobular arteries provide the smaller arterioles that penetrate the renal cortex and medulla (Fig. 22.3).

There are a number of variations in renal artery anatomy that warrant mention. The most common variant is the presence of an accessory renal artery, which occurs in up to 30% of individuals and refers to a second, generally smaller-caliber, renal artery that most commonly arises inferior to the main renal artery (Fig. 22.4). Accessory renal arteries typically arise from the abdominal aorta but may also arise from the common iliac, superior and inferior mesenteric, and right hepatic arteries. In some instances, the accessory renal artery may be of similar caliber to the main renal artery, thus supplying a large portion of the renal blood supply. In these circumstances, revascularization of stenosed accessory renal arteries has been performed.

A second anatomic variant is early subdivision of the main renal artery (Fig. 22.5). Normally, a main renal artery remains intact for several centimeters prior to dividing into a variable number of segmental branches. In some cases, a main renal artery may immediately subdivide into segmental branches just beyond its origin, thus making optimal percutaneous revascularization more challenging.

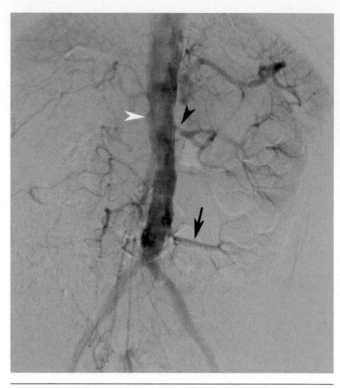

Figure 22.4 • Abdominal aortogram demonstrating accessory left inferior renal artery *(black arrow)*. This patient has a proximal lesion in the left upper renal artery *(black arrowhead)* and an occlusion of the right renal artery *(white arrowhead)*, most likely caused by atherosclerosis.

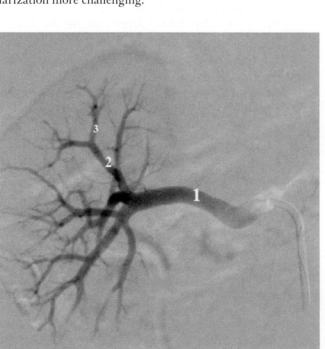

Figure 22.3 • Digital subtraction angiogram of right renal artery demonstrating *(1)* main renal trunk, *(2)* segmental artery, and *(3)* interlobar artery.

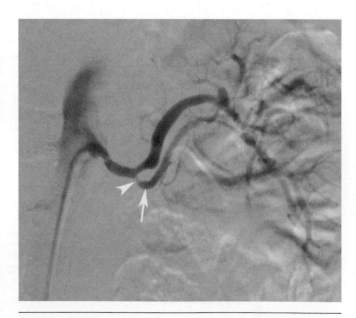

Figure 22.5 • Left renal artery digital subtraction angiogram demonstrating early origin of a segmental branch of the renal artery *(white arrow)*. There is a severe stenosis at the origin of this branch *(white arrowhead)*.

RENAL ARTERY INTERVENTION

Arterial Access

In most cases, arterial access for renal angiography is retrograde, via either common femoral artery, using a modified Seldinger technique to place a 4- to 6-Fr. arterial sheath. If there is moderately severe atherosclerotic disease in the iliofemoral vascular tree, a long sheath (i.e., about 35 cm) may be placed to avoid additional trauma to these vessels during catheter exchanges. In cases where there is severe bilateral aortoiliac disease, severely downgoing orientation of the proximal segment of the renal arteries, or when an abdominal aortic aneurysm is present, an antegrade approach via the brachial or radial artery may be performed.

Diagnostic Angiography

As a general rule, it is a good idea to obtain an abdominal aortogram prior to performing selective renal artery angiography (Fig. 22.6). The abdominal aortogram will provide important information regarding the location of the renal artery ostia, the presence of high-grade ostial stenosis, the presence of accessory

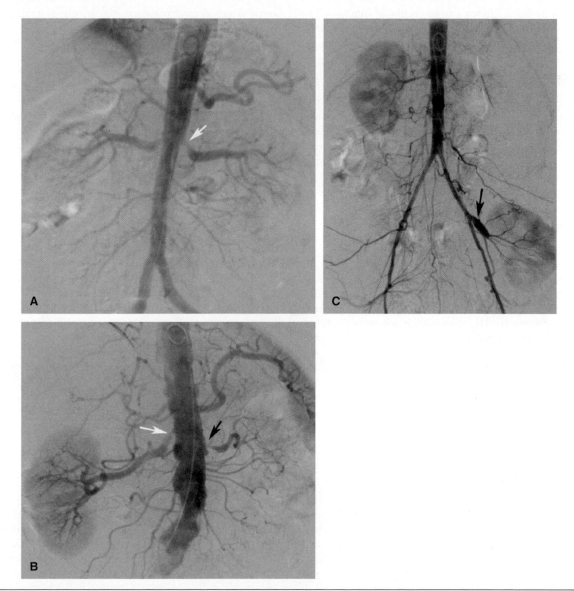

Figure 22.6 • Selection of abdominal aortograms highlighting the utility of this study prior to renal artery angiography.   **A:** Abdominal aortogram demonstrating a relatively smooth aortic lumen, a mild stenosis of the proximal right renal artery, and a severe stenosis at the origin of the left renal artery *(white arrow)*. **B:** Abdominal aortogram demonstrating an ostial left renal artery stenosis *(black arrow)* with a delayed left nephrogram, a mild to moderate proximal right renal artery stenosis *(white arrow)* with a normal right nephrogram, and diffuse irregularity of the lumen of the aorta consistent with significant atherosclerosis. **C:** Abdominal aortogram in a patient with known fibromuscular dysplasia. Prior left renal artery stenting resulted in occlusion of the vessel, necessitating surgical transposition of the kidney and its renal artery to the pelvis, where the renal artery was attached to the left common iliac artery *(black arrow)*. There is evidence of stenosis at the origin of the right renal artery.

renal arteries or other anomalies, the degree of aortic calcification and atherosclerotic disease adjacent to the renal artery ostia, and the presence and degree of aneurysmal dilation of the abdominal aorta. Frequently, an optimal image of the renal arteries may be obtained in a shallow (10° to 15°) left-anterior oblique or AP projection (17).

To engage the renal arteries selectively, the authors recommend the use of 4- to 6-Fr. diagnostic catheters. Commonly employed diagnostic catheters include the internal mammary (IMA), renal double curve (RDC), Judkins Right® (JR4), SOS®, and Cobra® catheters. Cineangiography should be performed long enough to allow visualization of contrast in the renal cortex (i.e., a nephrogram) in order to gain additional information on overall kidney size and regional function. The choice of contrast medium is at the discretion of the operator; however, low-osmolar and nonionic contrast media are recommended.

General Strategy

The goal of renal artery intervention is to achieve effective revascularization of the RAS with minimal manipulation of catheters within the aorta and the ostium of the renal artery. Balloon angioplasty, without stenting, is sufficient in most patients with FMD; however, atherosclerotic narrowing of the arteries, particularly that involving the ostium of the renal artery, requires stent placement to achieve an optimal result.

Intervention

In general, patients should receive full-dose aspirin (i.e., 325 mg) and intravenous hydration prior to arriving in the catheterization lab. Once arterial access has been obtained, heparin should be administered to achieve a goal-activated clotting time (ACT) of 250 to 275 seconds. The routine use of platelet glycoprotein IIb/IIIa inhibitors is not recommended; however, these agents may be useful in cases complicated by the development of acute thrombus or distal embolization. Following the intervention, patients should receive dual antiplatelet therapy with aspirin and clopidogrel, for at least 30 days. In patients receiving renal stents prior to major surgery, aspirin monotherapy is usually sufficient. It is hypothesized that the high flow rate to the renal arteries is the reason aspirin monotherapy in renal stenting has been associated with good outcomes (18).

Guide Catheter/Guide Sheath

A guide catheter or guide sheath is used to provide a conduit for delivery of equipment to the renal artery. A guide catheter is inserted through a conventional arterial sheath. A guide sheath refers to a long sheath whose tip is shaped as a guide. The major advantage of a guide sheath is the ability to use a small-caliber sheath in the groin. However, the major disadvantage of guide sheaths is the compromise in ease of manipulation of the sheath tip compared with the guide catheter tip. The choice of guide catheter/sheath shape depends upon several factors: the location of the stenosis, the angle at which the renal artery comes off the aorta, and operator preference. A 6-Fr. guide is used in most interventions, and commonly employed guide catheters include the IMA, JR4, renal standard curve (RSC), RDC, and hockey stick. There

are two basic techniques for guide-catheter engagement: direct engagement and telescoping engagement.

DIRECT ENGAGEMENT

The guide catheter is gently manipulated until it is seated in the ostium of the renal artery. This is a safe approach for most lesions; however, with high-grade ostial lesions or severe adjacent aortic disease, there is an increased risk of guide catheter–induced dissection, embolization, or abrupt closure, using this technique. A variation that may be safer is to use is the "no touch" technique, wherein a 0.035″ guidewire is positioned extending up the abdominal aorta, while the guiding catheter is manipulated toward the ostium of the renal artery. When the renal artery is approximated, the wire is retracted, allowing the guiding catheter to engage the artery.

TELESCOPING ENGAGEMENT

A long 4- or 5-Fr. diagnostic catheter is telescoped through a shorter 6-Fr. guide catheter. The diagnostic and guide catheters are advanced into the abdominal aorta over a 0.035″ guidewire, and the diagnostic catheter is used to engage the ostia of the renal artery. An interventional steerable guidewire is then advanced through the diagnostic catheter and across the stenosis. The guide catheter is then advanced over the diagnostic catheter/guidewire combination. The diagnostic catheter is then removed. This minimizes guide catheter manipulations within the aorta and the renal artery ostium.

Interventional Wires

The choice of wire is based, primarily, on operator preference. Renal interventions may be performed over 0.035″, 0.018″, or 0.014″ wires. Irrespective of diameter, the wire chosen to cross the stenosis should be one with torque capabilities, with a soft tip to minimize distal embolization and to avoid trauma to the lesion and vessel. Recent trends suggest a movement toward 0.014″ wires (e.g., Asahi Soft, Ashai Prowater; Abbott Vascular) for renal interventions. Emboli protection devices (EPDs) are being used more frequently in renal intervention, as will be discussed later, and these devices are generally mounted onto a 0.014″ wire.

Balloons and Stents

The choice of angioplasty balloon depends upon the size of the renal artery. The average diameter of a renal artery ranges from 5 to 7 mm; however, there may be a significant degree of variation from this average range. It is recommended that measurements be performed on a nonstenotic segment of vessel, free of poststenotic dilation, adjacent to the area of interest using the diagnostic or guide catheter as a reference diameter. Many operators suggest an initial balloon diameter that is approximately 1 mm less than the measured diameter of the vessel. As mentioned previously, optimal results are often obtainable with angioplasty alone for RAS caused by FMD; however, stent placement is typically required for patients with atherosclerotic RAS, particularly if the stenosis involves the ostium.

Ostial lesions are best managed with balloon-expandable stents, whereas consideration may be given to the use of self-expanding stents for stenoses that are in the mid portion of the vessel. After deployment of a stent for ostial RAS, the authors recommend "flaring" the ostium by retracting the balloon approximately one half the balloon's length and inflating it to a higher pressure. It is important to be sensitive to any pain (i.e., usually back pain) reported by the patient during either stent deployment or postdilation of the stent, as this reflects stretch of the renal artery, and further dilation may increase the risk of renal artery or aortic perforation.

Three stents are approved for use with failed renal artery angioplasty: the Palmaz® stent (Cordis), the Express SD® (Boston Scientific), and the Bridge Extra Support (Medtronic); however, many operators use other balloon-expandable stents, often those approved for biliary indications, for the purpose of renal artery revascularization (Fig. 22.7).

Embolic Protection

Balloon angioplasty or stent placement within an atherosclerotic lesion may result in embolization of particulate debris into the distal vasculature. During complex coronary cases (i.e., thrombus-laden lesions or saphenous vein-graft interventions), the risk of embolization is high, and myocardial necrosis or no reflow are common. Likewise, embolization during peripheral interventions may be associated with end-organ ischemia or infarction.

Several EPDs have recently been developed to reduce the embolic burden during endovascular procedures. These EPDs fall into one of the two categories: balloon occlusive devices (e.g., Percusurge Guardwire®; Medtronic) or filter devices (e.g., FilterWire® EZ; Boston Scientific). To date, these devices have only been approved for saphenous vein graft interventions; however, many investigators have employed these devices in an "off-label" use for peripheral interventions. Distal embolization during renal intervention may result in ischemic nephropathy, and thus result in a deterioration of renal function, rather than achieving the intended goals of improvement or stabilization of renal function.

The role for these devices in renal artery interventions has not been studied in a prospective manner; however, case reports suggest a high rate of technical success with significant particulate debris retrieved (19). The use of EPDs during renal artery intervention may be limited by the underlying anatomy. If the main renal artery has a proximal branch point, often one must choose the largest segmental artery in which to place the EPD, recognizing that full protection is not possible in that setting.

Complications

There are a number of complications that may arise during renal artery intervention (Table 22.2).

Damage to the renal artery in the form of dissection or abrupt closure may occur as a complication of guide catheter engagement, wiring, or balloon or stent deployment. In abrupt occlusions, attempts should be made to cross the occlusion with a wire. Dissections involving the renal artery ostium generally require stent placement, whereas focal dissections that occur more distally may respond favorably to balloon inflation (Fig. 22.8).

Aneurysmal renal arteries are felt to be at higher risk for perforation, though rare cases of perforation may occur in otherwise normal vessels from an oversized stent, aggressive stent postdilation, or spearing of calcium plaque through the vessel wall. Oftentimes these may be managed with prolonged balloon inflation with, or without, reversal of anticoagulation. In nearly all circumstances, a low-pressure inflation should be performed, often with an oversized balloon, simply to stop bleeding. In cases that do not respond to balloon inflation tamponade, consideration may be given to placing a stent graft (e.g., JOSTENT GraftMaster, Abbott Vascular or iCAST, Atrium); however, if percutaneous sealing cannot be achieved with these measures, emergency surgery may be necessary.

Wire perforations in the parenchyma of the kidney may respond to particle or coil embolization and reversal of anticoagulation. Distal embolization in renal artery interventions may result in renal infarction or worsening ischemic nephropathy. Recognizing the salutary effects of glycoprotein IIb/IIIa inhibitors on embolization during coronary interventions, some operators advocate the administration of these agents when there is evidence of renal artery embolization; however, supportive data are lacking for the use of these agents in renal artery intervention. In heavily atheromatous aortas, cholesterol embolization to the lower extremities and splanchnic vessels may occur, as a result of catheter manipulation. As with any interventional procedure, bleeding or access site difficulties are the complications most commonly encountered.

LONG-TERM OUTCOMES

Restenosis following angioplasty, in patients with FMD, is generally caused by elastic recoil and occurs in approximately 10% of the cases. These restenotic lesions often respond favorably to repeat balloon angioplasty. In-stent restenosis (ISR) caused by neointimal hyperplasia occurs in approximately 10% to 20% of renal interventions with stents (Fig. 22.9). The mainstay treatment for renal artery ISR has been balloon angioplasty. Some centers employed gamma brachytherapy, in an off-label use, as an adjunct to balloon angioplasty; however, this treatment modality is no longer readily available. The application of drug-eluting technology to peripheral vascular stents holds great promise for reducing the rate of restenosis, although a drug-eluting peripheral-vascular stent is not currently available.

LONG-TERM FOLLOW-UP MONITORING

After renal artery intervention, patients should be followed, long-term, by a physician knowledgeable in RAS and the syndromes of renovascular HTN and ischemic nephropathy. Patients may develop delayed renal dysfunction stemming from embolization, restenosis, or progression of other causes of nephropathy; therefore, long-term follow-up assessment of renal function is advisable. Similarly, those patients who present with HTN are certainly at risk for continued HTN, or recurrence of HTN if restenosis is encountered; therefore, regular BP monitoring is recommended.

Anatomic follow-up evaluation to detect restenosis is somewhat controversial. Some operators follow only BP and renal function, reserving anatomic evaluation for those patients with worsening of one or both parameters. Other clinicians perform a surveillance anatomic assessment at between 6 months and 1 year after treatment, to detect restenosis.

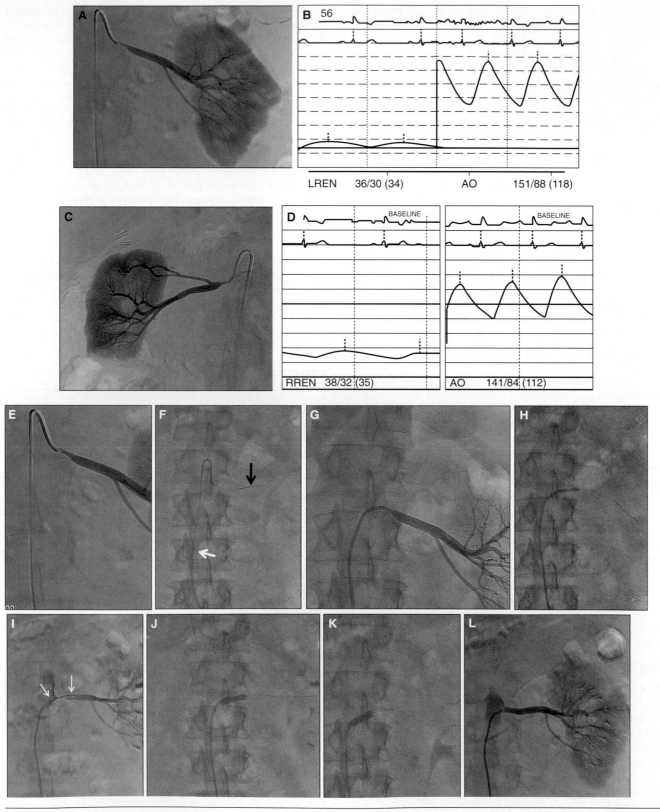

LREN   36/30 (34)   AO   151/88 (118)

RREN   38/32 (35)   AO   141/84 (112)

Figure 22.7 • *(See Legend on facing page)*

TABLE 22.2 Complications of Renal Artery Intervention

Complication
Renal infarction
Deterioration in renal function
Distal embolization to renal artery
Renal artery dissection

Cholesterol embolism
    To lower extremity circulation
    To mesenteric circulation

Renal artery/aortic perforation
Perinephric hematoma
Occlusion or thrombosis of renal artery
Bleeding complications
Stent embolization
Infection

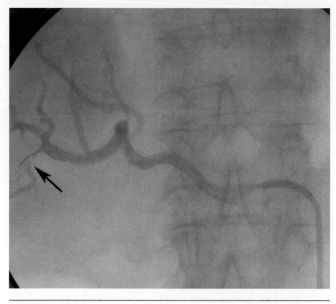

Figure 22.8 • Focal dissection compromising the vessel lumen in an interlobar branch of the renal artery caused by the interventional wire.

Currently, duplex ultrasonography with careful interrogation of velocities along the renal artery, from the aortic origin to the kidney proper, is the preferred strategy. It does not require contrast medium, involves no ionizing radiation, and may provide diagnostic data regarding the stented segment; however, not all centers are adept at this technology and some patients have body shapes that preclude adequate ultrasound evaluation. Under these circumstances, CT angiography is a reasonable alternative. MRA is of limited value in this instance, as metallic artifact compromises visualization of the stented segment.

KEY PRINCIPLES (PEARLS, DOS AND DON'TS)

Dos

1. Document clinical indications and results of noninvasive anatomic and functional testing, prior to proceeding with revascularization.
2. Administer periprocedural hydration and *N*-acetylcysteine in patients with documented renal insufficiency.
3. Confirm stent placement in optimal view before deployment, to avoid missing the ostium.

Figure 22.7 • Left renal artery intervention in a 53-year-old male with subacute deterioration in renal function from baseline Cr of 1.5 to 2.7 mg/dL. **A:** Baseline angiogram of left renal artery showing a critical ostial stenosis. **B:** Recording of pressure gradient across ostial stenosis with a drop in the mean gradient from 118 mm Hg in the aorta to 34 mm Hg in the left renal artery (using 4-Fr. Sos catheter). The left kidney had a vertical length of 9.9 cm and mild irregularity of the renal contour consistent with the presence of parenchymal disease. **C:** Baseline angiogram of right renal artery showing a critical ostial stenosis. **D:** Recording of pressure gradient across ostial stenosis with a drop in the mean gradient from 112 mm Hg in the aorta to 35 mm Hg in the right renal artery (using 4-Fr. Sos catheter). The right kidney had a vertical length of 8.8 cm and severe irregularity of the renal contour consistent with the presence of severe parenchymal disease. **E–L** Left renal artery intervention. Based on the findings outlined in A–D, the decision was made to proceed with revascularization of the left renal artery since the left kidney was felt to be the healthier of the two kidneys and that revascularization of that kidney was more likely to result in an improvement in renal function (i.e., the patient's primary clinical presentation). **E:** Baseline angiogram of the left renal artery using 4-Fr. Sos catheter. **F:** The Sos catheter was removed and telescoped through a 7-Fr. RDC guide catheter outside the body. The Sos catheter was then used to re-engage the left renal artery ostium with the tip of the RDC guide in the distal abdominal aorta (*white arrow*). A 0.014″ Asahi soft wire was inserted through the Sos catheter into the left renal artery (*black arrow*). **G:** The Sos catheter was then removed, and the RDC guide was railed over the Asahi soft wire to engage the ostium minimizing any manipulation of the guide in the aorta. **H:** The ostial lesion was then predilated with a 4 × 20-mm Maverick balloon (monorail). **I:** A 6 × 18-mm Express SD stent was then positioned across the lesion, being careful to cover the ostium of the renal artery (proximal and distal margins of stent indicated by white arrows). **J:** The stent was postdilated with a 6 × 20-mm Aviator balloon. **K:** The postdilation balloon was withdrawn and positioned with the proximal marker in the aorta and the distal marker in the mid portion of the stent to ensure flaring of the ostium of the stent. **L:** Final angiogram following left renal artery intervention. The patient's serum Cr returned to baseline within 7 days of this procedure.

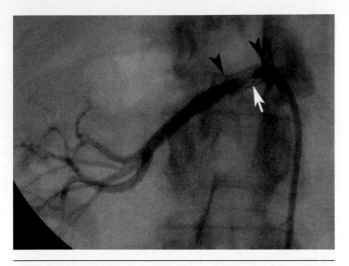

Figure 22.9 • Right renal artery angiogram demonstrating severe in-stent restenosis *(white arrow)* in a previously placed stent *(margins shown by black arrowheads)* in the proximal segment of the vessel.

Don'ts

1. Do not intervene routinely on stenoses discovered during incidental renal angiography obtained at the time of cardiac catheterization. Anatomic and functional testing is indicated prior to intervention.
2. Do not perform bilateral renal artery stenting during one procedure. There will be exceptions to this rule; however, in the vast majority of cases where bilateral renal stenting is indicated, the procedures should be performed in a staged manner.
3. Do not routinely stent lesions caused by FMD. Balloon angioplasty is equally efficacious and stenting should be reserved for use if dissection occurs.

References

1. Harding MB, Smith LR, Himmelstein SI, et al. Renal artery stenosis: prevalence and associated risk factors in patients undergoing routine cardiac catheterization. *J Am Soc Nephrol*. 1992;2:1608–1616.
2. Olin JW, Melia M, Young JR, et al. Prevalence of atherosclerotic renal artery stenosis in patients with atherosclerosis elsewhere. *Am J Med*. 1990;88:46N–51N.
3. Safian RD, Textor SC. Renal-artery stenosis. *N Engl J Med*. 2001;344:431–434.
4. Zierler RE, Bergelin RO, Isaacson JA, et al. Natural history of atherosclerotic renal artery stenosis: a prospective study with duplex ultrasonography. *J Vasc Surg*. 1994;19:250–258.
5. Wright JR, Shurrab AE, Cheung C, et al. A prospective study of the determinants of renal functional outcome and mortality in atherosclerotic renovascular disease. *Am J Kidney Dis*. 2002;39:1153–1161.
6. Suresh M, Laboi P, Mamtora H, et al. Relationship of renal dysfunction to proximal arterial disease severity in atherosclerotic renovascular disease. *Nephrol Dial Transplant*. 2000;15:631–636.
7. Hunt JC, Sheps SG, Harrison EG Jr, et al. Renal and renovascular hypertension. A reasoned approach to diagnosis and management. *Arch Intern Med*. 1974;133:988–999.
8. Weibull H, Bergqvist D, Bergentz SE, et al. Percutaneous transluminal renal angioplasty versus surgical reconstruction of atherosclerotic renal artery stenosis: a prospective randomized study. *J Vasc Surg*. 1993;18:841–852.
9. Rees CR, Palmaz JC, Becker GJ, et al. Palmaz stent in atherosclerotic stenoses involving the ostia of the renal arteries: preliminary report of a multicenter study. *Radiology*. 1991;181:507–514.
10. van de Ven PJ, Kaatee R, Beutler JJ, et al. Arterial stenting and balloon angioplasty in ostial atherosclerotic renovascular disease: a randomised trial. *Lancet*. 1999;353:282–286.
11. van Jaarsveld BC, Krijnen P, Pieterman H, et al. The effect of balloon angioplasty on hypertension in atherosclerotic renal artery stenosis. Dutch Renal Artery Stenosis Intervention Cooperative Study Group. *N Engl J Med*. 2000;342:1007–1014.
12. Webster J, Marshall F, Abdalla M, et al. Randomised comparison of percutaneous angioplasty vs continued medical therapy for hypertensive patients with atheromatous renal artery stenosis. Scottish and Newcastle Renal Artery Stenosis Collaborative Group. *J Hum Hypertens*. 1998;12:329–335.
13. Plouin PF, Chatellier G, Darne B, et al. Blood pressure outcome of angioplasty in atherosclerotic renal artery stenosis: a randomized trial. Essai Multicentrique Medicaments vs Angioplastie (EMMA) Study Group. *Hypertension*. 1998;31:823–829.
14. The Astral Investigators. Revascularization versus medical therapy for renal-artery stenosis. *N Engl J Med*. 2009;361:1953–1962.
15. White CJ. Kiss my astral: one seriously flawed study of renal stenting after another. *Catheter Cardiovasc Interv*. 2010;75:305–307.
16. Tan WA, Yadav JS, Wholey MH, et al. Endovascular options for peripheral arterial occlusive and aneurysmal disease. In: Topol EJ, ed. *Textbook of Interventional Cardiology*. 4th ed. Philadelphia, PA: Saunders; 2003:481–522.
17. Bates MC, Crotty B, Kavasmaneck C, et al. Renal artery angiography: "the right ipsilateral oblique" myth. *Catheter Cardiovasc Interv*. 2006;67:283–287.
18. Burket MW, Cooper CJ, Kennedy DJ, et al. Renal artery angioplasty and stent placement: predictors of a favorable outcome. *Am Heart J*. 2000;139:64–71.
19. Jaff MR, Olin JW. Atherosclerotic stenosis of the renal arteries: indications for intervention. *Texas Heart Inst J*. 1998;25:34–39.

CHAPTER 23

Mesenteric Vascular Intervention

Ross Kessler and Brian Funaki

Vascular interventions of the mesenteric vessels are typically performed to treat intestinal ischemia. Although acute mesenteric ischemia (AMI) and chronic mesenteric ischemia (CMI) differ in their clinical presentation, etiology, and management, both are a result of inadequate perfusion of the mesenteric vessels that can ultimately result in bowel infarction. It is essential that the treating vascular interventionalist should have a thorough knowledge of the current imaging modalities and endovascular therapies utilized in the diagnosis and management of mesenteric ischemia, respectively. This chapter will focus on the relevant anatomy, diagnostic evaluation, interventional techniques, and current research pertaining to mesenteric ischemia.

ANATOMIC CONSIDERATIONS

The small and large intestines are supplied by branches from three major arteries arising from the anterior surface of the abdominal aorta: the celiac trunk, the superior mesenteric artery (SMA), and the inferior mesenteric artery (IMA). Corresponding to their embryologic origins, the celiac trunk supplies the foregut region between the esophagus and the distal duodenum, the SMA supplies the midgut area between the proximal jejunum of the small intestine and the mid-transverse colon, and the IMA supplies the hindgut from the mid-transverse colon to the rectum (1). Within and across the vascular distributions, there is wide variability in normal individuals.

Arising at the level of T12, the celiac trunk is the first major branch of the abdominal aorta. In more than two thirds of cases, it courses anteriorly for 1 to 2 cm and bifurcates into the splenic and common hepatic arteries before giving rise to the left gastric artery (Fig. 23.1). In approximately one third of patients, the celiac trunk trifurcates into three main branches. In a very small percentage of cases, the origin of the celiac artery fuses with the SMA, creating a celiacomesenteric trunk (Fig. 23.2).

Typically, the splenic artery arises within 2 cm of the celiac trunk and has a torturous leftward and posterior course toward the hilum of the spleen. The first branch of the splenic artery is the dorsal pancreatic artery, which, as the name implies, supplies the posterior aspect of the pancreas and gives rise to the transverse pancreatic artery that perfuses the pancreatic body and tail. The dorsal pancreatic artery originates from the splenic artery in 39% of adults, but in the remaining 61% originates from another vessel such as the right hepatic artery, SMA, or celiac trunk (2). The distal splenic artery provides multiple short gastric arteries and the left gastroepiploic artery, which supply regions of the stomach and the greater omentum.

The common hepatic artery courses rightward and anteriorly, dividing into the proper hepatic artery and the gastroduodenal artery (Fig. 23.3). The proper hepatic artery subsequently divides into the right and left hepatic arteries; however, in 19% of patients, the right hepatic artery originates from the SMA and is referred to as a replaced right hepatic artery. Similarly, in less than 2% of cases, the entire common hepatic artery may arise from the SMA and is named a replaced common hepatic artery. In addition, the gastroduodenal artery, which provides branches to the stomach, pancreas, and proximal duodenum, arises from the common hepatic artery in 75% of patients but may originate from the left hepatic artery (11%) or right hepatic artery (8%) (3).

The SMA typically arises at the level of L1 and originates from the aorta approximately 1 cm inferior to the celiac trunk and superior to the renal arteries (Fig. 23.4). Its origin is posterior to the pancreas and splenic vein and the artery courses anteriorly toward the third portion of the duodenum. The SMA lies to the left of the superior mesenteric vein (SMV) as it crosses over the third portion of the duodenum and is usually posterior to the SMV as it enters the mesentery.

The SMA supplies several individual branches that arise sequentially from the right side of the main trunk including the inferior pancreaticoduodenal, middle colic, right colic, and ileocolic, and multiple jejunal (4–6) and ileal (8–12) branches that arise from the left side of the main trunk. The inferior pancreaticoduodenal artery, which anastomoses with branches from the gastroduodenal artery, may arise either as two separate branches or as a common single trunk. In succession, the middle colic artery and the right colic artery arise from the SMA and supply blood to the transverse and ascending colon, respectively. The right colic artery originates as a branch of the middle colic artery in 52% of cases (3). The ileocolic artery is the most constant branch of the SMA and can be used as an important landmark for angiographic interpretation. It provides collateral vessels to the terminal ileum, cecum, and first half of the right colon. Aberrant arteries arising from the SMA are a relatively common finding and include the hepatic artery, right hepatic artery, cystic artery, splenic artery, gastroduodenal artery, and left gastric artery (4).

The IMA typically arises at the level of L3 and is significantly smaller than either the celiac trunk or SMA (Fig. 23.5). The IMA courses to the left and provides branches to the distal transverse, descending, and sigmoid colon before it terminates

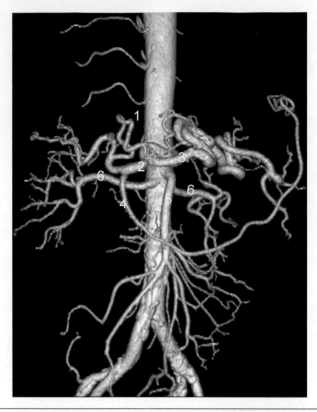

Figure 23.1 • CT angiogram of normal mesenteric arterial anatomy. Surface shaded reconstruction demonstrates typical anatomy. *(1)* Left gastric artery. *(2)* Common hepatic artery. *(3)* Splenic artery. *(4)* Gastroduodenal artery. *(5)* Superior mesenteric artery. *(6)* Renal arteries.

by dividing into two superior rectal (or hemorrhoidal) arteries. It gives origin to several branches from its left side, including the left colic artery, colosigmoid artery, and rectosigmoid artery. The left colic artery, the first and major branch of the IMA, travels adjacent to the inferior mesenteric vein (IMV) and bifurcates at the splenic flexure.

Collateral connections between the mesenteric vessels are well recognized and are essential for maintaining adequate perfusion when major mesenteric vessels are occluded or surgically ligated. An understanding of the collateral circulation is mandatory when performing endovascular revascularization procedures. Between the SMA and IMA, the major collateral arcade consists of the marginal artery of Drummond and meandering artery of Moskowitz, composed of branches of the ileocolic and right, middle, and left colic arteries (Fig. 23.6). In the absence of arterial occlusion, the marginal artery of Drummond may not be clearly visible on angiography, but it can enlarge significantly when the SMA or IMA is occluded. The arc of Riolan refers to a set of collaterals that communicates between the middle colic and left colic arteries at the splenic flexure. If the meandering artery of Moskowitz within this arc is visible on angiography, it is a strong indication that the SMA or IMA is occluded (Fig. 23.7) (5). The collateral circulation between celiac axis and SMA is predominantly via the pancreaticoduodenal arcade (Fig. 23.8). In some patients, persistence of a direct celiac and SMA communication may exist and is termed the arc of Buehler (Fig. 23.9).

In the mesenteric venous circulation, the SMV is typically a single vessel formed by a right and a left branch that receive blood from several veins (i.e., ileocolic, right colic, and middle colic veins). In other patients, the right and left branches may not form a single SMV, but instead join the splenic vein

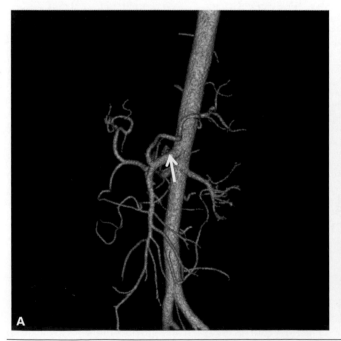

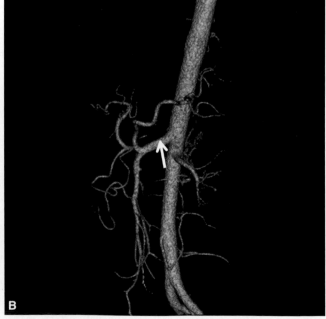

Figure 23.2 • Celiacomesenteric trunk. A,B: Shaded surface CTA reconstructions demonstrate celiacomesenteric trunk *(arrow)*.

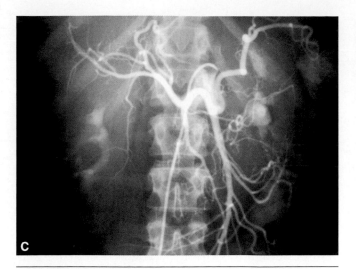

Figure 23.2 • *(Continued)* **C:** Conventional angiographic image shows celiacomesenteric trunk.

separately to form the portal vein. Similarly, the IMV may drain into the splenic vein or into the SMV after receiving blood from its mesenteric tributaries.

ACUTE MESENTERIC ISCHEMIA

AMI is a potentially fatal vascular emergency that necessitates early diagnosis and intervention to restore mesenteric blood flow and prevent bowel necrosis. Despite the development of modern treatment modalities, AMI remains a diagnostic challenge for clinicians due to its non-specific clinical presentation. The delay in diagnosis contributes to the high incidence of bowel infarction and the continued high mortality rate of 60% to 80% associated with this diagnosis (6).

The key to diagnosis of AMI is maintaining a high degree of clinical suspicion in high-risk individuals (see Table 23.1). Imaging may or may not be helpful. The utility

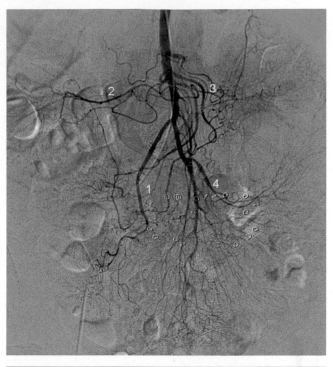

Figure 23.4 • **Anatomy of the superior mesenteric artery.** Selective angiogram of SMA shows conventional anatomy. *(1)* Ileocolic artery. *(2)* Right colic artery. *(3)* Jejunal branches. *(4)* Ileal branches.

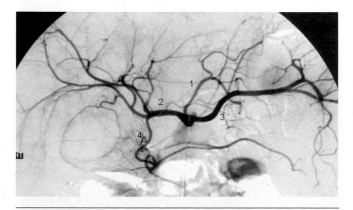

Figure 23.3 • **Anatomy of the celiac axis.** Selective angiogram of celiac trunk shows conventional celiac anatomy. *(1)* Left gastric artery. *(2)* Common hepatic artery. *(3)* Splenic artery. *(4)* Gastroduodenal artery.

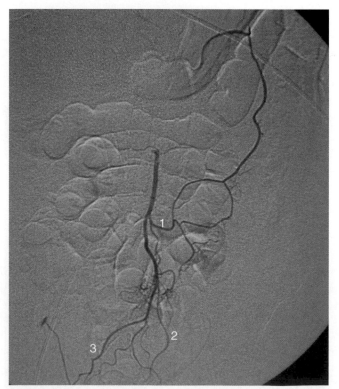

Figure 23.5 • **Anatomy of the inferior mesenteric artery.** Conventional inferior mesenteric angiogram showing perfusion of descending and sigmoid colon. *(1)* Left colic. *(2)* Sigmoid branches. *(3)* Superior rectal branch.

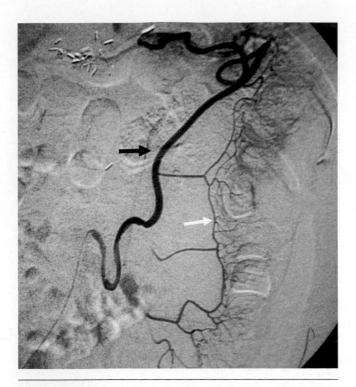

Figure 23.6 • Inferior mesenteric angiogram showing the meandering artery composed of ascending left colic branches *(black arrow)* and the marginal artery *(white arrow)*.

of plain radiographs is limited since findings of mesenteric thickening and thumbprinting are nonspecific and relatively late manifestations of the condition. The more specific findings of portal venous gas and intramural pneumatosis typically occur with bowel infarction and are associated with a poor prognosis. In addition, other noninvasive imaging modalities such as magnetic resonance angiography (MRA) and duplex ultrasound generally do not play an important role in the diagnostic workup of AMI because of its acute presentation. However, recent studies have shown that computed tomography angiography (CTA) has provided a noninvasive alternative to conventional angiography for the diagnosis of AMI (7–9). Multidetector CT scanners particularly with sagittal reformatting are capable of demonstrating the proximal mesenteric vessels very well. In one prospective study involving 62 patients undergoing biphasic multidetector row CT, AMI was identified as a possible diagnosis in all 26 who were ultimately determined to have mesenteric ischemia. Notably, only eight of these patients had arterial abnormalities seen on the CT angiogram, emphasizing the importance of associated bowel findings in making the diagnosis (7). CT findings of bowel wall thickening, intramural or portal venous gas, solid organ infarction, or lack of enhancement of bowel wall all aid in the diagnosis of mesenteric ischemia. However, it is important to recognize the limitations of CTA, as distal branches are not reliably evaluated compared with conventional angiography, and CTA is rarely able to diagnose nonocclusive mesenteric ischemia (NOMI).

Despite the recent interest in CTA, the gold standard for the diagnosis of AMI remains digital subtraction angiography. Because early diagnosis and treatment is critically important

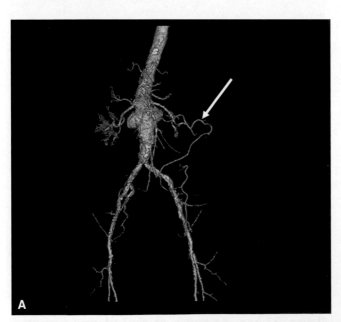

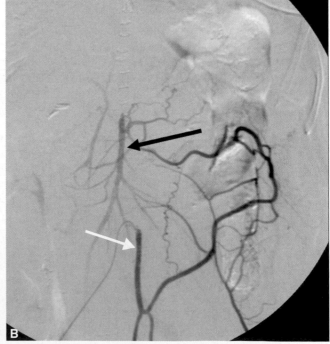

Figure 23.7 • **Hypertrophy of meandering artery of Moskowitz in patient with celiac and superior mesenteric artery occlusion.** **A:** Shaded surface CT angiogram shows enlarged meandering artery *(white arrow)*. **B:** Conventional selective inferior mesenteric artery (IMA) angiogram shows reconstitution of superior mesenteric artery *(black arrow)* via collateral from the IMA *(white arrow)*.

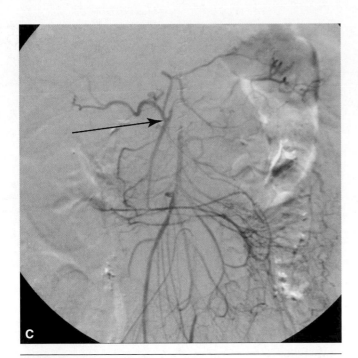

Figure 23.7 • *(Continued)* **C:** Delayed image from selective IMA angiogram shows reconstitution of the celiac axis *(black arrow)*.

supply and collaterals, the lateral view is better for visualizing the origins of the major visceral arteries.

Causes and Angiographic Appearance of Acute Mesenteric Ischemia

Although there are numerous causes of AMI (see Table 23.2), the four major etiologies are SMA embolism, NOMI, SMA thrombosis, and mesenteric venous thrombosis (MVT). By far, the most common cause of AMI is embolic occlusion of the SMA (Fig. 23.10), which accounts for 40% to 50% of all cases (10). Emboli are usually cardiac in origin and are associated with mural thrombi from cardiac hypokinesia, valvular vegetations, or arrhythmias in high-risk patients. While 15% of arterial emboli occur at the origin of the SMA, the majority lodge distal to the origin of the middle colic artery, which is the first major branch of the SMA (11). Due to the lack of collateral circulation in the setting of acute SMA obstruction, the onset of symptoms typically manifests as severe abdominal pain, fever, emesis, and diarrhea (sometimes bloody). The classic presentation is significant abdominal pain that is out of proportion to the patient's physical findings. However, it is not uncommon for a patient to present with an acute abdomen, including peritoneal signs and hypotension secondary to bowel infarction. Due to excessive fluid loss, laboratory findings include metabolic acidosis with elevated lactate levels, leukocytosis, and hemoconcentration. Angiographic findings of an acute embolus include the presence of a filling defect outlined by contrast, occlusion within a convex meniscus, and occlusion more than 3 cm distal to the origin of the SMA (12). In contrast, SMA thrombosis most commonly occurs in the setting of pre-existing stenotic disease at the origin of the vessel and usually spares distal arteries.

in AMI to avoid bowel infarction, angiography can provide rapid diagnostic information not available from CT and enables concurrent therapeutic treatment. Angiography begins with biplane abdominal aortography. While the anteroposterior view is best for demonstrating the distal mesenteric blood

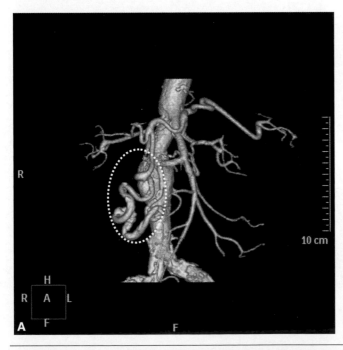

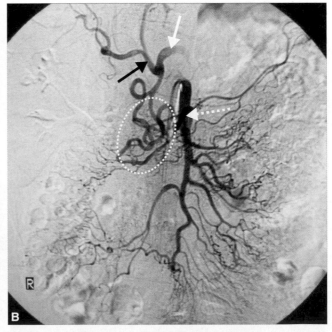

Figure 23.8 • Hypertrophy of pancreaticoduodenal arcade in patient with celiac axis occlusive disease. **A:** Shaded surface reconstruction CTA demonstrates hypertrophy of pancreaticoduodenal arcade *(within white circle)*. **B:** Conventional superior mesenteric artery *(interrupted white arrow)* angiogram showing retrograde flow through the pancreaticoduodenal arcade *(within white circle)* reconstituting common *(white arrow)* and proper *(black arrow)* hepatic arteries. *(Continued)*

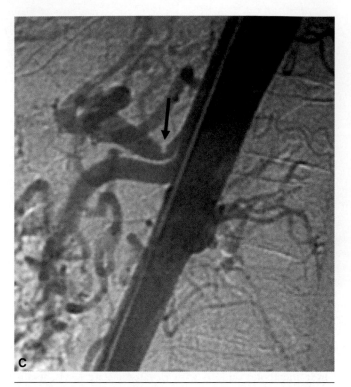

Figure 23.8 • *(Continued)* **C:** Lateral aortogram showing high-grade celiac stenosis *(black arrow)* in this patient.

NOMI accounts for 20% to 30% of all cases of AMI with a mortality rate of approximately 50% (13). The pathogenesis of NOMI is not clearly understood but involves a period of systemic hypotension associated with diffuse mesenteric vasoconstriction. In low-flow states, peripheral vasodilation may occur with shunting of blood away from the gut. This splanchnic vasoconstriction ultimately causes intestinal hypoxia and necrosis. Congestive heart failure, aortic insufficiency, hepatorenal disease, and vasoactive drugs such as cocaine, digitalis,

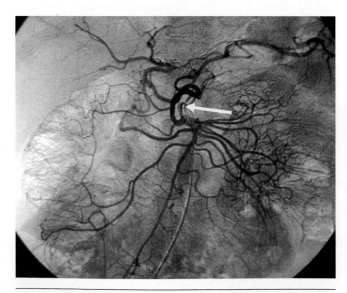

Figure 23.9 • Arc of Buehler. Conventional superior mesenteric angiogram shows communication between the superior mesenteric artery and celiac trunk via the arc of Buehler *(white arrow)*.

TABLE 23.1 Risk Factors for Acute Mesenteric Ischemia

Age >50 years

Cardiac disease
   Congestive heart failure
   Arrhythmias
   Recent or concurrent myocardial infarction
   Valvular disease
   Recent cardiac surgery
   Vasoconstrictor therapy

Hypovolemia

Hypotension

Sepsis

Hypercoagulable states

Prior arterial or venous emboli

Vasculitis

Trauma

TABLE 23.2 Causes of an Acute Mesenteric Ischemia

Arterial occlusion (50%)
   Embolus—usually to the superior mesenteric artery
   Thrombotic occlusion
   Aortic aneurysm
   Vasculitis
   Fibromuscular dysplasia
   Trauma

Nonocclusive ischemia (25–35%)
   Systemic hypotension
   Cardiac failure
   Septic shock
   Mesenteric vasoconstriction

Venous occlusion (10–15%)

Extravascular etiologies (<5%)
   Incarcerated hernia
   Volvulus
   Intussusception
   Adhesive disease

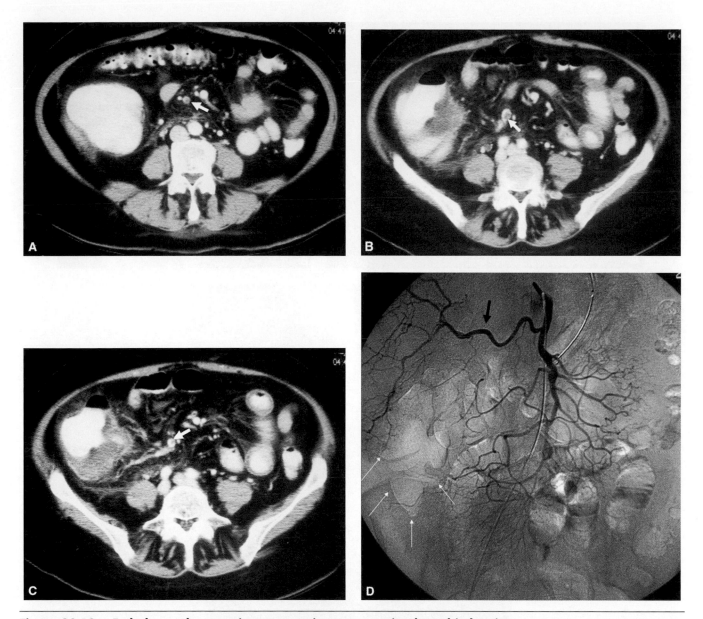

Figure 23.10 • Embolus to the superior mesenteric artery causing bowel ischemia. **A–C:** Axial enhanced CT images show marked bowel wall thickening of the cecum and distal small bowel and a round filling defect representing an embolus in the ileocolic branch of the superior mesenteric artery *(white arrow)*. **D:** Conventional superior mesenteric angiogram demonstrates no evidence of filling of the ileocolic branch with complete lack of perfusion to the cecum *(white arrows)*. Note replaced right hepatic artery *(black arrow)*.

and dopamine have all been shown to predispose patients to developing NOMI. Unlike patients with SMA embolism who have an acute onset of symptoms, those with NOMI typically have a more protracted clinical course. Because this condition frequently affects critically ill patients, some are unable to describe symptoms and instead undergo unexplained worsening in their clinical condition. More healthy patients may describe nonspecific abdominal pain. Angiographic findings of NOMI include diffuse arterial vasospasm, diminished arterial flow with reflux of contrast from the SMA into the aorta, and narrowing of peripheral mesenteric vessels or a pattern of alternating dilatation and narrowing (12).

Acute mesenteric thrombosis accounts for approximately 25% of all cases of AMI and occurs almost exclusively in the

setting of severe atherosclerotic disease (14). Although it can present acutely like a SMA embolism, most patients with SMA arterial thrombosis present with insidious symptoms of postprandial abdominal pain, nausea, and weight loss. Often patients with this condition can tolerate major mesenteric artery obstruction because the progressive nature of atherosclerosis allows the development of important collaterals. Reflecting the more chronic nature of the obstruction, angiographic findings reveal collateral vessels reconstituting distal SMA branches in many cases. The SMA is typically occluded proximally within 1 to 2 cm of its origin but reconstitutes distally via collateral circulation (Fig. 23.11) (12).

Usually located within the SMV, MVT accounts for less than 5% of cases of AMI (Fig. 23.12) (14). In the setting of acute

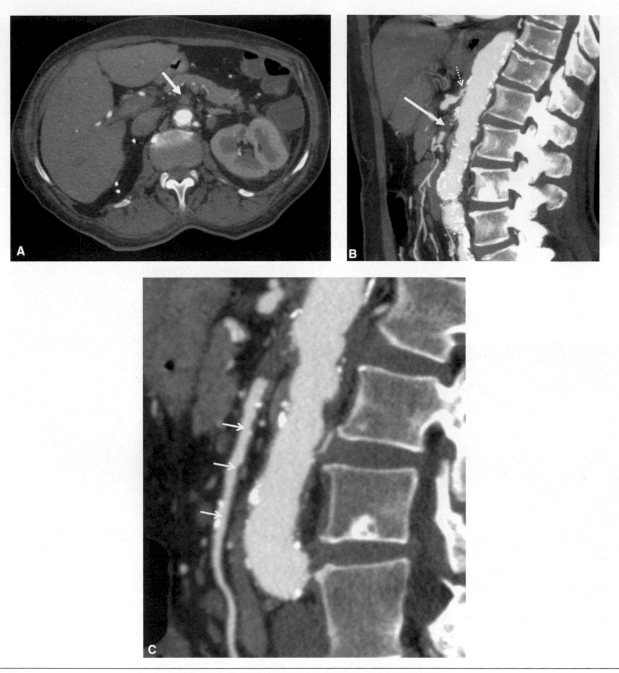

Figure 23.11 • Superior mesenteric artery thrombosis. **A:** Axial enhanced CT image shows thrombus *(white arrow)* in proximal superior mesenteric artery (SMA). **B:** Sagittal reformatted enhanced CT image shows proximal thrombus in SMA *(white arrow)* and high-grade stenosis of the celiac axis *(dashed white arrow)*. Note the presence of extensive calcification and atheroma in the abdominal aorta. **C:** Sagittal reformatted enhanced CT image shows distal SMA is patent without thrombus *(white arrows)*.

venous thrombosis without adequate collateral formation, intestinal mucosa edema develops and inhibits mesenteric arterial perfusion. Cases of MVT are commonly associated with hypercoagulable states, portal hypertension, oral contraceptives, and recent abdominal surgery (15). Except in the most severe cases, patients with MVT typically present late with nonspecific abdominal pain associated with anorexia, fever, and diarrhea. The angiographic findings of MVT include increased arterial resistance to flow, prolonged and intense mucosal staining of the bowel wall, vasospasm of the mesenteric arteries with persistence of the arterial phase, and lack of opacification of the mesenteric veins or portal vein (12).

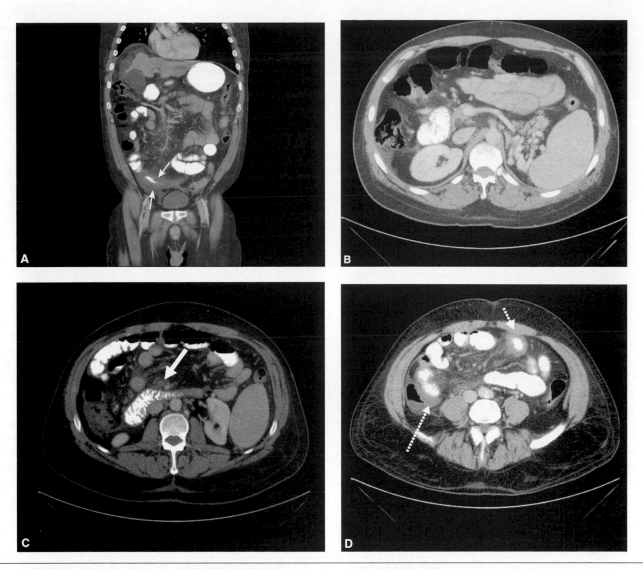

Figure 23.12 • Superior mesenteric vein thrombosis. **A:** Coronal reformatted CTA shows small bowel edema *(white arrows)* and fluid in the right lower quadrant. **B–D:** Axial CT images show thrombus in the superior mesenteric vein *(thick white arrow)* and bowel wall edema *(dashed white arrows)*.

Management of Acute Mesenteric Ischemia

Management of AMI is highly dependent on the underlying etiology and extent of the disease. Initial management in all cases involves adequate intravenous fluid resuscitation with crystalloids and blood products and should be initiated quickly to correct the volume deficit or systemic hypotension. In addition, empiric broad-spectrum antibiotics are recommended as ischemia leads to more frequent translocation of bacteria through the intestinal wall. Patients suspected of having AMI should undergo prompt diagnostic angiography in order to identify the extent of splanchnic occlusions and evaluate the overall mesenteric circulation. The presence of peritoneal signs

generally indicates bowel infarction rather than ischemia alone and necessitates emergency laparotomy. In a patient presenting with peritoneal signs, surgical procedures such as embolectomy or mesenteric bypass grafting are generally required in order to preserve remaining viable bowel and avoid certain mortality.

The role of endovascular therapy in the management of AMI may be either adjunctive or as the sole treatment modality in specific circumstances. In the setting of acute occlusive mesenteric ischemia (i.e., SMA embolism, arterial, or venous thrombosis), intra-arterial papaverine administration has been used before, during, and after surgery to prevent persistent mesenteric arterial vasoconstriction and minimize bowel infarction. In our hospital, this scenario is most common when AMI is diagnosed angiographically, enabling endovascular vasodilator therapy to mitigate the disorder while the patient is transported from the interventional radiology suite to the operating room. Several studies have reported lowered mortality rates of 45% to 50% and shorter bowel resections with coupled papaverine infusion compared to surgery alone (16). Furthermore, in the absence of peritoneal signs, endovascular thrombolytic therapy and balloon dilatation without surgery has been successful in recent reported cases of acute occlusive mesenteric ischemia. In terms of balloon dilatation, it is important to remember that macerating proximal clot will invariably lead to distal emboli that in some cases may worsen prognosis. While no data exist regarding the utility of distal embolic protection devices in this situation, it appears to be an ideal application of these devices. The inability to confidently exclude bowel infarction in many patients with mesenteric ischemia has limited widespread use of thrombolysis. Bowel infarction is an absolute contraindication to catheter-directed thrombolysis. While technically feasible, a recent review article identified published reports of thrombolytic therapy covering only a total of 43 patients and concluded that more evidence is needed to determine its effectiveness (17). If endovascular thrombolytic therapy is to be pursued without surgery, hemodynamically stable patients with comorbidities that present significant operative risk are prime candidates. Lastly, in patients with a small volume of arterial clot or MVT and minimal symptoms, anticoagulation and supportive therapy may be adequate.

In contrast to acute occlusive mesenteric ischemia, NOMI is typically treated without surgery unless peritoneal signs are present. The mainstay of therapy involves correcting the patient's underlying precipitating event, optimizing cardiovascular status, and endovascular intra-arterial infusion of papaverine for approximately 12 to 24 hours. The papaverine infusion is continued until all signs and symptoms of mesenteric ischemia have resolved. The administration of papaverine is contraindicated in the setting of systemic hypotension or hypovolemia due to the likelihood of causing a precipitous drop in systemic blood pressure.

Endovascular Treatment of NOMI with Intra-Arterial Papaverine

PATIENT SELECTION AND PREPARATION

Appropriate patients include individuals at risk for AMI with persistent abdominal pain lasting several hours. Typical resuscitative efforts should be instituted to restore an adequate circulating blood volume and address cardiac failure. Because cardiogenic shock and congestive heart failure may require systemic vasoconstrictor therapy for adequate management, this treatment may aggravate or precipitate mesenteric ischemia. Close multidisciplinary coordination is essential for management of these clinically complex patients.

ACCESS AND INTERVENTION

Femoral access is preferable and we usually begin with the right common femoral artery as the access site of choice. A 5- or 6-Fr. sheath is used to maintain vascular access and facilitate catheter exchange. Guiding catheters and sheaths are typically unnecessary. The authors preferentially use 0.035" guidewire

compatible systems. Frontal and lateral aortography is performed using approximately 30 to 40 mL of nonionic contrast injected at a rate of 15 to 20 mL/sec in each angiographic run. As noted above, the lateral projection best depicts proximal disease in the mesenteric vessels.

Selective catheterization of the visceral arteries should then be performed, to assess the adequacy of splanchnic blood flow and the extent of mesenteric vasoconstriction. The authors begin with an RC-1 curve catheter for celiac and SMA catheterization and RIM curve catheter for inferior mesenteric artery catheterization. If catheterization proves difficult, short recursive catheters such as Visceral Selective (VS)-1 may be helpful, especially in cases of proximal stenosis. For particularly challenging anatomy, hydrophilic catheters, guidewires, and using adjunctive catheterization techniques such as a Waltman's loop may be helpful but are usually unnecessary in the authors' experience.

Most typically, angiographic findings of NOMI include diffuse vasoconstriction of the mesenteric circulation with distal pruning and occasional areas of dilation and spasm in any given artery. When appropriate, papaverine infusion is initiated into the proximal SMA through the same 5-Fr. catheter used to engage the artery. The catheter tip should be positioned several centimeters distal to the origin of the artery to reduce the possibility of catheter disengagement. Papaverine, diluted in saline to 1 mg/mL, may be administered at a rate of 30 to 60 mL per hour, intra-arterially. A bolus of papaverine (30 to 60 mg) can also be given at the initiation of the infusion. The concentration may be changed depending on the patient's fluid status. Heparin should not be mixed with the infusion as it is incompatible with papaverine. Both sheath and catheter should be secured at the groin. At the authors' hospital, the sheath is typically sutured in place and tegaderm tape is used to secure the catheter. Because the infusion typically runs for greater than 12 hours, it is also helpful to mark the location on the shaft of the catheter where it enters the sheath with an ink pen so that inadvertent catheter retraction may be recognized at the bedside.

Therapy is best assessed with intermittent repeated angiography tailored by the time of day and the patients' condition. The dose may be tapered or saline may be substituted for papaverine immediately before repeated angiography and prior to cessation of therapy. Infusions lasting 24 hours are typical although in some patients therapy may be continued for up to several days.

COMPLICATIONS AND PROGNOSIS

AMI carries a high, associated mortality rate and papaverine infusion may be more suited as adjunctive rather than definitive therapy. With aggressive early intervention, survival rates approaching 50% have been reported. Potential complications include acute renal failure, secondary to contrast administration. Sudden systemic hypotension should alert physicians to possible catheter dislodgement with papaverine infusion into the aorta. A bedside plain radiograph should be immediately obtained to assess catheter position. There is a small chance of arterial thromboembolism, predominantly in the lower extremities. This risk increases in individuals with severe atherosclerotic disease of the aorta and iliac arteries. As this procedure is usually performed in conjunction with surgery, follow-up evaluation is usually tailored to the post-operative needs.

CHRONIC MESENTERIC ISCHEMIA

CMI is an infrequently occurring disease overwhelmingly caused by atherosclerotic stenosis or occlusion of the mesenteric arteries. Although atherosclerosis is relatively common, CMI is rare due to the rich mesenteric collateral circulation that progressively develops to perfuse the intestines. The bowel has an immense potential for vascular collateralization, as exemplified by the marginal artery of Drummond and the meandering artery of Moskowitz. While it is conventionally taught that occlusive disease must involve at least two of the three main mesenteric arteries (celiac trunk, SMA, IMA) in order to produce clinical symptoms, it is now commonly accepted that one or any combination of the three vessels can result in CMI. Decreased ability to form collaterals in the setting of diabetes or end-stage renal disease may explain why certain individuals develop symptoms with occlusion of one vessel while others are asymptomatic in the setting of three-vessel disease. In addition to atherosclerosis, other etiologies such as fibromuscular dysplasia, vasculitis, and post-radiation stenoses have been implicated as causes of CMI (18).

Due to its insidious onset, CMI can present a diagnostic challenge to clinicians. Classically, individuals present with post-prandial abdominal pain, diarrhea, sitophobia (food fear), and associated weight loss. While the mesenteric circulation is capable of supporting the metabolic demands of the resting gut, the diseased vasculature is unable to meet the increased metabolic needs of motility, secretion, and absorption that are induced by digestion. Patients typically present in the sixth and seventh decades of life and there is a slight female predominance. As expected, risk factors are associated with atherosclerosis and include hypertension, diabetes, hyperlipidemia, and a history of smoking (see Table 23.3). Moreover, physical examination may reveal an epigastric bruit in 48% to 63% of patients (19). The differential diagnosis of CMI includes a myriad of malabsorptive intestinal disorders, inflammatory bowel disease, aortic dissection, and numerous neoplastic etiologies such as pancreatic cancer or retroperitoneal lymphoma.

Noninvasive tests such as CTA, MRA, or duplex ultrasound should be the initial diagnostic imaging tests of choice for evaluation of CMI. Although angiography remains the gold standard for diagnosing CMI, it is currently reserved for the diagnosis of distal vessel disease or performed concurrently with endovascular treatment. Particularly, the development of multidetector CT scanners has permitted detailed analysis of the proximal mesenteric vessels and vascular flow. Using CTA, any projection or plane can be created to evaluate the degree of stenosis and the anatomic configuration of the vessel. Recent research has shown that mesenteric arterial stenosis is equally well detected by CTA and digital subtraction angiography (9,20). However, if the clinical suspicion of mesenteric ischemia is high, a negative CT should not preclude selective angiography, particularly if distal disease is a consideration.

In a patient with renal insufficiency or a history of severe reaction to iodinated contrast, duplex ultrasound of the mesenteric vessels is preferred over CT. Although results will vary considerably with operator expertise, patient body habitus, and presence of bowel gas, accuracy in detecting stenosis of the proximal mesenteric arteries has been reported to be greater than 90% (21). Peak systolic velocities greater than 275 cm/sec or end-diastolic velocities greater than 45 cm/sec have been shown to be highly sensitive for the presence of a stenosis greater than 70% (see Chapter 3) (22). In addition, MRA has recently gained interest as a diagnostic tool to evaluate CMI. Similar to ultrasound, MRA allows noninvasive imaging without exposure to radiation. Several reports have validated the use of gadolinium-enhanced MRA in the diagnosis of disease of the proximal mesenteric vessels, with a sensitivity and specificity exceeding 90% (23).

Management of Chronic Mesenteric Ischemia

Patients with symptoms consistent with CMI who have occlusion or hemodynamically significant stenosis in one or more of the mesenteric arteries should undergo revascularization. Left untreated, CMI may progress to bowel infarction and death. In the past, the primary treatment for CMI had been surgical revascularization via bypass grafting or endarterectomy. However, endovascular therapy has supplanted open surgical repair in recent years as the preferred therapy for mesenteric origin stenoses in patients without bowel infarction. Considerably less invasive than open surgery, endovascular therapies include percutaneous transluminal angioplasty (PTA) alone, or with stenting. Several studies have shown mortality and morbidity to be lower for endovascular interventions compared with open repair (24,25).

Although initial technical success rates following endovascular intervention are high (88% to 100%), patency rates at 1 year have been shown to decrease to 70% to 80% (19). In a recent Mayo clinic retrospective series of patients undergoing surgery or endovascular therapy, those undergoing endovascular revascularization were five times more likely to develop restenosis and four times more likely to undergo re-intervention (26). It has been hypothesized that stenting of mesenteric arteries offers more structural support to the arterial wall against elastic recoil when compared with PTA alone. In fact, a review of the literature shows a better patency rate for stented mesenteric arteries compared with balloon angioplasty alone (27). Lastly, a small body of literature also supports the use of endovascular recanalization of completely occluded mesenteric arteries in patients at relatively high risk for surgery (28). However, in such cases, embolization that can lead to bowel infarction is a major concern and embolic protection should be considered.

TABLE 23.3 Risk Factors for Chronic Mesenteric Ischemia

Age (older than 50)
Hypertension
Diabetes mellitus
Hyperlipidemia
Coronary artery disease
Renal disease
Smoking
Obesity
Sedentary lifestyle

Endovascular Revascularization in Chronic Mesenteric Ischemia

PATIENT SELECTION

Commonly, the diagnosis of CMI is one of exclusion. In most cases, patients should have weight loss, abdominal pain, sitophobia, or some combination of these symptoms with noninvasive image findings that confirm proximal mesenteric occlusive disease. In out institution, Doppler ultrasound studies are often used as a screening study and nearly all patients receive CTA to confirm the diagnosis. MRA may be substituted for CTA in some hospitals based on local practice patterns and expertise.

ACCESS AND INTERVENTION

The common femoral artery is punctured and a 30- to 45-cm long 6-Fr. guiding sheath (such as a Balkin or renal curve) is inserted. The sheath functions as both a "backbone" to facilitate crossing tight mesenteric artery stenoses and a port to perform contrast injections while balloons, wires, and stents are positioned across the stenosis. A brachial artery approach is sometimes necessary for severely downward pointing mesenteric arteries (a multipurpose angled curved sheath is then used). However, we start with a femoral approach initially due to the lower risk of brachial artery puncture site complications and rarely (less than 5% of the time) need to use a brachial approach. The sheath is advanced into the infrarenal aorta from the femoral artery approximately 10 to 15 cm below the mesenteric arteries.

In patients with normal renal function, an aortogram is performed in the lateral view at the level of the mesenteric arteries in the projection dictated by cross-sectional imaging to best depict the origin and proximal aspect of the artery of interest in its entirety. The image intensifier may need to be positioned in a slightly oblique view rather than straight lateral view to be orthogonal to the ostium of the mesenteric artery of interest. The correct angulation can be easily determined by reviewing CTA data. The image intensifier must be orthogonal to the lesion of interest that is usually at the origin of the artery. In patients with renal insufficiency, carbon dioxide may be used or aortography may be omitted altogether, especially if either CTA or MRA is available. If occlusive findings are confirmed on aortography, the appropriate vessel is targeted for revascularization. In most cases, the SMA is technically easier to treat although the choice of vessel must be individualized in each patient.

Five thousand units of heparin are administered intra-arterially. Some interventionalists prefer the "no-touch" method of catheterization and this technique is more appropriate if distal embolic protection devices are utilized. We favor use of reverse-curved catheters and have not routinely used distal embolic protection. A short reverse-curved catheter (e.g., visceral selective 1, Cook, Bloomington, IN) is advanced into the abdominal aorta and formed below the mesenteric artery orifice. If this catheter does not spontaneously form in the abdominal aorta, it can be advanced into the descending thoracic aorta where it will form near the arch. Unlike longer reverse-curved catheters such as a Simmons 2, this short recursive catheter reforms itself in the thoracic aorta, making it technically easier to manipulate. If formed near the arch, a soft-tipped guidewire

(e.g., Bentson) is advanced out of the end of the catheter and the catheter is retracted with the wire leading into the infrarenal abdominal aorta. The guidewire prevents inadvertent catheterization of more proximal arteries such as spinal arteries and dragging the catheter across aortic plaques.

The catheter–guidewire combination is then advanced cephalad (i.e., assuming that the catheter can be reshaped inferior to the mesenteric orifice) and pointed toward the mesenteric artery of interest until the wire engages the orifice of the target artery. The wire is gently rotated by the fingertips of the operator as the catheter is pulled caudal to cross the lesion. The "knee" or top curve of the catheter is positioned at the level of the mesenteric artery orifice (Fig. 23.13). In very severe stenoses or occlusions, a hydrophilic wire may be necessary and, rarely, longer reverse-curved catheters may be used (Fig. 23.14) prior to resorting to brachial access (Fig. 23.15). The guiding sheath is then advanced close to the orifice of the mesenteric artery to provide mechanical advantage. The guidewire is removed and a small volume of dilute contrast is injected into the reverse-curved catheter to confirm intraluminal location and to exclude the possibility of dissection. Contrast injection to confirm intraluminal catheter tip position is very important and should not be omitted even if the lesion is crossed in an atraumatic fashion. If necessary, a pressure measurement can be obtained at this point recognizing that the catheter will tend to exacerbate the degree of stenosis (i.e., if the pressure gradient is less than 10 mm Hg, it is unlikely that the lesion is hemodynamically significant). A rigid, short-tipped "working wire" is advanced into the distal mesenteric artery. We typically use either a 0.035″ Rosen wire or a 0.018″ McNamara wire (Fig. 23.16) as the working wire for the intervention.

The authors' practice is to stent all ostial lesions. With current pre-mounted stents, pre-dilation with sheath advancement across the sheath is typically unnecessary. By omitting the pre-dilation, we believe the incidence of distal plaque embolization is reduced (although this is arguable). On the other hand, rarely, pre-dilation proves difficult or impossible and alerts the operator that stent insertion should NOT be attempted. A pre-mounted 5- or 6-mm balloon-expandable stent (the authors typically use a 6 mm diameter × 17-mm long stent in most patients) is positioned with approximately 2 to 3 mm protruding into the aorta. A small amount of dilute contrast is injected into the sidearm of the sheath to ensure proper positioning. The balloon is then slowly inflated to deploy the stent. Both ends of the balloon should inflate initially (the balloon looks like a dumbbell) so the stent does not migrate proximal or distal during deployment. As in all arterial dilation procedures, the guidewire must be maintained across the lesion at all times. A final angiogram is then obtained through the sidearm of the sheath to assess the result and exclude dissection. If the result is adequate, the catheter and wire are removed.

In patients with both celiac and SMA stenoses, both lesions may be treated during the same procedure although in our experience, revascularization of one artery will often result in significant symptomatic improvement. Revascularization of the IMA is rarely performed. The sheath is removed

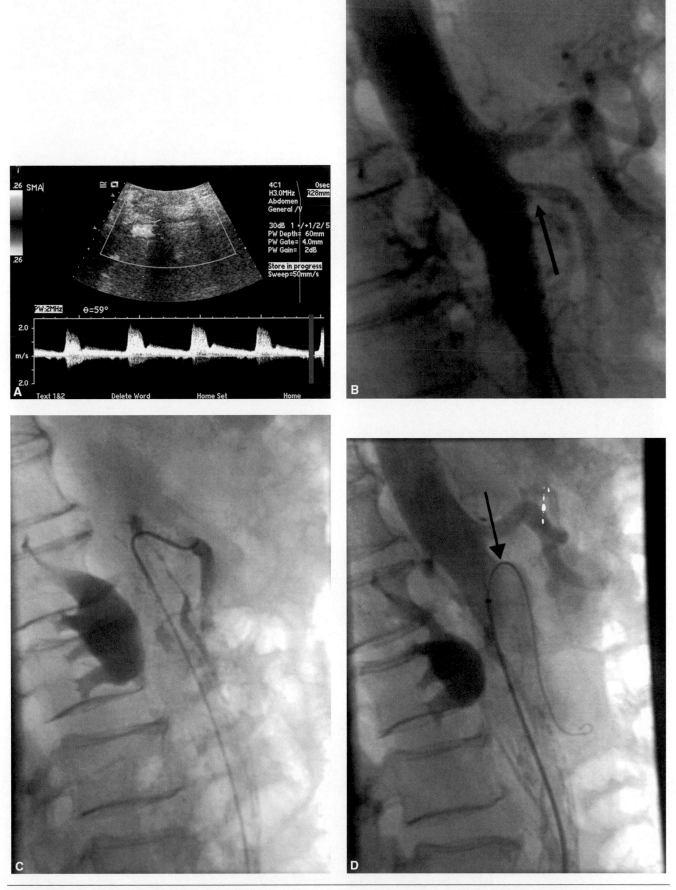

Figure 23.13 • Interventional treatment of high-grade superior mesenteric artery stenosis (SMA). A: Initial Doppler study demonstrating elevated peak systolic velocity of approximately 200 cm/min in the SMA. **B:** Lateral aortogram shows SMA stenosis en face *(black arrow)*. Trans-stenotic lesional gradient was greater than 35 mm Hg. **C:** Selective superior mesenteric angiogram after crossing the lesion with a reverse-curved catheter. **D:** 0.035″ wire has been advanced across the SMA stenosis. Aortogram obtained through the guiding sheath shows lesion *(black arrow)*. *(Continued)*

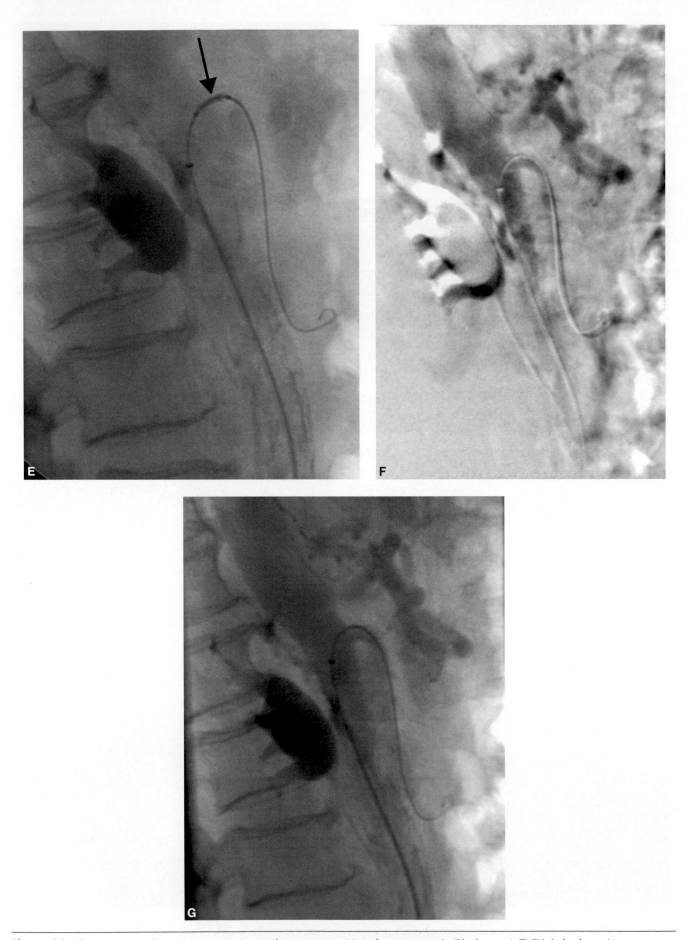

Figure 23.13 • *(Continued)* **E:** Fluoroscopic image shows stent positioned across stenosis *(black arrow)*. **F:** Digital subtraction aortogram via sheath following stenting. **G:** Unsubtracted aortogram shows wide patency of stent.

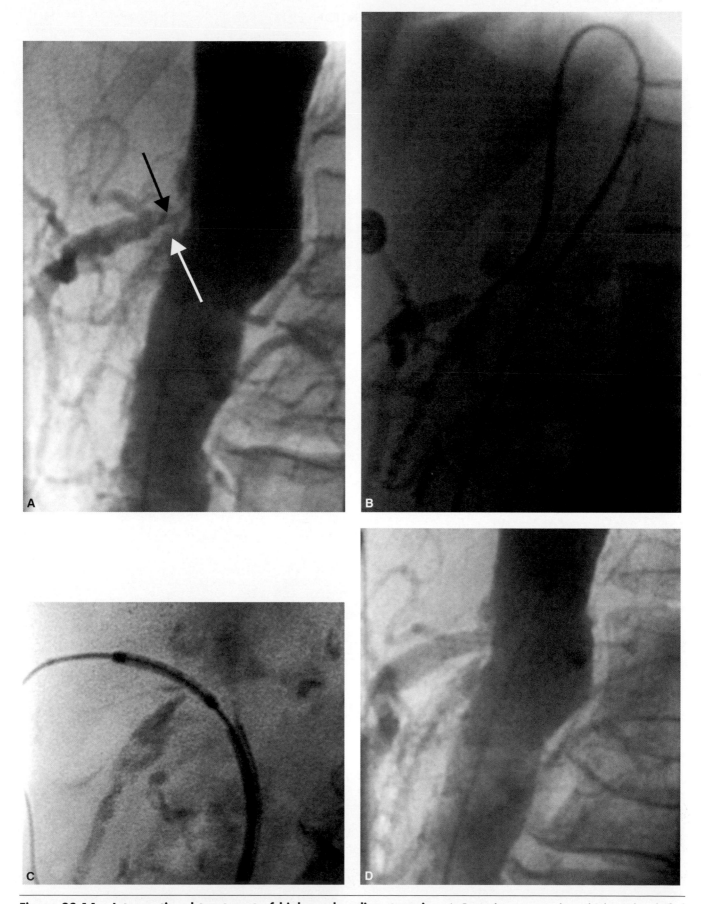

Figure 23.14 • Interventional treatment of high-grade celiac stenosis. **A:** Lateral aortogram shows high-grade calcified celiac *(black arrow)* and superior mesenteric artery (SMA) *(white arrow)* stenoses. **B:** Fluoroscopic image shows Simmons 2 catheter used to cross celiac stenosis. **C:** Fluoroscopic image shows stent positioning. **D:** Celiac angiogram after stent insertion shows relief of stenosis.

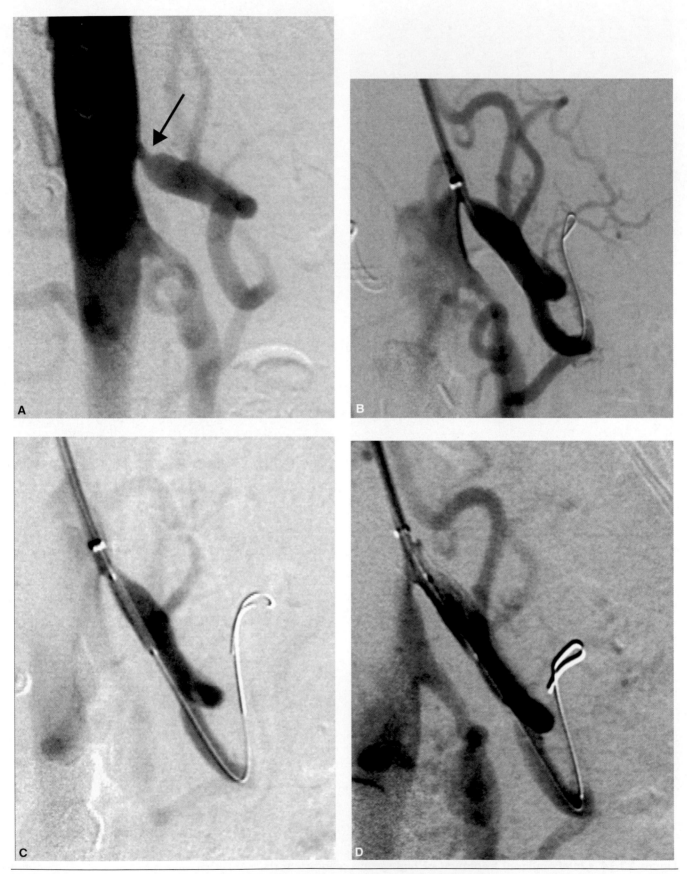

Figure 23.15 • Interventional treatment of celiac artery stenosis using brachial access. **A:** Lateral aortogram shows celiac stenosis *(black arrow)*. **B:** Angiogram via guiding sheath shows guidewire positioning. **C:** Angiogram via guiding sheath shows stent positioned too far into artery. **D:** Final angiogram via sheath following stent placement.

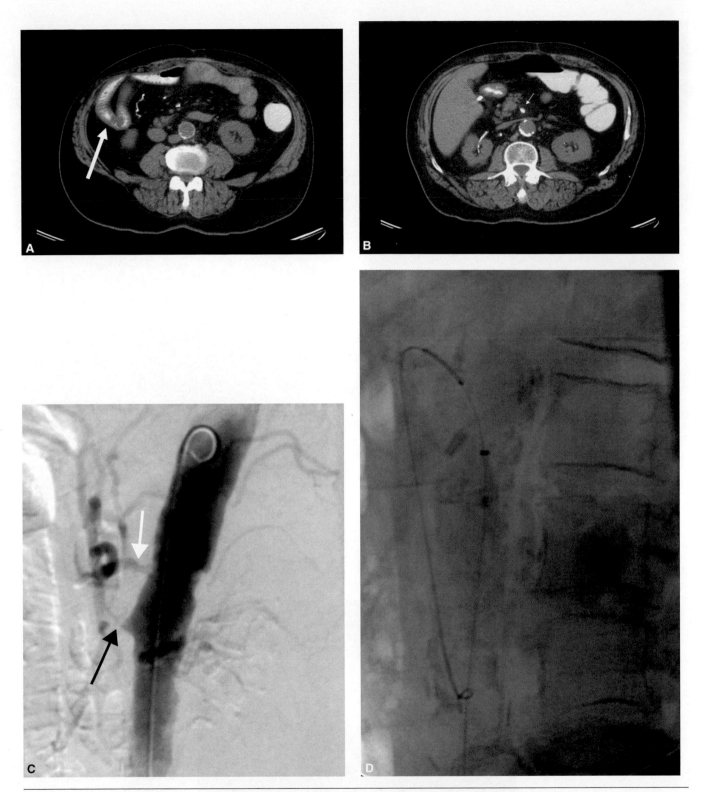

Figure 23.16 • Celiac stent insertion in patient with acute and chronic mesenteric ischemia. **A:** Axial CT image shows small bowel edema *(white arrow)*. **B:** Unenhanced CT image shows significant calcification in lumen of superior mesenteric artery (SMA). **C:** Lateral aortogram showing SMA occlusion *(black arrow)* and high-grade celiac stenosis *(white arrow)*. **D:** Fluoroscopic image shows stent positioning across celiac stenosis over 0.018″ guidewire. *(Continued)*

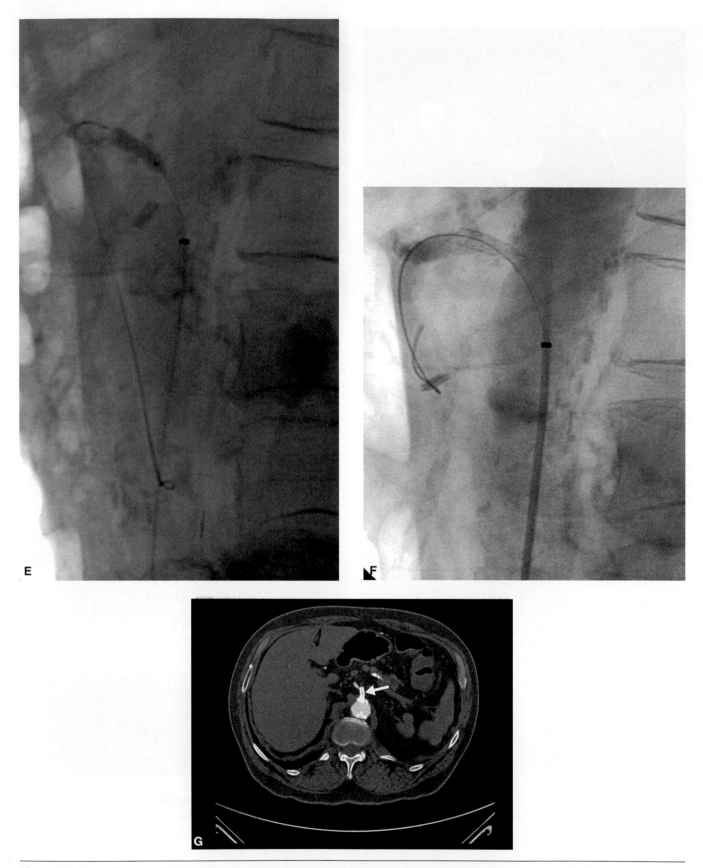

Figure 23.16 • *(Continued)* **E:** Fluoroscopic image shows stent deployment. **F:** Post-stent insertion aortogram via sheath shows patency of stent. **G:** Axial enhanced CT image obtained 1 year later shows continued patency of celiac stent *(white arrow)* with lateral calcified aortic plaque. The patient was asymptomatic at 1-year follow-up.

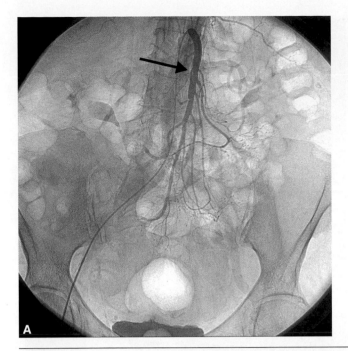
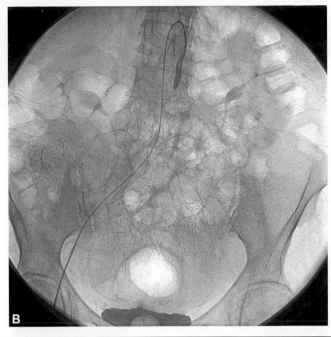

Figure 23.17 • Iatrogenic dissection of superior mesenteric artery. **A:** Superior mesenteric angiogram shows proximal spiral dissection in SMA (best seen at tip of *black arrow*). **B:** Delayed phase from superior mesenteric angiogram shows contrast stasis in false lumen of iatrogenic dissection.

when coagulation factors normalize or a closure device is used. We routinely admit patients overnight and they are discharged the morning after the procedure. They receive 3 to 6 months of clopidogrel (75 mg/day) and lifelong baby aspirin (81 mg/day).

FOLLOW-UP EVALUATION

A baseline duplex US evaluation is obtained to evaluate flow in the mesenteric circulation, at 6 months and yearly thereafter. CTA can also be used for periodic follow-up, particularly when vascular disease is present throughout multiple vascular territories.

COMPLICATIONS

Complications include access site hematoma, iatrogenic dissection, rupture, and distal embolization. Iatrogenic dissection is rare (Fig. 23.17) and if recognized may be treated with balloon angioplasty to tack the dissection flap down, stenting, or simply watchful waiting. The latter is appropriate if the dissection is not flow limiting. Overall, the complication rate is low, ranging between 0% and 10%, and is mostly related to access site complications (29).

MEDIAN ARCUATE LIGAMENT SYNDROME

The median arcuate ligament is a fibrous band connecting the right and left hemidiaphragms and is found in up to 20% of the population. Given the extensive collateral circulation between the celiac artery and the SMA, primarily via the pancreaticoduodenal arcade, existence of abdominal symptoms due to compression of the celiac artery by the median arcuate ligament is debatable. The compression has been postulated to limit blood flow to the bowel or irritate the celiac ganglion, both of which may result in abdominal pain. Angiography may be the best diagnostic modality to confirm the diagnosis of median arcuate ligament syndrome, in which dynamic compression of the celiac artery is demonstrated with a combination of inspiratory and expiratory images (19). However, compression of the celiac artery may also be a normal finding in asymptomatic patients and is well characterized (30). The diagnosis of median arcuate ligament syndrome should be considered in young patients who have unexplained abdominal pain, normal upper endoscopy, normal laboratory studies, and particularly in female patients with an abdominal bruit (from partially obstructed flow in the celiac artery). In terms of treatment, there is no current evidence that supports the use of angioplasty and stenting in the management of median arcuate ligament syndrome. Instead, surgical therapy with release of the median arcuate ligament should be the primary treatment of choice in these cases. Because chronic, repeated compression of the celiac axis may result in a fixed fibrotic stenosis, in patients with continued symptoms after ligament release, our practice is to perform angioplasty and stenting provided there is continued evidence of celiac narrowing (Fig. 23.18). Predictors for successful outcome following surgery are reported to include age between 40 and 60 (77% cured) and weight loss of 20 lb or more (67% cured) (31).

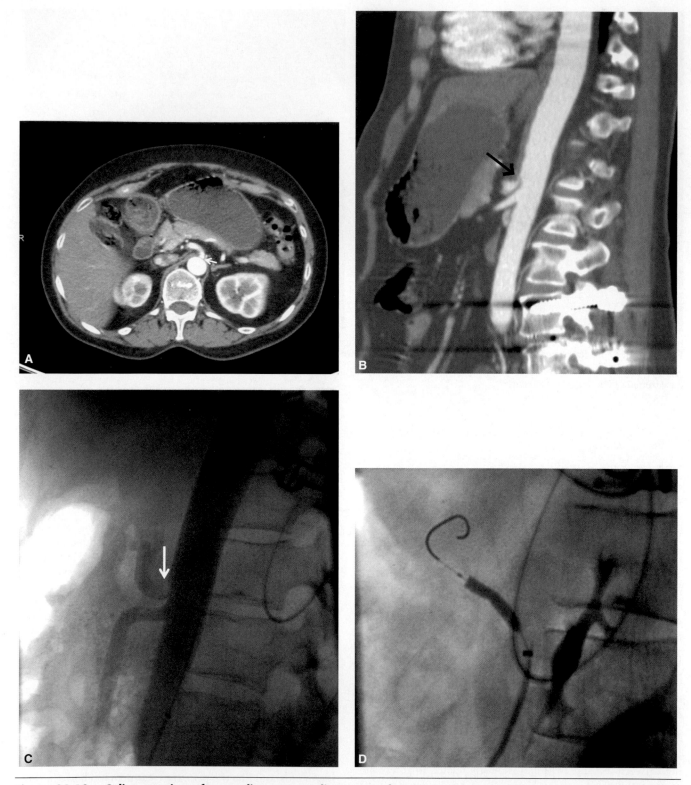

Figure 23.18 • Celiac stenting after median arcuate ligament release. **A:** Axial CT angiogram shows proximal band-like stenosis of celiac axis *(white arrow)*. **B:** Sagittal reconstruction of CT angiogram shows high-grade celiac stenosis *(black arrow)*. **C:** After laparoscopic ligament release, a lateral aortogram shows continued stenosis of the celiac axis *(white arrow)*. **D:** Fluoroscopic image shows stent deployment.

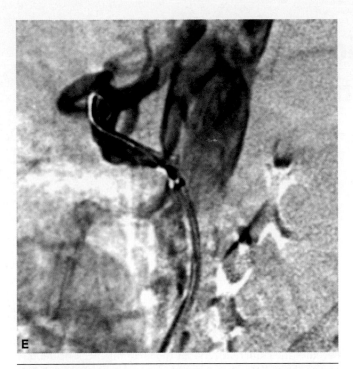

Figure 23.18 • *(Continued)* **E:** Subtraction aortogram obtained via the sheath shows improved flow through the proximal celiac artery with poststenotic dilation.

References

1. Sadler TW. *Langman's Medical Embryology*. Baltimore, MD: Williams & Wilkins; 1985.
2. Michels N. *Blood Supply and Anatomy of the Upper Abdominal Organs*. Philadelphia, PA: J.B. Lippincott; 1955.
3. Lin PH, Chaikof EL. Embryology, anatomy and surgical exposure of the great abdominal vessels. *Surg Clin North Am*. 2000;80:417–433.
4. Iannaccone R, Laghi A, Passariello R. Multislice CT angiography of mesenteric vessels. *Abdom Imaging*. 2004;29:146–152.
5. Connolly JE. The meandering mesenteric artery or central anastomotic artery. *J Vasc Surg*. 2006;43:1059.
6. Oldenburg WA, Lau LL, Rodenberg TJ, et al. Acute mesenteric ischemia: a clinical review. *Arch Intern Med*. 2004;164:1054–1062.
7. Kirkpatrick ID, Kroeker MA, Greenberg HM. Biphasic CT with mesenteric CT angiography in the evaluation of acute mesenteric ischemia: initial experience. *Radiology*. 2003;229:91–98.
8. Lee R, Tung HK, Tung PH, et al. CT in acute mesenteric ischemia. *Clin Radiol*. 2003;58:279–287.
9. Stueckle CA, Haegele KF, Jendreck M, et al. Multislice computed tomography angiography of the abdominal arteries: comparison between computed tomography angiography and digital subtraction angiography findings in 52 cases. *Australas Radiol*. 2004;48:142–147.
10. Kaleya RN, Sammartano RJ, Boley SJ. Aggressive approach to acute mesenteric ischemia. *Surg Clin North Am*. 1992;72:157–182.
11. Stoney RJ, Cunningham CG. Acute mesenteric ischemia. *Surgery*. 1993;114:489–490.
12. Baum S, Pentecost MJ, eds. Abrams' *Angiography: Interventional Radiology*. 2nd ed. Philadelphia, PA: Lippincott Williams & Wilkins; 2006.
13. Trompeter M, Brazda T, Remy CT, et al. Non-occlusive mesenteric ischemia: etiology, diagnosis, and interventional therapy. *Eur Radiol*. 2002;12:1179–1187.
14. Mansour MA. Management of acute mesenteric ischemia. *Arch Surg*. 1999;134:328–330.
15. Hassan H, Raufman JP. Mesenteric venous thrombosis. *South Med J*. 1999;92:558–562.
16. Boley SJ, Feinstein FR, Sammartano R, et al. New concepts in the management of emboli of the superior mesenteric artery. *Surg Gynecol Obstet*. 1981;153:561–569.
17. Schoots IG, Levi MM, Reekers JA, et al. Thrombolytic therapy for acute superior mesenteric artery occlusion. *J Vasc Interv Radiol*. 2005;16:317–329.
18. Cognet F, Ben Salem D, Dranssart M, et al. Chronic mesenteric ischemia: imaging and percutaneous treatment. *Radiographics*. 2002;22:863–879.
19. Herbert H, Steele S. Acute and chronic mesenteric ischemia. *Surg Clin North Am*. 2007;87:1115–1134.
20. Cademartiri F, Raaijmakers RH, Kuiper JW, et al. Multidetector row CT angiography in patients with abdominal angina. *Radiographics*. 2004;24:969–984.
21. Harward TR, Smith S, Seeger JM. Detection of celiac axis and superior mesenteric artery occlusive disease with use of abdominal duplex scanning. *J Vasc Surg*. 1993;17:738–745.
22. Perko MJ. Duplex ultrasound for assessment of superior mesenteric artery blood flow. *Eur J Vasc Endovasc Surg*. 2001;21:106–117.
23. Meaney JF, Prince MR, Nostrant TT, et al. Gadolinium-enhanced MR angiography of visceral arteries in patients with suspected chronic mesenteric ischemia. *J Magn Reson Imaging*. 1997;7:171–176.
24. Brown DJ, Schermerhorn ML, Powell RJ, et al. Mesenteric stenting for chronic mesenteric ischemia. *J Vasc Surg*. 2005;42:268–274.
25. Matsumoto AH, Angle JF, Spinosa DJ, et al. Percutaneous transluminal angioplasty and stenting in the treatment of chronic mesenteric ischemia: results and longterm followup. *J Am Coll Surg*. 2002;194(suppl 1):S22–S31.
26. Oderich GS, Sullivan TM, Bower TC, et al. Open vs endovascular revascularization for chronic ischemia: risk-stratified outcomes. Paper presented at: Society for Vascular Surgery Annual Meeting; June 3, 2006; Philadelphia, PA.
27. Landis MS, Rajan DK, Simson ME, et al. Percutaneous management of chronic mesenteric ischemia: outcomes after intervention. *J Vasc Interv Radiol*. 2005;16:1319–1325.
28. Sarac TP, Altinel A, Kashyap V, et al. Endovascular treatment of stenotic and occluded visceral arteries for chronic mesenteric ischemia. *J Vasc Surg*. 2008;47:485–491.
29. Schaefer PJ, Schaefer FK, Muller-Huelsbeck S, et al. Chronic mesenteric ischemia. Stenting of mesenteric arteries. *Abdom Imaging*. 2007;32:304–309.
30. Lee VS, Morgan JN, Tan AG, et al. Celiac artery compression by the median arcuate ligament: a pitfall of end-expiratory MR imaging. *Radiology*. 2003;228:437–442.
31. Reilly LM, Ammar AD, Stoney RJ, et al. Late results following operative repair for celiac artery compression syndrome. *J Vasc Surg*. 1985;2:79–91.

CHAPTER 24

Subclavian, Brachiocephalic, and Upper Extremity Intervention

Leslie Cho, Ivan P. Casserly, and Mark H. Wholey

Brachiocephalic or subclavian artery obstruction accounts for about 15% of symptomatic, extracranial, cerebrovascular disease. Rapid advances in technology and evolution in technique over the last decade have resulted in percutaneous revascularization techniques supplanting surgery as the therapy of choice for the treatment of these lesions. Owing to the predilection of atherosclerosis for these sites, and the relative sparing of more distal upper extremity vessels, brachiocephalic and subclavian artery intervention comprise the majority of upper extremity endovascular procedures and will form the major focus of this chapter. Additional, less common vascular pathologies encountered during angiography of the upper extremity arterial circulation will also be highlighted.

ANATOMY

The subclavian arteries originate from the bifurcation of the brachiocephalic artery on the right, and directly from the aortic arch as the third, and final, of the great vessels on the left (Fig. 24.1A).

In approximately 0.5% of patients, the right subclavian artery arises anomalously, as the terminal vessel from the descending thoracic aorta, and courses toward its normal distribution to the right upper extremity (Fig. 24.1B).

Rarely, the right subclavian artery and right common carotid arteries have a separate origin as the first and second of the great vessels, respectively, from the arch (Fig. 24.1C).

Additional variations in arch anatomy that are important during upper extremity angiography include common origin of the innominate and left common carotid artery (CCA) from the arch (about 15%) (Fig. 24.1D), and bovine origin of the left CCA from the innominate artery (about 10%) (Fig. 24.1E).

In healthy young individuals, the great vessels arise from the horizontal portion of the arch. With increasing age and atherosclerotic disease, this portion of the arch descends into the thoracic cavity together with the origin of the great vessels, such that they appear to arise from the ascending portion of the arch (Fig. 24.1F,G).

The most important branches of the subclavian artery arise from the first segment of the artery (i.e., medial to the scalenus anterior muscle) (Fig. 24.2A). The vertebral and internal mammary artery branches of the subclavian artery are remarkably constant in their origin and course, arising as the first and second branches, respectively. These branches supply the posterior cerebral circulation and the anterior chest wall, respectively. In 1% to 5% of patients, the left vertebral artery had a direct origin from the aortic arch, typically between the origins of the left CCA and the left subclavian artery (Fig. 24.2B).

In contrast, the thyrocervical trunk, which arises as the third branch, demonstrates significant variation in both the pattern and size of its various branches (i.e., inferior thyroid, suprascapular, ascending cervical, transverse cervical).

At the lateral margin of the first rib, the subclavian artery becomes the axillary artery. At the anatomic neck of the humerus, the axillary artery changes name to become the brachial artery (Fig. 24.2C).

In the arm, the brachial artery supplies the deep brachial branch that runs posteriorly (and is relatively small in caliber compared with its counterpart in the thigh), and the superior and inferior ulnar collateral arteries that supply collateral flow to the elbow region. Opposite the neck of the radius, the brachial artery typically divides into the radial and ulnar arteries (Fig. 24.2D).

The ulnar artery is usually the larger of the terminal branches of the brachial artery. Just distal to its origin, it gives off the anterior and posterior ulnar recurrent arteries that supply collateral flow to the elbow, and then gives off its major branch, the common interosseous. Thereafter, the ulnar artery descends on the medial side of the forearm. The radial artery supplies a radial recurrent branch to the elbow, and descends on the lateral side of the forearm. In some cases, the radial artery may originate high from the axillary or upper brachial artery. This is an important anatomic variant, as it may cause significant confusion during diagnostic angiography if its presence is not appreciated.

The arterial anatomy of the hand is extremely variable, and deviations from the classic patterns are common (Fig. 24.2E,F).

The ulnar artery supplies the superficial palmar arch and the radial artery supplies the deep palmar arch. In 10% of the population, the anterior interosseous or median artery persists and supplies the deep palmar arch. Typically, the superficial arch is dominant and lies distal to the deep arch. The princeps pollicis and radialis indicis arteries arise from the radial artery and supply the thumb and index finger. The superficial palmar arch gives off three or four common palmar digital arteries, and the deep arch gives off the palmar metacarpal arteries. At the bases of the proximal phalanges, adjacent metacarpal vessels from each arch join and then immediately divide into proper digital arteries, which supply the fingers (1,2).

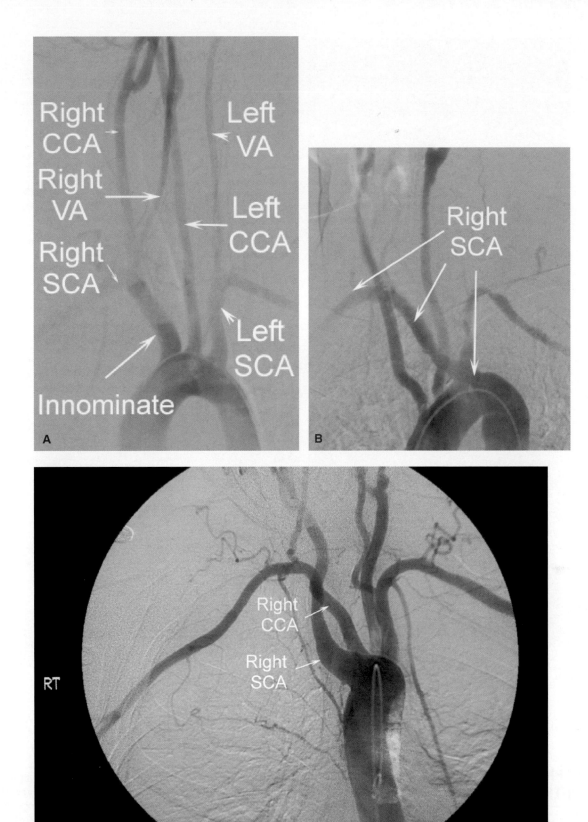

Figure 24.1 • Normal and variant anatomy of the aortic arch.   **A:** Arch aortogram in LAO projection demonstrating normal angiographic anatomy. **B:** Anomalous origin of right SCA as terminal great vessel off aortic arch. **C:** Separate origin of right SCA and CCA from aortic arch demonstrated in aortogram in RAO projection. *(Continued)*

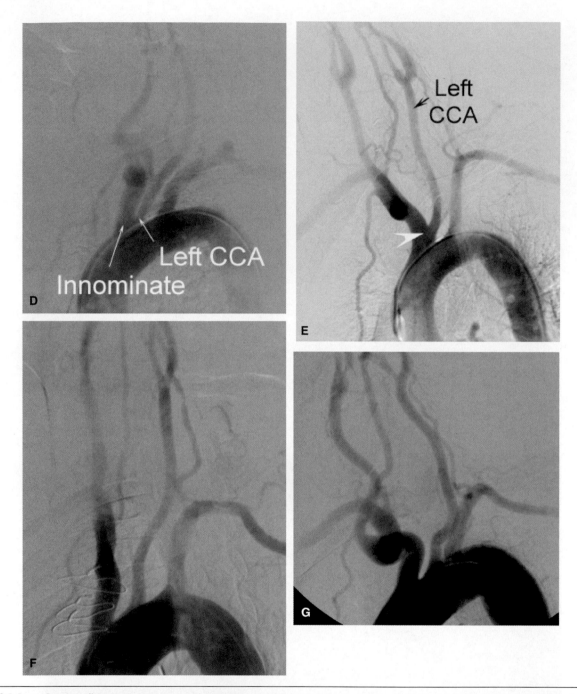

Figure 24.1 • *(Continued)* **D:** Common origin of innominate and left CCA from aortic arch. **E:** Bovine origin of left CCA from innominate artery *(arrowhead)*. **F:** Type II aortic arch. **G:** Type III aortic arch. CCA, common carotid artery; VA, vertebral artery; SCA, subclavian artery.

BRACHIOCEPHALIC AND SUBCLAVIAN ARTERY INTERVENTION

Patient Selection

As in all endovascular procedures, careful patient selection is absolutely crucial to the success of the intervention (Table 24.1).

With some exceptions, intervention is generally reserved for patients with symptomatic subclavian or brachiocephalic disease. It is worth emphasizing that most patients with angiographic evidence of subclavian or brachiocephalic artery stenosis are asymptomatic. When symptoms are present, they may be attributable to ischemia of the upper extremity muscle groups that is precipitated by upper extremity activity. Alternatively, symptoms may be attributable to "steal" of blood flow from the posterior cerebral circulation toward the upper extremity, via retrograde flow along the ipsilateral vertebral artery, caused by significant proximal brachiocephalic/subclavian stenosis or obstruction (Fig. 24.3) (3,4). When symptomatic (i.e., subclavian steal syndrome), patients present with symptoms of posterior circulation ischemia including

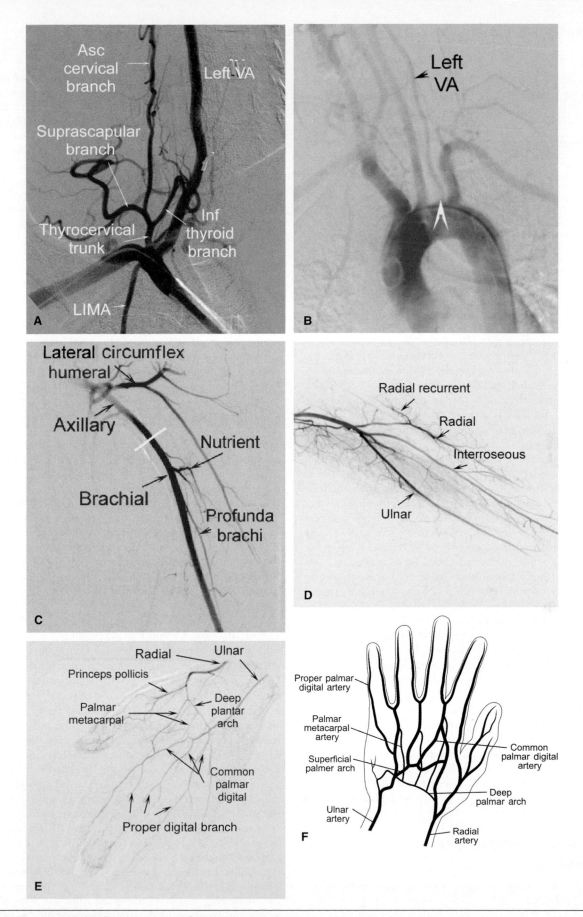

Figure 24.2 • Angiographic anatomy of upper extremity. **A:** Angiography of right subclavian artery demonstrating origin and course of the major branches from the first segment of the vessel. **B:** Arch aortogram demonstrating anomalous origin of left vertebral artery from typical location on aortic arch *(arrowhead)*. **C:** Angiography of left axillary and brachial artery. **D:** Angiography of distal left brachial artery and ulnar and radial branches. **E:** Angiography of right hand of a patient with small-vessel vasculitis involving the proper digital branches. **F:** Schematic illustration of typical arterial anatomy in the hand. VA, vertebral artery; Inf, inferior; Asc, ascending; LIMA, left internal mammary artery.

TABLE 24.1 Indications for Subclavian Artery or Innominate Artery Revascularization

Vertebrobasilar Insufficiency
Symptomatic subclavian steal syndrome
Disabling upper extremity claudication
Preservation of flow to in situ LIMA or RIMA grafts
Preservation of inflow to axillary graft or dialysis conduit
Embolization to the fingers from subclavian disease

dizziness, diplopia, nystagmus, ataxia, and visual symptoms associated with upper extremity activity. Again, it is worth emphasizing that the presence of retrograde flow along the vertebral artery is most commonly asymptomatic, and is referred to as the "subclavian steal phenomenon."

In patients with prior bypass surgery involving "in situ" right internal mammary artery (RIMA) or left internal mammary artery (LIMA) grafts, coronary "steal" may also occur as a result of retrograde flow along the graft from the coronary circulation toward the distal subclavian artery, precipitating coronary ischemia (Fig. 24.4) (5).

Typically, these "steal" syndromes are worsened by upper extremity activity. Specific to brachiocephalic artery lesions, ischemia in the distribution of the right internal carotid artery (ICA) may be the presenting symptom, on the basis of atherothrombotic embolization from the lesion, or hemodynamic compromise of flow. In asymptomatic patients, subclavian or brachiocephalic artery intervention may be performed to protect the inflow to a variety of surgical grafts including axilloaxillary, axillofemoral, subclavian–carotid, and IMA–coronary.

The dominant contraindication to subclavian/brachiocephalic percutaneous intervention is the presence of fresh thrombus. Embolization to the vertebral artery or right ICA during subclavian and brachiocephalic artery intervention is an important complication in this circumstance. There are significant technical challenges to the use of embolic protection devices (EPDs) for these procedures that further add to the risk in this setting. Therefore, with thrombotic lesions, the authors recommend either thrombolysis, or 2 to 4 weeks of anticoagulation, prior to proceeding with intervention. If the lesion must be dealt with immediately, use of a glycoprotein IIb/IIIa inhibitor, in addition to the use of embolic protection devices, is recommended.

Upper Extremity Angiography
AORTOGRAM

The major indications for upper extremity angiography are listed in Table 24.2.

Prior to selective angiography of the upper extremity, it is prudent to always perform an arch aortogram (40° LAO projection). Our practice is to use a multisidehole pigtail catheter (Fig. 24.5A) for this purpose.

The arch aortogram facilitates the detection of important anomalies, as outlined earlier, and anatomic features (e.g., tortuosity of brachiocephalic or proximal subclavian artery, type III aortic arch) that influence the choice of equipment used to perform angiography and intervention, and increase the technical complexity of these procedures. An RAO view is rarely helpful, except in circumstances where there is significant overlap of vessels in the LAO view. Ideally, rotational angiography would be the gold standard, allowing a complete 3D assessment of the arch and the origins of the great vessels.

When selective angiography of the entire upper extremity is required, it is advisable to adopt a systematic, stepwise approach, starting proximally and working distally. This approach facilitates the prompt detection of anomalies, such as the high origin of either the radial or ulnar artery from the brachial artery, or the origin of the radial artery from the axillary artery. Failure to adopt this approach may result in an erroneous diagnosis of vessel occlusion. Iodixanol, an iso-osmolar nonionic contrast agent, is the preferred contrast medium for use in upper extremity angiography because of its excellent tolerability. By using hand injections of 5 to 10 mL of contrast agent with digital subtraction angiography (DSA), adequate visualization of all major vessels is achieved (2,6).

SUBCLAVIAN AND BRACHIOCEPHALIC ARTERY ANGIOGRAPHY

Selective engagement of the brachiocephalic artery and left subclavian artery may generally be achieved using a JR4 diagnostic of Berenstein catheter (Fig. 24.5B). For patients with unfolding of the aortic arch (i.e., type III arches), alternative catheters may be required (e.g., Vitek, Simmons, Headhunter-1) (Fig. 24.5C–E). The appropriate use of these catheters is important. In the case of the Vitek catheter, the practice is to advance the catheter to the descending thoracic aorta, where advancement of the catheter will usually allow the catheter to form its pre-formed shape. Further advancing the catheter over the arch will usually result in the tip of the catheter engaging the origin of the great vessels sequentially.

Safe removal of the Vitek catheter is accomplished by advancing the catheter into the ascending aorta, passing a long wire through the catheter beyond the tip to straighten the curve, and then removing the catheter and wire in unison. This technique minimizes trauma to the arch from the catheter tip. Owing to the larger primary curve of the Simmons catheter, it is more challenging to use because of the difficulty in reshaping the catheter in the aortic arch. The author's preferred method for reshaping a Simmons catheter is to use a diagnostic catheter to engage the left subclavian artery and advance an exchange length wire (i.e., 260–300 cm) into the left subclavian artery. The diagnostic catheter is removed and the Simmons catheter is advanced over the wire and its tip is positioned in the proximal segment of the left subclavian artery. The wire is then withdrawn close to the tip of the catheter and the Simmons catheter is advanced forward resulting in prolapse of the catheter into the arch assuming its preformed shape. A similar removal technique for the Simmons catheter is employed, as described, for the Vitek catheter.

Following selective engagement of the left subclavian artery and brachiocephalic artery, angiography is performed in orthogonal oblique projections. The bifurcation of the brachiocephalic artery and origin of the right subclavian artery is well delineated in the RAO projection. The origins of the

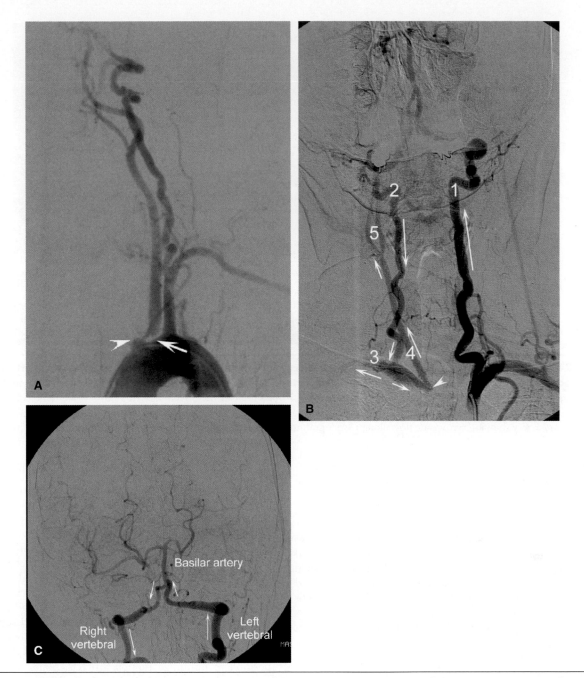

Figure 24.3 • Demonstration of subclavian artery steal from vertebrobasilar circulation in a patient with innominate artery occlusion. **A:** Arch aortogram demonstrating innominate artery occlusion *(arrowhead)* and ostial left common carotid artery (CCA) stenosis *(arrow)*. **B:** Left subclavian artery angiography demonstrating antegrade flow along left vertebral artery *(1)*, and retrograde flow along right vertebral artery *(2)*, toward the right subclavian artery *(3)*, and right CCA *(4)*. *Arrows* indicate the direction of flow. *(5)* Right CCA bifurcation. **C:** Selective angiography of left vertebral artery showing that flow from the left to right vertebral artery occurs at the level of the vertebrobasilar junction. *Arrows* indicate the direction of flow.

right vertebral artery and RIMA are usually best visualized in the LAO projection. For the left subclavian artery, the origins of the left vertebral artery and LIMA are usually best visualized in the RAO projection. Subclavian artery angiography is performed with the patient's arm adducted at the patient's side (i.e., neutral position). In the specific circumstance when thoracic-outlet syndrome causing arterial compression is suspected, angiography is performed in the posteroanterior (PA) projection with the arm in neutral position, and repeated with

the shoulder in full abduction, external rotation, and retroversion (i.e., the throwing position).

AXILLARY AND BRACHIAL ARTERY ANGIOGRAPHY

Selective angiography of the axillary or brachial arteries requires delivery of the diagnostic catheter into the distal subclavian artery, beyond the brachiocephalic/left subclavian artery ostium. Following the initial engagement of the respective ostia with the diagnostic catheter, a long (i.e., 300 cm) soft-tipped, 0.035"

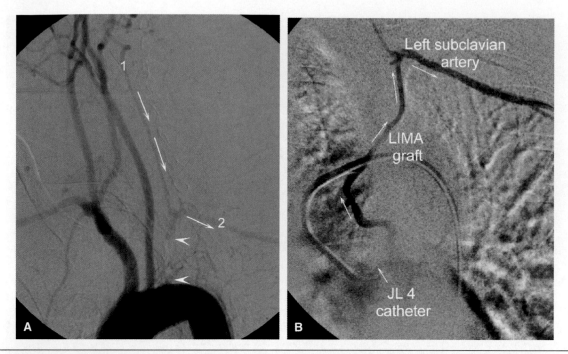

Figure 24.4 • Demonstration of subclavian artery steal from coronary circulation in patient with left subclavian artery occlusion and prior left internal mammary artery (LIMA) graft to left anterior descending artery graft. **A:** Arch aortogram demonstrating left subclavian artery occlusion. *Arrows* indicate the direction of flow; *arrowheads* delineate the proximal and distal extent of the left subclavian artery occlusion. *(1)* Left vertebral artery. *(2)* Left subclavian artery. **B:** Selective angiography of left main coronary artery showing retrograde flow along LIMA graft toward the left subclavian artery. *Arrows* indicate the direction of flow.

wire (e.g., Wholey/Magic Torque®) is advanced into the brachial artery, using the DSA road-mapping function, and then the diagnostic catheter is advanced over this wire. This is a straightforward maneuver when the diagnostic catheter is a JR4, Berenstein, or angled glide catheter. When a Vitek or Simmons catheter is required to engage the respective ostia, an alternative strategy is usually required. In this circumstance, a soft-tipped wire, or stiff-angled glide wire, is advanced into the brachial artery, and the Vitek or Simmons catheter is then exchanged for a "friendly" diagnostic catheter (e.g., angled glide catheter or multipurpose catheter) (Fig. 24.5F,G). The angled glide wire is very steerable but care is required so as not to cause vessel dissection. Additionally, catheter exchanges over this wire are difficult and must be performed with great care so as not to loose wire position. Axillary artery angiography is performed with the arm in the neutral position or slightly abducted, whereas brachial artery angiography is performed with the arm abducted, and the forearm placed supine on an arm board.

TABLE 24.2	Indications for Upper Extremity Angiography
Acute upper extremity ischemia	
Arm claudication	
Blue digit syndrome	
Severe digital ischemia	
Blunt trauma with signs of vascular injury	
Penetrating trauma with signs of vascular injury	

FOREARM AND HAND ANGIOGRAPHY

Adequate angiography of the forearm and hand requires that the diagnostic catheter be advanced to the level of the mid-distal brachial artery, over an appropriate wire (e.g., angled glidewire, Wholey). Liberal administration of vasodilators (e.g., nitroglycerin, calcium channel antagonists) is recommended, because of the propensity of the brachial artery to spasm, and vasodilators may also improve visualization of the digital vessels.

Appropriate positioning of the forearm and hand is important. The forearm and hand must be placed supine on an arm board; the fingers of the hand are splayed, and the thumb is abducted. It is advisable to tape the digits and thumb in this position to minimize motion artifacts. Some operators will wrap the hands with warm cloths to promote vasodilatation and improve visualization of the digital vessels. Angiography is usually performed in the PA projection, although angulated views sometimes may be helpful. For example, during forearm angiography, an ipsilateral oblique projection may help separate the course of the ulnar, interosseous, and radial arteries.

Interventional Technique

Although subclavian and brachiocephalic artery interventions are often pooled together, brachiocephalic artery intervention presents a number of unique, technical challenges that are not encountered in subclavian artery intervention. Therefore, a description of the technique for subclavian artery intervention is first described, and building on the fundamental principles of that technique, a description of the approach to brachiocephalic artery intervention follows.

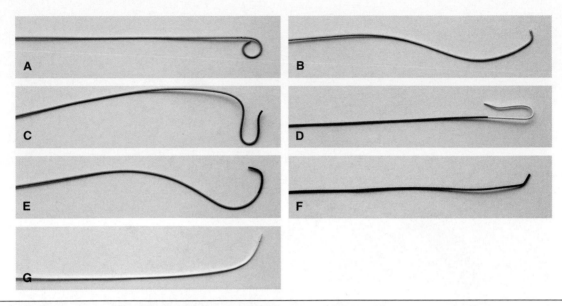

Figure 24.5 • Diagnostic catheters used during upper extremity angiography.   **A:** Pigtail. **B:** JR4. **C:** Vitek. **D:** Simmons-1. **E:** Cobra. **F:** Angled glide. **G:** Multipurpose.

SUBCLAVIAN ARTERY INTERVENTION

The vast majority of subclavian artery stenoses are caused by atherosclerotic disease. In most series, the incidence of left subclavian artery stenosis far exceeds that of right subclavian artery stenosis. Stenoses typically involve the first portion of the subclavian artery and occur proximal to the origin of the vertebral artery (Fig. 24.6). Occlusions generally extend from the ostium of the subclavian artery to the origin of the vertebral artery (Fig. 24.4A).

Prior to embarking on a subclavian intervention, a high-quality arch aortogram, and selective angiography of the brachiocephalic/right subclavian and left subclavian arteries, is required, using the technique described earlier. For the right subclavian artery, the relation of the proximal extent of the lesion to the innominate and right CCA is critical. Similarly, for the left subclavian artery, assessment of the involvement of the true ostium of the vessel off the aortic arch is an important factor. For both vessels, it is necessary to demarcate the relation of the lesion to the origin of its two critical branches (vertebral and IMA). By defining the arch anatomy and the anatomy of the lesion, the interventional strategy may be planned.

PHARMACOLOGY

For patients undergoing planned brachiocephalic or subclavian artery intervention, pre-procedural aspirin (325 mg daily) and clopidogrel (300-mg bolus, 75 mg daily for 2 to 3 days) is administered. Currently, all of our procedures are performed using unfractionated heparin to achieve an activated clotting time (ACT) of approximately 250 to 300 seconds. Use of the direct thrombin inhibitor, bivalirudin, is gaining popularity but data to support its use are still preliminary.

ACCESS

The choice of access site for subclavian artery intervention is strongly influenced by the nature of the obstructive lesion.

Stenoses are almost always approached using common femoral artery (CFA) access, since crossing the lesion is generally straightforward, and the antegrade approach offers an advantage in visualizing the ostium of the vessel. Additionally, the CFA access site is associated with fewer access site complications. For occlusions, and particularly for flush occlusions, most operators prefer an approach from involved dual access from the ipsilateral brachial artery and CFA. In such circumstances, the CFA access is useful to help identify the origin of the vessel, and guide successful crossing of the lesion with the wire from the brachial access. For patients with severe aortoiliac disease, the brachial access is the preferred access site for both stenoses and occlusions. Radial artery access is also a reasonable alternative to brachial artery access where upper extremity access is required, assuming the patient has a negative Allen's test in that extremity.

CFA ACCESS SITE STRATEGY

When using the CFA access site, a 6-Fr. sheath (80-cm long) or 7- to 8-Fr. guide-based system may be used (Fig. 24.7). The advantage of the guide-based system is that it provides more support and flexibility during the procedure, although support is generally only an issue for occlusive lesions. In patients with significant peripheral vascular disease, the use of the smaller 6-Fr. sheath system may offer some advantage. The goal is to deliver the sheath or guide proximal to the lesion without causing atheroembolism. A telescoping technique is employed to achieve this.

GUIDE-BASED SYSTEM

A long (i.e., 125 cm) diagnostic catheter (JR4, Vitek) is advanced through a guide (e.g., JR4, H-1, Multipurpose) (Fig. 24.8) and is engaged in the origin of the subclavian or brachiocephalic artery. A heavy support 0.014″ (e.g., GrandSlam, Abbott Vascular), 0.018″ (Flex T, Covidien), or a soft-tipped 0.035″ wire is advanced into the proximal brachial artery. In general, the authors recommend using 0.035″ wires to perform subclavian

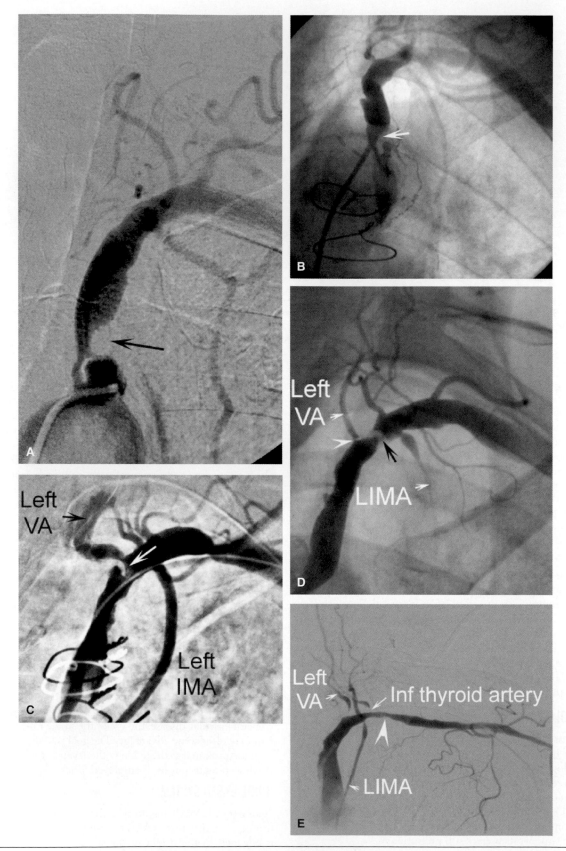

Figure 24.6 • Variation in location of left subclavian artery stenosis. **A:** Typical proximal location *(black arrow)*. **B:** Ulcerated lesion in typical proximal location *(white arrow)*. **C:** Shelf-like lesion adjacent and proximal to the left vertebral artery (VA). IMA, internal mammary artery. **D:** Calcified lesion between the origin of the left VA and left internal mammary (LIMA) arteries. **E:** Atypical smooth subclavian stenosis *(white arrowhead)* distal to the LIMA associated with ostial stenoses in the left VA and inferior thyroid branches in a patient with temporal arteritis.

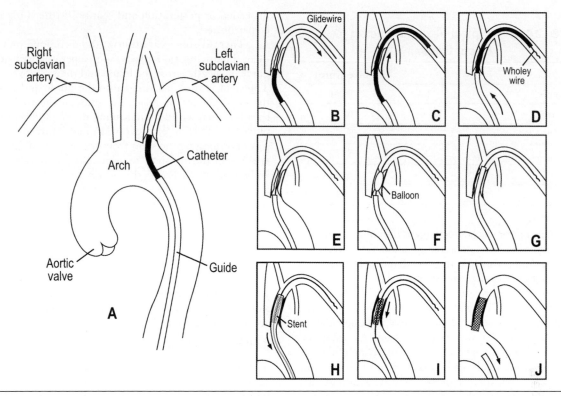

Figure 24.7 • Interventional technique employed for subclavian artery stenosis when using common femoral artery access. See text for details. (Reproduced with permission from Casserly IP, Kapadia SR. Subclavian artery and upper extremity intervention. In: Bhatt DL, ed. *Guide to Peripheral and Cerebrovascular Intervention*. London: Remedica Publishing; 2004.)

intervention. Ideally, the guide is then advanced over the diagnostic catheter and torqued (e.g., usually counterclockwise) into the ostium, with subsequent removal of the catheter. Occasionally, the wire will not provide sufficient support for this maneuver, and the diagnostic catheter may have to be advanced across the lesion, prior to advancing the guide. This should not be attempted if the lesion is critical and the risk of atheroembolism with this maneuver is perceived to be high. In this circumstance, the safest option is to approximate the guide as close to the ostium as possible.

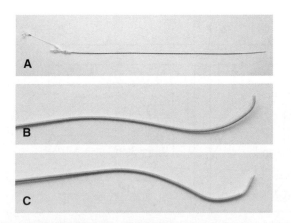

Figure 24.8 • Sheaths and guides used during subclavian and innominate artery intervention. **A:** Shuttle sheath. **B:** JR4 guide. **C:** H-1 guide.

SHEATH-BASED SYSTEM

When employing a sheath (Fig. 24.8), remove the sheath dilator and telescope the long diagnostic catheter through the sheath. The ostium of the brachiocephalic or left subclavian is engaged with the diagnostic catheter, and a 0.035″ wire is passed distally into the proximal brachial artery, as before. The diagnostic catheter is then removed and the sheath dilator combination is advanced proximal to the lesion. It is unlikely that a 0.014″ or 0.018″ wire will provide enough support to allow delivery of the sheath dilator.

ANGIOPLASTY

Currently, balloon angioplasty, alone, is rarely performed, as stenting achieves such excellent and predictable results. Angioplasty is generally performed prior to stenting to facilitate stent delivery, as most lesions are heavily calcified. It may also provide some confirmation of the estimated vessel size and length of the lesion. The risk of dissection is minimized by using a conservative approach to balloon sizing, using a balloon diameter approximately 70% of the estimated diameter of the vessel. For most patients this will be approximately 5 to 6 mm.

STENTING

Subclavian stenoses proximal to the vertebral artery are usually treated with balloon-expandable stents, owing to the need for accurate stent placement and strong radial force in this location. It should be appreciated that the proximal subclavian artery is an intrathoracic structure and that perforation in this location

TABLE 24.3 Typical Vessel Diameters in Upper Extremity

Vessel	Size (mm)
Innominate	8–11
Subclavian	6–8
Axillary	5–7
Brachial	5–7
Radial	3–4
Ulnar	3–4

may result in intrathoracic hemorrhage and significant morbidity or mortality. Therefore, stent sizing should be relatively conservative to minimize this risk. In general, most patients will be treated with 6- to 8-mm-diameter stents (Table 24.3).

Ostial lesions require attention so that the ostium is fully covered by the stent. This will usually result in 1 to 2 mm of free stent in the aortic arch. The ipsilateral oblique view will generally be optimal for this determination. As mentioned above, the use of a CFA approach is particularly helpful in this setting, as it is very difficult to visualize the ostium when using the brachial approach. Before deployment, it is important to confirm that the origins of the vertebral and IMA branches are not impinged by the stent, which is generally best defined in the contralateral oblique view. During inflation of the balloon-expandable stent, the patient should be actively questioned as to the presence or absence of pain. Onset of pain is a sign that further expansion may be associated with an increased risk of

dissection or perforation and that no further inflation should be performed.

There is some variation in the technique of stent placement. Following angioplasty, some operators will advance the guide or sheath across the lesion and then remove the balloon. The stent is then delivered into the guide and positioned at the site of the lesion, inside the guide or sheath. The guide or sheath is then withdrawn, leaving the stent in position for deployment. This method evolved in an effort to minimize the risk of dislodging the stent from the balloon of the stent delivery system during stent manipulations and subsequent stent embolization. Typically, this occurs when an undeployed stent is withdrawn into the guide or sheath. In our experience, the use of a 0.035″ compatible stent delivery system over a 0.014″ wire increases the risk of stent dislodgement. Therefore, use of the appropriately sized wire for the stent delivery system employed is recommended.

For stenoses distal to the vertebral artery, self-expanding stents are generally used. Accurate placement in this location is less critical, and the transition of the subclavian artery into the axillary artery is a flexion point where self-expanding stents are most appropriate.

BRACHIAL ARTERY ACCESS SITE STRATEGY

The retrograde brachial artery access approach is the preferred strategy for the treatment of the subclavian artery occlusions, which present a significantly greater technical challenge, as compared with that required for the treatment of stenoses (Figs. 24.9 and 24.10).

A 6-Fr. sheath (35 to 55 mm in length) is advanced with its tip just distal to the occlusion. These occlusions are generally difficult to cross and will require the use of a 0.035″

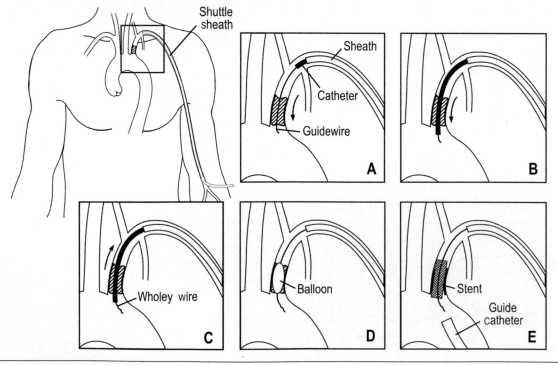

Figure 24.9 • Interventional technique employed for subclavian artery occlusions when using brachial artery access. See text for details. (Reproduced with permission from Casserly IP, Kapadia SR. Subclavian artery and upper extremity intervention. In: Bhatt DL, ed. *Guide to Peripheral and Cerebrovascular Intervention.* London: Remedica Publishing; 2004.)

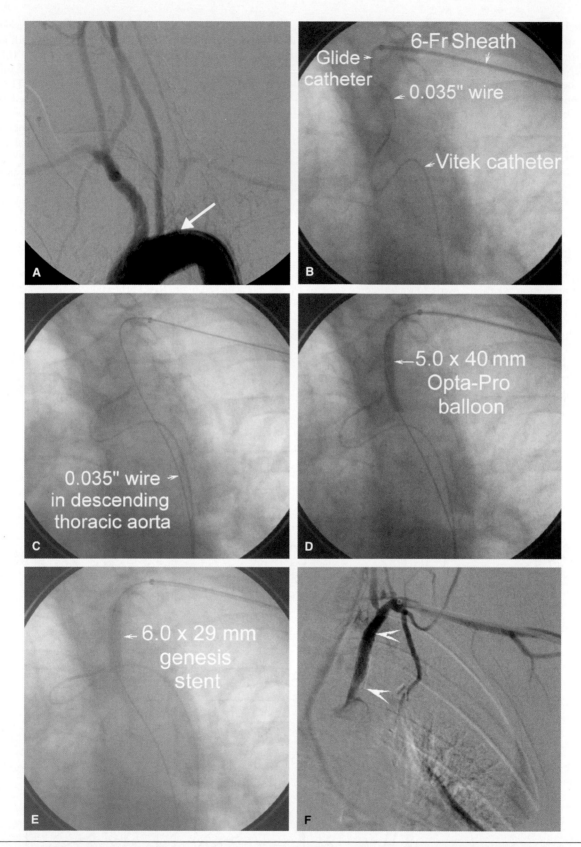

Figure 24.10 • Illustrative case of left subclavian artery occlusion treated using technique outlined in Figure 24.9.
A: Arch aortogram showing flush occlusion of left subclavian artery *(arrow)*. **B:** A Vitek catheter from the right common femoral artery access site is used to engage the ostium of the left subclavian artery to help direct the wire advanced across the lesion from the brachial access toward the true lumen. **C:** Wire has successfully crossed lesion and is in descending thoracic aorta. **D:** Balloon angioplasty. **E:** Stent deployment. **F:** Final angiography. *Arrowheads* indicate the proximal and distal extent of the stent.

stiff-angled glide wire supported by a glide or multipurpose catheter, or an over-the-wire balloon. Occasionally, a stiff 0.014″ wire (e.g., Confianza®, Abbott, Vascular) supported by an over-the-wire balloon may have some utility in crossing these occlusions because these wires have a high degree of directional control. Placement of a diagnostic catheter in the stump of the occlusion may aid in directing the wire toward the true lumen. Finding the true lumen at the ostium of the left subclavian artery is crucial, as dissection at this point will involve the aortic arch and may compromise flow in the other arch branches. Having crossed the lesion, the technique is similar to that outlined earlier for nonocclusive stenoses. Accurate positioning of the stent at the ostium of the vessel is again facilitated by injection of contrast agent, via the femoral access site catheter.

Brachiocephalic Artery Intervention

Brachiocephalic artery intervention is more complicated than subclavian artery intervention, owing to the potential for embolization to the anterior cerebral circulation via the right CCA (Fig. 24.11).

The threshold for using embolic protection is, therefore, significantly lowered compared to that of subclavian intervention. Additionally, ensuring patency of both limbs of the brachiocephalic bifurcation, with continued antegrade access, may present a significant technical challenge for true bifurcation lesions.

If the use of an EPD is planned, right brachial artery access is obtained and a 35 to 55 cm sheath is placed. In addition, CFA access with a short 8-Fr. sheath is obtained. A 6-Fr. IMA guide is advanced through the brachial sheath over a 0.035″ soft-tipped wire and positioned at the ostium of the right CCA. Through the guide, a filter wire is advanced and the filter positioned in the distal cervical portion of the ICA, replicating the position employed during ICA bifurcation interventions. The intervention is then performed from the CFA access site, using a similar technique described above.

For ostial brachiocephalic artery lesions, extra care is required during guide catheter manipulation. Typically, one may employ a multipurpose guide with the intention of staying outside of the ostium of the vessel. Preservation of access to the right CCA will generally take priority, and the wire from the CFA guide is usually passed toward the right external carotid artery (ECA). Balloon-expandable stents should always be used in this location, and accurate positioning of the stent, with respect to the bifurcation, is usually achieved in the RAO projection. Stent sizes used are typically between 8 and 10 mm, in this location (Table 24.3).

OUTCOMES

As with most peripheral vascular interventions, there are no randomized data comparing endovascular and surgical revascularization techniques. In addition, there are no randomized

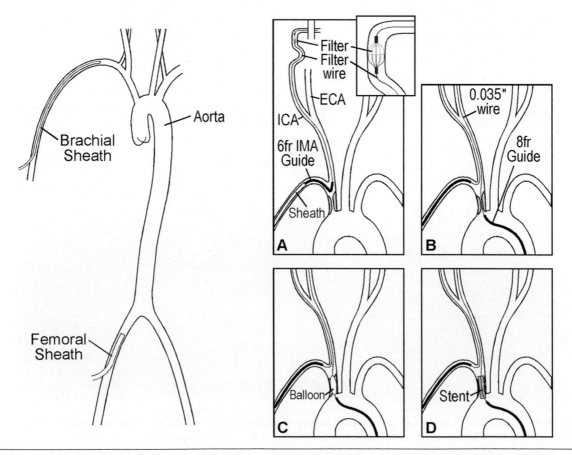

Figure 24.11 • Interventional technique employed for innominate artery stenosis/occlusion when emboli protection is planned. See text for details.

TABLE 24.4 Observational Comparison of Endovascular versus Surgical Revascularization for Innominate and Subclavian Artery Intervention

	Endovascular (n = 108) (%)	Surgery (n = 2496) (%)
Technical success	97 (88–100)	96 (75–100)
Stroke	0	3 (0–14)
Death	0	2 (0–11)
Complications	6 (0–14)*	16 (0–43)†
Recurrence	3 (0–12)	16 (0–50)

Numbers refer to mean percent (range).
*Vascular assess complications and stent dislodgement.
†Stroke/transient ischemic attack, Horner syndrome, delayed wound healing or infection, graft thrombosis, chylothorax, pneumonia, and pleural effusion.
(Adapted from Hadjipetrou P, Cox S, Piemonte T, et al. Percutaneous revascularization of atherosclerotic obstruction of aortic arch vessels. *J Am Coll Cardiol.* 1999;33:1238–1245.)

data comparing different endovascular strategies. An assessment of the technical success, efficacy, and morbidity and mortality associated with the procedure is derived exclusively from a number of retrospective case series (7–21). These series are now somewhat outdated, in that in some cases angioplasty, alone, was the treatment strategy, or when stents were used, older balloon-expandable (i.e., Palmaz®) and self-expanding (Wallstent®, Strecker®) stents were deployed.

Hadjipetrou et al. reviewed the experience with surgical and endovascular (using stents) revascularization for brachiocephalic and subclavian artery disease (Table 24.4) (10). Despite the limitations of such an observational comparison, the data suggest that endovascular revascularization has equal effectiveness, and is associated with fewer complications, supporting the use of percutaneous revascularization as the therapy of choice for such lesions.

In contemporary series, the technical success for the endovascular treatment of subclavian and brachiocephalic artery stenosis approaches 100%. Previously, the success rate for total occlusions in these vessels was significantly less (70% to 80%) (14), but recent series have reported a significant improvement (greater than 90%) attributable to improved technology and the evolution in technique by experienced operators (7,20,21).

The major risk of these procedures is distal embolization. This may occur in the arm (i.e., usually to the digits) or in the posterior cerebral circulation, via the vertebral artery during subclavian or brachiocephalic artery intervention. Embolization to the anterior circulation via the right CCA may occur during brachiocephalic intervention. Fortunately, the cumulative rate of significant embolization to these territories has consistently been less than 1% in most series. Previous studies have demonstrated that there is a significant delay (i.e., up to 20 minutes) in the re-establishment of antegrade flow in the vertebral artery following relief of a proximal stenosis (22).

This likely explains the low rate of posterior cerebral circulation embolization. It is worth noting that when cerebral events occur, operators have reported a greater relation to manipulation in the aortic arch than to angioplasty or stenting of the subclavian or innominate artery, itself.

Access site complications are the most common complication reported (0% to 7%). The major risk factor for these events is the use of brachial artery access and highlights the need for particular care when using this access site. Complications include hematoma formation, thrombosis, and pseudoaneurysm formation.

Stent migration is reported in 0% to 6% of case series. This term is often not defined but likely describes both malpositioning of the stent and the rare occurrence of stent dislodgement from the balloon of the stent delivery system. Stent malposition may be a problem if critical branch vessels are covered (i.e., vertebral, IMA). Stent dislodgement will require either percutaneous or surgical retrieval. Alternatively, the dislodged stent is occasionally compressed against the vessel wall in a benign location (e.g., common iliac artery).

Prior to the introduction of stents, patients treated with angioplasty, alone, had a reported restenosis rate of 15% to 20% for brachiocephalic or subclavian artery intervention (16,23). The advent of stenting has reduced this figure to less than 10% (7,20,21).

A variety of options exist for the management of restenosis, depending largely on the presumed etiology. In cases where restenosis represents a failure to cover the ostium of the vessel adequately, angioplasty of the restenosed area and repeat stenting of the ostium are required. If inadequate stent expansion is suspected, based on the angiographic appearance of the stent or the findings by intravascular ultrasound, more aggressive dilation of the stent may be attempted. If this proves inadequate, restenting may be required. If neither of these factors appears operative, repeat angioplasty with gamma-brachytherapy is a reasonable option. Drug-coated stents with a diameter adequate to treat subclavian or brachiocephalic artery stenosis are not available and are unlikely to be available for the foreseeable future. When endovascular techniques fail, surgical revascularization is an option. Currently, an extrathoracic approach (i.e., carotid–subclavian, axilloaxillary) is the technique employed, owing to the lower morbidity associated with this type of surgical revascularization (Fig. 24.12) (24).

POST-PROCEDURAL CARE AND FOLLOW-UP MONITORING

Most patients undergoing subclavian or innominate artery intervention are discharged within 6 to 8 hours of completion of the procedure. High-risk patients are generally admitted overnight for observation. All patients receive prescriptions for lifelong aspirin therapy (162 to 325 mg daily) and clopidogrel (75 mg daily) for at least 4 weeks. Prior to discharge, blood pressure measurements in both arms should be carefully documented to provide an accurate baseline against which future changes may be compared. During follow-up monitoring, the patients should be assessed for recurrence of symptoms, and any change in upper extremity blood pressure measurements. A duplex ultrasound exam may be performed when these

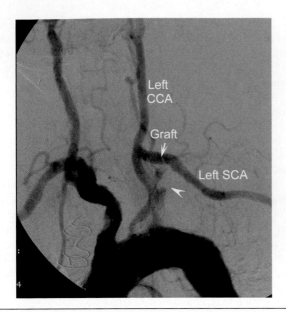

Figure 24.12 • Arch aortogram demonstrating extrathoracic left common carotid artery (CCA) to left subclavian artery (SCA) graft. This patient had a prior stent placed in the left SCA that had occlusive restenosis *(arrowhead)*.

indices suggest recurrence. Early detection of stenosis before progression to occlusion is an important factor in maintaining secondary patency rates above 90% to 95%.

THORACIC OUTLET SYNDROME

Thoracic outlet syndrome is a term used to describe the spectrum of clinical presentations caused by compression of the neurovascular structures of the upper extremity (i.e., subclavian artery, subclavian vein, brachial plexus) in the region of the thoracic outlet. In the majority of cases (greater than 90%), symptoms are caused by compression of the brachial plexus and related nerves (25). Arterial and venous compression account for less than 10% of cases but are responsible for most of the serious morbidity and mortality associated with the condition (26).

Arterial compression in the thoracic outlet usually occurs in the scalene triangle (i.e., bordered by the first rib, scalenus anterior, and scalenus medius muscles) or the subcoracoid space (i.e., bordered by the pectoralis minor muscle, ribs, and coracoid process) and is the least common manifestation of thoracic outlet syndrome. Extrinsic arterial compression at these sites is typically caused by cervical ribs and congenital fibromuscular bands, and less commonly by anomalies of the first rib, muscular hypertrophy, or excess callus formation following prior clavicular fractures.

Recurrent, chronic, arterial compression leads to intimal and medial vessel injury, producing localized stenosis or occlusion and post-stenotic dilation, or occasionally, aneurysmal formation. The formation of collaterals usually minimizes the occurrence of upper extremity ischemia. Distal thromboembolism is the most typical clinical presentation. Patients are generally young or middle-aged adults.

Angiography is the gold standard for diagnosing extrinsic arterial compression in the thoracic outlet. It should be performed in the neutral position and repeated in whatever position reproduces the patient's symptoms. Traditionally, these positions will include one or more of the following: depression of the shoulder with the head turned to the symptomatic side (i.e., Adson maneuver), shoulder hyperflexion (i.e., military position), hyperabduction of the arm, and hands above the head (i.e., surrender position). Angiography may reveal normal, smooth, arterial anatomy and compression only with provocative maneuvers (Fig. 24.13).

In addition, angiography may reveal additional features, such as post-stenotic dilation, aneurysm formation, thrombosis, or evidence of distal embolization.

The treatment of the subclavian arterial compression type of thoracic outlet syndrome is reserved for patients who are symptomatic or who have evidence of embolization. Surgical decompression of the artery is required and will generally

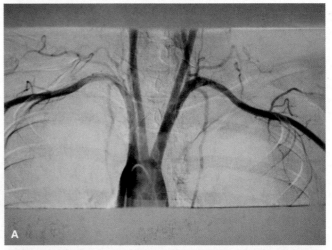

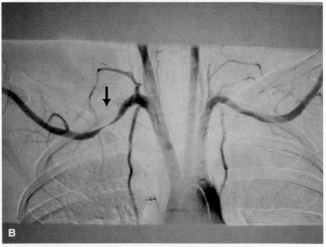

Figure 24.13 • Diagnostic angiography from patient with symptoms of thoracic outlet syndrome. A: Arch aortogram with arms in neutral position demonstrating normal angiographic appearance of right subclavian artery. **B:** Arch aortogram from same patient with right arm abducted, externally rotated, and retroverted showing compression of the subclavian artery *(arrow)*.

involve resection of the first rib and release of any muscular or ligamentous abnormality. Structural abnormalities of the artery (e.g., aneurysms) are surgically repaired, concomitantly. The presence of unilateral disease should always prompt a search for contralateral involvement and occasionally, prophylactic surgical intervention may be warranted.

References

1. Moore KL. The upper limb. In: *Clinically Oriented Anatomy*. 2nd ed. Baltimore, MD: Williams & Wilkins; 1985:626–793.

2. Kadir S. Arteriography of the upper extremities. In: *Diagnostic Angiography*. Philadelphia, PA: Saunders; 1986:172–206.

3. Jaeger HJ, Mathias KD, Kempkes U. Bilateral subclavian steal syndrome: treatment with percutaneous transluminal angioplasty and stent placement. *Cardiovasc Intervent Radiol*. 1994;17: 328–332.

4. Chan-Tack KM. Subclavian steal syndrome: a rare but important cause of syncope. *South Med J*. 2001;94:445–447.

5. Elian D, Gerniak A, Guetta V, et al. Subclavian coronary steal syndrome: an obligatory common fate between subclavian artery, internal mammary graft and coronary circulation. *Cardiology*. 2002;97:175–179.

6. Zeitler E, Huttl K, Mathias KD. Subclavian and brachial artery diseases. In: Zeitler E, ed. *Radiology of Peripheral Vascular Diseases*. New York, NY: Springer-Verlag; 2000:591–623.

7. Al-Mubarak N, Liu MW, Dean LS, et al. Immediate and late outcomes of subclavian artery stenting. *Catheter Cardiovasc Interv*. 1999;46:169–172.

8. Angle JF, Matsumoto AH, McGraw JK, et al. Percutaneous angioplasty and stenting of left subclavian artery stenosis in patients with left internal mammary–coronary bypass grafts: clinical experience and long-term follow-up. *Vasc Endovascular Surg*. 2003;37:89–97.

9. Gonzalez A, Gil-Peralta A, Gonzalez-Marcos JR, et al. Angioplasty and stenting for total symptomatic atherosclerotic occlusion of the subclavian or innominate arteries. *Cerebrovasc Dis*. 2002;13:107–113.

10. Hadjipetrou P, Cox S, Piemonte T, et al. Percutaneous revascularization of atherosclerotic obstruction of aortic arch vessels. *J Am Coll Cardiol*. 1999;33:1238–1245.

11. Henry M, Amor M, Henry I, et al. Percutaneous transluminal angioplasty of the subclavian arteries. *J Endovasc Surg*. 1999; 6:33–41.

12. Kumar K, Dorros G, Bates MC, et al. Primary stent deployment in occlusive subclavian artery disease. *Catheter Cardiovasc Diagn*. 1995;34:281–285.

13. Martinez R, Rodriguez-Lopez J, Torruella L, et al. Stenting for occlusion of the subclavian arteries. Technical aspects and follow-up results. *Tex Heart Inst J*. 1997;24:23–27.

14. Mathias KD, Luth I, Haarmann P. Percutaneous transluminal angioplasty of proximal subclavian artery occlusions. *Cardiovasc Intervent Radiol*. 1993;16:214–218.

15. McNamara TO, Greaser LE III, Fischer JR, et al. Initial and long-term results of treatment of brachiocephalic arterial stenoses and occlusions with balloon angioplasty, thrombolysis, stents. *J Invasive Cardiol*. 1997;9:372–383.

16. Millaire A, Trinca M, Marache P, et al. Subclavian angioplasty: immediate and late results in 50 patients. *Catheter Cardiovasc Diagn*. 1993;29:8–17.

17. Motarjeme A. Percutaneous transluminal angioplasty of supra-aortic vessels. *J Endovasc Surg*. 1996;3:171–181.

18. Motarjeme A. PTA and stenting of subclavian and innominate arteries. In: White RA, Fogarty TJ, eds. *Peripheral Endovascular Interventions*. 2nd ed. New York, NY: Springer-Verlag; 1999:413–422.

19. Nomura M, Kida S, Yamashima T, et al. Percutaneous transluminal angioplasty and stent placement for subclavian and brachiocephalic artery stenosis in aortitis syndrome. *Cardiovasc Intervent Radiol*. 1999;22:427–432.

20. Rodriguez-Lopez JA, Werner A, Martinez R, et al. Stenting for atherosclerotic occlusive disease of the subclavian artery. *Ann Vasc Surg*. 1999;13:254–260.

21. Sullivan TM, Gray BH, Bacharach JM, et al. Angioplasty and primary stenting of the subclavian, innominate, and common carotid arteries in 83 patients. *J Vasc Surg*. 1998;28:1059–1065.

22. Ringelstein EB, Zeumer H. Delayed reversal of vertebral artery blood flow following percutaneous transluminal angioplasty for subclavian steal syndrome. *Neuroradiology*. 1984;26:189–198.

23. Becker GJ, Katzen BT, Dake MD. Noncoronary angioplasty. *Radiology*. 1989;170:921–940.

24. Paty PS, Mehta M, Darling RC 3rd, et al. Surgical treatment of coronary subclavian steal syndrome with carotid subclavian bypass. *Ann Vasc Surg*. 2003;17:22–26.

25. Novak CB. Thoracic outlet syndrome. *Clin Plast Surg*. 2003;30:175–188.

26. Hood DB, Kuehne J, Yellin AE, et al. Vascular complications of thoracic outlet syndrome. *Am Surg*. 1997;63:913–917.

CHAPTER 25

Complications of Endovascular Interventions

Subhash Banerjee and Tony S. Das

The last two decades have seen a dramatic increase in the number of endovascular procedures performed, due to expansion to treatment in all vascular territories and the use of novel techniques and devices (1). Vascular complications are encountered in 5% to 6% of endovascular procedures and result in significant morbidity and mortality (2). As a result, knowledge of these complications and the ability to anticipate and manage them are crucial for any endovascular specialist. In this chapter, we will review in detail the most commonly encountered access site complications, and briefly discuss other complications common to most endovascular procedures including distal embolization, dissections, perforations, and retrieval of foreign bodies.

ACCESS SITE COMPLICATIONS

Vascular access site complications are some of the most common complications encountered during endovascular procedures. These include:

1. Bleeding
2. Pseudoaneurysm formation
3. Arteriovenous fistula (AVF) formation

Bleeding

The femoral artery is most commonly accessed artery during endovascular procedures (3). Major bleeding complications related to femoral arterial access occur in 1% to 2% of cases and are more common than with brachial and radial artery access. Obesity (body mass index >25), female sex, use of glycoprotein (GP) IIb/IIIa inhibitors, hypertension, chronic kidney disease, and diabetes are the most consistent predictors of localized bleeding (4). High femoral artery puncture along with numerous procedural factors such as performance of interventions, duration of procedure, sheath size, and concomitant venous access have also been identified as predictors of hemorrhagic complications in numerous studies (5).

The most serious bleeding complication is that of retroperitoneal hemorrhage or hematoma (RPH), and has been reported in 0.5% of patients following endovascular procedures. Puncture of the femoral artery above the middle third of the femoral head and insertion of the sheath above the inguinal ligament is associated with RPH. In half of the cases of RPH, the puncture site of the common femoral artery is below the level of the inguinal ligament. RPH in such cases is related to the puncture of the posterior arterial wall, the inferior epigastric artery, and/or multiple access attempts with

passage of blood along the facial planes into the superiorly located retroperitoneal space.

The initial symptoms and signs of RPH are nonspecific and may include back, abdominal, or groin pain and lower quadrant tenderness ipsilateral to the femoral puncture site (6). In nearly 50% of patients, the diagnosis is made after significant blood loss has occurred leading to hemodynamic compromise and hypovolemic shock, manifest by tachycardia and hypotension. Almost 75% of cases present within 3 hours of the procedure and thus hypotension during this interval following an endovascular procedure should prompt a compulsive search for a retroperitoneal source of bleeding (7). It is imperative to understand that the diagnosis of RPH is a clinical one, and that when suspected on the basis of the clinical symptoms, and signs, appropriate management should be instituted immediately. This includes the following measures:

a. Apply pressure at and slightly proximal to the femoral puncture site.
b. Stop any anticoagulant or antiplatelet infusions.
c. Obtain robust IV access (minimum of two 16- to 18-Fr. peripheral IV access sites or central venous access) and administering wide-open IV normal saline (i.e., two separate 1-L normal saline bags wrapped in pressure bags).
d. Send blood for emergency type and cross of 3 to 6 units of blood based on the clinical circumstance.
e. Consider the need for platelet infusion if the patient has received abciximab (non-competitive GP IIb/IIIa inhibitor) during the procedure (Table 25.2).
f. Consider the need for reversal of any residual anticoagulant effect of IV heparin using protamine (Table 25.2).
g. If these measures do not result in prompt resuscitation of the patient, localization of the exact site of bleeding by selective iliac artery angiography from upper extremity or contralateral femoral access should be performed (8). If there is evidence of ongoing bleeding, slightly oversized balloon can be used to occlude the source of bleeding. Failed balloon tamponade can be rescued by administration of thrombin, placement of a covered stent graft, or referral for an open surgical repair. Surgical intervention is required in only 12% of cases and is associated with significant morbidity (7).

Imaging studies may be used to confirm the diagnosis and assess the anatomic extent of the RPH, but only following stabilization of the patient (Fig. 25.1). Nearly all patients require transfusion of blood products and have an extended hospital stay associated with increased costs. RPH is a strong

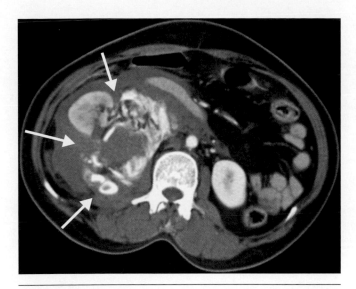

Figure 25.1 • Retroperitoneal hematoma. A large right-sided retroperitoneal hematoma is indicated by the *white arrows.*

predictor of in-hospital and long-term mortality (9). Mortality from RPH occurs in ~4% of patients. Associated complications of RPH include femoral nerve neuropathy, which occurs in up to 24% to 54% of patients, and deep vein thrombosis secondary to inferior venous cava compression, which occurs in 2% to 10% of cases (10).

Given the morbidity and mortality associated with RPH, it is important to be aware of measures that prevent its occurrence and bleeding complications in general. These include the use of micropuncture needles to gain arterial access and the performance of femoral access using fluoroscopic landmarking and/or under ultrasound (US) guidance. Additional measures include the use of weight-adjusted unfractionated heparin (or bivalirudin in appropriate patients), early removal of arterial sheaths, avoidance of concomitant femoral venous access where possible, and meticulous post-procedural care. Evidence regarding the use of access-closure devices and the incidence of hemorrhagic complications following percutaneous coronary intervention has been discrepant, which likely relates to differences in patient populations, variation in closure devices, and the absence of randomized data. For endovascular intervention, the authors' bias is to avoid closure devices due to a clinical impression of higher rates of ischemic complications with these devices in the patient population with peripheral artery disease.

Pseudoaneurysm Formation

The incidence of pseudoaneurysms after femoral access for endovascular procedures is estimated to be between 0.6% and 6%. Larger catheters, anticoagulant use, and simultaneous catheterization of the femoral artery and vein are predictors of pseudoaneurysm formation. Some studies have indicated that puncture of the superficial femoral artery (SFA) may lead to a higher risk of pseudoaneurysm formation than with puncture of the common femoral artery (11). The most common clinical scenario in which a pseudoaneurysm is diagnosed is in a patient who has some evidence of post-procedural bleeding, followed by marked pain and swelling at the

groin site. Clinical examination reveals a new systolic bruit. Additional complications may occur as a result of compression by the pseudoaneurysm of the adjacent common femoral nerve (nerve palsy) and/or common femoral vein (deep venous thrombosis). Compartment syndrome of the lower extremity and distal embolization of clot formed in the sac of the pseudoaneurysm that migrates through the neck of the pseudoaneurysm to the distal circulation are very rare complications. Prompt recognition and management is the key to prevention of significant morbidity (12). Pseudoaneurysms are best-visualized and diagnosed using US and adjunctive Doppler and color Doppler assessment. An echogenic mass, with systolic flow signals at the neck of the sac alongside the femoral artery is diagnostic.

The management of femoral artery pseudoaneurysms is largely driven by the diameter measurement of the aneurysm by ultrasound (Fig. 25.2). Small pseudoaneurysms (i.e., <2 cm) will often resolve with conservative treatment (13). Larger pseudoaneurysms (i.e., >2 cm) usually require intervention. Although prompt surgical repair was formerly the mainstay of pseudoaneurysm treatment, this has been largely replaced by US-guided compression of the pseudoaneurysm neck and/ or by thrombin injection (13). The neck of the pseudoaneurysm is located and mechanical pressure is applied at that site using the US transducer for ~20 minutes initially. This should be performed under conscious sedation because of the severe pain associated with this maneuver. Subsequent compression is often required to assure complete cessation of flow, detected with color Doppler, in the pseudoaneurysm neck. A follow-up US examination is suggested in 24 hours to confirm a durable result. Success rates of around 86% have been reported in patients on anticoagulants.

Thrombin injection into the pseudoaneurysm sac under US guidance is often used as part of an initial strategy with US-guided compression of the neck or following a failed attempt to occlude the pseudoaneurysm neck with manual compression alone (14). Approximately 300 IU of thrombin is injected slowly into the pseudoaneurysm sac for over 10 to 15 minutes. The injecting needle is directed to the base of the sac, away from the neck of the pseudoaneurysm. Cessation of Doppler flow within the pseudoaneurysm signals successful treatment. Post-procedure bed rest is advised. If residual flow is detected, additional doses of thrombin may be injected. A follow-up US examination after successful treatment is often performed at 24 hours and again in 1 week. Excess or rapid injection of thrombin may result in parent vessel thrombosis and distal embolization. During thrombin injection of multiloculated pseudoaneurysms or those with neck diameters >5mm, balloon occlusion of the parent artery during thrombin injection is advised to prevent distal embolization. The success rate for thrombin injection in the treatment of femoral pseudoaneurysms is >96%. In extreme situations, coil embolization of the pseudoaneurysm sac and exclusion of the pseudoaneurysm neck with a stent graft can also be employed. When nonsurgical measures are unsuccessful or are contraindicated (e.g., evidence of infection in pseudoaneurysm), surgical pseudoaneurysm repair should be performed (Table 25.1).

Complications related to nonsurgical treatment of femoral pseudoaneurysms include acute enlargement or rupture of the pseudoaneurysm, vasovagal syncope (most commonly

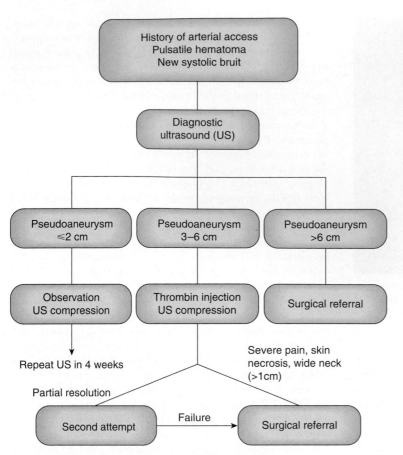

Figure 25.2 • Management of femoral artery pseudoaneurysm.

related to pain), and deep vein thrombosis. Distal embolization may occur in about 4% of cases using this strategy and may be related to escape of thrombin from the pseudoaneurysm sac or embolism of preformed thrombus within the sac. The treatment of distal embolization associated with thrombin injection of a femoral artery pseudoaneurysm is managed according to the clinical situation, but will generally require emergent angiography (using contralateral retrograde femoral or ipsilateral antegrade femoral access), followed by mechanical thrombectomy and/or intra-arterial thrombolysis.

TABLE 25.1 Indications for Surgical Repair of Pseudoaneurysms

Rapid expansion of the pseudoaneurysm

Recurrence of pseudoaneurysm

Skin necrosis, distal ischemia, or embolization and femoral nerve palsy

Infected pseudoaneurysm, especially "mycotic" (rapid enlargement with subsequent rupture or septic emboli)

Failure of percutaneous intervention

Arteriovenous Fistula

AVF formation refers to an abnormal communication that is created between the femoral artery and femoral vein following placement of arterial and/or venous access in the groin. The result is a continuous (i.e., in both systole and diastole) shunt from the femoral artery to the femoral vein, which clinically manifests as a continuous bruit. The reported incidence of AVF formation following femoral access is between 0.2% and 2.1% (15). AVF are more common when both arterial and venous sheaths are placed on the same side, when multiple puncture attempts are made, and with the use of anti-coagulants or intravenous GP IIb/IIIa inhibitors. Most patients with an AVF are asymptomatic. They are identified following a clinical exam that reveals a new continuous bruit, or following common femoral angiography during a subsequent procedure. In rare circumstances, a large AV fistula may present with ipsilateral arterial insufficiency, congestive heart failure, or an ipsilateral swollen lower extremity. The natural history of stable AVF is benign and frequently results in spontaneous resolution, but the diagnosis can be confirmed by a Doppler US examination. The pathognomonic finding is that of arterialization of the femoral venous waveform (Fig. 25.3). If symptomatic (a rare circumstance), AVF can be treated with US compression with a 75% reported success rate, or surgical repair. Prevention of AVF formation is predicated on careful access technique.

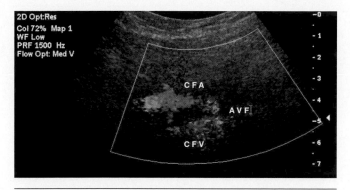

Figure 25.3 • Femoral arteriovenous fistula. AVF, right groin arteriovenous fistula; CFA, common femoral artery; CFV, common femoral vein. (Courtesy of Dr. Michael Jaff)

PERFORATION

Vascular injury leading to disruption of the vascular wall integrity and leakage of blood into the perivascular space is a serious complication of endovascular procedures. The key determinants of patient outcome include the location of bleeding and the speed of recognition (16). For example, bleeding as a consequence of perforation of thoracoabdominal and pelvic vessels can be a potentially life-threatening emergency due to the fact that bleeding occurs into low-pressure spacious chambers that can accommodate large volumes of blood. In contrast, perforation of infrainguinal vessels which are located in muscular compartments results in hemorrhage that is rarely life-threatening because hemorrhage is associated with an abrupt rise in the pressure of the compartment (leading to a risk of compartment syndrome), which results in tamponade of the bleeding source (Fig 25.4). Perforation of the

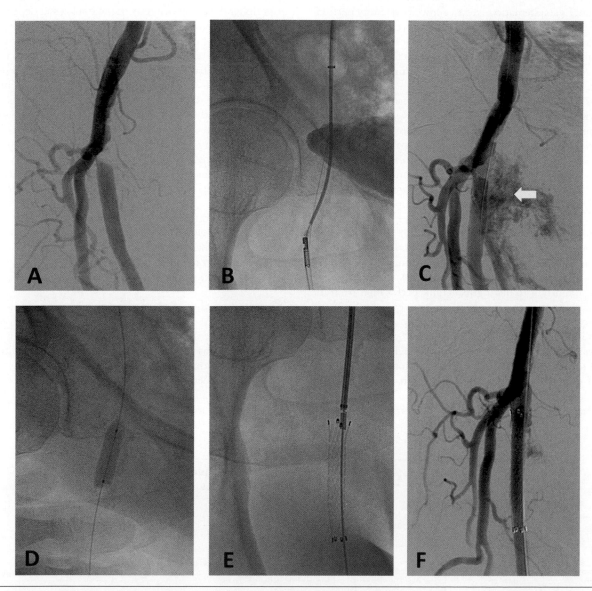

Figure 25.4 • Perforation of the proximal right superficial femoral artery (SFA). Right SFA ostial stenosis **A:** treated with SilverHawk atherectomy **B:** perforation of the proximal right SFA indicated by a *white arrow* **C:** treated with initial balloon occlusion **D:** followed by covered stent implant (Fluency) **E:** and successful hemostasis **F.**

carotid artery can be life-threatening due to compression of the airway rather than the volume of blood loss.

Wire perforations are the most common type of perforation, occur in the distal vascular bed, and are generally minor. Stiff, straight-tip, and hydrophilic wires are the most common culprits. These types of perforations can usually be managed conservatively, except in certain vascular beds such as the kidney or brain.

Vessel rupture following balloon angioplasty or stent deployment is much less frequent, but is often serious and typically requires specific treatment. Laplace's law indicates that the risk of perforation with overstretching and dilation of a vascular wall increases with its diameter. Thus, larger arteries have a higher relative risk of perforation with overstretching compared to smaller caliber vessels. Pain during balloon dilation or stent deployment in large arteries should be considered a sign of overstretching of the vascular wall and serve as a sign to refrain from further significant balloon inflation or stent expansion. In a systematic review of lower extremity perforations in patients with critical limb ischemia, vessel calcification, and decreased vessel compliance in diabetics were consistent predictors of perforation. It is also important to emphasize that heavily calcified vessels are more likely to rupture at nominal inflation pressures.

It is impossible to describe the specific management for perforation in all vessel locations. However, some general comments can be made. For infrainguinal lower-limb arterial perforations, management usually consists of prolonged balloon tamponade and reversal of anticoagulation (Fig. 25.5). Table 25.2 illustrates reversal strategies of anticoagulants and antiplatelet drugs commonly used in interventional practice.

For frank perforation of the femoropopliteal artery that does not respond to these measures, placement of covered self-expanding stents is indicated (e.g., Viabahn). Similarly, frank perforation of tibial vessels that does not respond to first-line measures should be treated with coronary-type covered balloon-expandable stents (i.e., Graftmaster).

It is important to distinguish frank perforation from the irregular tears that commonly occur between the SFA and the adjacent femoral vein following angioplasty, particularly in the subintimal plane. These perforations will often resolve over time and can be managed conservatively (Fig. 16.25). If deemed significant at the time of intervention, they will often respond to placement of a bare-metal self-expanding stent (Fig 16.26). The major risk of frank perforation in the infrainguinal arteries is the subsequent development of compartment

syndrome that is manifest by the complaint of increasing leg pain, which may be associated with neurologic symptoms. Although measurement of compartment pressures can be helpful, if compartment syndrome is suspected clinically, fasciotomy should generally be performed to avoid the risk of limb loss.

For large vessel perforations of the pelvic, thoracic, and abdominal vessels, immediate recognition is essential in achieving a successful clinical outcome. Watching for subtle signs such as localized eccentric expansion of a stent, indicating a tear in the adventitia, and careful observation of hemodynamic parameters following angioplasty and stent deployment will aid in this regard. As with infrainguinal perforations, the cornerstone of treatment includes the reversal of anticoagulant agents and relevant IV GP IIb/IIIa agents (i.e., Abciximab). Table 25.3 illustrates large vessel occlusion balloons, commonly used in interventional practice for the treatment of aortic perforations. Iliac perforations may be occluded using these large caliber balloons deployed in the distal abdominal aorta, or peripheral balloons directly in the iliac vessel depending on the specific circumstance. If these measures fail, covered stents will be required (summarized in Table 25.4). Aortic perforations should be treated with aortic grafts, whereas iliac perforations may be treated using self-expanding covered stents or the iCAST-balloon-expandable covered stent. It is important to be aware of the sheath-size requirements of these stents, understanding that they require larger sheath sizes compared with bare-metal stents, and that the iCAST stent is remarkably stiff, which requires that the strategy for delivery be carefully planned (e.g., using a stiff wire for stent delivery, placing the sheath across the treatment site and then retracting the sheath following successful delivery of the stent to the desired location).

It is imperative for endovascular specialists to have an appropriate inventory of these types of covered stents and be familiar with their deployment so that they can successfully deal with these rare but serious events (17).

Dissections

Arterial dissections occur commonly during endovascular intervention. At the angioplasty treatment site, dissections that involve the intima and media are ubiquitous. In a small percentage of cases, these dissections can be flow limiting and mandate additional treatment, typically involving placement of a stent. In locations where stent placement is not desired (e.g., common femoral artery), alternative treatments including athrectomy may be required.

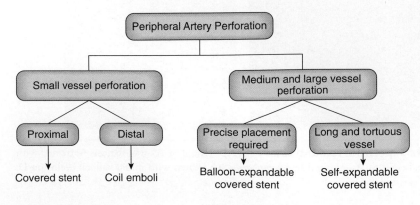

Figure 25.5 • Treatment strategy of arterial perforations with stent implants and coil embolization.

TABLE 25.2 Summary of Agents Used to Reverse the Effect of Anti-coagulant, Anti-platelet, and Fibrinolytic Agents Used During Peripheral Vascular Intervention

Drug	Reversal Agent(s)	Test	Comments
Warfarin	Vitamin K PO, SQ, IV 3-factor PCC 4000 IU rFVIIa (15–90 mg/kg)	PT/INR	Route of administration dependent on clinical situation Monitor PT/INR every 6 hr for 24 hr
Unfractionated heparin	Stop infusion Protamine sulfate 1 mg for each 100 units	PTT	FFP contraindicated May use slow IV infusion of protamine 5 mg/min to avoid hypotension and bronchoconstriction
Low molecular weight heparin (LMWH)	Protamine sulfate 1 mg for each 1 mg of LMWH Consider rFVIIa	Anti-Xa assay	Partial reversal with protamine
Direct thrombin inhibitors	DDAVP 0.3 µg/kg Consider cryoprecipitate Consider rFVIIa	PTT	No specific antidote
Pentasaccharide	rFVIIa 30–90 µg/kg	Anti-Xa assay	
Aspirin, clopidogrel, ticlopidine, prasugrel	IU platelet transfusion Consider DDAVP 0.3 µg/kg rFVIIa 30–90 µg/kg	Consider platelet aggregometry	DDAVP may cause hyponatremia, elevated ICP, and seizures
Glycoprotein IIb/IIIa inhibitor			
Abciximab	Platelet transfusion –6 units	Consider platelet aggregrometry	Produces partial reversal of effect
Tirofiban	N/A		Effect of drug wears off after ~ 4 hours
Eptifibatide	N/A		Effect of drug wears off after ~ 4 hours
Fibrinolytics	Fresh frozen plasma 15ml/Kg Cryoprecipitate 1 bag/10Kg Aminocaproic acid PO/IV–5mg during first hour, 1-1.25mg/hr for 8 hours or until bleeding stops		First line therapy First line therapy Second line therapy

PTT, partial thromboplastin time; PT, prothrombin time; INR, international normalized ratio; rFVIIa, recombinant factor VIIa, 3-factor PCC, three-factor prothrombin complex concentrate; ICP, intracranial pressure; DDAVP-desamino d-arginine vasopressin,.

Arterial dissections caused by wire, catheter, or sheath manipulation or during device delivery are much less common (18). In such situations, the management of the dissection is determined by the direction of the dissection with respect to blood flow and whether the dissection is flow limiting. Retrograde dissections (e.g., dissection of the external iliac artery following retrograde advancement of a wire) that are not flow limiting can usually be managed conservatively, since antegrade flow will usually maintain the vessel lumen and limit further propagation of the dissection, and facilitate subsequent healing of

TABLE 25.3 Covered Stent Options for Vascular Perforations

	Reliant Balloon	Boston XXL Balloon	Cook CODA Balloon	Boston Equalizer Balloon
Minimum introducer sheath	12 Fr.	7–8 Fr.	14 Fr.	14–16 Fr.
Shaft diameter	8 Fr.	5–6 Fr.	10 Fr.	7 Fr.
Usable catheter length	100 cm	75, 120 cm	100, 120 cm	65, 100 cm
Balloon material	Polyurethane	Latex	Polyurethane	Latex
Maximum balloon diameter	46 mm	18 mm	40 mm	40 mm
Compliant balloon	Yes	No	Yes	Yes

the dissection flap. Antegrade dissections are more concerning since they can be propagated forward due to antegrade blood flow leading to extension of the dissection plane and compromise of the vessel lumen and antegrade blood flow. The goal in these cases is to obtain and maintain wire access distally within the true lumen. In the treatment of arterial dissection, uncovered stent placement over the dissection entry point serves to reapproximate the intima, media, and adventitia, preventing continued flow into the false vessel lumen.

Foreign Body Retrieval

The loss of objects in the peripheral circulation during endovascular intervention is estimated to occur in 0.1% of cases. This may be an underestimate of the actual incidence in the current era of expanding arterial and venous endovascular procedures. Migrated polyurethane catheters account for over 80% of all reported arterial and venous foreign body embolization, followed by trapped guide wires and stent or implantable device embolizations. Patient outcomes are related to the site of final lodgment (19). Intracardiac, intracerebral, and occlusive peripheral arterial embolizations are associated with the

greatest risk of serious complications and even death. A serious morbidity and mortality rate of 21% to 27% and 23.7% to 27%, respectively, have been reported with foreign body embolization. Most serious complications have been reported with intracardiac embolization leading to ventricular arrhythmias, myocardial infarction, perforation, pericardial tamponade, thromboembolism, and myocarditis. The overall rates of foreign body embolization in the arterial circulation are less common than in the venous circulation. Objects in the venous circulation often embolize to their final location and secondary embolization is rare, as is passage from one caval system to another.

Surgical retrieval of foreign objects is associated with a high risk of adverse events and carries a mortality rate of 10%, which is significantly higher than with percutaneous retrieval. Percutaneous retrieval techniques are clearly favored where possible. The loop-snare technique requires a guidewire introduced through a catheter and folded back through the exit port to create a loop that can be maneuvered into different sizes and lengths. Pre-formed loop snares are custom-made and most commonly used. Nitinol Goose neck snares offer a particular advantage given the shape memory of the nitinol loop and the

TABLE 25.4 Covered Stent Options for Treatment of Vascular Perforations

Device	Type	Sheath Size (Fr.)	Diameter (mm)	Length (mm)
Viabahn	Self-expandable	7–12	5–13	25, 50, 100, 150
Wallgraft	Self-expandable	9–12	6–14	20, 30, 50, 70
Fluency	Self-expandable	8–9	5–12	30, 40, 60, 80, 100, 120
Jostent	Balloon-expandable	4Fr	3, 3.5, 4, 4.5, 5	12, 16, 19, 26
iCAST	Balloon-expandable	6–7	5–10	16, 22, 38, 59

ability to generate variable force on the loop. The Microneva Goose neck snare is one of the more common ones used in published literature to remove free-floating intravascular foreign objects with over 90% success rates. A three-dimensional retrieval snare (Entrio-snare™, Bard, and Murray Hill, NJ) has three interlaced nitinol loops, which provides good vessel coverage, torque control, flexibility, and kink resistance for use in small, medium, and large vessels.

Small snare wires (2 to 4 mm, 3-Fr. compatible) are used primarily for small vessels. Larger, 9 to 15 mm, 6-Fr. compatible snares are most frequently employed for peripheral arterial retrievals. The largest, 27 to 45 mm, 7-Fr. compatible snares are often used for retrievals form large vessels like the superior or inferior vena cava and cardiac chambers. The three-dimensional snares should be advanced through accompanying delivery catheters to avoid entrapment especially in intracardiac structures.

The choice of the snare system is based on the vessel size, size of the snare loop, and adaptability of the snare to the foreign object dimension and orientation. The dimension of the sheath is also an important variable to consider (20). Most polyurethane catheters can be retrieved through 6-Fr. sheath compatible snares even if the dislodged foreign body is up to 8 Fr., in size given its flexibility and ability to fold on itself. If the object gets blocked at the sheath tip during extraction attempts, it may result in laceration of the artery or vein. To avoid such complications the operator has to anticipate this and use larger introducer sheaths from the beginning of the retrieval procedure. A surgical cutdown should be performed if the device cannot be removed through the sheath.

References

1. Anderson PL, Gelijns A, Moskowitz A, et al. Understanding trends in inpatient surgical volume: vascular interventions, 1980–2000. *J Vasc Surg*. 2004;39:1200–1208.
2. Matsi PJ, Manninen HI. Complications of lower-limb percutaneous transluminal angioplasty: a prospective analysis of 410 procedures on 295 consecutive patients. *Cardiovasc Intervent Radiol*. 1998;21:361–366.
3. Lin PH, Dodson TF, Bush RL, et al. Surgical intervention for complications caused by femoral artery catheterization in pediatric patients. *J Vasc Surg*. 2001;34:1071–1078.
4. Shammas NW, Allie D, Hall P, et al. Predictors of in-hospital and 30-day complications of peripheral vascular interventions using bivalirudin as the primary anticoagulant: results from the APPROVE Registry. *J Invasive Cardiol*. 2005;17:356–359.
5. Sherev DA, Shaw RE, Brent BN. Angiographic predictors of femoral access site complications: implication for planned percutaneous coronary intervention. *Catheter Cardiovasc Interv*. 2005;65:196–202.
6. Lauer MA, Karweit JA, Cascade EF, et al. Practice patterns and outcomes of percutaneous coronary interventions in the United States: 1995 to 1997. *Am J Cardiol*. 2002;89:924–929.
7. Farouque HM, Tremmel JA, Raissi Shabari F, et al. Risk factors for the development of retroperitoneal hematoma after percutaneous coronary intervention in the era of GP IIb/IIIa inhibitors and vascular closure devices. *J Am Coll Cardiol*. 2005;45:363–368.
8. Gonzalez C, Penado S, Llata L, et al. The clinical spectrum of retroperitoneal hematoma in anticoagulated patients. *Medicine (Baltimore)*. 2003;82:257–262.
9. Quint LE, Holland D, Korobkin M, et al. Role of femoral vessel catheterization and altered hemostasis in the development of extraperitoneal hematomas: CT study in 44 patients. *Am J Roentgenol*. 1993;160:855–858.
10. Sreeram S, Lumsden AB, Miller JS, et al. Retroperitoneal hematoma following femoral arterial catheterization: a serious and often fatal complication. *Am Surg*. 1993;59:94–98.
11. Kiemeneij F, Laarman GJ, Odekerken D, et al. A randomized comparison of percutaneous transluminal coronary angioplasty by the radial, brachial and femoral approaches: the access study. *J Am Coll Cardiol*. 1997;29:1269–1275.
12. Hu ZJ, Wang SM, Li XX, et al. Tolerable hemodynamic changes after femoral artery ligation for the treatment of infected femoral artery pseudoaneurysm. *Ann Vasc Surg*. 2010;24:212–218.
13. Coley BD, Roberts AC, Fellmeth BD, et al. Postangiographic femoral artery pseudoaneurysms: further experience with US-guided compression repair. *Radiology*. 1995;194:307–311.
14. Morgan R, Belli AM. Current treatment methods for postcatheterization pseudoaneurysms. *J Vasc Interv Radiol*. 2003;14:697–710.
15. Johnson LW, Esente P, Giambartolomei A, et al. Peripheral vascular complications of coronary angioplasty by the femoral and brachial techniques. *Catheter Cardiovasc Diagn*. 1994;31:165–172.
16. Lewis DR, Bullbulia RA, Murphy P, et al. Vascular surgical intervention for complications of cardiovascular radiology: 13 years' experience in a single centre. *Ann R Coll Surg Engl*. 1999;81:23–26.
17. Yeo KK, Rogers JH, Laird JR. Use of stent grafts and coils in vessel rupture and perforation. *J Interv Cardiol*. 2008;21:86–99.
18. Prasad A, Compton PA, Roesle M, et al. Incidence and treatment of arterial access dissections occurring during cardiac catheterization. *J Interv Cardiol*. 2008;21:61–66.
19. Tateishi M, Tomizawa Y. Intravascular foreign bodies: danger of unretrieved fragmented medical devices. *J Artif Organs*. 2009;12:80–89.
20. Fisher RG, Ferreyro R. Evaluation of current techniques for nonsurgical removal of intravascular iatrogenic foreign bodies. *Am J Roentgenol*. 1978;130:541–548.

Venous Intervention

CHAPTER 26

Central Venous Obstruction

Michael Wholey and William C. S. Wu

Central venous obstruction encompasses the varied disorders that result in the compression and occlusion of the venous structures in the chest. These include diseases related to the superior vena cava (SVC) as well as those affecting its contributing branches.

CENTRAL VENOUS ANATOMY

The SVC is formed from the union of the right and left brachiocephalic/innominate veins (Fig. 26.1). Each brachiocephalic vein is formed from the union of the respective internal jugular and subclavian veins. The subclavian veins represent the continuation of the brachial and axillary veins from each upper extremity. The anatomic structure delineating the transition from axillary to subclavian vein is the first rib.

ETIOLOGY OF CENTRAL VENOUS OBSTRUCTION

Central venous obstruction is typically divided into two broad categories based on the anatomic location of the obstruction—that is, the SVC or the axillary and subclavian veins. Brachiocephalic obstructions are inconsistently included in either of these groups.

SVC obstruction, which frequently involves the brachiocephalic branches, results in the SVC syndrome. Malignant causes, particularly carcinoma of the bronchus, are now responsible for in excess of 90% of cases of SVC syndrome (1–5). Squamous cell carcinoma of the bronchus is more commonly associated with SVC syndrome than non-squamous cell-type cancers. Less common malignancies associated with SVC syndrome include lymphoma, metastatic disease, and thymoma.

Axillary/subclavian venous occlusion may be due to primary or secondary causes. The dominant primary cause is Paget–von Schroetter syndrome (PSS) (also referred to as effort thrombosis thoracic outlet syndrome [TOS]) (6). This syndrome most commonly occurs in the dominant arm (~70%) of males (~70%) and is related to repetitive or unusual arm activity. There is a high incidence of associated anatomic abnormalities that lead to compression of the thoracic outlet (7,8) (Fig. 26.2). In 1821, Sir Astley Cooper first described axillary/subclavian artery symptoms due to compression from a cervical rib (9). In 1875, James Paget described the clinical symptoms resulting from subclavian vein thrombosis (arm swelling and pain). In 1884, von Schroetter correctly attributed these upper extremity venous symptoms to thrombosis or compression of the subclavian vein at the thoracic outlet (7–9). Consequently, venous thrombosis at the thoracic outlet became known as venous TOS or PSS.

Axillary/subclavian venous occlusion is most commonly caused by secondary etiologies such as indwelling central venous catheters or pacemaker leads, underlying malignancy, hypercoagulability, trauma, or infection. Several investigators have shown that venous obstruction after pacemaker implantation may be observed in approximately 31% to 50%, though it may be closer to 20% when pre- and post-lead studies are reviewed (10). These secondary causes also frequently result in central venous obstruction of the SVC.

DIAGNOSIS

Axillary/subclavian venous occlusion is supported by the presence of upper extremity swelling, venous engorgement, and pain. Secondary causes such as pacemaker leads or central venous catheters will usually be clinically obvious. These signs and symptoms, in association with radiologic documentation of venous compression at the thoracic outlet, confirm the diagnosis of TOS/PSS. Sometimes, venous compression cannot be demonstrated, and the diagnosis is made clinically by the pattern of venous thrombosis.

Signs and symptoms of SVC occlusion include difficulty breathing, swollen neck and chest wall veins, bilateral arm/neck/facial swelling, hoarseness, and headache. CTA and other noninvasive imaging modalities (including multiplanar fast MR imaging) are very helpful in diagnosing central venous obstruction (Fig. 26.3). Digital subtraction angiography (DSA) remains the gold standard and typically reveals the site of occlusion and the development of collateral pathways. An obstructed SVC initiates collateral venous return to the heart from the upper half of the body through four principal pathways (Fig. 26.4). The first and most important pathway is the azygous venous system, which includes the azygous vein, the hemiazygous vein, and the connecting intercostal veins. The second pathway is the internal mammary venous system plus tributaries and secondary communications to the superior and inferior epigastric veins. The long thoracic venous system, with its connections to the femoral veins, and the vertebral veins provide the third and fourth collateral routes, respectively. Despite these collateral networks, venous pressure is almost always elevated in the upper chest in the presence of SVC obstruction (Fig. 26.5A–C).

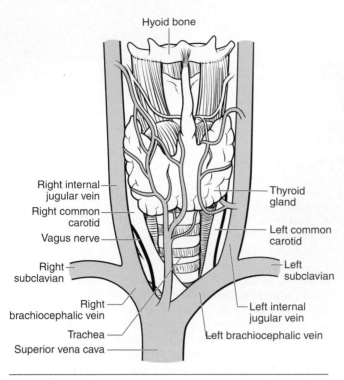

Figure 26.1 • Schematic illustration of central venous anatomy.

MANAGEMENT

Recanalizing Central Venous Obstruction

In managing patients with central venous obstruction, heparinization is often the first step in relieving symptoms from the thrombosis; although it does not lyse the clot, it will help increase collateral flow to reduce the edema experienced by many patients. Second, if there is an offending mechanical factor contributing to thrombosis/obstruction (i.e., central line and pacemaker lead), it should be removed if possible. Unfortunately, many lines and wires cannot be removed.

Before interventional options are considered, recanalization must first be achieved. Once femoral and/or jugular venous access is achieved with ultrasound guidance, the authors typically place a large sheath and deliver either diagnostic catheters, such as a 5-Fr. vertebral or multipurpose, or a 6- or 7-Fr. guide catheter to the site of the occlusion. We frequently use a 0.035″ glidewire to cross the occlusion, starting with the floppy glidewire and moving to the stiff shaft glidewire if necessary. Sometimes, recanalization is the most difficult part of the procedure as the clot may be chronic and organized. Failure to cross central venous occlusions can account for 15% of the technical failures (11). Flush occlusion of the central vein increases the risk of failure.

If the vessel is partially occluded, then thrombolysis prior to an attempted intervention may be an option. Thrombolysis has a rate of complete lysis of 76% to 84% for primary axillary/subclavian occlusions (12–14). Unfortunately, urokinase (formerly Abbott Pharmaceuticals, Abbott Park, IL) was more effective in treating older thrombus than the currently available thrombolytic agent, tissue plasminogen activator (tPA) (Figs. 26.6 to 26.8).

Managing Axillary/Subclavian Venous Disease

Patients with primary (i.e., PSS) and secondary thrombotic occlusion of the axillary/subclavian veins have distinct management strategies. In patients with PSS, the thrombotic occlusion is typically crossed and thrombolytic therapy is administered in the hopes of achieving recanalization and some restoration of venous flow. For occlusions older than 10 to 14 days, the chances of successful thrombolysis are poor. Some studies have found residual lesions in as many as 100% of these patients following thrombolysis (15,16). Regardless of the outcome following thrombolysis, prompt surgical correction of the underlying anatomic abnormality is required. Typically, the surgery will involve resection of the first rib, division of the costoclavicular ligament, and division and resection of the anterior scalene muscle. This surgical approach has proved to be an effective treatment (15). The timing of surgical decompression following thrombolysis is controversial: most surgeons wait at least 4 weeks before performing a decompressive procedure.

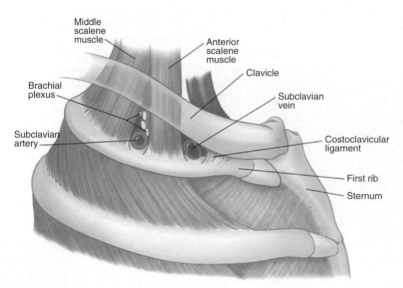

Figure 26.2 • Schematic illustration of the normal anatomy of the thoracic outlet. Note the relationship of the subclavian vein to the anterior scalene muscle posteriorly, the costoclavicular ligament anteriorly, the clavicle superiorly, and the first rib inferiorly. (From Urschel HC Jr, Patel AN. Surgery Remains the Most Effective Treatment for Paget-Schroetter Syndrome: 50 Years' Experience. *Ann Thorac Surg.* 2008;86:254–260).

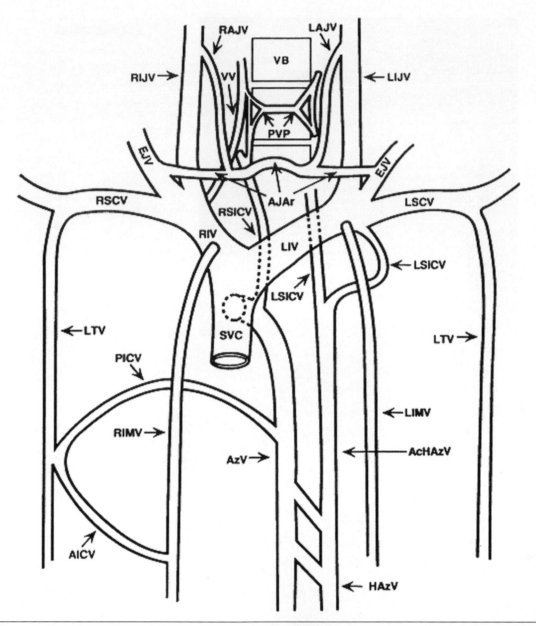

Figure 26.3 • Schematic illustration of major collateral networks that compensate for the presence of central venous obstruction. Ac-HAzV, accessory hemiazygos vein; AICV, anterior intercostal vein; AJAr, anterior jugular arch; AzV, azygos vein; EJV, external jugular vein; HAzV, hemiazygos vein; LAJV, left anterior jugular vein; LIJV, left internal jugular vein; LIMV, left internal mammary vein; LIV, left innominate vein; LSICV, left superior intercostal vein; LSCV, left subclavian vein; LTV, lateral thoracic vein; PICV, posterior intercostal vein; PVP, paravertebral plexus; RAJV, right anterior jugular vein; RIJV, right internal jugular vein; RIMV, right internal mammary vein; RIV, right innominate vein; RSCV, right subclavian vein; RSICV, right superior intercostal vein; SVC, superior vena cava; VB, vertebral body; VV, vertebral vein. (Reprinted from Chasen MH, Charnsangavej C. Venous chest anatomy: clinical implications. *Eur J Radiol.* 1998;27:2–14, with permission from Elsevier.)

In patients with secondary occlusion of the brachiocephalic, subclavian, and/or axillary venous segment(s), the most common treatment options include angioplasty and/or stent placement: angioplasty with 0.035″-compatible balloon catheters with diameters ranging from 5 to 15 mm (Figs. 26.5 and 26.6). Non-compliant balloon catheters are preferred. Most operators size the balloon to the vessel being dilated. Cutting balloon catheters should be considered for resistant lesions. In general, endovascular therapy with PTA or cutting balloon catheters for central venous stenosis is safe, with low rates of technical failure.

However, patency rates with balloon angioplasty are poor with reported 12-month primary and secondary patency rates of 22% to 29% and 63% to 73%, respectively (17,18). As a result, multiple additional interventions are the rule with both treatments. Cutting balloon angioplasty has not been shown to improve patency rates compared with PTA and does not add to the longevity of ipsilateral hemodialysis access sites (18).

If angioplasty fails, we will consider stent placement. For lesions in the brachiocephalic, axillary, or subclavian veins, self-expandable stents (e.g., Wallstent) are recommended

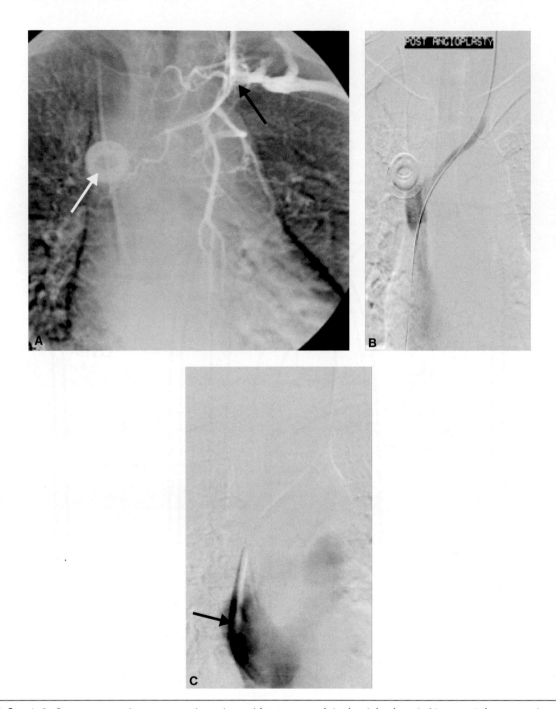

Figure 26.4 • **A:** Left upper extremity venogram in patient with a port-a-cath in the right chest *(white arrow)* demonstrating an occlusion of the left brachiocephalic and subclavian veins *(black arrow)* which has resulted in the formation of numerous collateral vessels in the left chest and shoulder. **B:** The occlusion was successfully recanalized using left internal jugular venous access and angioplasty was performed. **C:** This allowed the placement of a hemodialysis catheter from a left internal jugular approach with the catheter tip in the right superior vena cava *(black arrow)*.

(Fig. 26.9). General rules for stent choice and placement include the following: avoid undersizing the stent, avoid placing brachiocephalic or subclavian stents across the internal jugular vein junction, and avoid placing brachiocephalic stents across the junction with the SVC. By blocking these key junctions makes future central venous catheter placement, particularly of large diameter hemodialysis catheters, very difficult (19). Patency rates following stenting of subclavian/axillary veins is highly variable, with 6- to 12-month

patency rates of 29% to 88% being reported in the literature (19–21).

There has been some discussion of the use of covered stents in these venous segments. Overall, results have not been impressive (22). There have been small series that report problems of stent fracture and poor patency (29% primary at 12 months) (23,24).

Less often used treatment modalities included laser ablation or mechanical atherectomy. These have not been well

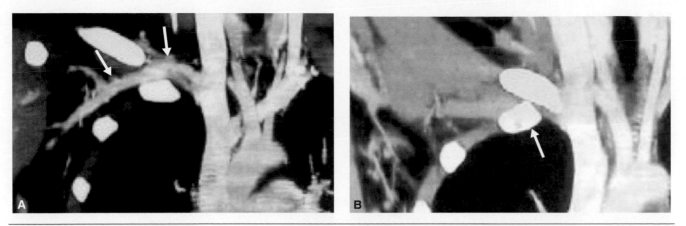

Figures 26.5 • **A:** CT angiogram with the right arm in the adducted position demonstrating wide patency of the right subclavian vein *(white arrows)*. **B:** CT angiogram from the same patient with the arm in the abducted and external rotated position demonstrating compression of the axillary/subclavian vein at the junction of the first rib *(white arrow)* and the clavicle. This is diagnostic for thoracic outlet syndrome (TOS).

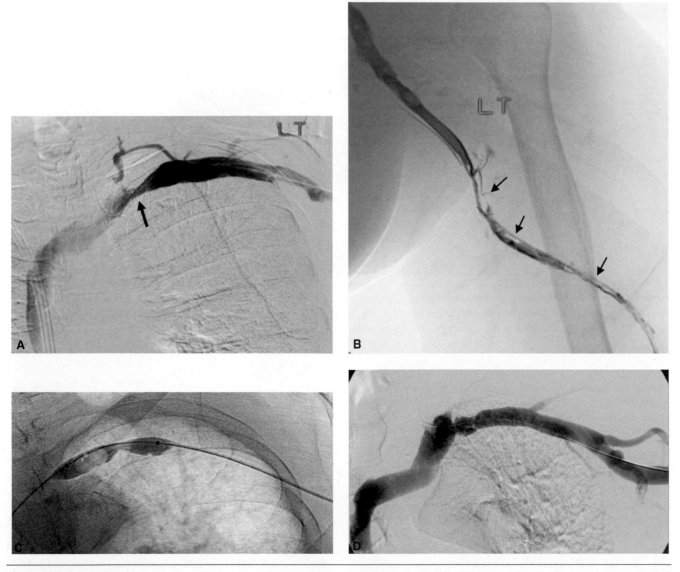

Figure 26.6 • **A,B:** Left upper extremity venography in a patient on chronic hemodialysis demonstrating significant stenosis in the left subclavian vein *(black arrow)* which resulted in decreased flow and thrombosis in the left brachial vein *(black arrows)*. **C:** Thrombolytics were administered into the brachial vein in the arm. Next, angioplasty with 10- and 14-mm balloon catheters was performed resulting in improved flow through the stenosed subclavian vein lesion. **D:** Final venography demonstrating residual stenosis in left sublavian with sufficient venous flow to allow hemodialysis.

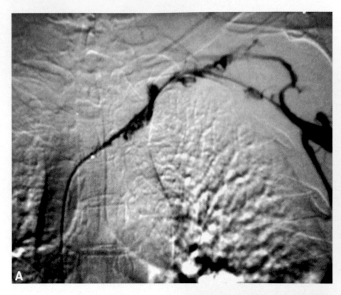
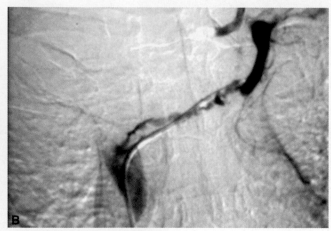
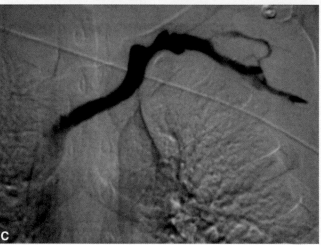

Figure 26.7 • **A:** Left upper extremity venography demonstrating subtotal occlusion of the left subclavian and brachiocephalic veins. **B:** Following initial angioplasty, residual thrombus was seen. Overnight thrombolysis was administered. **C:** Venography following thrombolysis demonstrating resolution of the majority of the thrombus burden. No additional angioplasty was required.

received in treating venous strictures due to the risk of vessel rupture and entanglement with indwelling catheters and/or devices. In addition, restenosis rates appear to be no better than with angioplasty alone (25).

Managing Superior Vena Cava Disease

Many of the cases of superior vena disease and occlusion are due to malignant obstruction, requiring stent placement to maintain patency, while chemotherapy or radiation treatment for tumor management is instituted. Often, thrombolytic therapy or mechanical thrombectomy is required beforehand to deal with the large thrombus burden and reduce the risk of embolization of thrombus to the pulmonary circulation.

Balloon-expandable (Palmaz) and self-expanding (Wallstent, Guanturco Z) stents have been used in the SVC. Use of balloon-expandable stents is preferred where precise placement of the stent is required. Due to the large size of most SVCs (i.e., >10 mm), it is typical to have to hand mount the Palmaz stent onto the appropriately sized noncompliant balloon (i.e., matching the diameter of the SVC). The Wallstent self-expanding stent must be carefully centered across the stenosis/occlusion due to significant shortening that occurs with stent deployment and the tendency of the stent to migrate from the narrowest point toward the normal venous segment (Fig. 26.10). In situations where both brachiocephalic veins and the SVC are obstructed, it is generally sufficient to stent either the right or left brachiocephalic vein and SVC. Overall, stenting is associated with high technical success, primary patency rates of >80%, and clinical success rates of 68% to 100% (26–29). Stents do not interfere with subsequent anti-tumor treatments and provide urgently needed relief of symptoms. The response is immediate with the disappearance of symptoms within

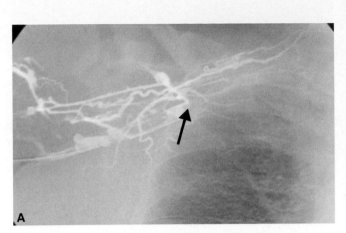
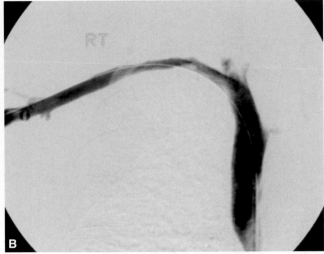

Figure 26.8 • **A:** Baseline venography in patient with right subclavian vein occlusion *(black arrow)*. **B:** Venography following treatment with Medrad Possis Angiojet in addition to angioplasty.

24 to 72 hours (26). Percutaneous implantation of stents appears fully justified in terminally ill patients (irrespective of their life expectancy) because of the rapid relief of clinical symptoms, which eliminates the protracted waiting time of 3 to 4 weeks that would be required with chemotherapy and/or radiotherapy treatment without stenting. Bypass surgery often requires a sternotomy and is associated with significant post-operative morbidity. As a result, it is not justified because of the near-terminal status of many of these patients (27).

Those patients with SVC syndrome due to non-tumor causes may be treated using angioplasty or stenting (Fig. 26.11). It is the author's practice to perform angioplasty for SVC stenoses and stenting for occlusions, especially those that are chronic. Primary and secondary patency for stent placement in this cohort are ~67% and 100%, respectively (20,28,29).

Complications

Fortunately, complications from angioplasty and stent placement of the central veins are infrequent, with minor (e.g., access site hematoma) and major (e.g., rupture of the SVC, pericardial tamponade, pulmonary embolus, and stent migration) complications occurring in 3% to 7% of all cases.

Rupture can occur in 1% to 5% of cases and is the most catastrophic complication encountered. It is typically recognized at the time of the procedure, but some case reports of delayed rupture (between 15 minutes to 6 months post-procedure) do exist. The risk of rupture emphasizes the need to always maintain wire access across the treatment site and to typically deliver the PTA balloon/stent using a large sheath from the common femoral vein, which allows for easier delivery of a covered stent if required (25).

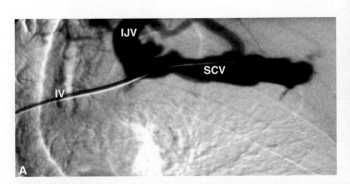
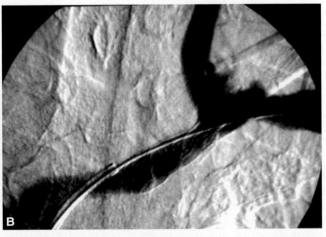

Figure 26.9 • **A:** Baseline venography demonstrating chronic total occlusion of the left brachiocephalic vein that was successfully crossed using common femoral venous access. IJV, internal jugular vein; SCV, subclavian vein; IV, innominate vein. **B:** Venography following placement of a self-expandable nitinol stent due to significant recoil following angioplasty.

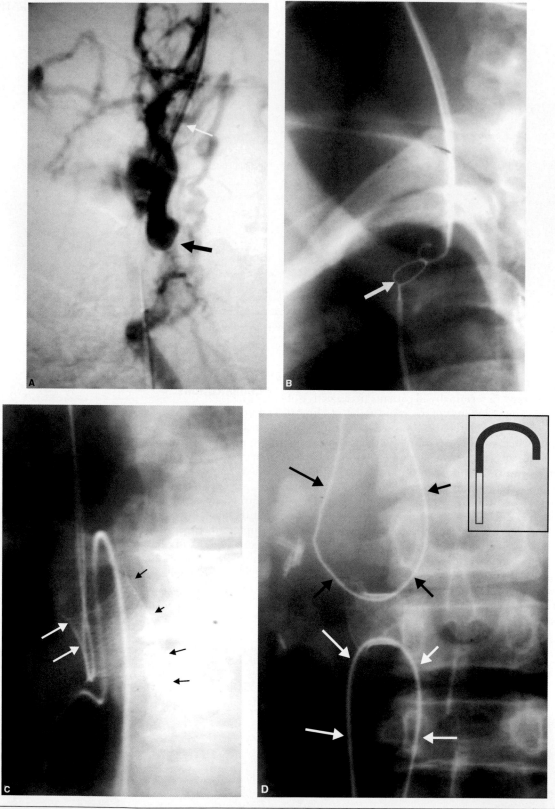

Figure 26.10 • A: Baseline venography in a patient with superior vena cava (SVC) syndrome from right internal jugular venous (IJV) access *(white arrow)* demonstrating complete occlusion of the right brachiocephalic and SVC *(black arrow)*. **B:** Snare *(white arrow)* advanced from right common femoral vein (CFV) access used to snare wire which had been advanced across the occlusion from the right IJV access. **C:** Angioplasty was then performed from the right IVJ access site, but significant residual stenosis required stent placement. A 16-mm diameter Wallstent was deployed from right IJV access site into the SVC but the stent jumped forward into the right atrium *(white and black arrows outlining the right and left border of the stent, respectively)*. When it moved into the right atrium, its diameter increased and could not be captured with a snare. **D:** This required the use of two RIM (Rosch inferior mesenteric) catheters (see inset for illustration of catheter shape) to allow dual wire control in which the IJV wire went through the center of the stent and back or retrograde along the outside the stent back to the IJV *(black arrows)*. A similar technique was performed from the CFV access *(white arrows)*. This allowed the careful pull of the migrated stent back down the IVC to the femoral vein where it was removed.

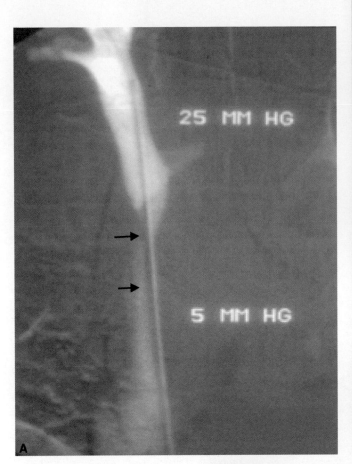

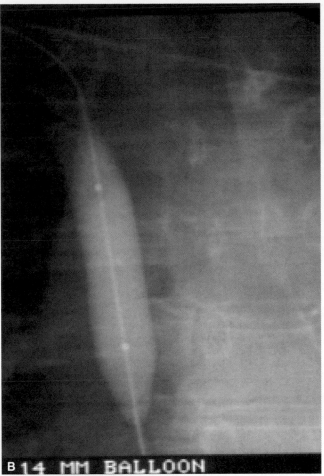

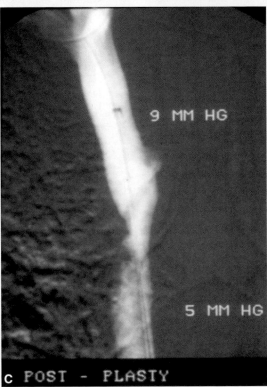

Figure 26.11 • Patient with superior vena cava (SVC) syndrome from benign cause (pacemaker leads). A: Venogram following crossing of SVC from inferior vena cava (IVC) approach demonstrating high-grade stenosis *(black arrows)* with significant pressure gradient (20mmHg) and no evidence of thrombus. After PTA with 14-mm balloon catheter (**B**), the gradient was reduced to 4 mm with resolution of symptoms (**C**).

Special attention must be given to patients with heart disease. Peri-procedural hemodynamic monitoring (e.g., using a Swan–Ganz catheter) may be useful to prevent complications related to heart failure and pulmonary edema after stent placement (26).

References

1. Ahmann FR. A reassessment of the clinical implications of the superior vena caval syndrome. *J Clin Oncol*. 1984;2:961–969.
2. Hassikou H, Bono W, Bahiri R, et al. Vascular involvement in Behçet's disease. Two case reports. *Joint Bone Spine*. 2002;69:416–418.
3. Hunter W. The history of an aneurysm of the aorta with some remarks on aneurysms in general. *Med Obs Enq*. 1757;1: 323–357.
4. Salsali M, Cliffton EE. Superior vena caval obstruction in carcinoma of lung. *N Y State J Med*. 1969;69:2875–280.
5. Rice TW, Rodriguez RM, Light RW. The superior vena cava syndrome: clinical characteristics and evolving etiology. *Medicine (Baltimore)*. 2006;85:37–42.
6. Abe M, Ichinohe K, Nishida J. Diagnosis, treatment, and complications of thoracic outlet syndrome. *J Orthop Sci*. 1999;4:66–69.
7. Feugier P, Chevalier JM. The Paget-Schroetter syndrome. *Acta Chir Belg*. 2005;105:256–264.
8. Oktar GL, Ergul EG. Paget-Schroetter syndrome. *Hong Kong Med J*. 2007;13:243–247.
9. Bauer G C. Sir Astley Cooper. Prototype of the modern day academic orthopedist. *Clin Orthop Relat Res*. 1987:247–254.
10. Oginowawa O, Abe H, Nakashima Y. The incidence and risk factors for venous obstruction after implantation of transvenous pacing leads. *Pacing Clin Electrophysiol*. 2002;25:1605–1611.
11. Crowe MT, Davies CH, Gaines PA. Percutaneous management of superior vena cava occlusions. *Cardiovasc Intervent Radiol*. 1995;18:367–72.
12. Machleder HI. Evaluation of a new treatment strategy for Paget-Schroetter syndrome: spontaneous thrombosis of the axillary-subclavian vein. *J Vasc Surg*. 1993;17:305–315.
13. Lau KY, Tan LT, Wong WW, et al. *Ann Acad Med Singapore*. 2003;32:461–465.
14. Beygui RE, Olcott C IV, Dalman R. *Ann Vasc Surg*. 1997;11: 247–255.
15. Fugate MW, Rotellini-Coltvet L, Freischlag JA. Current management of thoracic outlet syndrome. *Curr Treat Options Cardiovasc Med*. 2009;11:176–183.
16. Sharafuddin MJ, Sun S, Hoballah JJ. Endovascular management of venous thrombotic diseases of the upper torso and extremities. *J Vasc Interv Radiol*. 2002;13:975–990.
17. Nael K, Kee ST, Solomon H, et al. Endovascular management of central thoracic veno-occlusive diseases in hemodialysis patients: a single institutional experience in 69 consecutive patients. *J Vasc Interv Radiol*. 2009;20:46–51.
18. Bakken AM, Protack CD, Saad WE, et al. Long-term outcomes of primary angioplasty and primary stenting of central venous stenosis in hemodialysis patients. *Vasc Surg*. 2007;45:776–783.
19. Crowe. Percutaneous management of superior vena cava occlusions. *Cardiovasc Intervent Radiol*. 1995;18:367–372.
20. Bornak A, Wicky S, Ris HB, et al. Endovascular treatment of stenoses in the superior vena cava syndrome caused by non-tumoral lesions. *Eur Radiol*. 2003;13:950–956.
21. Nazarian. Venous recanalization by metallic stents after failure of balloon angioplasty or surgery: four-year experience. *Cardiovasc Intervent Radiol*. 1996;19:227–233.
22. Gianfranco Butera GM. Use of radiofrequency energy and covered stents in patients with an occluded superior vena cava and requiring endocardial pace. *J Invas Card*.
23. Phipp LH, Scott DJ, Kessel D, et al. Subclavian stents and stent-grafts: cause for concern. *J Endovasc Surg*. 1999;6:223–226.
24. Farber A, Barbey MM, Grunert JH, et al. Access-related venous stenoses and occlusions: treatment with percutaneous transluminal angioplasty and Dacron-covered stents. *Cardiovasc Intervent Radiol*. 1999;22:214–218.
25. Savader S, Trerotola SO. *Venous Interventional Radiology: With Clinical Perspective*. New York, NY: Thieme Medical Publishing; 2000:254–258.
26. Yamagami T, Nakamura T, Kato T, et al. Hemodynamic changes after self-expandable metallic stent therapy for vena cava syndrome. *Am J Roentgenol*. 2002;178:635–639.
27. Lanciego C, Chacón JL, Julián A, et al. Stenting as first option for endovascular treatment of malignant superior vena cava syndrome. *Am J Roentgenol*. 2001;177:585–593.
28. Nagata T, Makutani S, Uchida H, et al. Follow-up results of 71 patients undergoing metallic stent placement for the treatment of a malignant obstruction of the superior vena cava. *Cardiovasc Intervent Radiol*. 2007;30:959–967.
29. Dinkel HP, Mettke B, Schmid F, et al. Endovascular treatment of malignant superior vena cava syndrome: is bilateral wallstent placement superior to unilateral placement? *J Endovasc Ther*. 2003;10:788–797.

CHAPTER 27

Management of Deep Vein Thrombosis

Mitchell J. Silver and Jayme Rock-Willoughby

Venous thromboembolism, which comprises deep vein thrombosis (DVT) and pulmonary embolism (PE), is a leading cause of morbidity and mortality. In the United States, it is the third leading cause of cardiovascular death after myocardial infarction and stroke (1). Moreover, approximately 600,000 cases of venous thromboembolism have been estimated to occur annually in the United States (2).

DVT is a process that can affect each one of the deep veins in the body, but is more frequently present in the deep veins of the lower extremity. If undiagnosed and left untreated, both acute and chronic complications can occur. PE is the acute complication that occurs most frequently. Clinical PE occurs in 26% to 67% of patients with untreated proximal deep venous thrombosis and is associated with a mortality rate of 11% to 23% if not treated (3). It is estimated that 40% to 50% of patients with proximal DVT will suffer from silent PE (4).

Phlegmasia cerulea dolens is another rare but serious acute complication of DVT, developing in 1% of patients with iliofemoral thromboses (5). This occurs in the setting of an extensive iliofemoral DVT. Symptoms include acute massive edema, cyanosis, and severe pain. Risk factors for the development of phlegmasia cerulea dolens include underlying advanced malignancy, severe infections, surgery, fractures, etc. Potentially devastating complications include PE that occurs in up to one third of patients, and lower extremity gangrene due to compartment syndrome that occurs as frequently as 50% in some reports (2). Endovascular treatment for this condition and decreasing the risk of PTS will be discussed below.

Post-thrombotic syndrome (PTS) is the major chronic complication of lower extremity DVT. Persistent venous outflow obstruction leads to venous hypertension, which is estimated to occur in over half of patients with ileofemoral DVT and one third of patients with calf vein thrombosis (6). Risk factors for PTS include proximal location of DVT, male gender, and high D-dimer levels despite anticoagulation. Typical symptoms include leg pain and swelling. Symptoms of venous claudication may occur and are exacerbated by standing and physical activity, and are relieved with rest and elevation of the lower extremities. Venous claudication occurs most commonly in patients treated for ileofemoral DVT with standard anti-coagulation, as the majority of ileofemoral DVT will fail to recanalize with routine anti-coagulation. This persistent proximal venous obstruction leads to reduced outflow of blood, causing increased pressure with muscle contractions that occur with ambulation. Patients who develop PTS are at an increased risk of recurrent venous thromboembolism when compared to patients with uncomplicated infra-inguinal DVT. Finally, lower extremity ulceration, typically over the medial aspect of the lower leg, is a late manifestation of post-thrombotic syndrome.

ANATOMIC CONSIDERATIONS

Veins are larger in caliber and more numerous than arteries. The venous system has a much greater volume capacity than the arterial system. In the lower extremity, the venous circulation can be divided into three distinct systems that include the deep venous system, the superficial venous system, and the perforating or communicating system (See Fig. 30.3). The deep veins include anterior and posterior tibial, peroneal, popliteal, femoral, and iliac veins. These veins can be divided into regions: iliofemoral including iliac and femoral veins, femoral–popliteal including femoral and popliteal veins, and infrapopliteal including peroneal, anterior, and posterior tibial veins. These deep veins supply 90% to 95% of venous outflow from the lower extremity (3).

Valves exist along the entire length of the deep veins of the lower extremity, with the exception of the common iliac veins. They are more numerous and closely situated in the smaller, more distal veins, where the force of gravity is the greatest. The main function of these valves is to ensure antegrade flow of blood and to prevent backflow away from the heart. Blood flow is normally diminished around valves in the venous vasculature, and typically most venous thrombi form behind valve pockets, where the vein wall is slightly dilated behind each of the leaflets.

PATHOPHYSIOLOGY

In 1856 Rudolph Virchow, a German pathologist, postulated three factors precipitating venous thrombosis: venous stasis, endothelial damage to the vessel wall, and hypercoagulability. The main conditions contributing to the formation of venous thrombus in the deep veins of the legs are related to these three basic risk factors described by Virchow and include advanced age, prolonged bed rest, and major surgery. The rate for venous thromboembolism among elderly patients is approximately 20 times that of young adults, making advanced age an important risk factor (1). Major abdominal and orthopedic (e.g., total hip and knee replacement) surgeries are associated with the highest risk. Additional risk factors include: previous venous thrombosis, malignancy, trauma, chronic venous insufficiency, pregnancy and the postpartum period, use of contraceptive pills, and primary and secondary hypercoagulable states. Finally, obesity is also becoming another important risk factor, given the epidemic of this disorder in the United States. Obese individuals have a two to three times likelihood of developing venous thromboembolism (7).

NATURAL HISTORY

Deep venous thrombosis most often originates in the venous sinuses of the calf muscles, but occasionally originates in the proximal veins of the lower extremity (8,9). Sometimes, the thrombi propagate from the calf veins to the proximal veins. Specifically, 25% of untreated calf thrombi extend into the proximal veins, which is where they are more likely to embolize (7). PE occurs in up to 50% of patients with proximal deep venous thrombosis (8,9). Conversely, calf vein thrombosis rarely leads to significant PE (8).

DIAGNOSTIC TESTING

Unfortunately, the clinical diagnosis of lower extremity DVT is extremely inaccurate, with the classic signs and symptoms of DVT being as common in patients without DVT as they are in those with confirmed DVT. Therefore, if DVT is suspected, objective confirmation is mandatory.

D-dimer is a byproduct in the degradation of cross-linked fibrin by plasmin. In the setting of acute DVT, levels of D-dimer are typically elevated. Nonetheless, D-dimer levels are also increased by conditions such as recent major surgery, hemorrhage, trauma, pregnancy, malignancy, or acute arterial thrombosis. As a result, D-dimer assays are sensitive but not specific. The high sensitivity makes it possible to exclude DVT as a diagnosis, but the low specificity and positive predictive value force confirmatory non-invasive testing after a positive result.

Historically, ascending venography was the gold standard for the diagnosis of acute DVT. However, it is an invasive test, not easily repeatable, and impossible to perform or interpret in 9% to 14% of patients. Ascending venography also fails to visualize all venous segments in 10% to 30% of studies. Interobserver disagreements occur in 4% to 10% of studies. Because of these limitations, ascending venography has been replaced by venous duplex ultrasonography as the most widely used diagnostic test for acute DVT.

The sensitivity and specificity of venous ultrasonography for the diagnosis of symptomatic proximal DVT are 97% and 94%, respectively (10). A complete ultrasound evaluation of the lower extremities includes an assessment of venous compressibility, the presence of intraluminal echoes, venous flow characteristics, and luminal color filling. Venous incompressibility, or failure to completely coapt the venous walls with gentle probe compression, is the most widely used diagnostic criterion for acute DVT. Adjunctive gray-scale findings include the appearance of echogenic thrombus within the vein lumen and dilation of an acutely thrombosed segment. Normal flow in the proximal veins should be spontaneous and should vary with respiration (increasing during expiration and decreasing during inspiration).

Other non-invasive imaging techniques for the diagnosis of lower extremity DVT include magnetic resonance venography (MRV) and CT angiography. These studies are comparable to venography, but they cannot be performed at the bedside. In addition, CT angiography carries the risk of contrast allergy and radiation exposure, whereas MRV requires the use of gadolinium, which limits its applicability in patients with renal insufficiency. Both studies are more expensive than venous duplex ultrasonography.

A combined strategy using an assessment of clinical probability, D-dimer testing, and venous duplex ultrasonography provides the greatest diagnostic potential to confirm or reject the diagnosis of DVT. The negative predictive value of this approach is almost 100% in outpatients with a low pretest clinical probability for DVT.

TREATMENT

There are four generally accepted goals for the treatment of lower extremity DVT: (1) diminish the severity and duration of lower extremity symptoms, (2) prevent PE, (3) minimize the risk of recurrent venous thrombosis, and/or (4) prevent PTS. It is uniformly agreed upon that anti-coagulation is required to prevent thrombus growth and PE. Intravenous unfractionated heparin was historically the medication of choice, but low-molecular-weight heparin (LMWH) has emerged as the anti-coagulant of choice in the management of DVT. While both agents are effective and relatively safe in lower extremity DVT management, LMWH is suitable for outpatient therapy because of improved bioavailability and more predictable anticoagulant response. Serious potential complications of heparin therapy, such as heparin-induced thrombocytopenia and osteoporosis (with long-term use), occur less commonly with LMWH. Either unfractionated heparin or LMWH is used as a bridge to warfarin therapy, which should ideally be initiated within 24 hours of the diagnosis of DVT. The ideal international normalized ratio (INR) is 2.0 to 3.0. The optimal duration of warfarin therapy is controversial and dependent on the clinical situation: 6 to 12 weeks for a symptomatic isolated calf vein thrombosis, 3 months for the first DVT event with a known reversible or time-limited risk factor for venous thromboembolic disease, such as trauma or surgery, at least 6 months for the first episode of idiopathic venous thromboembolic disease, and at least 12 months to lifelong therapy for recurrent idiopathic venous thromboembolic disease or permanent risk factor such as thrombophilia (11). It is likely that there will be a major shift in recommendations for the treatment of DVT following the recent approval of the oral direct thrombin inhibitor, dabigatran. This agent, which appears to be equal in efficacy to warfarin for the prevention in stroke for patients with atrial fibrillation has the advantage of not requiring routine monitoring, and is not influenced by diet. On that basis, it is likely to replace warfarin as the default chronic therapy for DVT.

Although medical therapy with anti-coagulation is the mainstay of the initial management of lower extremity DVT, many patients, particularly those with large proximal iliofemoral DVT, have persistent leg edema, pain, and difficulty ambulating. These symptoms arise from venous hypertension caused by outflow obstruction. Relief of outflow obstruction is one of the primary goals of therapy for lower extremity DVT, but this is typically not accomplished with anti-coagulation alone. Thrombus regression occurs in only 50% of patients with ileofemoral DVT (3). Endovascular techniques, including catheter-directed thrombolysis (CDT), mechanical thrombectomy, and stenting, offer practical options in treating ileofemoral DVT.

Catheter-Directed Thrombolysis

In the early 1990s, Semba and Drake (12) first reported the feasibility of CDT for iliofemoral thrombosis as an alternative

TABLE 27.1 Catheter-Directed Thrombolysis for Deep Vein Thrombosis (Single-Center Case Studies)

Authors	N	Agent	Outcome (% lysis)	Hemorrhage (%)	
				Major	Minor
Molina et al.	12	UK	95	0	0
Comerota et al.	7	UK	71	0	0
Semba and Drake	27	UK	92	0	0
Bjarnason et al.	87	UK	86	6.9	14
Patel et al.	10	UK	100	0	0
Ouriel et al.	11	rPA	73	0	0
Castaneda et al.	25	rPA	92	4	4
Chang et al.	10	tPA	90	0	0
Horne et al.	10	tPA	90	0	30
Razavi et al.	36	TNK	83	2.7	8.3

UK, Urokinase; rPA, recombinant tissue plasminogen activator; tPA, tissue plasminogen activator; TNK, tenecteplase.

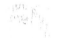

to systemic anticoagulation, systemic thrombolysis, or surgical venous thrombectomy.

CDT, or the delivery of thrombolytic agents directly into the thrombus, offers significant advantages over systemic therapy, which may fail to reach and penetrate an occluded venous segment. Because thrombolytic agents activate plasminogen within the thrombus, the delivery of the drug to that site enhances its effectiveness. CDT allows the delivery of higher concentrations of the drug to the treatment site, resulting in improved lysis rates, reduced duration of treatment, and reduced complications associated with exposure of the patient to systemic thrombolytic therapy. After successful CDT, it is hoped that preservation of valvular function and removal of the obstructing thrombus will result in a lower incidence of PTS. In addition, this endovascular approach allows for the detection and correction of any underlying venous obstructive lesions with balloon angioplasty and/or stents that should help reduce the rate of recurrent events.

Currently, no thrombolytic agents have been approved for CDT for the treatment of DVT by the US Food and Drug Administration (FDA). Therefore, the use of thrombolytic agents in CDT for venous thrombosis constitutes an "off-label" use. There are five thrombolytic agents available in the United States that can be used during CDT for venous thrombosis. Although the various agents have unique properties that might theoretically imply superiority of one over another, there is no peer-reviewed consensus on a superior or "best choice" agent for CDT for venous thrombosis. The literature on CDT for venous thrombosis has a paucity of prospective randomized comparative trials. Therefore, the choice of thrombolytic agent is usually individualized based on the physician's discretion.

The largest published experience with CDT has come from the National Venous Thrombolysis Registry (12) that included 287 patients treated with urokinase and monitored for up to 1 year. Overall, 71% of the patients were treated for iliofemoral DVT. Complete dissolution of thrombus was achieved in 31% of cases, and partial thrombus dissolution

was reported in an additional 52%. Primary patency at 1 year was 60%. Preservation of valvular competence was demonstrated in 72% of the patients with complete thrombolysis. Table 27.1 reviews the available clinical experience for CDT in the treatment of DVT.

The decision to perform CDT for lower extremity DVT must be individualized to each case based on a risk-benefit analysis. The CDT technique for lower extremity DVT is not standardized; however, the primary goal is to deliver the lytic agent directly into venous clot.

Access

The location of the lower extremity DVT and the patients' symptoms determine the specific venous access site chosen. For most cases of iliofemoral DVT, the ipsilateral popliteal vein is favored if the clinical situation allows. With the patient prone on the angiographic table, the venous access site should be accessed under ultrasound guidance with a small-gauge echogenic needle (e.g., 21-gauge micropuncture needle). Should the popliteal vein be thrombosed, the ipsilateral posterior tibial vein can be cannulated. After popliteal vein cannulation, a 5 Fr. short sheath is introduced, through which all subsequent catheters are exchanged. Next, a baseline venogram is obtained using the venous sheath, and then a combination of 0.035″ straight and curved glidewires is used to cross the occluded venous segment. After wire and then catheter traversal of the occluded venous segment, venography is repeated to confirm the intraluminal position of the catheter. The catheter is then exchanged for a 5 Fr. infusing coaxial system, consisting of a proximal multiside-hole infusion catheter (e.g., Cragg–McNamara, ev3) and a distal infusion wire (ProStream, ev3). The Cragg–McNamara infusion catheter comes in 4 and 5 Fr. sizes, and varies in both the entire length of the catheter (40 to 135 cm) and the active infusion length (5 to 50 cm). Similarly, the ProStream infusion wire varies in the entire length of the wire (145 to 175 cm) and the active infusion length (6 to 12 cm).

It is essential to position the system directly into the thrombus to maximize plasminogen activation at the site of obstruction.

Indications for placement of an IVC filter during CDT for lower extremity DVT fall within the same spectrum as that for routine prophylactic IVC filter placement (Table 29.1). The use of IVC filters during lower extremity venous thrombolysis has always been controversial because of the low incidence of complications that occur when lysis is performed without filter protection. With the advent of retrievable IVC filters, the authors' practice is to implement them routinely when performing CDT for iliofemoral DVT. This seems particularly reasonable for patients in whom the venogram defines a true "free-floating" iliac vein thrombus or for those with a documented pulmonary embolus and limited cardiopulmonary reserve for additional emboli.

Following placement of the infusion catheter/wire and/or IVC filter placement, the patient is monitored in the interventional recovery unit as the thrombolytic agent is infused. It is quite common, particularly with extensive thrombus burden, for the duration of therapy to exceed 24 hours. Follow-up venography should be performed every 12 hours to assess and/or reposition the infusion catheter and/or wire directly into any remaining thrombus. Weighing the risk versus the benefit of lytic therapy, the infusion should be continued until adequate lysis is achieved.

If venous patency has been restored and there is no underlying stenotic/occlusive lesion, thrombolysis is discontinued and anticoagulation is initiated. Hemodynamically significant lesions that are uncovered in the iliac veins should be considered for endovascular stenting, although the long-term benefits of venous stenting are not known. However, if left untreated, a significant iliac vein stenosis appears to be a significant risk of early rethrombosis (Fig. 27.1).

Use of metallic stents has been associated with good outcomes in central veins such as the IVC and iliac veins (13,14). If an underlying stenosis after successful CDT is believed to be secondary to iliac vein compression, stent deployment is required, because vein compression typically does not respond to stand-alone angioplasty. This iliac vein compression, or May–Thurner syndrome, typically involves extrinsic compression of the left common iliac vein by the crossing right common iliac artery, at the iliocaval junction (Fig. 27.2). Self-expanding stents are usually preferred because of their longitudinal flexibility and ability to conform to various venous configurations. In the iliac veins, we usually utilize self-expanding stents between 10 and 16 mm in diameter, with 12- to 14-mm-diameter stents being the most commonly used. Post-dilation angioplasty should be performed and should be gauged to the patient's perception of pain during balloon inflation. A significant limitation of using undersized stents and balloons is the high rate of restenosis and thrombotic reocclusion. Therefore, appropriate sizing of both stents and balloons is essential to achieve favorable outcomes. Care should be exercised to avoid stenting across the common femoral vein, particularly at the saphenofemoral junction.

Percutaneous Mechanical Thrombectomy (PMT)

Important limitations of CDT for lower extremity DVT include the time required to achieve lysis, need for intensive care monitoring, hemorrhagic risks, and cost. With these issues in mind, PMT is conceptually attractive because such a technique may result in a shorter time to vein patency, shorter length of

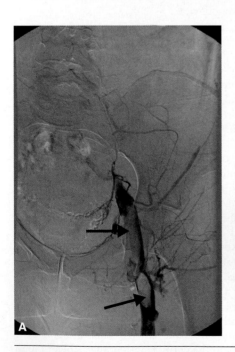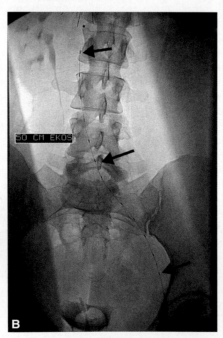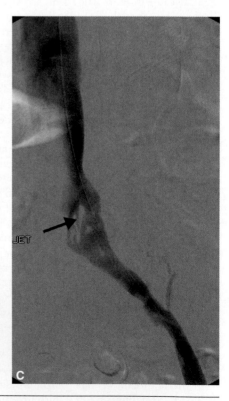

Figure 27.1 • Interventional management of thrombotic occlusion of left common femoral and iliac vein. **A:** 4 Fr. micropuncture sheath was placed in the left popliteal vein with the patient in the prone position. Diagnostic venography revealed a large occlusive thrombus left common femoral and iliac veins *(arrows)*. **B:** Placement of 50-cm EKOS catheter *(indicated by arrows)* from left common femoral vein to inferior vena cava (IVC). **C:** Small residual thrombus in left common iliac vein *(arrow)* following EKOS therapy and adjunctive AngioJet thrombectomy with expedior catheter.

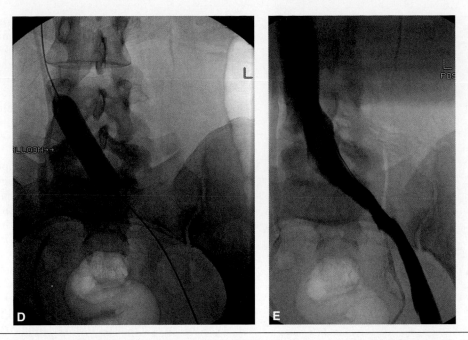

Figure 27.1 • *(Continued)* **D:** Angioplasty of left common iliac vein using 12 × 40 mm Cordis P3 balloon. **E:** Finishing venogram with no pressure gradient in left common iliac vein.

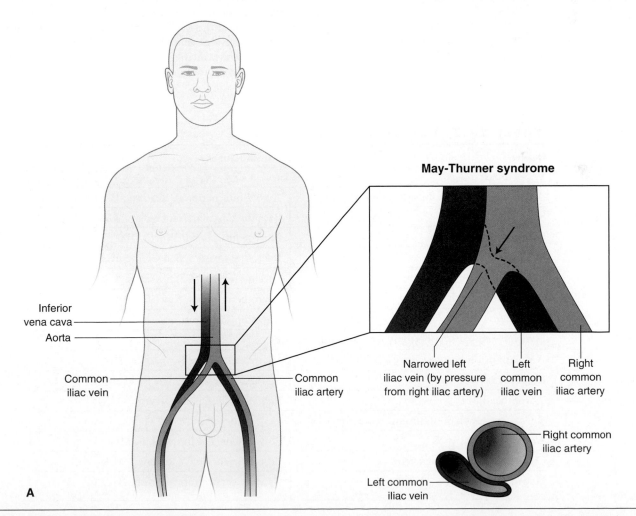

Figure 27.2 • **May–Thurner syndrome.** **A:** Schematic illustration of typical anatomic abnormality underlying May–Thurner syndrome where there is extrinsic compression of the left common iliac vein by the right common iliac artery. *(Continued)*

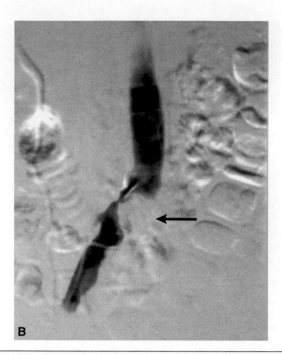

Figure 27.2 • *(Continued)* **B:** Venogram in patient with May–Thurner syndrome. Note that the patient is in the prone position. Severe narrowing of the proximal left common iliac vein indicated by *arrow*.

hospital stay, reduction in hemorrhagic risk, and overall cost savings because of reduced hospitalization and elimination or reduction in use of thrombolytic drugs.

From a mechanistic standpoint, PMT devices can be categorized as rotational, hydrodynamic, or ultrasound-facilitated. Table 27.2 outlines the currently available mechanical thrombectomy devices. In addition, with some of these PMT devices, simultaneous administration of thrombolytic therapy can be performed; this is known as pharmacomechanical thrombectomy.

Rotational thrombectomy devices employ a high-speed rotating basket or impeller to pulverize or fragment the thrombus. Pre-clinical evaluation of these devices focused on clot removal and assessment of potential valve injury. In one such study, the Arrow-Trerotola (Arrow) percutaneous thrombectomy device did not cause physiologically significant damage to veins 7 mm or larger in diameter (15). In several cases, small particles have been documented to embolize to the pulmonary circulation during rotational thrombectomy (15,16). Because these rotational thrombectomy devices have the potential of damaging the endothelial lining of the vein, the Bacchus Fino device (Bacchus Vascular) was designed to use a rotating Archimedes screw that is protected from vessel wall contact by a helically oriented nitinol framework. The screw fragments the thrombus, extracting much of it into a sheath through rotational motion.

Hydrodynamic or "rheolytic" recirculation devices have become a common treatment modality for lower extremity DVT. One of the PMT devices that has been shown to be effective in removal of acute thrombus is the AngioJet (Possis Medical) system. The principle of this device is based on the Venturi effect, whereby aspiration of adjacent thrombus is achieved by

TABLE 27.2 Current Mechanical Thrombectomy Devices

Device	Manufacturer
Wall contact devices	
Arrow percutaneous thrombectomy device	Arrow International, Reading, PA
Solera	Bacchus Vascular, Santa Clara, CA
Cleaner	Rex Medical, Forth Worth, TX
MTI-Castaneda Brush	Microtherapeutics, San Clemente, CA
Fino	Bacchus Vascular, Santa Clara, CA
Cragg Brush	Microtherapeutics, San Clemente, CA
Prolumen	Datascope, Maheah, NJ
Hydrodynamic thrombectomy fragmentation devices	
Amplatz thrombectomy device (ATD/Helix)	Microvena, White Bear Lake, MN
Rotarex catheter	Straub Medical, Wamgs, Switzerland
Thrombex PMT	Edwards Lifesciences, Irvine, CA
Rheolytic (flow-based) thrombectomy devices	
AngioJet	Possis Medical, Minneapolis, MN
Oasis Thrombectomy System	Boston Scientific, Watertown, MA
Hydrolyser	Cordis Corporation, Warren, NJ

the suction effect of rapidly flowing saline jets that are directed backward from the tip of the device to outflow channels in a coaxial fashion. This generates a vacuum force that draws the thrombus into the catheter (Fig. 14.6). One major advantage of this PMT device is that the thrombectomy catheter can be delivered through a 6 Fr. introducer sheath, which reduces access site complications. Devices based on "rheolytic" recirculation might possibly produce less valvular or endothelial damage than PMT devices that employ rotational thrombectomy, although these two mechanisms of thrombus removal have not been directly compared. Examples of other "rheolytic" recirculation devices include the Hydrolyser (Cordis Corporation) and the Oasis Thrombectomy System (Boston Scientific). The Hydrolyser system uses a conventional contrast power injector to inject saline solution through an injection lumen. The resultant pressure reduction at the nozzle tip creates a 360-degree vortex that fragments and aspirates thrombus into an exhaust lumen. The thrombotic material is then discharged through the exhaust lumen into a collection bag. The Oasis Thrombectomy System operates similarly to the AngioJet, using a Venturi effect with thrombus fragmentation. However, the AngioJet system now has a "large vessel" (DVX) catheter that has the ability to extract a large amount of thrombus.

Despite great advances in PMT technologies, complete thrombus resolution rarely occurs, so adjunctive thrombolytic therapy is often required. In an effort to improve thrombus resolution, an ultrasound-based infusion system, the EkoSonic Endovascular System (EKOS Corporation), was developed. The EKOS System combines high-frequency, low-power ultrasound with simultaneous CDT to accelerate clot dissolution. The exposure of thrombus to non-fragmenting ultrasound has no lytic effect on its own. However, the combination of directed ultrasound with local lytic infusion accelerates the thrombolytic process (17). The mechanism for accelerated thrombolysis is that the delivery of high-frequency, low-power ultrasound loosens the fibrin matrix to increase clot permeability and allow the thrombolytic agent reach deep into the thrombus for better drug distribution. In addition, the ultrasound energy penetrates venous valves and facilitates clearing of thrombus associated with them.

The EKOS System consists of a 5.2 Fr., multi-lumen drug delivery catheter with one central lumen and three separate infusion ports (Fig. 27.3). Each catheter has a matched ultrasound core wire that is placed in the central lumen that delivers the ultrasound energy evenly along the entire infusion pathway. After the catheter is positioned in the thrombus, an infusion

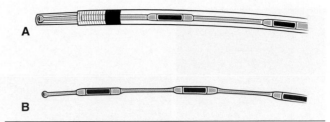

Figure 27.3 • EkoSonic Endovascular System. A: Drug delivery catheter (DDC). B: Ultrasound core catheter that is delivered through the central lumen of the DDC.

of lytic agent is started, along with saline to serve as a coolant. Ultrasound is then started and delivered simultaneously with the lytic agent infusion.

Another ultrasound-based technology, the OmniSonics Resolution Endovascular System (OmniSonics Medical Technologies), is based on ultrasound ablation of thrombus. Currently, ultrasound technology is routinely used for disintegration of renal and urethral calculi, aortic valve decalcification, and cataract phacoemulsion procedures. In regard to thrombus dissolution, there are many hypotheses regarding the mode of action of ultrasonic energy. In the case of intravascular ultrasound delivery catheters, cavitation, microstreaming, and mechanical effects are the primary modes of action of thrombolysis (18).

The OmniSonics Resolution Endovascular System utilizes OmniWave Technology, which enables the creation of a standing transverse wave on the distal section of a small profile wire (Fig. 27.4) (19). The transverse wave creates ultrasonic energy circumferentially around the wire using very low power. The proprietary wire design converts the longitudinal motion to traverse motion in the treatment zone, producing an extended region of ultrasonic activation. The system has a pump that irrigates fluid down the catheter to ensure the system does not produce a temperature greater than 41°C. The Resolution Endovascular System is currently FDA approved for declotting hemodialysis grafts. It is being tested in large animal models in iliofemoral arteries and veins.

Pharmacomechanical thrombectomy, or the simultaneous administration of thrombolytics during PMT, represents true "combination therapy." This form of PMT has been reported with the AngioJet (Possis Medical) and the Trellis (Bacchus Vascular) (Fig. 27.5) devices.

In a small series, Uppot et al. (20) reported a technique of mixing the thrombolytic drug in the AngioJet saline infusion

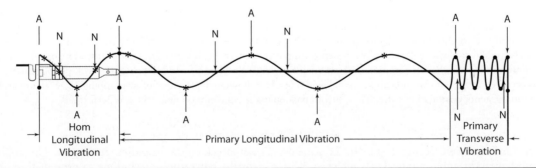

Figure 27.4 • OmniSonics OmniWave technology enables the creation of a standing transverse wave on the distal section of a small profile wire. This produces an extended region of ultrasonic activation.

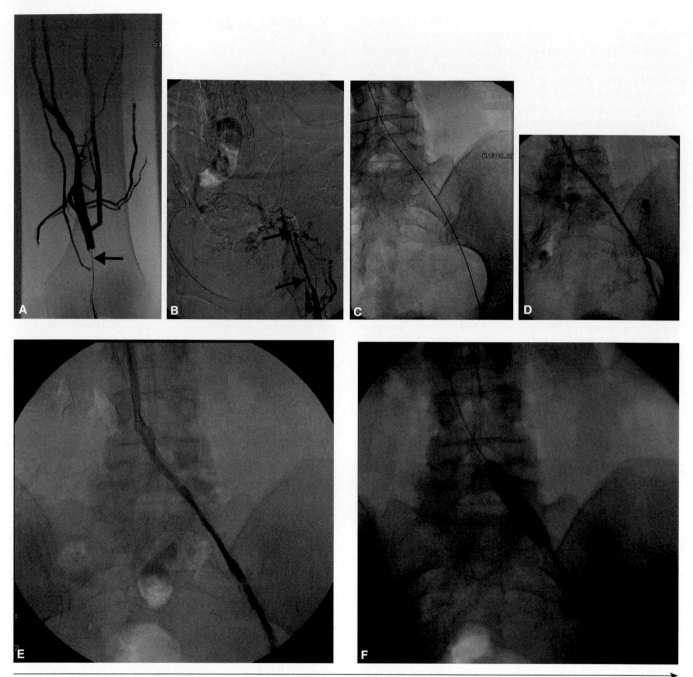

Figure 27.5 • Interventional treatment of left ileofemoral deep venous thrombosis. A 46-year-old female presented with an extensive left-sided ileofemoral deep venous thrombosis 10 weeks prior. She had persistent left lower extremity pain and swelling with prolonged standing, and presented for interventional therapy. **A:** The patient was placed prone on the angiographic table. Using ultrasound guidance, a 4 Fr. micropuncture sheath *(arrow)* was inserted into the left popliteal vein. **B:** Venography from the left popliteal vein demonstrates extensive thrombotic occlusion of the left common and external iliac veins *(arrows)*. **C:** Utilizing an Expeditor AngioJet catheter, a total of 5 U of retavase was delivered via "pulse spray" to the left common and external iliac veins. **D:** After a 10-minute dwell period, venography now shows venous outflow via the left common and external iliac veins. **E:** After a further 20-minute dwell period, further resolution of thrombosis has occurred in the left common and external iliac veins. **F:** Following deployment of overlapping 12 × 60 mm and 12 × 30 mm self-expanding nitinol stents, postdilation with a 12 × 40 mm balloon to the left common iliac vein was performed.

bag for direct administration during PMT. In 24 patients, complete or substantial thrombus removal was achieved. With more experience, this technique has been refined to develop the "power pulse technique." This technique involves placement of a stopcock on the AngioJet return port. The stopcock is closed for the power pulse technique to prevent thrombus and lytic drug aspiration. With the outflow port occluded, the AngioJet catheter effectively becomes a one-way infusion system with

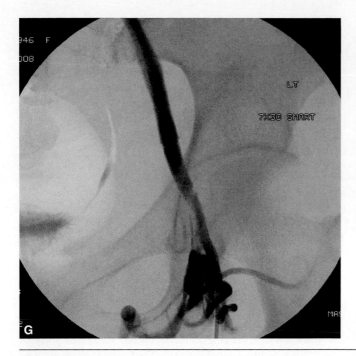
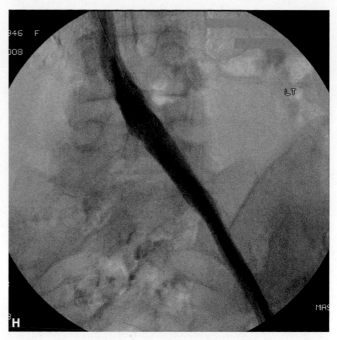

Figure 27.5 • *(Continued)* **G:** Completion venogram of the left external iliac vein. **H:** Completion venogram of the left common iliac vein. Post-procedure: The patient was placed on IV unfractionated heparin 1 hour after sheath removal. The left lower extremity swelling was completely resolved within 24 hours, and the patient was discharged with an INR of 2.7. Compression stockings were prescribed, and the patient has continued to do well post-procedure.

dilute lytic agent pulsed into the clot. The newest generation AngioJet console does have a "pulse-spray" option obviating the need for a stopcock on the return port. After delivery of the lytic agent throughout the thrombus, a period of up to 30 to 45 minutes is allowed to elapse, permitting time for the clot to lyse. After this period, the AngioJet is activated in a normal fashion, with the outflow port open to allow aspiration of thrombus.

The Bacchus Trellis (Bacchus Vascular) consists of a catheter with proximal and distal occlusion balloons (Fig. 14.10), and a sheath designed to aspirate contents between the balloons. A sinusoidal nitinol wire placed within the catheter is rotated to mix the blood between the balloons. The Trellis device, which combines a high concentration of thrombolytic medication with mechanical disruption of thrombus, has been used with success to treat patients with DVT (21). The occlusive balloons limit leakage of thrombolytic agent into the systemic circulation, potentially reducing the risk of bleeding complications, whereas the central balloon is intended to reduce embolization of particulate matter to the pulmonary circulation.

These exciting combination strategies continue to be developed and investigated, and with further follow-up will be better defined for their efficacy and role in PMT for DVT.

POSTPROCEDURE MANAGEMENT

After completion of the venous intervention, the venous access sheath is removed in the post-intervention unit as soon as the clinical decision to stop thrombolysis is made. With well-trained staff, and meticulous access site management, the rate of access site complications has been exceedingly low in our venous practice (i.e., less than 2% even without interrupting anti-coagulation). If a sheath larger than 6 Fr. is used for the procedure, we do hold heparin for 1 hour before sheath removal.

After sheath removal, anti-coagulation with unfractionated heparin is used to achieve an activated partial thromboplastin time of 1.5 to 2.5 times control to bridge patients until the optimal INR is achieved using warfarin. The optimal INR and duration of warfarin anti-coagulation depend on the location and etiology of the DVT, and the individual clinical situation (11).

Patients' symptoms and leg swelling typically subside within 24 hours after restoring flow and allowing for 24 hours of leg elevation. Patients who do not experience relief of symptoms and resolution of leg swelling should be restudied for any evidence of early rethrombosis and need for repeat intervention. Follow-up should include a work-up for hypercoaguable conditions and duplex ultrasound at 3, 6, and 12 months. We routinely follow patients on an annual basis for 3 to 5 years or as symptoms develop.

A critical part of post-procedure care at home is the use of graduated compression stockings that has been shown to reduce the risk of PTS in this high-risk population of patients (22).

References

1. Brotman DJ, Jaffer AK. Prevention of venous thromboembolism in the geriatric patient. *Cardiol Clin*. 2008;26:221–234.
2. Nair DG, Dodson TF. Surgical treatment of carotid and peripheral vascular disease. In: Foster V, O'Rourke RA, Walsh RA, et al., eds. *Hurst's The Heart*. 12th ed. China: McGraw-Hill; 2008:2392–2395.

3. Silver M, Ansel G. Venous intervention. In: Topol EJ, ed. *Textbook of Interventional Cardiology*. 5th ed. Philadelphia: Saunders; 2007:795–812.

4. Meignan M, Rosso J, Gauthier H, et al. Systematic lung scans reveal a high frequency of silent pulmonary embolism in patients with proximal DVT. *Arch Intern Med*. 2000;160:145–146.

5. Bulger CM, Jacobs C, Patel NH. Epidemiology of acute deep vein thrombosis. *Tech Vasc Interv Radiol*. 2004;7:50–54.

6. Ginsberg JS. Management of venous thromboembolism. *N Engl J Med*. 1996;335:1816–1828.

7. Goldhaber SZ. Pulmonary embolism. In: Braunwald E, Lippy P, Bonow R, et al., eds. *Braunwald's Heart Disease: A Textbook of Cardiovascular Medicine*. 8th ed. Philadelphia, PA: Saunders; 2008:1863–1881.

8. Bates SM, Ginsberg JS. Treatment of deep-vein thrombosis. *N Engl J Med*. 2004;351:268–277.

9. Tapson VF. Acute pulmonary embolism. *N Engl J Med*. 2008; 358:1037–1052.

10. Zierler BK. Ultrasonography and diagnosis of venous thromboembolism. *Circulation*. 2004;109(suppl 1):I-9–I-14.

11. Kearon C, Kahn SR, Agnelli G, et al. Antithrombotic therapy for venous thromboembolic disease: American College of Chest Physicians evidence-based clinical practice guidelines, 8th ed. *Chest*. 2008;133(suppl 6):454S–545S.

12. Semba CP, Drake M. Iliofemoral deep vein thrombosis: aggressive therapy using catheter-directed thrombolysis. *Radiology*. 1994;191:487–494.

13. O'Sullivan GO, Semba CP, Bittner CA. Endovascular management of iliac vein compression (May–Thurner) syndrome. *J Vasc Interv Radiol*. 2000;11:823–826.

14. Razavi M, Hansch E, Kee S. Endovascular treatment of chronically occluded inferior vena cava. *Radiology*. 2000;214:133–138.

15. McClennan G, Trerotola S, Davidson D, et al. The effects of a mechanical thrombolytic device on normal canine vein valves. *J Vasc Interv Radiol*. 2001;12:89–94.

16. Delomez M, Beregi JP, Willoteaux S, et al. Mechanical thrombectomy in patients with deep venous thrombosis. *Cardiovasc Intervent Radiol*. 2001;24:42–48.

17. Braaten JV, Goss RA, Francis CW. Ultrasound reversibly disaggregates fibrin fibers. *Thromb Haemost*. 1997;78:1063–1068.

18. Altar S, Rosenschein U. Perspectives on the role of ultrasonic devices in thrombolysis. *J Thromb Thrombolysis*. 2004;2:107–114.

19. Hallisey MJ. Ultrasonic energy treatment of deep vein thrombosis. *J Endovasc Today*. 2006;4:80–82.

20. Uppot RN, Garcia MJ, Roe C, et al. Management of deep venous thrombosis using the AngioJet rheolytic thrombectomy system. *J Vasc Interv Radiol*. 2002;13(S):S116.

21. Ramaiah V, Del Santo PB, Rodriguez-Lopez JA, et al. Trellis thrombectomy system for the treatment of iliofemoral deep venous thrombosis. *J Endovasc Ther*. 2003;10:585–589.

22. Brandjes DP, Buller HR, Heijboer H. Randomized trial of effect of compression stockings in patients with symptomatic proximal vein thrombosis. *Lancet*. 1997;349:759–762.

CHAPTER 28

Management of Hemodialysis Access

Rajan K. Gupta

In 2006, approximately 350,000 patients were managed on dialysis programs in the United States alone, and this number is estimated to increase to 530,000 by 2020 (1,2). Almost 93% of these individuals are managed with hemodialysis (1,2). This has created an enormous cost and resource burden on the health care system. A large component of care of the dialysis-dependent patient involves the creation and maintenance of appropriate access for adequate hemodialysis. In the past several decades, interventional practitioners have assumed an increasingly important role in the evaluation and treatment of access dysfunction. Percutaneous intervention is now generally accepted as first-line treatment for the majority of access management.

Although this chapter focuses on the interventional practice of dialysis access management, the importance of a team approach to these patients cannot be overemphasized. Dialysis patients are complex and require coordination between multiple services including nephrologists, surgeons, interventionalists, and dialysis centers. Local expertise in various treatment modalities plays an important role in selection of the most appropriate management strategy. Multidisciplinary conferences and close communication between services that care for dialysis patients will lead to better patient outcomes (3).

LONG-TERM HEMODIALYSIS ACCESS

The two main types of long-term hemodialysis access are native fistulas and synthetic dialysis grafts (Fig. 28.1). These are surgically created connections between arteries and veins that create a long-term, high-flow conduit to allow for hemodialysis. The National Kidney Foundation's Kidney Disease Outcome Quality Initiative (NKF-KDOQI) guidelines have recommended that fistulae be the primary access created in hemodialysis patients given their higher long-term patency, lower risks of infection, and lower cost of maintenance (4). Although fistula placement is increasing in frequency in the United States, dialysis grafts remain the most common long-term access.

Creation of dialysis access is performed first in the upper extremities, beginning in the non-dominant arm distally near the wrist and progressing more centrally to the upper arm to preserve the useable "venous capital" required for the creation of long-term access. When a single arm is exhausted of sites, the opposite arm is utilized in a similar fashion. When upper extremity sites for potential access have been exhausted, the lower extremities are utilized, although there is a greater risk of infection and lower long-term patency.

The most common fistula is the Brescia–Cimino fistula, which is an end-to-side anastomosis of the cephalic vein with the radial artery at the level of the wrist. A brachiocephalic fistula is the next most common fistula access, which is an end-to-side anastomosis of the cephalic vein to the brachial artery at the level of the elbow. Creation of these types of fistulae requires mobilization of a short venous segment, and most side branches of the normal venous anatomy are left intact. This is in contrast with transposed fistulae where a long segment of vein is exposed, the side branches are ligated, and the vein may be superficialized in a staged procedure for ease of cannulation. Fistulae need a period of time, typically 6 to 12 weeks, to dilate and mature before they can be used for hemodialysis. A significant number of fistulae (20% to 50%) fail to mature and may need further interventional evaluation and management. Percutaneous interventions on the arterial anastomosis should not be performed for at least 4 weeks due to the risk of perforating the surgical anastomosis.

Synthetic grafts are most commonly created out of polytetrafluoroethylene (PTFE) and may be either looped or straight in configuration. Looped grafts are preferred. Grafts tend to have lower patency rates, although they can be used within 2 weeks of creation for dialysis. The most common forearm graft is a loop graft from the brachial artery to the brachial vein. When upper extremity access has been exhausted, grafts in the thigh are most often constructed from the common femoral artery to the common femoral vein in a loop configuration. Grafts frequently develop stenosis at the graft-venous anastomosis. They tend to be technically easier to declot as they are a single conduit without side branches.

EVALUATION OF SHUNT DYSFUNCTION

The primary goal of monitoring programs is to identify possible stenoses that may be contributing to inadequate dialysis and predispose to access thrombosis (5). Early detection of access dysfunction can decrease patient morbidity associated with poor dialysis, prevent thrombosis, avoid the need for temporary access, and allow for new access planning in a more timely fashion.

Many parameters are monitored by a dialysis center and include static and dynamic pressures, flow rates, and recirculation rates (4,5). Additionally, clinical factors such as increased bleeding time or an abnormal bruit or thrill may raise suspicion of access dysfunction (4,5).

Access History

The first step in evaluation and treatment of any patient referred for percutaneous evaluation is to review the access

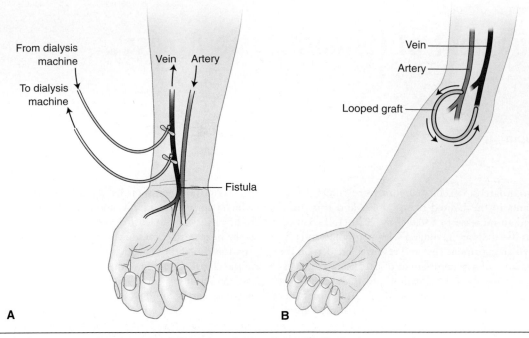

Figure 28.1 • Schematic representation of the two primary hemodialysis access types.   **A:** Arteriovenous fistula between radial artery and cephalic vein (i.e., Brescia-Cimino fistula). **B:** Arteriovenous graft.

history. This includes a combination of review of the medical record and a conversation with the patient. Review of the relevant operative report, previous venography, and prior percutaneous interventions will provide a great deal of important information. Particularly important is the age of the access, size of a graft, previous areas of stenosis, size and type of previous balloons used, and durability of the previous intervention. This information can also direct the physical exam and help guide the best site to access for diagnosis and therapy.

Physical Exam

All physicians performing interventions on dialysis access should be familiar with the basic physical exam of hemodialysis access. This will help predict the site of stenosis, direct the location of access for evaluation and therapy, and allow the operator to assess for changes after therapy. The anastomosis can be easily located by finding the surgical scar. Normally, a fistula has a soft, easily compressible pulse, a continuous thrill and low pitched bruit at the arterial anastomosis (6). An AV graft tends to be less compressible and has a thrill evident along a broader area (6,7). With a venous stenosis, the proximal pulse becomes firm with a water-hammer quality, often causing enlargement of a fistula and loss of the thrill (5,6). Central to a stenosis (i.e., on the venous side), there may be a caliber change in a fistula, a systolic predominant thrill and high-pitched bruit at the point of stenosis, and a diminished distal pulse (5,6).

Central obstruction can manifest as arm swelling or with dilated chest wall collaterals. Pseudoaneurysms are easily visualized and palpated. Skin breakdown over aneurysm sites is also important to note as it may signify impeding rupture or infection.

With intervention, it is important to know which way venous outflow is directed. This is obvious with AV fistulae, but may not be obvious with a looped AV graft. Grafts are typically constructed with the arterial limb medially and the vzenous limb laterally, although anatomy may dictate that this is reversed in certain patients. Patients are often aware of which limb is arterial and asking the patient is helpful. Compression of the mid-graft will also define the direction of flow, as pulsation should only be subsequently felt in the arterial limb (6). With experience, physical exam can be accomplished within several minutes, often during the consent process.

Angiographic Evaluation

Angiographic evaluation of dialysis access is critical to diagnosis and treatment. The entire circuit from the arterial anastomosis through the right atrium should be evaluated. Most evaluations can be performed via the graft or fistula safely without the need for arterial puncture. Exceptions include evaluation of suspected steal syndrome, evaluation of the nonmaturing fistula, and evaluation of high-grade anastomotic stenoses that cannot be crossed from the venous side. In these cases, brachial arterial puncture may be very helpful.

Many clues can direct the operator to the most appropriate site for the initial puncture to avoid multiple sites of access. The first clue is the indication for the intervention. High venous pressure and increased bleeding time suggest a venous stenosis, while low flow or high recirculation rates can imply either arterial or venous problems. Physical exam and real-time evaluation of the access with sonography can also reliably detect stenotic or thrombosed segments. Additionally, review of the medical record can demonstrate areas of previous stenosis, which are likely to recur.

In the absence of other clues, access should be made in the fistula/graft near the arterial anastomosis directed to venous outflow, as the majority of stenoses occur in the venous circuit. Buttonhole access points (i.e., specific points that are constant

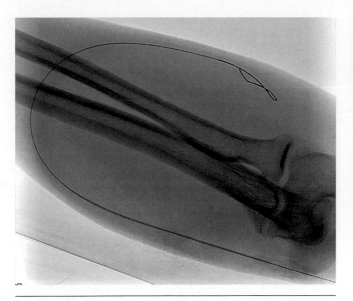

Figure 28.2 • Typical micropuncture of hemodialysis access visualized under fluoroscopy. The wire follows the expected course of the access and passes smoothly.

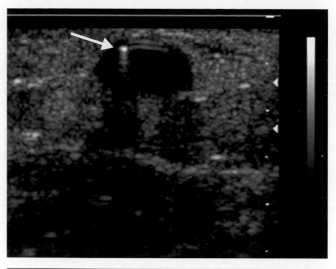

Figure 28.3 • Ultrasound guidance of hemodialysis access. Ultrasound easily demonstrates that access wire (*white arrow*) is appropriately within the vessel target.

and used to provide access for dialysis) should be avoided as percutaneous intervention at or near these sites may compromise future use. Pseudoaneurysms should also be avoided as access at these sites may promote expansion and eventual perforation. In the loop graft, access can be made near the graft apex directed to venous outflow to maintain a straight path for the treatment of lesions centrally.

Micropuncture access with manual palpation or ultrasound guidance is recommended, as it is the least traumatic. For graft access, trapping the graft between two fingers during access is helpful. The fibrotic nature of grafts will yield a popping sensation as the needle penetrates the graft and pulsatile flow is observed. Access of fistulae is similar, although it may be more difficult if the fistula is poorly developed or there is low flow. Use of upper arm tourniquets and real-time ultrasound is particularly useful. The passage of the guidewire should be observed with fluoroscopy to ensure passage of the wire within the access (Fig. 28.2). Appropriately adjusting the patient under the image intensifier prior to access is advisable to prevent dislodging the needle during patient movement. Typically, the wire will pass easily without resistance and follow the expected course of the access. Any resistance should prompt evaluation of possible extravascular placement. This is easily accomplished with ultrasound (Fig. 28.3) and fluoroscopic evaluation.

Diagnostic venography can then be performed through the 5-Fr. micropuncture transitional dilator used for access. Use of extension tubing and a one-way stopcock can decrease operator exposure during filming. The entire access circuit should be evaluated from the arterial anastamosis to the right atrium. The presence of collaterals is an important clue to a hemodynamically significant stenosis. Visualization of the arterial anastomosis can be accomplished by occlusion of the outflow during injection of contrast so that contrast refluxes across the anastamosis. This can be performed by manual compression of the outflow or during balloon angioplasty of a venous stenosis by injection of the sheath side port (Fig. 28.4).

The latter method decreases the radiation dose to the operator. Multiple obliquities are often needed to define the arterial anastomosis optimally. If the initial access is unacceptable for treatment, a new access is made in a similar fashion.

TREATMENT OF STENOSIS OF AV GRAFT OR MATURE AV FISTULA

Treatment of an angiographic stenosis in a graft or mature fistula is indicated when there is greater than 50% angiographic narrowing and some associated clinical or physiologic abnormality (low flow, elevated venous pressure, increased bleeding time, bruit, etc.) (4). The presence of venous collaterals is an important clue to hemodynamic significance and their resolution after successful angioplasty is further evidence that treatment is successful. Treatment is generally defined as successful if there is less than 30% residual stenosis.

After a diagnostic angiogram has been performed, a 6-Fr. sheath is placed, which will accommodate the majority of balloon sizes for the arm veins. The stenosis is crossed with an angled catheter and hydrophilic wire, utilizing roadmap technique if the stenosis is tight. The hydrophilic wire is replaced with a steel wire for the treatment as this simplifies exchanges and minimizes the risk of losing access. It is important to ensure that there is an adequate amount of wire purchase in the central vasculature to maintain access across the stenosis during device exchanges in case rupture occurs. The balloon diameter is typically mildly oversized to the adjacent normal vein by 10% to 15%. In the case of a graft, the balloon is sized to the graft diameter or oversized by 1 mm.

Balloon Selection

It is generally accepted that hemodialysis-related venous stenoses are resistant to balloon dilation. Many stenoses will respond to moderate-pressure (15 atm) angioplasty, although a subset of

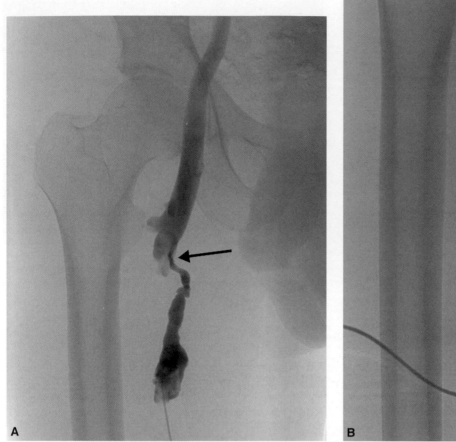

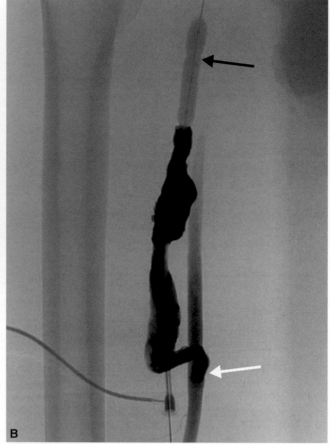

Figure 28.4 • Evaluation of the arterial anastomosis during balloon treatment of venous stenosis in a patient with a prior right thigh transposition fistula. **A:** A right thigh transposition fistula venogram demonstrates a high-grade venous anastomotic stricture *(black arrow)*. **B:** During balloon inflation *(black arrow)*, a reflux venogram is performed through the sheath side port to demonstrate the arterial anastomosis *(white arrow)*.

stenoses will require high pressures (30 atm). A routinely used high-pressure balloon is the Conquest balloon (Bard Vascular, Tempe, AZ). Trerotola et al. found that almost 20% of stenoses in native fistulae and 10% of stenoses in grafts required pressures greater than 20 atm (8). Given the greater cost of high-pressure balloons, the choice of the initial balloon is left to the operator, although in the face of recurrent stenosis, a high-pressure balloon may be a better initial choice. Typically, 4-cm-long balloons are used, although 2-cm-long balloons are helpful in areas of tortuosity, such as at the arterial anastomosis. Given the pressures required, an inflation device with a pressure gauge is mandatory. The balloon should be centered over the lesion and inflated under fluoroscopic guidance and the inflation pressure titrated to the patient's response. Discomfort, pressure, and pain are common and dilation should be accompanied by conscious sedation. If the patient experiences significant pain, inflation should be stopped temporarily as this may indicate rupture. Gauging the patient's pain response comes with experience, and frequent intermittent venography is recommended for dilation in the patient with significant pain. The stenosis will appear as a waist in the balloon and will slowly efface with increasing pressure. Watermelon seeding, where the balloon tends to push forward or backward on the wire, is common and should be guarded against. Inattention to this phenomenon may increase the risk

of rupture. Once the balloon is at profile, it is typically safe to increase the pressure to the rated maximum burst pressure without an increase in the rupture rate or significantly changing the patient's perceived pain. Inflations of 60 to 120 seconds are typically performed, although several prolonged inflations of up to 5 minutes may be necessary to dilate resistant stenoses. During this inflation period, it is common to see the pressure on the inflation gauge drop as the elastic stenosis is being dilated. Maintaining inflation to the maximal burst pressure may be helpful to dilate resistant stenoses during these episodes of prolonged inflation. When the dilation is complete, the balloon is completely deflated by fluoroscopy and removed from the sheath. The balloon is left on the wire in case extravasation is detected and rapid balloon occlusion is required. Follow-up venography is performed through the sheath side port and assessment of success is judged by degree of residual stenosis and resolution of collateral veins. Treatment is generally defined as successful if there is less than 30% residual stenosis associated with a reduction of collateral filling (4). If there is a persistent narrowing that requires treatment, two to three prolonged additional inflations with the same balloon or changing to a higher-pressure balloon is recommended.

Elastic stenoses are defined as stenoses that persist after the waist has been completely effaced with balloon angioplasty. With appropriate oversizing (10% to 15%), use of high-pressure balloons (up to 30 atm), and prolonged inflation (2 to 5 minutes), resistant stenoses are rare. In these cases, cutting balloons or stents may be utilized.

Cutting Balloon Angioplasty

Cutting balloons were first introduced in 1991. Vorwerk first described their use in the venous circulation in 1995 (9). Peripheral cutting balloons (Boston Scientific, San Diego, CA) have four small linear blades infolded into the balloon that create controlled incisions on the vascular wall (9). This differs from the irregular intimal injury caused by standard angioplasty. The working height of the blades when the balloon is fully expanded is only 0.007". The controlled intimal injury created by cutting balloons allows for dilation of stenoses at lower atmospheric pressures and has been shown to reduce the inflammatory response in the vascular wall. This has been theorized to reduce intimal hyperplasia and potentially reduce the risk of restenosis.

The literature regarding cutting balloon angioplasty for dialysis access is sparse. Most studies are retrospective and many are confounded by the concurrent use of standard balloon angioplasty either before or after the use of cutting balloons. The only prospective study by Vesely and Siegel compared primary cutting balloon angioplasty (without concurrent standard percutaneous transluminal angioplasty (PTA)) to standard balloon angioplasty in hemodialysis grafts and found no significant differences in 6-month patency (10). The cutting balloon, therefore, does not seem to improve patency when all stenoses in grafts are considered. However, a study by Guiu et al. suggests that primary cutting balloon angioplasty may have improved patency in long segment stenoses in fistulae (>2 cm), although the patient population in this study was small and the data have not been confirmed in larger prospective series (11).

Given their increased cost and a lack of compelling data, cutting balloons cannot be routinely recommended as first-line treatment for most stenoses. They may, however, be most effective for treating long segment stenoses in fistulae and for treating elastic stenoses resistant to standard balloon angioplasty.

It is important to note that the technique of using cutting balloons differs from standard PTA in several ways. First, care must be taken not to grasp the balloon itself during insertion and withdrawal, as the operator may injure themselves on the blades. Cutting balloons are used over a 018" wire system, and 5 to 8 mm diameter sizes are deliverable through a 7-Fr. sheath. Nominal inflation pressure is 6 atm, and the burst pressure is 10 atm. Given a theoretically higher risk of perforation, these balloons should not be oversized by more than 10%. Cutting balloons are inflated and deflated at a much slower rate than standard balloons, with the goal of allowing appropriate unfolding (during inflation) and refolding (during deflation) of the blades. When the balloon is brought to profile, it does not need to be brought to maximal pressure as the scoring of the vessel surface has already occurred. The balloon is maximally deflated and under negative pressure prior to sheath withdrawal, as the sheath may be cut if appropriate care is not taken. In general, pain with cutting balloon angioplasty is minimally reduced compared to standard PTA.

Specific Areas of Stenosis

Graft-Vein Anastamosis

AV grafts most commonly develop stenoses at the graft-vein anastomosis, although more central venous stenoses are also common. AV grafts are typically tubular and commonly measure 6 mm in diameter, although tapered grafts are used in many centers and can taper in diameter from 7 to 4 mm. Review of the operative note is helpful. Typically, it is best to size the balloon to the graft size or oversize it by 1 mm.

Juxta-Anastomotic Stenosis

Stenosis in the proximal several centimeters of a fistula is common and thought to be related to turbulent flow and some element of ischemia despite excellent surgical technique. These are known as juxta-anastomotic strictures (Figs. 28.5 and 28.6) and may be a common cause of failure of a fistula to mature.

Figure 28.5 • Juxta-anastomotic stricture. **A:** A juxta-anastomotic stricture *(black arrow)* is present in an upper arm fistula. The venous collaterals are due to compression of the venous outflow and not from an underlying stenosis. **B:** The balloon waist *(black arrow)* is demonstrated during dilation. **C:** Post-angioplasty, there is complete resolution of the stenosis.

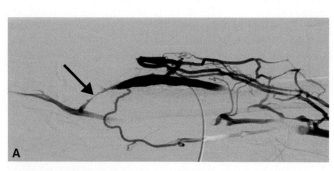

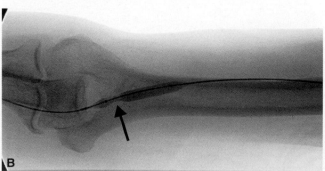

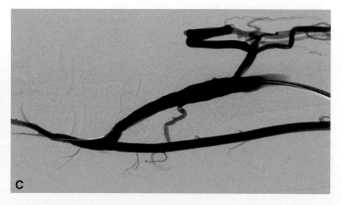

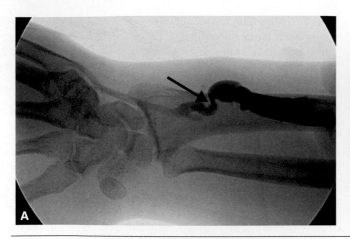
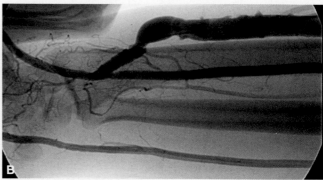

Figure 28.6 • Juxta-anastomotic stricture. **A:** A juxta-anastomotic stricture *(black arrow)* is present in a Brescia–Cimino fistula. **B:** Post-angioplasty, there is near complete resolution of the stenosis.

Balloon angioplasty remains the primary treatment modality, although surgical revision with a neoanastomosis or jump graft provides a good alternative with excellent patency.

Cephalic Arch Stenosis

Brachiocephalic upper arm fistulae tend to have worse patency compared to radiocephalic fistulae. A significant component of this is felt to be due to the higher prevalence of cephalic arch stenosis (Fig. 28.7), which is present in an estimated 40% to 55% of brachiocephalic fistulae versus 2% to 7% of radiocephalic fistulae (12,13). Cephalic arch stenosis is thought to be caused by several factors including higher turbulent flow and altered shear stress related to the mechanics of the curve of the cephalic arch, external compression of the clavicopectoral and pectoralis facia, and a high number of venous valves (12,13). The shorter segment of venous capacitance present in upper arm fistulae is thought to make cephalic stenosis more common in upper arm fistulae. Additionally, these lesions have a higher reported rupture rate (6% to 15%) and have lower primary patency rates at 1 year (20%) (12,13). No literature has yet compared cutting balloon angioplasty with standard balloon angioplasty in the treatment of cephalic stenoses. In the case of rupture, careful stent placement is required to prevent future

compromise of the subclavian vein (Fig. 28.8). It is prudent to ensure that a properly sized covered stent is available prior to treatment.

Central Venous Stenosis

Central venous stenosis is a well-recognized problem in the dialysis population. It is associated with central venous catheter use (particularly subclavian lines and left internal jugular vein lines—Fig. 28.9), pacemaker wires (Fig. 28.10), and previous peripherally inserted center catheter (PICC) placement. The first-line therapy is endovascular as this area is difficult to surgically access. It is increasingly recognized that percutaneous balloon angioplasty and primary stent placement have similar patency rates and both require frequent reintervention to maintain patency. Balloon angioplasty (Fig. 28.11) is therefore recommended as first-line therapy. In fact, a retrospective study by Levit et al. demonstrated that asymptomatic stenoses that undergo treatment may progress more rapidly than those that are left untreated (14). For these reasons, central venous stenoses should only be treated in asymptomatic patients if they are deemed to be the culprit lesion for shunt dysfunction. For instance, if there is a significant upper arm stenosis and an additional central venous stenosis, the upper arm stenosis should be

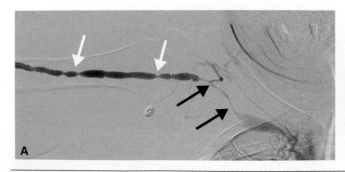
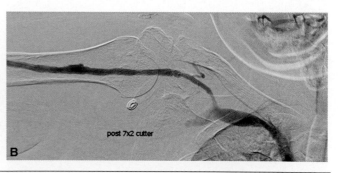

Figure 28.7 • Cephalic arch stenosis. **A:** Long-segment (>2 cm) stenosis of cephalic arch *(black arrows)*. Multiple additional short segment venous stenoses *(white arrows)* are present in the cephalic vein. **B:** Technical success after treatment with a peripheral cutting balloon (Boston Scientific). A cutting balloon was chosen due to the presence of a long segment stenosis in the fistula.

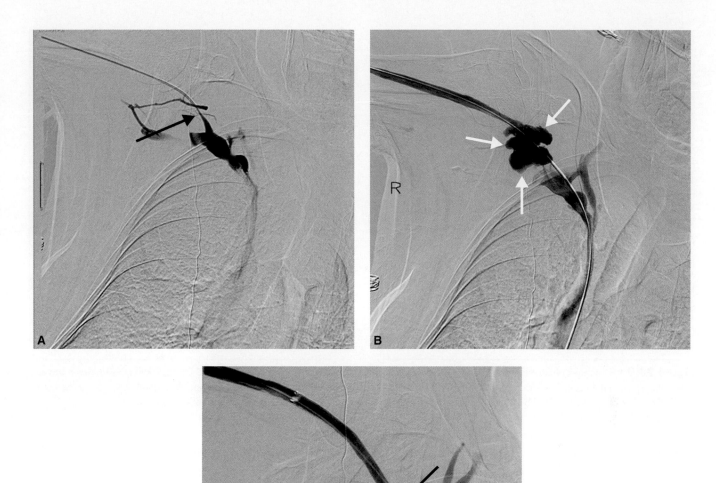

Figure 28.8 • Rupture of cephalic arch during treatment of stenosis. **A:** High-grade cephalic arch stenosis *(black arrow)*. **B:** Obvious extravasation secondary to rupture after balloon angioplasty. **C:** Venogram following placement of Fluency covered stent graft (Bard). Note the careful distal positioning of the stent to prevent compromise of the axillary venous flow (distal margin of stent indicted by *black arrow*).

treated first and the central stenosis should only be treated if low dialysis flow or symptoms such as upper extremity edema persist. If there is a frequently recurring stenosis (i.e., more than two interventions in 3 months), stent placement (Figs. 28.12 and 28.13) may be considered, although repeat angioplasty is a viable alternative with similar results. The optimal stent type for treatment of central venous stenosis is controversial and many operators are moving toward self-expanding nitinol stents, although compelling evidence in the literature is lacking.

If stent placement is chosen, it is important not to "jail" other tributary veins such as the internal jugular or contralateral brachiocephalic vein, which can eliminate future access options. Dedicated venography of the internal jugular vein may be necessary to assess patency. Central venous stents should be moderately oversized to prevent stent migration.

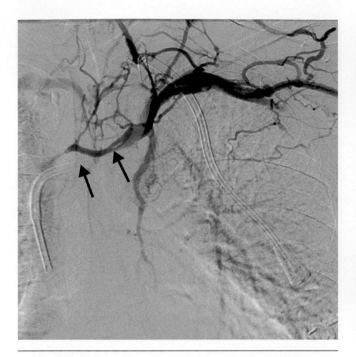

Figure 28.9 • Brachiocephalic venous occlusion following placement of a left internal jugular central venous catheter *(black arrows)*. Multiple collaterals are present. The incidence of venous occlusion is higher with left-sided catheters.

Figure 28.10 • Occlusion of the left subclavian vein *(white arrows)* following permanent pacemaker placement *(generator indicated by black arrow)*. Note the presence of multiple collaterals.

Indications for Stenting

In general, stents in the hemodialysis access circuit should be avoided, particularly at sites of puncture (Fig. 28.14). The most compelling indication for stent placement is a rupture that does not resolve in response to prolonged balloon inflation. Uncovered, self-expanding stents are typically adequate to seal small/moderate leaks although covered stents may be used for larger or central ruptures. In general, self-expanding

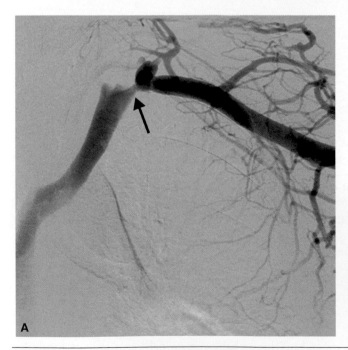

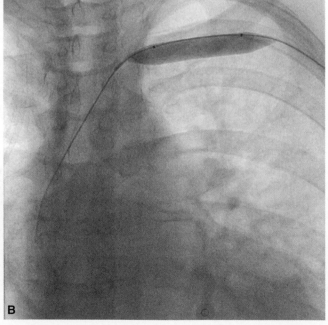

Figure 28.11 • Treatment of left subclavian vein stenosis. **A:** Venogram demonstrating a high-grade stenosis in the left subclavian vein *(black arrow)* and numerous collaterals in the left chest wall. **B:** A prolonged (3-minute) balloon inflation is performed.

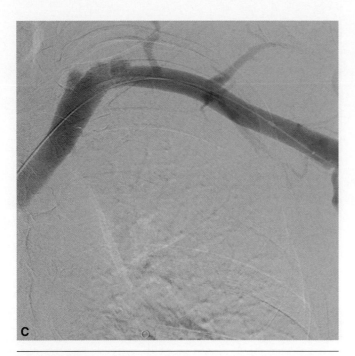

Figure 28.11 • *(Continued)* **C:** Post-angioplasty, there is angiographic resolution of the stenosis and resolution of the patient's symptoms. Note the marked reduction in collateral filling.

nitinol stents are preferred and seem to have better patency compared to balloon-expandable stents. Additional selected indications for stent placement include recurrent stenoses, elastic lesions unresponsive to high-pressure or cutting-balloon angioplasty (rare with current technology), and the treatment of aneurysms/pseudoaneurysms where the patient is not a surgical candidate. It is advisable to confer with vascular surgery prior to elective stent placement as stent placement may preclude surgical options such as revision with patch angioplasty or new fistula or graft creation.

Complications

Complications with treatment of shunt stenosis are rare, occurring with a frequency of 2% to 3% if good technique is utilized. The main complication is venous rupture. This can typically be managed with prolonged low-pressure balloon inflation across the area of extravasation for several minutes. Use of the minimal pressure to achieve occlusion is recommended to prevent further tearing of the vessel. If the rupture persists after balloon occlusion, then stent placement is indicated. Typically, uncovered self-expanding stents are adequate for small ruptures, although larger or central ruptures may require placement of a covered stent. Venous rupture may also result in hematomas or pseudoaneurysms, which may compress the access and cause thrombosis. Other complications such as contrast reaction or medication allergy are similar to other endovascular procedures.

FAILURE OF FISTULA TO MATURE

DOQI guidelines recommend evaluation of a fistula 6 weeks after placement if adequate maturation has not occurred to

support dialysis (4). Generally, blood flow of at least 500 mL/min and a diameter of at least 4 mm are needed to support dialysis, although the goal is the "rule of sixes" (15). The fistula should have a flow of at least 600 mL/min, be 6 mm in diameter, and be no more than 6 mm deep (15). Fistulae that are inadequate for dialysis within the first 3 months of creation are termed early failures. Early failures can occur up to 20% to 50% of the time and require interventional therapy to treat (16–19).

Early failures can be due to many causes. Arterial problems are responsible for only a minority of cases (6%) (19). Venous stenosis is generally the underlying cause of maturation failure, with the majority of venous stenoses (>50%) being juxta-anastomotic (19). Some have advocated for embolization or ligation of competitive venous outflow (Fig. 28.15). This issue is particularly controversial, as collaterals due to venous stenosis may often appear to be competitive veins. In general, the presence of an underlying venous stenosis is the rule rather than the exception, although embolization/ligation of competitive venous channels may be helpful in select circumstances.

In the case of failure to mature, evaluation of the entire circuit may require arterial access. Reflux venography is often extremely confusing and identification of the arterial anastomosis may be impossible (Fig. 28.16A). It is often difficult to evaluate which is the major outflow pathway and where stenosis may be occurring, particularly if venous spasm is encountered. In these cases, evaluation from the arterial side is quite helpful (Fig. 28.16B). Brachial access is obtained with ultrasound guidance and micropuncture technique. The 3-Fr. inner dilator can be used to perform arteriography to minimize the arterial access size and possible complications. In the majority of cases, a venous stenosis will be identified and can

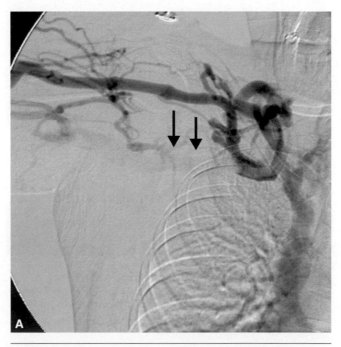

Figure 28.12 • Treatment of right subclavian venous occlusion. A: Occlusion of the right subclavian vein *(arrows)* with multiple right chest collaterals. *(Continued)*

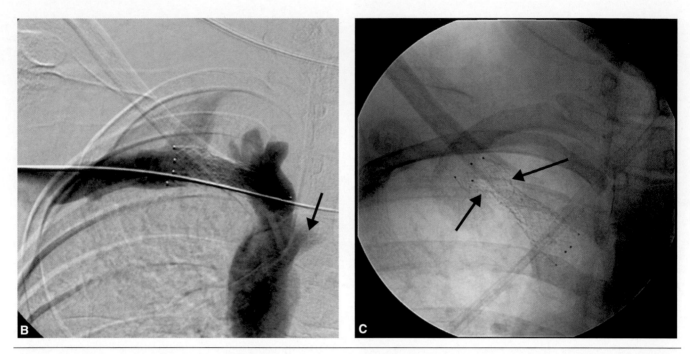

Figure 28.12 • *(Continued)* **B:** Venous recanalization and nitinol stent placement result in resolution of collaterals. Care has been taken not to cover the left innominate vein *(position indicated by arrow)*. **C:** This stent fractured (fractures indicated by *black arrows*) and reoccluded in less than 3 months. It was not possible to recross the stenosis.

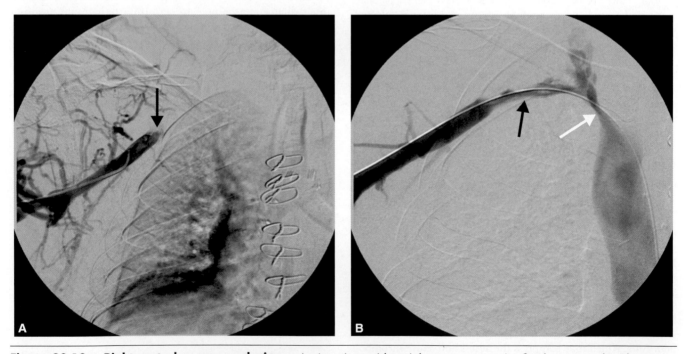

Figure 28.13 • **Right central venous occlusion.** **A:** A patient with a right upper extremity fistula presented with massive upper extremity swelling. A fistulogram demonstrates complete obstruction of the right subclavian vein *(arrow)* with numerous chest wall collaterals. **B:** After prolonged balloon dilation, there is resolution of collateral flow although there is significant residual stenosis in the subclavian vein *(black arrow)* and right innominate vein *(white arrow)*. The patient had no resolution of symptoms and reoccluded within 2 days.

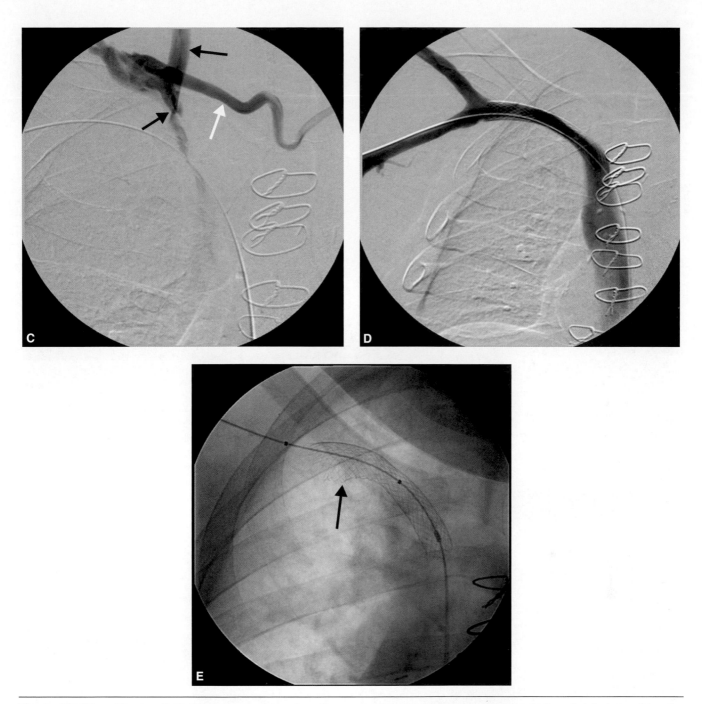

Figure 28.13 • *(Continued)* **C:** Given the necessity of stenting across the right internal jugular vein, dedicated right internal jugular venography *(internal jugular vein indicated by long black arrow)* was performed. A high-grade right brachiocephalic stenosis *(short black arrow)* was demonstrated with drainage via a large venous collateral *(white arrow)*. **D:** A Wallstent was placed that did not "jail" the left innominate vein. This resulted in rapid resolution of patient symptoms. **E:** This patient required repeat balloon angioplasty every 2 months following stent placement. Fracture of stent struts *(black arrow)* was noted after the second re-intervention.

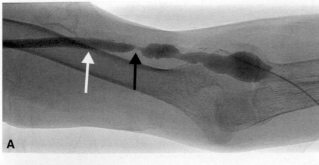

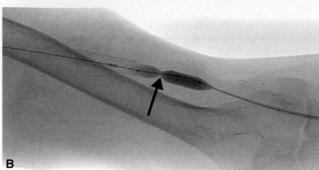

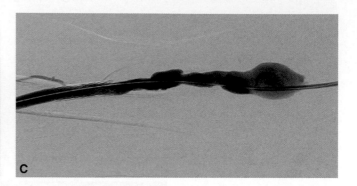

Figure 28.14 • Venous stenosis following prior stent placement in hemodialysis access. **A:** An upper arm fistula has a hemodynamically significant stenosis *(black arrow)* adjacent to a previously placed stent *(white arrow)* in an area of cannulation. The stent is in the area of cannulation which should be avoided when possible. **B:** The waist *(black arrow)* of the balloon is demonstrated. **C:** Post-angioplasty, there is resolution of the stenosis.

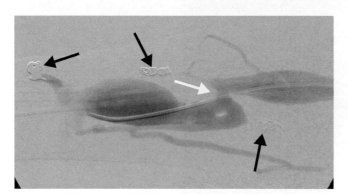

Figure 28.15 • Failure of maturation of fistula due to competitive veins and venous stenosis. Multiple "competitive outflow" veins have been coil embolized *(black arrows)* in this fistula that has not matured although the underlying problem of a venous stenosis *(white arrow)* persists.

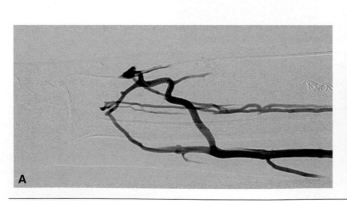

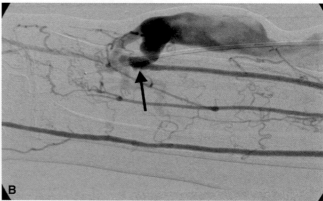

Figure 28.16 • Assessment of hemodialysis fistula access that has failed to mature. **A:** Reflux venography is confusing without demonstration of the arterial anastomosis due to multiple outflow venous channels. **B:** Brachial arteriography with a high frame rate (4 to 6 fps) demonstrates the arterial anastomosis *(black arrow)*.

be treated with a second puncture of the appropriate venous channel.

In the case of juxta-anastomotic strictures, evaluation with physical exam and sonography can appropriately direct treatment. Due to a patent anastomosis, these patients frequently have a short segment of pulsatile vein just distal to the anastomosis with a subsequent venous stenosis associated with a thrill. The downstream vein is typically flat from low flow. In this case, retrograde puncture of the fistula directed to arterial inflow with PTA of the lesion is appropriate. Retrograde puncture of the fistula can be aided by distending veins with a tourniquet and using ultrasound guidance for access. Long segment, often multiple, high-grade stenoses are also somewhat common and may require several sequential, staged dilations to minimize rupture and allow for maturation (Fig. 28.17). If they are resistant to dilation, surgical revision is a viable approach.

Clark et al. reported that the presence of a strong thrill was the single best predictor of patency after intervention (17). Collateral/accessory veins frequently disappear after treatment of the culprit lesion. In the case that they do not resolve and flow remains inadequate, consideration should be given to embolization of accessory veins to maximize flow through the main outflow channel (16). Several techniques have been described including coil embolization, surgical cut down for ligation, and percutaneous ligation with sutures (16,18).

Use of Contrast Agents During Hemodialysis Access Management

A unique problem sometimes occurs in the pre-dialysis patient population. Often a fistula is placed in anticipation of dialysis that has not yet begun. If this fistula fails to mature, evaluation of the access requires the use of contrast agents in the very patients who are at highest risk of contrast nephropathy. Historically, gadolinium contrast agents have been used in this population, although recent evidence demonstrates that this population (GFR < 30) is at highest risk for nephrogenic systemic fibrosis, a debilitating scleroderma-like illness, and gadolinium use can no longer be routinely recommended. CO_2 venography also carries risk. While it is safe in primary venography in the absence of a fistula, reflux in the arterial system and up the vertebral or carotid artery can have devastating consequences including seizure or stroke. Dilution of iodinated contrast agents with saline (4:1 or 5:1) in combination with high-quality digital subtraction is the best strategy to prevent contrast nephropathy. Monitoring the contrast dose and staging the procedure if the dose is escalating are also recommended.

THROMBOSIS OF FISTULA OR GRAFT

Thrombosis of dialysis access is almost universally caused by an underlying stenosis. Treatment of the clot can be accomplished by many techniques including purely mechanical methods, purely pharmacologic methods, and pharmacomechanical methods. There are numerous available devices and only the techniques that are commonly used in our practice will be discussed. In general, grafts are technically easier to declot than fistulae, and many interventionalists historically have abandoned thrombolysis of fistulae. Recent experience, however, shows that thrombolysis of fistulae may have more durable outcomes than graft thrombolysis and can therefore be more rewarding and beneficial for long-term patient outcome (4).

Several concepts are important to keep in mind with any declotting procedure. There is almost always one or more venous stenoses that need treatment. There is almost universally a segment of resistant thrombus near the arterial anastomosis that needs to be mechanically dislodged in order to re-establish adequate flow. The re-establishment of flow in a timely fashion is a priority.

History

Infection is an absolute contraindication to intervention, as septic pulmonary emboli will cause rapid clinical deterioration. A history of fever and chills or an elevated white cell count should prompt further evaluation. A review of the access history is important. Thrombosis of the access within the first month of creation or multiple repeated episodes of thrombosis (recurrent thrombosis within 1 month) suggest that surgical revision will be necessary. An estimation of the suspected duration of thrombosis is also helpful. This can be assessed by determining when the access was last successfully used. It is optimal to declot access within several days of the onset of thrombosis. Fistulae tend to be easiest to declot within 1 week, and grafts can often be opened several weeks after the onset of thrombosis. In general, the longer the access has been clotted, the lower the likelihood of successful intervention and long-term patency.

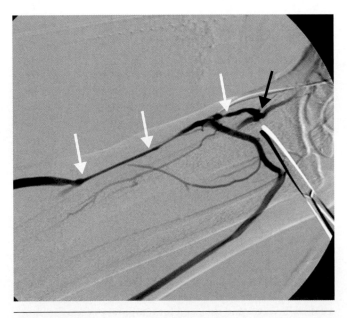

Figure 28.17 • Venography of this Brescia–Cimino fistula demonstrates a long segment stenosis (*white arrows*) that is best treated by sequential dilation. Venous spasm can look quite similar. The arterial anastomosis (*black arrow*) is patent.

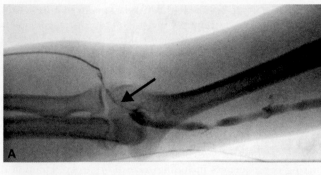

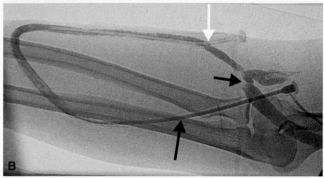

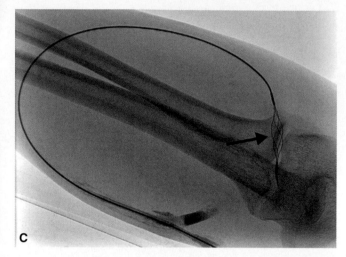

Figure 28.18 • Right forearm loop graft declot. **A:** A last image hold of a pullback venogram (using sheath inserted into graft toward venous outflow) demonstrates thrombosis at the expected location of the venous anastomosis *(black arrow)* with a patent venous system centrally. **B:** Dual sheaths have been placed for this graft declot. The initial sheath *(long black arrow)* is placed near the arterial anastomosis directed toward the venous outflow. The second sheath *(white arrow)* is directed toward the arterial inflow. Note that the sheaths do not overlap. The venous anastomosis *(short black arrow)* is well demonstrated. **C:** The Arrow Treratola basket *(black arrow)* is being used to mechanically macerate clot in the graft. The Arrow basket contacts the wall and helps remove adherent clot.

It is also important to assess whether the patient can tolerate the anticipated intervention. If dialysis has not been performed at a normal interval, the patient may be volume overloaded, have hyperkalemia, and may not be able to tolerate conscious sedation. In this case, a temporary line to allow dialysis may be required before an attempt at lysis. A review of contraindications for thrombolytics is prudent if their use is anticipated.

Physical Exam

The first thing to assess is whether the access is actually thrombosed. It is relatively common to have low flow in an access that is actually patent. Ultrasound is particularly helpful and can define the segment of thrombosed access along its length with relative ease. Non-compressibility, lack of color flow, and internal echogenic debris are the hallmarks of clot.

The next step in evaluation is to determine there is any indication of infection. Hemodialysis patients are relatively immunosuppressed and signs of infection may be subtle. Erythema, fluctuance, and purulent discharge are strong signs of infection and are absolute contraindications to a declot procedure. In cases of significant infection in a graft, explantation may be indicated. In a fistula, however, superficial thrombophlebitis manifesting as mild tenderness and redness is common and is not a contraindication to intervention.

The size of the thrombosed segments and the presence of pseudoaneurysms are also important. Grafts have a regular size and the overall clot volume is relatively low. In contrast, however, fistulae may be large in diameter with significant pseudoaneurysms that may contain a large volume of clot. These may require more aggressive pharmacologic lysis in order to prevent clinically significant pulmonary embolism.

Another potential complication of a declot procedure is arterial embolism. Assessment of the distal pulse exam, temperature of the hand, and capillary refill is critical to establish a baseline exam and to manage complications if they arise.

Laboratory Evaluation

Unlike evaluation of the dysfunctional access in those undergoing routine dialysis, patients with thrombosed access may not have had recent dialysis. Evaluation of the potassium and basic electrolytes is important for triage. In the patient with moderate or severe hyperkalemia, obtaining an EKG to evaluate for peaked T-waves and the need for temporary access for immediate dialysis can prevent sedation-related complications. Since thrombolytics and anti-coagulants are often administered, assessment of baseline coagulation parameters is also important to mitigate the bleeding risk. Although absolute numbers are not well defined, an INR of <2 and a platelet count >50 are generally safe.

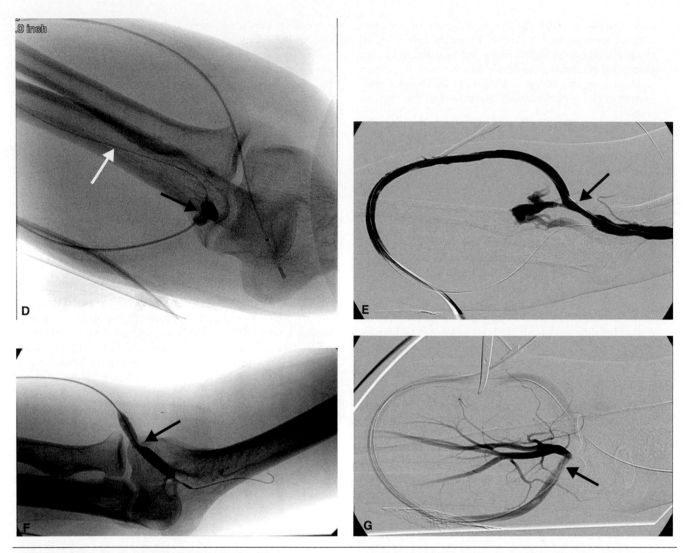

Figure 28.18 • *(Continued)* **D:** A 0.025″ wire has been placed into the artery *(white arrow)* and a Fogarty balloon has been used to dislodge the arterial plug. The balloon is seen to be deformed as it crosses into the arterial anastomosis *(black arrow)*. **E:** Venography of the outflow can be performed when flow has been re-established. A mild venous anastomotic stricture *(black arrow)* is present and represents the cause of thrombosis. **F:** Balloon angioplasty of the venous stenosis demonstrates a waist *(black arrow)*. **G:** Compression of the venous outflow with a hemostat for reflux venography allows evaluation of the arterial anastomosis. Narrowing of the proximal graft *(black arrow)* represents the resistant platelet plug, which must be disrupted often with multiple Fogarty balloon passes.

Technique for a Graft Declot

See Figure 28.18.
1. Establish that the patient is a candidate for a declot procedure and exclude infection.
2. Obtain access using micropuncture technique. Access should be near the arterial anastomosis and directed toward the venous outflow. Place a short 6-Fr. sheath.
3. If desired and there are no contraindications, infuse 2 to 4 mg tissue plasminogen activator (tPA) while compressing the arterial anastomosis (to prevent reflux of clot into the artery). This is referred to as a "lyse and go" technique.
4. Obtain micropuncture access directed toward the arterial inflow using a similar technique and place a second short 6-Fr. sheath. Avoid overlapped crossed sheaths, which can obstruct flow. Some operators will declot

the graft and aspirate thrombus prior to obtaining the second access. However, obtaining access is markedly easier when the graft is filled with thrombus and is non-compressible.
5. Use an angled 5-Fr. catheter and hydrophilic wire to navigate centrally along the venous outflow. It is common to have difficulty passing the venous anastomosis, as this is often the site of underlying stenosis that caused thrombosis.
6. Perform a pullback venogram to define the distal area of thrombosis where the suspected venous stenosis is present. This should correlate with ultrasound findings performed prior to intervention.
7. Administer dose-adjusted IV heparin.
8. Treat the presumed venous stenosis identified on pullback venography.

9. Mechanically macerate the clot in the graft. In our practice, we tend to use the Arrow Treratola device within the graft. Although approved for use in native veins, the possibility of catching the device on a venous valve deters us from using this device in AV fistulae and balloon maceration of clot is preferentially performed in that circumstance.

10. At this point, aspirate clot from the graft with both sheaths. You may have to remove the sheaths over a wire, clean them, and re-insert them.

11. Use a hydrophilic wire and angled catheter to cross into the artieral system from the retrograde access. Exchange for a 0.025″ soft tipped steel wire.

12. Pull the "arterial plug." Place a 4.5-Fr. Fogarty OTW balloon into the artery from the retrograde access. Gently inflate the balloon in the artery taking care not to overdistend the balloon and injure the native artery. Under fluoroscopic observation, pull the balloon back into the graft. The balloon will deform upon reaching the anastomosis. When the balloon is within the graft, balloon pressure may be increased and clot can be pulled into the mid-graft. Several passes of the balloon may be needed to dislodge the plug and establish good arterial inflow.

13. Gentle injection into the side port of the venous-directed sheath is performed to confirm antegrade flow. If there is antegrade flow, venography is performed taking care to minimize reflux into the arterial limb and therefore minimize the risk of arterial embolization. If the flow is stagnant, additional mechanical debulking or angioplasty of the venous outflow may be necessary.

14. Any venous stenosis(es) is treated with standard PTA. During PTA of the venous anastomosis, a reflux arteriogram can be performed to visualize the arterial anastomosis. Additional clearing of the "arterial plug" may be necessary with the Fogarty OTW balloon.

15. Palpation of a strong thrill indicates a good end point.

16. Hemostasis can be obtained with purse-string sutures at the completion of the procedure.

Technique for a Fistula Declot

Thrombolysis of the native fistula is more technically challenging. There are many methods available for the management of the thrombosed fistula. A simple method of declotting a fistula that should be considered is the pulse-spray technique. This was initially described for AV grafts but is equally applicable to AV fistulae. In this method, crossed infusion catheters are placed into the fistula across the entire length of the thrombosed segment and small aliquots of thrombolytics (0.2 to 0.4 mg) are infused with moderate force every 30 seconds until flow is re-established. No more than 15 mg of tPA should be used. This technique is technically simple and safe although dislodging of the arterial plug and treatment of venous stenoses will need to be performed as well. Declotting of a fistula can be accomplished with a similar technique as for a graft as previously described. Unlike graft declotting, repetitive boluses of heparin may be necessary to keep the activated clotting time (ACT) > 200 seconds as the procedure may be prolonged. Balloon maceration of clot is technically simple for those operators who are unfamiliar with other devices, although it is less successful at removing clot adherent to the vessel wall.

Many other mechanical devices are available and are too numerous to review. More recently, purely mechanical declotting of fistulae with thin-walled non-tapered aspiration

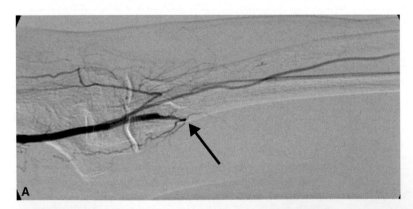

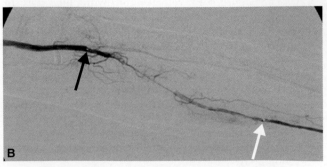

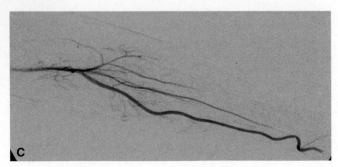

Figure 28.19 • Arterial embolization during declot procedure. A: Arterial embolism to the ulnar artery (*black arrow*) is a complication of a declotting procedure. **B:** An infusion catheter has been placed across the clot as the patient was symptomatic. The proximal (*black arrow*) and distal (*white arrow*) ends of the infusion catheter demonstrate that the infusion catheter is appropriately placed across the entire length of the clot. **C:** Following overnight lytic infusion, there is complete resolution of the clot.

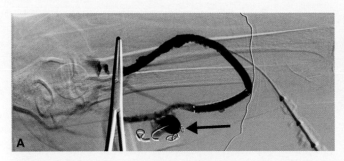 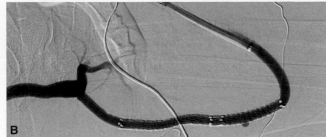

Figure 28.20 • Treatment of pseudoaneurysm of hemodialysis graft with covered stent. **A:** An enlarging pseudoaneurysm (*black arrow*) required treatment due to enlargement and risk of rupture. **B:** The pseudoaneurysm has been treated with two overlapping covered stents. In this case, Bard Fluency stent grafts were used.

sheaths (7 to 8 Fr.)has also been described with high rates of technical success.

Complications

Although pulmonary embolism likely occurs in most patients, the clot burden is small and few are symptomatic. Care should be taken with patients with large pseudoaneurysms where the clot burden may be substantial. In these cases, overnight thrombolysis with a crossed infusion catheter technique may be prudent.

Embolization of clot into the arterial circulation is infrequent if appropriate technique is used. It is either detected by patient symptoms of hand pain or numbness, or during the reflux arteriogram. If asymptomatic, it may not require treatment and may lyse on its own. If symptomatic, there are several methods for treatment. Fogarty OTW balloons may be used to pull the clot into the access, aspiration thrombectomy may be performed using various catheters, or pharmacologic lysis (Fig. 28.19) may be performed. Other complications are similar to the treatment of dysfunctional access.

Obtaining Hemostasis

The most common method for obtaining hemostasis after percutaneous intervention is the use of a purse-string suture. This suture is placed superficially in the epidermis, most often with a 3-O non-absorbable monofilament suture and is tightened upon sheath removal. Care must be taken not to puncture the graft or fistula. Placement of small segments of tubing through a loop in the purse-string suture can help facilitate removal by dialysis nurses at the time of next dialysis. Alternatively, compression dressings may be used.

PSEUDOANEURYSMS

Degenerative changes in a graft or fistula, combined with repetitive venopuncture and outflow stenosis, can result in pseudoaneurysm formation. Pseudoaneurysm formation can limit cannulation sites, cause skin necrosis or infection, and can rupture and cause massive hemorrhage. Primary treatment of pseudoaneurysms in fistulae or grafts is surgical revision. Several small series have demonstrated that exclusion of pseudoaneurysms with covered stent grafts is technically

feasible and safe (Fig. 28.20). Primary patency is poor, however, with a reported 20% to 25% patency at 6 months. Wallgraft (Boston Scientific, Natick, MA), Viabahn (Gore), Hemobahn (Gore), and Fluency stent grafts (Bard) have all been used with success.

References

1. Gilbertson DT, Liu J, Xue JL, et al. Projecting the number of patients with end-stage renal disease in the United States to the year 2015. *J Am Soc Nephrol.* 2005;16:3736–3741.
2. U.S. Renal Data System. *USRDS 2008 Annual Data Report: Atlas of Chronic Kidney Disease and End-Stage Renal Disease in the United States.* Bethesda, MD: National Institutes of Health, National Institute of Diabetes and Digestive and Kidney Diseases;. 2008.
3. Flu H, Breslau PJ, Krol-van Straaten JM, et al. The effect of implementation of an optimized care protocol on the outcome of arteriovenous hemodialysis access surgery. *J Vasc Surg.* 2008;48:659–668.
4. KDOQI Advisory Board. Clinical practice guidelines for hemodialysis adequacy, update 2006. *Am J Kidney Dis.* 2006;48 (Suppl 1):S2–S90.
5. Roberts A, Valji K. Screening and assessment of dialysis graft function. *Tech Vasc Interv Radiol.* 1999;2:186–188.
6. Beathard GA. Physical examination of the dialysis vascular access. *Semin Dial.* 1998;11:231–236.
7. Trerotola SO, Scheel PJ Jr, Powe NR, et al. Screening for dialysis access graft malfunction: comparison of physical examination with US. *J Vasc Interv Radiol.* 1996;7:15–20.
8. Trerotola SO, Kwak A, Clark TW, et al. Prospective study of balloon inflation pressures and other technical aspects of hemodialysis access angioplasty. *J Vasc Interv Radiol.* 2005;16: 1613–1618.
9. Carrafiello G, Laganà D, Mangini M, et al. Cutting balloon angioplasty for the treatment of haemodyalisis vascular accesses: midterm results. *Radiol Med.* 2006;111:724–732.
10. Vesely TM, Siegel JB. Use of the peripheral cutting balloon to treat hemodialysis-related stenoses. *J Vasc Interv Radiol.* 2005;16:1593–1603.
11. Guiu B, Loffroy R, Ben Salem D, et al. Angioplasty of long venous stenoses in hemodialysis access: at last an indication for cutting balloon? *J Vasc Interv Radiol.* 2007;18:994–1000.
12. Kian K, Asif A. Cephalic arch stenosis. *Semin Dial.* 2008; 21:78–82.
13. Rajan DK, Clark TW, Patel NK, et al. Prevalence and treatment of cephalic arch stenosis in dysfunctional autogenous hemodialysis fistulas. *J Vasc Interv Radiol.* 2003;14:567–573.

14. Levit RD, Cohen RM, Kwak A, et al. Asymptomatic central venous stenosis in hemodialysis patients. *Radiology*. 2006;238:1051–1056.

15. Mercado C, Salman L, Krishnamurthy G, et al. Early and late fistula failure. *Clin Nephrol*. 2008;69:77–83.

16. Beathard GA, Arnold P, Jackson J, et al. Aggressive treatment of early fistula failure. *Kidney Int*. 2003;64:1487–1494.

17. Clark TW, Cohen RA, Kwak A, et al. Salvage of nonmaturing native fistulas by using angioplasty. *Radiology*. 2007;242:286–292.

18. Faiyaz R, Abreo K, Zaman F, et al. Salvage of poorly developed arteriovenous fistulae with percutaneous ligation of accessory veins. *Am J Kidney Dis*. 2002;39:824–827.

19. Turmel-Rodrigues L, Mouton A, Birmelé B, et al. Salvage of immature forearm fistulas for haemodialysis by interventional radiology. *Nephrol Dial Transplant*. 2001;16:2365–2371.

CHAPTER 29

Inferior Vena Cava Filters

Rajan K. Gupta

Pulmonary embolism (PE) as a complication of deep venous thrombosis of the lower extremity (and rarely of the upper extremity) is a widely recognized clinical problem causing an estimated 240,000 deaths per year in the United States alone (1). Caval filtration is designed to prevent clinically significant PE in high-risk patients. The use of inferior vena caval (IVC) filters has seen a dramatic increase in the past several decades with nearly 140,000 filters placed worldwide in 2003 (2).

Despite widespread use and acceptance, there remain little prospective data on long-term outcome of filters. Knowledge of anatomy, indications for placement, and techniques for removal are essential for optimal management of patients.

HISTORY OF CAVAL INTERRUPTION

Caval interruption was first suggested by Trousseau in 1868 (3–5). The first IVC ligation was performed in the 1940s. This was followed by IVC compartmentalization with sutures, staples, and serrated clips (1,4). These techniques were complicated by high rates of caval thrombosis, clinically significant lower extremity swelling, recurrent PE, and significant mortality (1,4). The first surgically implanted endovascular filter was the Mobin-Uddin umbrella filter in 1967, which suffered from high rates of IVC thrombosis (1,6). The next major advance in IVC filtration was the design of the Greenfield filter in 1973 (1,4,7). This filter had a conical design and a high packing efficiency allowing 70% to 80% of the filter to be filled with clot without inducing a significant pressure gradient or altering blood flow across the filter. Initially placed surgically, the Greenfield filter became the first standard in IVC filter technology. The first percutaneous Greenfield IVC filter was placed in 1984 (1,8). The past several decades have shown an explosion in filter technology, design, and usage.

ANATOMY

Normal Anatomy

The IVC is formed by the confluence of the common iliac veins at the L5 vertebral level (Fig. 29.1). The right common iliac vein is shorter and more vertical. The right common iliac artery passes over the left common iliac vein and may cause physiologically important obstruction (Fig. 29.2). The IVC ascends in the retroperitoneal space adjacent to the spine to the

right of the aorta. It receives major drainage from iliac, lumbar, gonadal, renal, and hepatic veins (9).

Four pairs of lumbar veins collect blood from the abdominal wall and posterior musculature and drain into the IVC (9). They are joined by vertically oriented ascending lumbar veins that anastamose with paravertebral veins more centrally (Fig. 29.3). Ascending lumbar and paravertebral veins are important sources of collateral flow in IVC obstruction. Above L2, the ascending lumbar veins continue to become the azygos vein to the right of spine and the hemiazygos vein to the left of spine (9). The hemiazygos vein typically drains into the azygos vein at approximately T8, which then drains into the superior venal cava (SVC) at the level of the aortic arch (9) (Fig. 29.4).

The renal veins enter at the L1/2 level (Figs. 29.5 and 29.6). The right renal vein is typically slightly lower than the left. Several clinically important variations of renal vein anatomy are common and will be discussed below. The right gonadal vein drains directly into the IVC and its course parallels the IVC (9). The left gonadal vein typically drains into the left renal vein.

The hepatic veins enter immediately inferior to the diaphragm on the right anterior aspect of the IVC (Fig. 29.7). The IVC then drains into posterior aspect of the right atrium. Accessory hepatic veins are common and enter the right side of the IVC between the renal veins and main hepatic venous confluence (Fig. 29.8). Phrenic veins and adrenal veins are typically small and are not usually clinically significant to filter placement.

Variant Anatomy

Congenital anomalies of renal veins occur in up to 30% of individuals (10–12). They are clinically relevant to caval filtration, as IVC filters should be placed below the level of the lowest renal vein to prevent thrombus bypassing the filter through major collateral pathways. Multiple right renal veins, circumaortic left renal vein (Fig. 29.9), and retroaortic left renal vein are the most common variants (Fig. 29.10) (11,13).

Congenital anomalies of the IVC are less common with an incidence of 2% to 3% (11,13). They are also clinically relevant to placement of IVC filters and result from the complex embryogenesis of IVC development (13). The most common variations are duplicated IVC, left IVC, and interrupted IVC with azygos/hemiazygos continuation (13). A duplicated IVC is present when each common iliac vein drains into its own vena cava, with the left IVC typically draining into the left renal vein. The left renal vein then crosses anterior to the aorta and joins the right IVC to form a normally oriented suprarenal

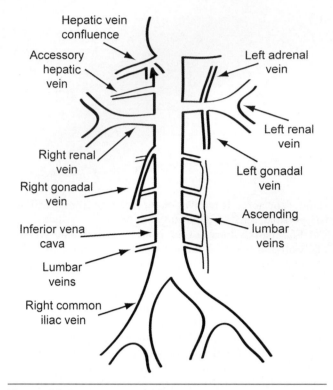

Hepatic vein confluence

Accessory hepatic vein

Left adrenal vein

Left renal vein

Right renal vein

Left gonadal vein

Right gonadal vein

Inferior vena cava

Ascending lumbar veins

Lumbar veins

Right common iliac vein

Figure 29.1 • Normal anatomy of the inferior vena cava (IVC).

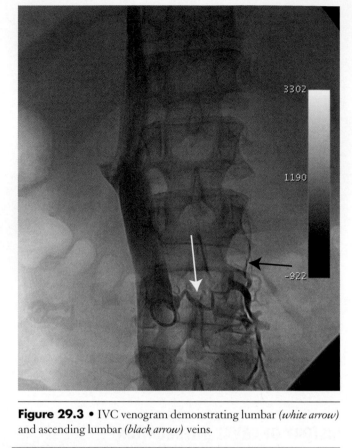

Figure 29.3 • IVC venogram demonstrating lumbar *(white arrow)* and ascending lumbar *(black arrow)* veins.

Figure 29.2 • Physiologic compression of left common iliac vein (CIV) by right common iliac artery (CIA). **A:** IVC venogram demonstrating the physiologic compression *(black arrow)* of the right CIA on the left CIV. If this causes deep venous thrombosis of left lower extremity, it is known as May–Thurner syndrome. **B:** Axial CT demonstrating physiologic compression of the right CIA *(white arrow)* on the left CIV *(black arrow)*.

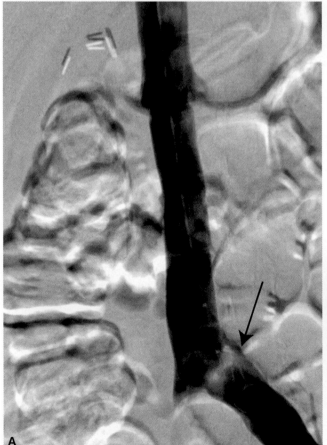

A

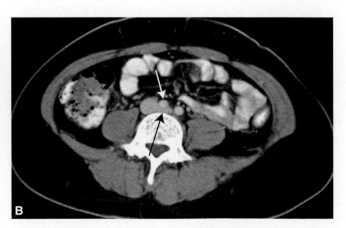

B

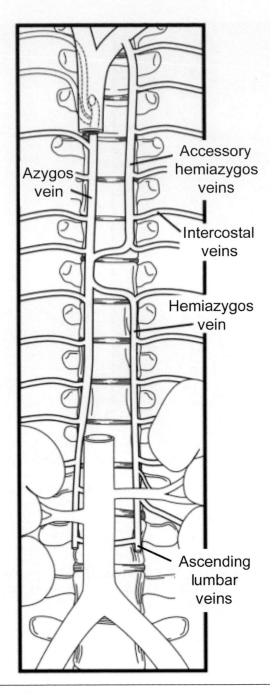

Figure 29.4 • Normal anatomy of azygos/hemiazygos system.

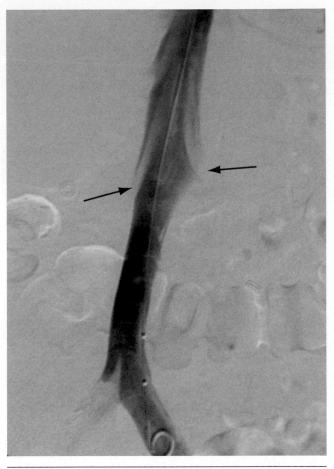

Figure 29.5 • A typical IVC venogram with streaming inflow from renal veins (*arrows*). Note the marker pigtail catheter for IVC sizing.

This anomaly is associated with congenital heart disease and polyspenia/asplenia syndromes. Congenital absence of the IVC is rare and is present when there is no infrarenal IVC and all abdominal venous drainage is via the ascending lumbar and paravertebral veins (Fig. 29.12).

INDICATIONS FOR IVC FILTER PLACEMENT

IVC filtration is designed to prevent clinically significant PE by trapping venous clot before it reaches the lungs. It does nothing to treat or prevent venous thrombosis and is not a substitute for therapeutic anti-coagulation, which remains the standard medical therapy for venous thromboembolism. For optimal treatment of thromboembolic disease, therapeutic anti-coagulation should be resumed as soon as possible (14,15).

Caval filters are used for two primary indications: (1) the prevention of PE in patients with known deep venous thrombosis (DVT) or pulmonary embolism where standard medical therapy is contraindicated, ineffective, or has to be interrupted and (2) for prophylaxis in patients without known venous thromboembolism when the risk for the

IVC. In patients with a left-sided (transposed) IVC, the infrarenal cava is located to the left of the aorta (Fig. 29.11). The left-sided cava typically drains into the left renal vein, which then crosses anterior to the aorta and joins with the right renal vein forming a normally oriented suprarenal IVC. Azygos continuation of the IVC is present when the IVC is interrupted between the hepatic and renal veins. Drainage of the infrarenal IVC is through the azygos/hemiazygos systems. The hepatic segment forms an IVC stump and drains into the right atrium.

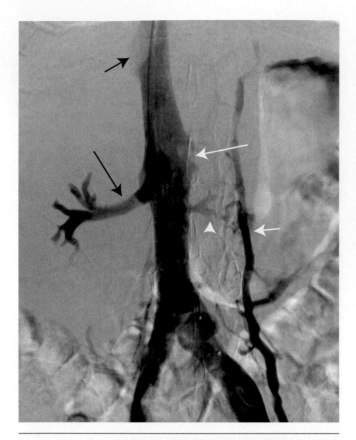

Figure 29.6 • IVC venogram demonstrating many aspects of normal anatomy not typically seen. The right renal vein *(long black arrow)* is lower than the left and is nearly fully opacified. The left renal vein *(long white arrow)* appears as streaming inflow as do the hepatic veins *(short black arrow)*. A lumbar vein *(white arrowhead)* connects to the left ascending lumbar vein *(short white arrow)*.

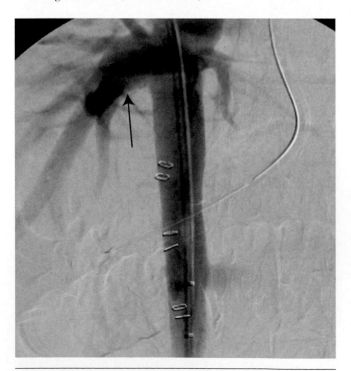

Figure 29.7 • Normal IVC venogram with opacification of the hepatic venous confluence *(black arrow)*.

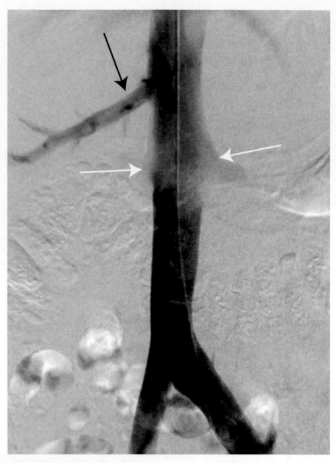

Figure 29.8 • IVC venogram demonstrating a typical appearance of an accessory right hepatic vein *(black arrow)*. Normal renal veins are demonstrated with *white arrows*.

development of DVT/PE is high and medical therapy is contraindicated. Table 29.1 lists common indications for filter placement (1,4,15,16).

CONTRAINDICATIONS

The only absolute contraindication to filter placement is an inability to place a filter due to IVC thrombosis or thrombosis of all available access vessels. Patients with an uncorrectable coagulopathy should be treated with caution, although control of access site bleeding is typically not problematic. A temporary central venous catheter may be left in place to tamponade bleeding at the insertion site as an alternative in critically ill patients who may benefit from additional access. Sepsis is no longer considered to be a contraindication to filter placement (1,16,17).

LOCATION OF FILTER PLACEMENT

Infrarenal IVC Filter Placement

The most common placement for an IVC filter is in the infrarenal vena cava. Ideal placement is with the filter apex at the level of the lowest renal vein (Fig. 29.13). Placement at this

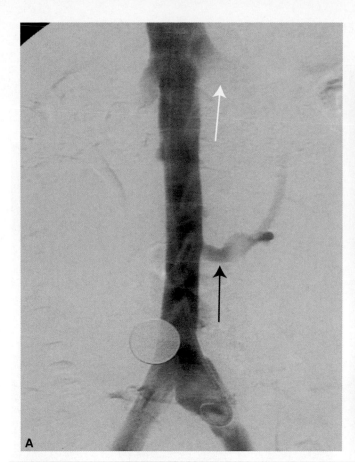

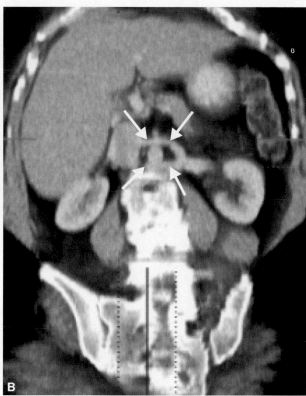

Figure 29.9 • Left circumaortic renal vein. **A:** IVC venogram demonstrating a circumaortic left renal vein *(black arrow)*. The left renal vein draining the superior segment of the left kidney is indicated with a *white arrow*. **B:** Oblique CT maximum intensity projection (MIP) demonstrating a left circumaortic renal vein (different patient).

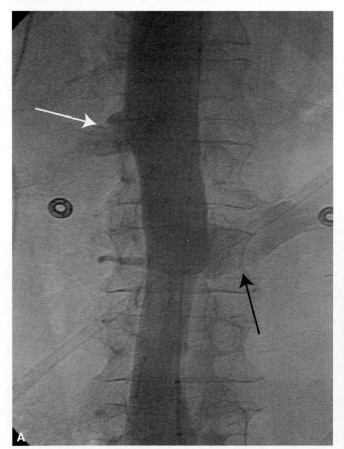

Figure 29.10 • Left retroaortic renal vein. **A:** IVC venogram demonstrating abnormally low insertion of a left renal vein *(black arrow)*. This is a typical appearance of a retroaortic left renal vein. The right renal vein is indicated with a *white arrow*. **B:** Axial CT correlate demonstrating the appearance of a retroaortic left renal vein *(black arrows)*. Note the low insertion onto the cava (axial level at the inferior pole of the kidneys).

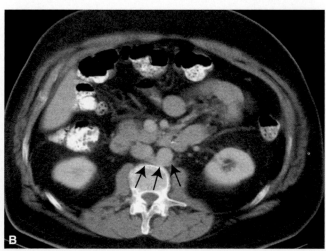

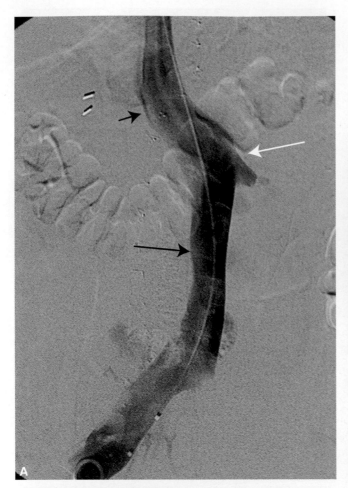
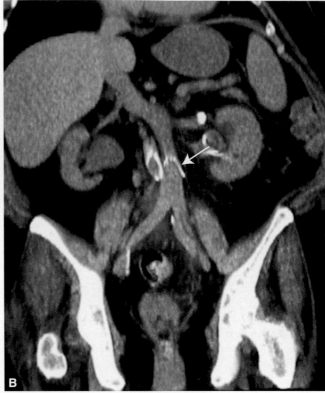

Figure 29.11 • Left-sided IVC. **A:** IVC venogram demonstrating a typical appearance of left-sided IVC *(long black arrow)* that joins the left renal vein *(white arrow)*. Right renal venous inflow is also demonstrated *(short black arrow)*. **B:** Curved CT multiplanar reconstruction (MPR) demonstrating a patient with a left-sided IVC and a filter *(white arrow)* in place.

level prevents clot from bypassing the filter through circumaortic or accessory renal veins. Placement of the filter apex at or near the lowest renal vein reduces the dead space above the filter. If the filter is placed low in the IVC, clot may form in the IVC between the level of the filter and the lowest renal vein, which may embolize unprotected to the lungs.

Suprarenal Filter Placement

Occasionally, placement of an IVC filter above the renal veins is necessary (Fig. 29.14). The main indications for placement of a filter in the suprarenal location are listed in Table 29.2. Suprarenal filters perform similarly to infrarenal filters in terms of effectiveness and complications based on limited data (18,19). If suprarenal filter placement is required, a Bird's Nest filter should be avoided as the wires may prolapse into the heart. Classic teaching is to place a suprarenal filter in pregnant patients to avoid the effects of uterine compression on the infrarenal IVC, which may make penetration of the IVC wall by the filter legs more likely with possible injury to the uterus, although there is little evidence to support this (18,19). When placing an IVC filter during pregnancy, a jugular approach with pelvic shielding is preferred to minimize radiation dose to the fetus.

SVC Filter Placement

Occasionally, upper extremity thrombosis and clinically significant PE will necessitate placement of an SVC filter. While limited literature suggests that SVC filter placement is safe and effective, it should be performed only in carefully selected patients with appropriate precautions (4,20,21).

Anatomic considerations for SVC filter placement include a short overall length of the SVC (approximately 7 cm), inflow from the azygos vein, and close proximity to the heart and great vessels, which induces cardiac motion (20). Pericardial tamponade is an additional risk of SVC filter placement secondary to filter leg perforation into the superior pericardial reflection, which is in close association with the SVC (20,21). Males younger than 60 years are felt to be at higher risk, for unclear reasons (21). Placement of the filter apex into the right atrium should be avoided to prevent arrhythmias and cardiac wall injury. The risk of prolapse of the wires from a Bird's Nest filter (Cook) into the right atrium makes this filter a less optimal choice for this location.

Existing central venous catheters must be removed or retracted out of the deployment area during placement. High-quality venography, careful sizing, and accurate

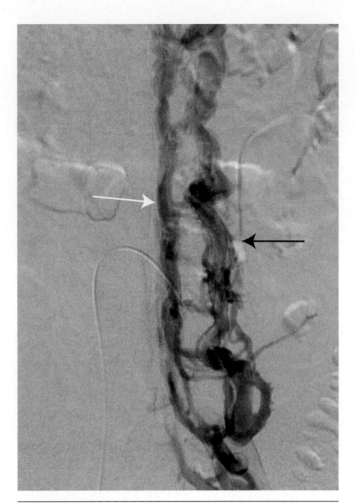

TABLE 29.1 Indications for IVC Filter Placement

Classic/widely accepted indications
Documented DVT/PE with:
1. Contraindication to anti-coagulation
2. Complication of anti-coagulation
3. Failure of therapeutic anti-coagulation
Relative indications
Documented DVT/PE with:
1. Poor cardiopulmonary reserve
2. Free-floating IVC thrombus ("widow-maker" clot)
3. High risk for anti-coagulation (frequent falls, ataxia)
4. Non-compliant patient or inability to maintain therapeutic anticoagulation
5. Planned pharmacomechanical thrombolysis of ilio-caval DVT
Prophylactic indications
No DVT/PE and anti-coagulation contraindicated:
1. Multiple trauma
2. History of DVT/PE with high-risk surgery (bariatric surgery, hip replacement, etc.)

IVC, inferior vena cava; DVT, deep venous thrombosis; PT, pulmonary embolus.

Figure 29.12 • Congenital absence of IVC. In this patient with congenital absence of the IVC, all venous drainage is through the hypertrophied ascending lumbar veins (*black arrow*) and more central paravertebral veins (*white arrow*). IVC obstruction may have a similar appearance.

placement are required to prevent complications. Most of the available data for SVC filtration are with permanent filters, although the use of retrievable filters may be considered, particularly when the anticipated duration of filtration is considered to be short. There is a paucity of data regarding the safety of retrieval.

Adequate documentation of SVC filter placement in the medical record is advisable, as these filters may be displaced by attempts at central line placement. Subsequent lines should ideally be placed under fluoroscopic guidance.

DEVICES

Filter Types

Filters can be classified into three categories: permanent, retrievable (optional), and temporary (Table 29.3; Figs. 29.15 and 29.16). Permanent filters cannot be repositioned or removed and are left in place as lifelong devices. There are many available permanent filters with a variety of designs and delivery systems.

Retrievable (optional) filters are designed for removal or repositioning at a later time, although they can be left in place as permanent devices. All retrievable filters in the United States are first Food and Drug Administration (FDA) approved as permanent devices. Currently, there are five filters approved by the FDA for retrieval: the Günther-Tulip (Cook), Celect (Cook), the G2 (Bard), the G2 Express (Bard), and the OptEase (Cordis).

Temporary filters are attached to a tethering device left outside the body or buried subcutaneously for later retrieval. They must be removed or repositioned. In the United States, there are currently no FDA-approved temporary filters, although there are devices available in Europe.

Filter Selection

The data on IVC filters are based on small case series, retrospective reviews, and single-center experiences (1,4,15,22). There are little prospective data on filter use and consequently there are no rigorous or compelling data that the various permanent or retrievable filters perform significantly differently. Selection is often based on anatomic considerations (caval size, length of available IVC), device availability, and operator preference. A retrievable filter should be placed when either the risks of DVT/PE will be of limited duration (peri-operative, trauma, thrombolysis, etc.) or therapeutic anti-coagulation will be resumed within a reasonable time period. Some authors advocate that retrievable filters should be placed in all patients, although there are less long-term data available for retrievable devices (2).

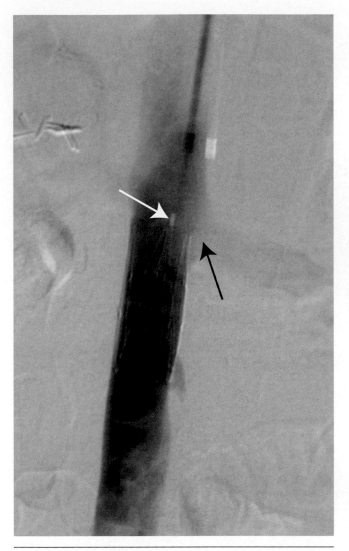

Figure 29.13 • IVC filter placement. IVC venogram demonstrating an optimally placed permanent IVC filter (Vena Tech LP, Braun) with apex *(white arrow)* at the level of the lowest (**left** in this case) renal vein *(black arrow)*. The "dead space" where clot may form above the filter if IVC thrombosis occurs is minimized.

DEVICE PLACEMENT

1. A review of all available imaging to assess anatomy is essential. Patients referred for filter placement often have prior abdominal computed tomography (CT) scans available for review. Anomalous anatomy can be difficult to identify with IVC venography and review of cross-sectional imaging can provide substantial information on patient anatomy. Duplicated IVC, retroaortic renal veins, circumaortic renal veins, and accessory renal veins may be visualized on cross-sectional imaging. The expected level of the lowest renal vein can be assessed and compared to bony landmarks (vertebral levels) and anticipated on the IVC venogram. Additionally, the IVC diameter can be gauged, although it is important to realize that IVC diameter changes substantially with hydration status and respiration.

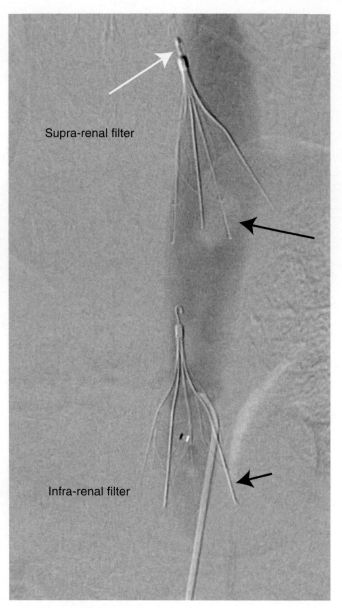

Supra-renal filter

Infra-renal filter

Figure 29.14 • Suprarenal filter placement. In this patient, a suprarenal Günther-Tulip (Cook) filter was placed during thrombolysis of complete IVC thrombosis that occurred with a pre-existing infrarenal filter in place.   A filling defect *(long black arrow)* depicts clot trapped against the caval wall after thrombolysis. There is significant tilting of the suprarenal filter with the retrieval hook *(white arrow)* located against the caval wall. This filter was removed by deflecting the filter hook off the caval wall from a femoral approach with subsequent jugular retrieval. If this filter were not retrieved in a short time window, the hook would likely become incorporated into the IVC wall precluding removal. The infrarenal filter was indwelling for several years and left in place after thrombolysis. Note the leg penetration of the caval wall *(short black arrow)*.

TABLE 29.2 Indications for Suprarenal IVC Filter Placement

1. Renal/gonadal vein thrombosis
2. IVC thrombus precluding infrarenal filter placement
3. Thrombus above an infrarenal filter
4. Continued PE through existing filter (lower extremity source) without room for additional infrarenal filter
5. IVC filter placement in pregnancy

2. Choose an access route. The internal jugular vein (IJV) and common femoral vein (CFV) are the most common access routes, although smaller introducer sheaths and more flexible filter designs allow for other access points including the antecubital or upper arm veins. The right IJV and CFV are preferred over the left IJV and CFA since it provides a straighter course to the IVC or SVC. If there is bilateral lower extremity DVT, placement from an IJV approach is preferable. If placing a Günther-Tulip, Celect, G2, or G2 Express, a potential advantage of jugular placement is the ability to reposition the device from the same access if needed, since the hook is at the cranial aspect of the device.

3. Verify access route patency. Prior to a sterile prep, ultrasound should be used to verify that the intended access route is indeed patent and free of clot. This is particularly important if femoral access is chosen, as DVT frequently involves the femoral veins.

4. Perform an IVC venogram. This is typically done with a 5-Fr. marker pigtail catheter for accurate sizing of the vena cava. If placement is from the IJV, the preferred pigtail placement is in the proximal left common iliac vein, as most IVC anatomic variants will be more readily identified from that location as opposed to a right-sided injection. In fact, inability to place a pigtail into the left common iliac vein and subsequent nonvisualization of left iliac venous inflow may be the only clue to the IVC anatomic variant of duplicated IVC. A test hand injection should always be performed to ensure that the catheter is not embedded in thrombus prior to power injection to prevent clot disruption and embolization. Imaging should be performed using breath hold DSA technique. Typically an injection rate of 15 to 25 cc/sec for 2 seconds is performed while imaging at 4 to 6 fps. Choose a field of view that covers from the upper pelvis through the lower thoracic vertebrae. If the patient has renal insufficiency, imaging with CO_2 provides reasonable results, although visualization of renal vein inflow and caval thrombus may be difficult (23). A CO_2 venogram should not be performed in those with known right-to-left shunts (23). Whenever there is doubt about caval

TABLE 29.3 Common IVC Filters

Filter	Maximum IVC Diameter (mm)	Access Route	Retrieval Route	Length (mm)	Material
Retrievable					
Celect (Cook)	30	J/F	J	45–50	Conichrome
Günther-Tulip (Cook)	30	J/F	J	45–50	Conichrome
G2 (Bard)	28	J/F	J	40	Nitinol
G2 Express (Bard)	28	J/F	J	40	Nitinol
OptEase (Cordis)	30	J/F/AC	F	54–67	Nitinol
Permanent					
Simon Nitinol (Bard)	28	J/F/AC	N/A	45	Nitinol
Vena Tech LGM (Braun)	28	J/F	N/A		Phynox
Vena Tech LP (Braun)	28 (35 mm in Europe)	J/F/AC	N/A	43	Phynox
Bird's Nest (Cook)	40	J/F	N/A	>70	Stainless steel*
TrapEase (Cordis)	30	J/F/AC	N/A	54–67	Nitinol
Titanium Greenfield (Boston Scientific)	28	J/F	N/A		Titanium
12 Fr OTW Greenfield (Boston Scientific)	28	J/F	N/A	49	Stainless steel*

*Stainless steel filters are not MRI compatible.
J, jugular; F, femoral; AC, antecubital or upper arm vein ; N/A, not applicable.

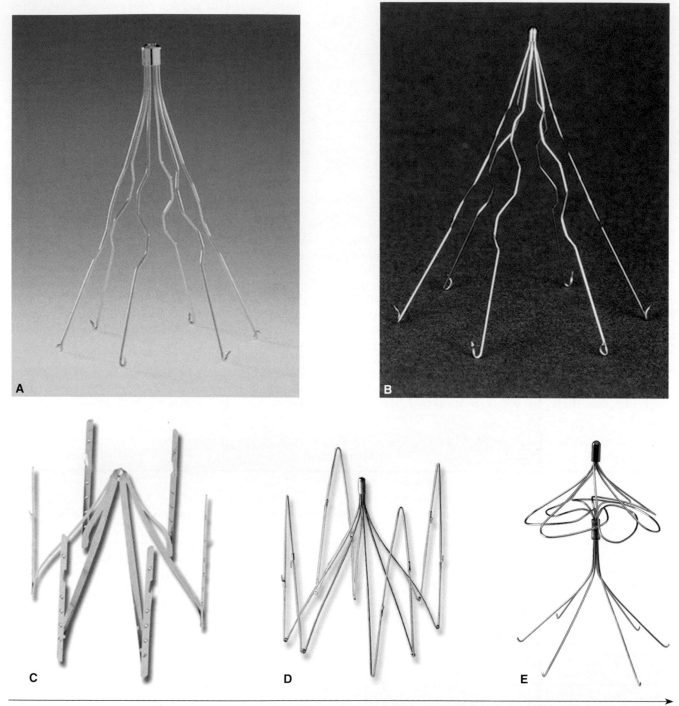

Figure 29.15 • Permanent IVC Filters.   **A:** Stainless steel over-the-wire Greenfield filter (Boston Scientific). **B:** Titanium Greenfield (Boston Scientific). **C:** Vena Tech LGM (Braun). **D:** Vena Tech LP (Braun). **E:** Simon Nitinol (Bard).

or side branch anatomy, selective venography should be performed with a hooked catheter such as a multipurpose, Cobra 2, or Kumpe catheter. Historically, gadolinium was utilized to image the IVC in patients with renal insufficiency; the risk of nephrogenic systemic fibrosis in patients with renal insufficiency has largely eliminated this strategy. Intravascular ultrasound (IVUS) may also be used to assess venous anatomy and caval thrombus if necessary.

5. Choose a device appropriate to the anatomy. All available devices can be placed in a vena cava with a diameter of 28 mm or less. In the presence of a mega cava (i.e., IVC larger than 30 mm), placement of a Bird's Nest filter (in IVC up to 40-mm diameter) or Vena Tech LP (in IVC up to 35 mm in diameter) is required. Placement of the Vena Tech LP filter in caval sizes of 31 to 35 mm has been approved in Europe although its use in the United States

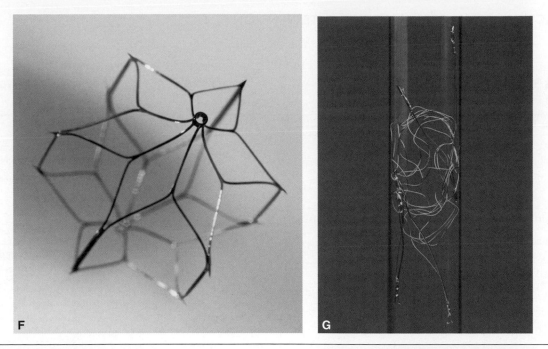

Figure 29.15 • *(Continued)* **F:** TrapEase (Cordis). Note that barbs are present on both superior and inferior ends of the longitudinal struts. Compare with the OptEase where barbs are present only on the cranial aspect (Fig. 29.16C). **G:** Bird's Nest (Cook).

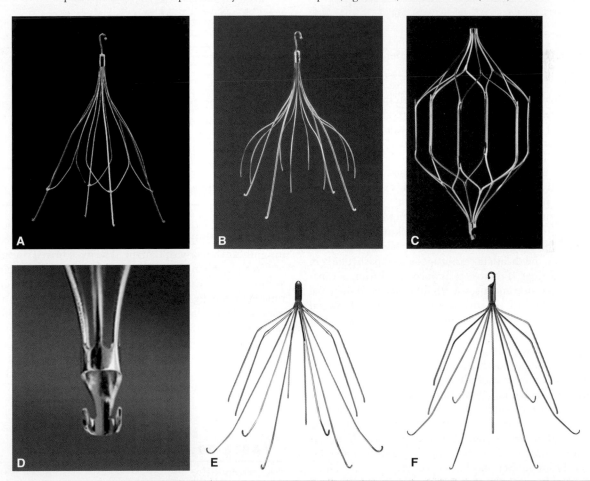

Figure 29.16 • Retrievable IVC filters. **A:** Günther-Tulip (Cook): Note the retrieval hook at the cranial end of the filter. This filter has four "petals," each with one anchoring strut. **B:** Celect (Cook): Note the retrieval hook at the cranial end of the filter. The Celect is a redesigned Günther-Tulip that has curved secondary struts designed to improve centering. **C:** OptEase (Cordis): Note the retrieval hook at the inferior aspect of the filter. The barbs are present only at the cranial aspect of the filter. This filter should only be placed in the IVC with the hook oriented down. If placed incorrectly with the hook superiorly, the lack of barbs on this aspect of the filter can cause superior migration. **D:** OptEase (Cordis): close-up view of retrieval hook. **E:** G2 (Bard): This filter must be removed with the Recovery cone system (see Fig. 29.20). **F:** G2 Express (Bard): Note the addition of a hook to the cranial aspect of the filter. This allows retrieval with either the Recovery cone or a standard snare device.

TABLE 29.4 Anatomic Considerations for Filter Placement

Anatomic Issue	Potential Solution(s)
Mega cava (IVC > 30 mm)	Vena-Tech LP up to 35 mm (off-label)
	Bird's Nest up to 40 mm
	Single filter in each CFV
IVC thrombus	Infrarenal filter above thrombus if room
	Suprarenal filter
Duplicated IVC	1 filter in each IVC
Accessory, circumaortic, retroaortic renal veins	Infrarenal filter below lowest renal if room
	Suprarenal filter
Pregnancy	Suprarenal filter

CFV, common femoral vein; IVC, inferior vena cava.

TABLE 29.5 Technical Problems during Filter Placement

Technical Problem	Potential Solution(s)
Sheath kinking	Advance sheath/filter several centimeters as unit to pass kink
	Beware of filter penetration of sheath
	Different access
	Different device
Incomplete expansion/crossed legs	Venography to assess, typically leave alone
	Place second filter above if: Concern for migration Concern for inadequate PE protection
	Reposition with care
Filter completely fails to open	Venogram to assess
	Place second filter above
	Rarely retrieve

PE, pulmonary embolus.

is technically off-label. Anatomic considerations for filter placement are given in Table 29.4.

6. Place the appropriate filter sheath. The sheath tip will typically have a radiopaque band, which should be placed distal to the desired location of the filter. It is important not to pull the sheath back and readvance it without a wire, particularly when placing the filter from a jugular approach. This may cause the sheath to inadvertently select the right gonadal vein if appropriate care is not exercised as this vein parallels the IVC. This is an important reason for non-expansion of the filter.

7. Load the filter into the sheath and advance it to the desired location—beware of sheath kinking. A kinked sheath can promote filter leg penetration of the sheath, which can occur when the sheath takes abrupt curves, particularly in an obese patient. If there is resistance met during advancing the filter, stop and assess with fluoroscopy. If there is a kink in the sheath, try advancing the filter/sheath several centimeters as a unit to pass the kink, although care must be exercised when advancing sheaths without a wire/dilator. If a filter leg has penetrated the sheath, it is best to remove the damaged filter and replace the sheath with an intact one. In the case of filters deployed using a pushing device, the sheath may have to be partially removed and cut to remove the indwelling filter and preserve access. Holding the system as straight as possible and choosing the straightest access route helps to prevent kinking. If kinking cannot be overcome, choosing a different access site or different filter may be necessary.

8. Place the filter with the apex at the level of the lowest renal vein. Of note, the OptEase filter can only be deployed with the retrieval hook placed inferiorly (for IVC placement). If the hook is placed superiorly, migration is likely. See Table 29.5 for technical difficulties in filter placement.

9. Document filter placement with a single fluoroscopic image or follow-up IVC venography through the sheath.

10. If retrieval is planned, schedule the patient for follow-up removal at the time of placement. This cannot be overemphasized, as a major reason for lack of retrieval is a patient who has been "lost to follow-up."

COMPLICATIONS/OUTCOMES

There are many reported complications with IVC filter placement (Table 29.6) (1,4,5,15,16). In general, most are clinically insignificant and asymptomatic. The most feared complication of filter placement is migration into the heart or pulmonary arteries, which can be fatal. Filter migration of several centimeters cranially or caudally is common, although the vast majority of significant migration is due to inadequate sizing of the device, incorrect placement, or placement without adequate imaging guidance. The use of fluoroscopic guidance, high-quality venography, knowledge of devices, and careful technique can greatly minimize these errors. Partial thrombosis of the access site is common, although it is rarely clinically

TABLE 29.6 Outcomes/Complications

Recurrent PE	5%
Symptomatic IVC thrombosis	5–10%
Clinically significant filter penetration	<1%
Clinically significant migration	<1%
Mortality	<1%

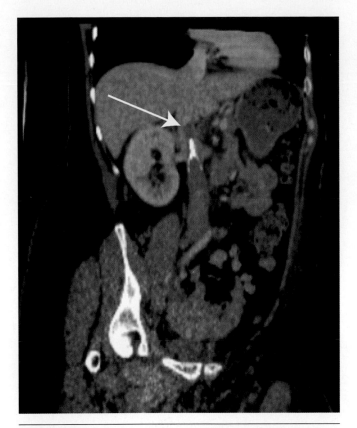

Figure 29.17 • CT MPR demonstrating complete IVC thrombosis. A minimal amount of clot extends above the IVC filter *(white arrow)*. This patient was clinically symptomatic and was treated with pharmacomechanical thrombolysis after placement of a second retrievable suprarenal filter (See Fig. 29.14).

TABLE 29.7	Managing Specific Filter Complications
Complication	**Management**
Migration into the heart	Attempt retrieval if feasible and experienced operator
	Consult for surgical removal
Asymptomatic IVC thrombosis	Do nothing
Symptomatic IVC thrombosis	Pharmacomechanical thrombolysis if able
	Leg elevation and compression stockings
Clinically significant filter penetration	Surgical referral
PE through indwelling IVC filter	Anticoagulate if no contraindications
	Additional IVC filter below existing infrarenal filter if room, suprarenal filter if no room
	Consider alternate sources (renal, gonadal veins)
	Suprarenal filter
	Consider alternate sources (upper extremity) SVC filter if clinically indicated

symptomatic. Filter leg penetration of the IVC wall is common (Fig. 29.14) and is rarely of clinical significance, although penetration into small bowel and the aorta does rarely occur. The generally accepted rate of filter failure with recurrent PE is approximately 5% and the rate of clinically significant IVC thrombosis is 5% to 10% (Fig. 29.17) and likely increases with dwell time. Table 29.7 lists ways to manage specific complications of filter placement.

RETRIEVAL

Filter retrieval is indicated when an optional device is in place in a clinically stable patient and either therapeutic anti-coagulation has been resumed or the risks of PE have resolved. There is no role for filter removal in the unstable patient or those with continued DVT/PE who cannot be therapeutically anti-coagulated (15).

Filter retrieval can be safely accomplished with the patient fully anticoagulated (24). Retrieval is device specific and is accomplished from a jugular approach for all retrievable filters except the OptEase, which is retrieved via a common femoral approach. The major reasons for inability to retrieve filters include a large thrombus burden in the filter, tilting of the filter precluding capturing of the retrieval hook, and incorporation of the filter legs or retrieval hook into the caval wall (15,25–29).

A very important reason for failure to remove retrievable filters is lack of follow-up. With the known incidence of clinically significant caval thrombosis and clinically significant filter penetration of the caval wall, it is incumbent on the operator to ensure that filters placed for relative or prophylactic indications are removed, particularly in young patients. Maintaining a database of retrievable filters that are intended to be removed, scheduling patients for filter removal at the time of placement, and informed consent are the best strategies to ensure removal before patients are lost to follow-up and the filter becomes incorporated into the IVC wall.

The timing of attempted retrieval is considered to be one of the most important factors affecting success and safety of removal. When a filter is placed, tissue ingrowth and endothelialization begin to occur. Over time, the filter legs incorporate and can substantially penetrate the IVC wall (Fig. 29.14). These factors make retrieval progressively more difficult. Early animal studies demonstrated that filters became incorporated into the IVC wall as early as 3 weeks (2). This led to the initial practice of filter repositioning at 10 to 14 days to extend the retrieval window. More recent animal studies and clinical reports have led to substantially longer retrieval intervals with some filters removed years after placement (2). Currently, there are no FDA regulations on the timing of removal and the removal window is left to operator preference and manufacturer's recommendations.

The window of optimal retrieval continues to evolve and remains somewhat device dependent. In general, the OptEase filter, which has greater IVC wall contact, tends to become incorporated at an earlier time and is generally considered to have a shorter retrieval window of 3 to 4 weeks. This is balanced with the fact that the OptEase filter centers quite well in the IVC and the retrieval hook generally remains centered and easy to grasp, infrequently becoming incorporated into the wall from device tilting, which may occur with the other retrievable filters. The Günther-Tulip, Celect, and G2/G2 Express filters have longer retrieval windows with reports in the literature of removal at greater than 1 year. These filters are considered to have an indefinite dwell time. In general, however, removal at extended time intervals requires greater force and must be tempered with the risks of IVC damage. Retrieval of these devices at 6 to 8 weeks is typically safe and successful without requiring excessive force.

STEPS IN FILTER RETRIEVAL

1. Assess if removal is indicated. Removal can be accomplished safely with the patient fully anticoagulated (24).
2. Determine the length of time that the filter has been in place. This will affect the chances of successful removal.
3. Determine which device is present by review of clinical records and radiographs. The G2, G2 Express, Günther-Tulip, and Celect filters need to be retrieved from an internal jugular approach. The OptEase filter needs to be removed from a femoral approach.
4. Obtain appropriate access, perform an IVC venogram with the pigtail catheter several centimeters below the filter, and assess the position and integrity of the filter. If placing a pigtail from a jugular approach, it is best to use an angled catheter and soft wire to cross through the filter before advancing the pigtail past the filter to prevent displacing or tilting the filter. Perform an IVC venogram with similar technique as previously described, although magnification on the filter may be helpful as general IVC anatomy and anatomic variants are no longer the subject of interest. Evaluate the venogram for retained thrombus, which will appear as a radiolucent filling defect (Fig. 29.18). Assessing filter tilt may require several oblique views. It is particularly important to assess for evidence of incorporation of the filter hook on the IVC wall as this may preclude filter removal. Filter leg or strut penetration of the caval wall and the presence of fractures in the filter should also be evaluated. Although there are no standard criteria for removal, many operators will attempt removal if the filter is intact, filled with a small amount (i.e., less than 30%) of thrombus, and if the filter hook is not embedded in the IVC wall. If there is a large amount of retained thrombus, continued therapeutic anti-coagulation and a re-attempt at removal in 2 to 3 weeks is recommended. If the filter has fractured or the hook has incorporated into the IVC wall, it is generally best to leave the filter in place as a permanent device.
5. Attempt removal per manufacturer's recommendations; see below for device-specific instructions. If there is difficulty engaging the hook, it is likely that the filter is tilted and an oblique venogram will be helpful to define the

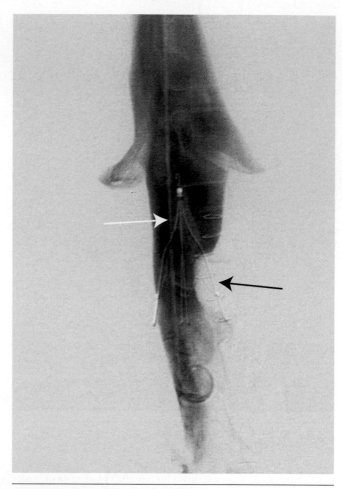

Figure 29.18 • Filter thrombus. Retained clot appears as a radiolucent filling defect *(white arrow)*. This is a relatively small amount of clot and should not prevent filter removal. IVC stenosis is present *(black arrow)* as well.

filter anatomy. Techniques for difficult removal are discussed below.
6. Perform a follow-up venogram through the sheath to assess for caval injury.

Günther-Tulip and Celect Filters

These filters are removed from an internal jugular approach (Fig. 29.19). A 10-Fr. sheath is placed several centimeters above the filter apex, and a snare device is used to grasp the retrieval hook at the cranial aspect of the filter. A Günther-Tulip retrieval set is available for this purpose, although a standard 10-Fr. sheath and a variety of snares may be used as well. The snare should be sized to the IVC (25-mm diameter snares work well). The snare is used to grasp the hook, and the sheath is advanced over the filter to collapse the filter. It is important to ensure that the snare grasps only the retrieval hook (not the metal band inferior to the hook; Fig. 29.19A) prior to resheathing the filter. If the metal band is grasped, advancing the sheath over the hook is often not possible. These filters are removed by resheathing the filter. Do not pull the filter into the sheath as this may increase the chances of damaging the IVC wall.

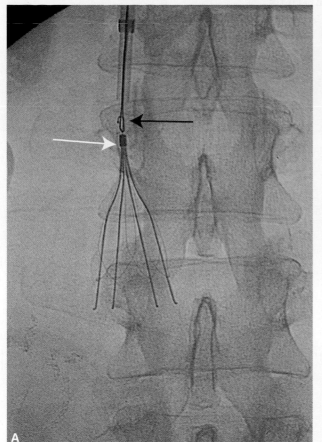

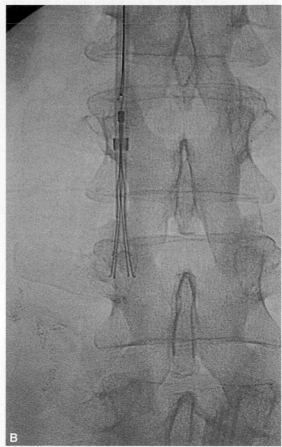

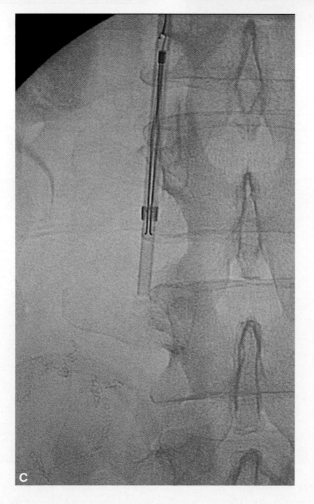

Figure 29.19 • Günther-Tulip filter removal. **A:** The metallic band inferior to the filter hook *(white arrow)* may be initially snared although resheathing is often not possible. Slightly open the snare until the filter hook alone *(black arrow)* is captured prior to attempting removal. **B:** The filter is held in place as it is resheathed. Note that this is different from G2/G2 Express removal, where the filter is pulled into the sheath. **C:** The filter is completely constrained in the filter and removed.

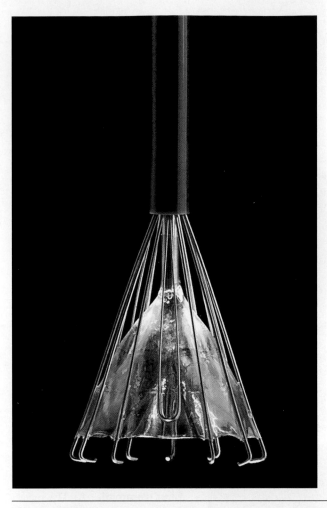

Figure 29.20 • Recovery Cone. The Recovery cone is designed for removal of the Recovery filter (discontinued), G2, and G2 Express filters. It is used over the wire. It is advanced over the top of the filter, constrained to capture the filter tip, and the filter is pulled into the sheath.

G2

This filter is removed from an internal jugular approach with the Recovery Cone (Fig. 29.20) Removal System. This is an over-the-wire cone-shaped grasping device. The sheath is placed several centimeters above the filter apex and the cone is deployed. The cone is then advanced over the filter apex, and then collapsed to capture the filter. The filter is removed by pulling the filter into the sheath as opposed to being resheathed.

G2 Express

This filter is identical to the G2, except that it also has a retrieval hook at the cranial aspect of the filter. This filter can be retrieved with either a snare (Fig. 29.21) or the Recovery cone. Removal is otherwise the same as the G2 removal, with the filter being pulled into the sheath.

OptEase

This filter must be removed from a femoral approach with a 10-Fr. sheath and a snare device (Fig. 29.22). Using standard technique, a snare is used to grasp the caudal hook. The sheath is advanced to the hook, and the filter is pulled into the sheath for removal. Do not push the sheath over the filter, as it may damage the IVC wall.

TECHNIQUES FOR DIFFICULT RETRIEVAL

A common difficulty with filter retrieval is the inability to grasp the retrieval device due to filter tilting. Many techniques have been reported to overcome this problem in the literature. Yamagami et al. described the concurrent use of a femoral angled sheath to push on the filter legs to tilt the filter into a position to permit simultaneous retrieval from a jugular approach (26). This is useful although it requires an additional access. Kuo et al. described a snare-over-guidewire technique (Fig. 29.23) for removal of tilted Günther-Tulip filters. This

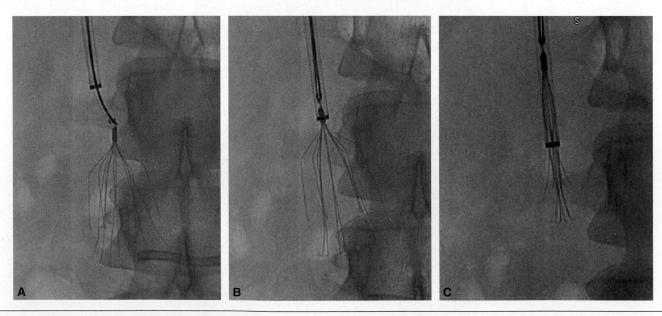

Figure 29.21 • **G2 Express filter removal.** **A:** A 25-mm snare is used with a long 10-Fr. sheath to snare the cranial hook of the G2 Express. **B:** The sheath is held in place and the filter is pulled into the sheath. **C:** Most of the filter has been recaptured. The filter should be pulled entirely into the sheath prior to removal.

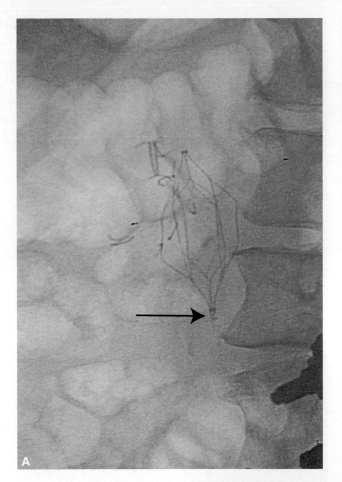

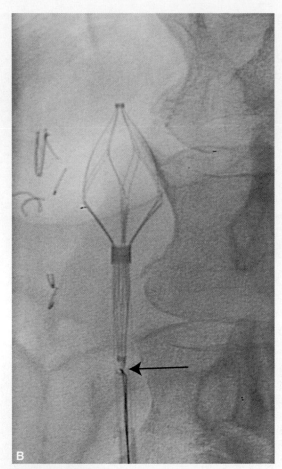

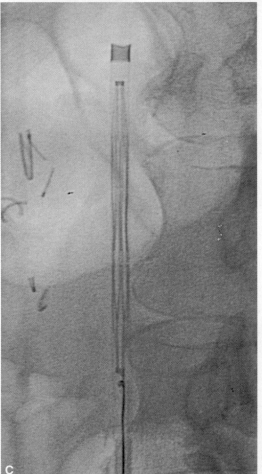

Figure 29.22 • OptEase filter retrieval. **A:** The retrieval hook *(black arrow)* for the OptEase is at the inferior aspect of the filter. **B:** The OptEase hook has been engaged with a snare *(black arrow)*. While holding the sheath in place, the filter is pulled into the sheath. **C:** The filter is completely constrained in the filter and removed.

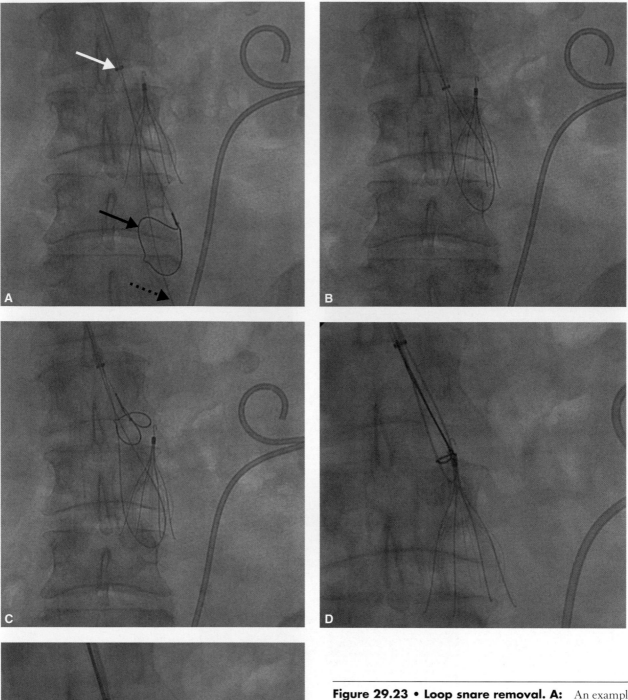

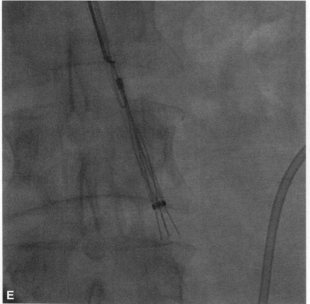

Figure 29.23 • Loop snare removal. A: An example of the snare-over-guidewire technique described by Kuo et al. A 10-Fr. sheath is placed above a Celect retrievable filter. A 5-Fr. 25-mm Gooseneck snare is advanced through the filter interstices and opened below the filter. An exchange-length glidewire is advanced side by side with the snare in the sheath. It is passed through the interstices of the filter and the tip is snared. In nearly all cases, the snare and glidewire will pass through different interstices. **B:** Simultaneously advance the back end of the glidewire while pulling the snared end of the glidewire though the sheath. This results in through-and-through wire access through separate interstices of the filter as depicted here. **C:** At this point, both the proximal and distal ends of the glidewire are outside of the body. Replace the snare over both ends of the glidewire and advance it through the sheath. **D:** Gentle tension on the looped glidewire will straighten the filter and the loop should easily advance over the hook guided by the wire loop. If the filter hook cannot be captured using this method, it is likely that the hook is embedded in the IVC wall. **E:** The filter can then be resheathed in standard fashion.

technique is easy, quite elegant, and has been very helpful in retrieving tilted filters. It involves obtaining through-and-through guidewire access through separate filter struts and subsequently advancing a snare over both ends of the guidewire to facilitate snare and sheath passage over the hook (25). A similar loop technique has been described by Rubenstein et al. (29). Use of a tip deflecting wire has been described by Hagspiel et al. to facilitate engaging the Recovery cone on the Recovery or G2 filters (28). The tip deflecting wire is used to put traction on the filter, which can then be engaged with the Recovery cone.

A greater technical difficulty exists when the hook becomes embedded in the caval wall. In this case, the previously described techniques will be ineffective. Most operators will leave these filters as permanent devices. Stavropoulos et al., however, have described a method using endobronchial forceps for removal of filters with embedded hooks (27). Although technically feasible, this technique is somewhat aggressive and should be used with caution, and only by experienced operators, as caval damage and filter fracture are more likely.

In all cases of difficult retrieval, caution should be made not to damage the indwelling filter with overly aggressive attempts at removal. All retrievable filters are designed to be permanent devices. Clinical judgment and experience should guide attempts at challenging removal.

References

1. Kinney TB. Update on inferior vena cava filters. *J Vasc Interv Radiol*. 2003;14:425–440.
2. Berczi V, Bottomley JR, Thomas SM, et al. Long-term retrievability of IVC filters: should we abandon permanent devices? *Cardiovasc Intervent Radiol*. 2007;30:820–827.
3. Trousseau A. Phlegmasia alba dolens. In: Trousseau A, ed. Clinique Medicale de l'Hotel-Dieu de Paris. Vol. 3. Paris: Balliere; 1865:654–712.
4. Hann CL, Streiff MB. The role of vena caval filters in the management of venous thromboembolism. *Blood Rev*. 2005;19:179–202.
5. Decousus H, Leizorovicz A, Parent F, et al. A clinical trial of vena caval filters in the prevention of pulmonary embolism in patients with proximal deep-vein thrombosis. Prevention du Risque d'Embolie Pulmonaire par Interruption Cave Study Group. *N Engl J Med*. 1998;338:409–415.
6. Mobin-Uddin K, Smith PE, Martines LO, et al. A vena caval filter for the prevention of pulmonary embolus. *Surg Forum*. 1967;18:209–211.
7. Greenfield LJ, McCrudy JR, Brown PP, et al. A new intracaval filter permitting continued flow and resolution of emboli. *Surgery*. 1973;73:599–606.
8. Tadavarthy SM, Castañeda-Zuñiga W, Salomonowitz E, et al. Kimray-Greenfield vena cava filter: percutaneous introduction. *Radiology*. 1984;151:525–526.
9. Standring S. *Gray's Anatomy: The Anatomical Basis for Clinical Practice*. 39th ed. Edinburgh; New York: Elsevier Churchill Livingstone, 2005.
10. Kaufman, JA, Waltman AC, Rivitz SM, et al. Anatomical observations on the renal veins and inferior vena cava at mgnetic resonance angiography. *Cardiovasc Intervent Radiol*. 1995;18:153–157.
11. Beckrnann CF, Abrams HC. Renal venography: Anatomy, technique, applications. Analysis of 132 venograms, and a review of the literature. *Cardiovasc Intervent Radiol*. 1980;3:45–70.
12. Kadir S. Kidneys. Atlas of normal and variant angiographic anatomy. Philadelphia: Saunders; 1991:387–428.
13. Bass JE, Redwine MD, Kramer LA, et al. Spectrum of congenital anomalies of the inferior vena cava: cross-sectional imaging findings. *Radiographics*. 2000;20:639–652.
14. Buller HR, Agnelli G, Hull RD, et al. Antithrombotic therapy for venous thromboembolic disease: the seventh ACCP conference on antithrombotic and thrombolytic therapy. *Chest*. 2004;126:401S–428S.
15. Kaufman JA, Optional vena cava filters: what, why, and when. *Vascular*. 2007;15:304–313.
16. Kaufman JA, Kinney TB, Streiff MB, et al. Guidelines for the use of retrievable and convertible vena cava filters: report from the Society of Interventional Radiology multidisciplinary consensus conference. *J Vasc Interv Radiol*. 2006;17:449–459.
17. Greenfield LJ, Proctor MC, Vena caval filter use in patients with sepsis: results in 175 patients. *Arch Surg*. 2003;138:1245–1248.
18. Greenfield LJ, Proctor MC.Suprarenal filter placement. *J Vasc Surg*. 1998;28:432–438; discussion 438.
19. Matchett WJ, Jones MP, McFarland DR, et al. Suprarenal vena caval filter placement: follow-up of four filter types in 22 patients. *J Vasc Interv Radiol*. 1998;9:588–593.
20. Mir MA. Superior vena cava filters: hindsight, insight and foresight. *J Thromb Thrombolysis*. 2008;26:257–261.
21. Usoh F, Hingorani A, Ascher E, et al. Long-term follow-up for superior vena cava filter placement. *Ann Vasc Surg*. 2009;23: 350–354.
22. Girard P, Stern JB, and Parent, F. Medical literature and vena cava filters: so far so weak. *Chest*. 2002;122:963–967.
23. Dewald CL, Jensen CC, Park YH, et al. Vena cavography with CO_2 versus with iodinated contrast material for inferior vena cava filter placement: a prospective evaluation. *Radiology*. 2000;216:752–757.
24. Hoppe H, Kaufman JA, Barton RE, et al. Safety of inferior vena cava filter retrieval in anticoagulated patients. *Chest*. 2007; 132:31–36.
25. Kuo WT, Bostaph AS, Loh CT, et al. Retrieval of trapped Gunther Tulip inferior vena cava filters: snare-over-guide wire loop technique. *J Vasc Interv Radiol*. 2006;17:1845–1849.
26. Yamagami T, Kato T, Nishimura T. Successful retrieval of a Gunther tulip vena cava filter with the assistance of a curved sheath introducer. *J Vasc Interv Radiol*. 2005;16:1760–1762.
27. Stavropoulos SW, Dixon RG, Burke CT, et al. Embedded inferior vena cava filter removal: use of endobronchial forceps. *J Vasc Interv Radiol*. 2008;19:1297–1301.
28. Hagspiel KD, Leung DA, Aladdin M, et al. Difficult retrieval of a recovery IVC filter. *J Vasc Interv Radiol*. 2004;15:645–647.
29. Rubenstein L, Chun AK, Chew M, et al. Loop-snare technique for difficult inferior vena cava filter retrievals. *J Vasc Interv Radiol*. 2007;18:1315–1318.

CHAPTER 30

Interventional Management of Varicose Veins

Raghu Kolluri

Dilatation of the superficial veins and/or venules of the leg, referred to as varicose veins, is the most common disorder of the superficial venous system of the lower extremity. This is a highly prevalent disorder, particularly in industrialized countries, with estimates of prevalence varying from 2% to 56% for males and 1% to 73% for females. Despite these facts, superficial venous disease receives relatively little attention in medical school curricula and during residency training (1–3). This chapter will summarize the anatomy of the superficial venous system, describe the pathogenesis of varicose veins, and provide an overview of the interventional therapies for the treatment of superficial venous disease.

LOWER EXTREMITY VENOUS ANATOMY

The venous system of the lower extremity can be divided into three different systems (Fig. 30.1):

1. the deep venous system that runs close to the tibia and the femur in the deep compartments;
2. the superficial venous system that runs in the superficial compartments;
3. the perforating veins or communicating veins that connect the superficial venous system to the deep venous system.

The deep venous system within the calf is composed of paired anterior tibial, posterior tibial, and peroneal veins that run parallel to the respective arteries. Soleal and gastrocnemius veins are the sinusoidal veins within the muscular compartment of the calf. All the calf veins drain into the popliteal vein below the level of the knee. The popliteal vein then ascends to become the femoral vein (previously called the "superficial femoral vein," a term that has been abandoned) (4). The profunda femoral vein joins the femoral vein to become the common femoral vein below the inguinal ligament.

The superficial system is mainly composed of the great saphenous vein (GSV) and the small saphenous vein (SSV) (4). These start on the medial and lateral aspects of the superficial dorsal venous arch of the foot, respectively. The GSV courses anterior to the medial malleolus on to the medial aspect of the calf and knee and then to the anteromedial thigh to join the common femoral vein just below the inguinal ligament. Proximal to the confluence of the GSV and the saphenofemoral junction, the anterior accessory saphenous vein (AASV) and posterior accessory saphenous vein (PASV) collecting the blood from the anterior thigh and posterior thigh, respectively, drain into the GSV. There is variability in the anatomy of this confluence. This anatomy is important to understand in order to avoid complications

during endoluminal ablative procedures. The SSV courses behind the lateral malleolus and ascends posterior in the calf to join the popliteal vein behind the knee. Intersaphenous anastomoses can connect the GSV and SSV networks in the thigh or the leg, as illustrated in Figure 30.2. The most common of these is the Giacomini vein, which is found in the thigh and represents an extension of the SSV that joins the GSV.

The perforating veins connect the superficial venous system to the deep venous system. There are several perforators connecting the GSV and SSV to the deep venous system. There are medial ankle, calf, and thigh perforators connecting GSV to the deep veins and lateral calf perforators connecting the SSV to the deep veins.

NORMAL VENOUS BLOOD FLOW

Deoxygenated blood is collected from the skin and subcutaneous tissues by an extensive subpapillary vein network. This network drains into the reticular veins, which in turn drain into the larger superficial veins such as the GSVs and the SSVs. These veins lie in the low-pressure chamber of the superficial compartment of the leg and flow is directed proximally toward the saphenofemoral and saphenopopliteal junctions, respectively. The deep veins lie in the high-pressure deep compartment of the leg due primarily to the pumping action of the calf muscles directing blood back to the heart. Perforator veins penetrate the muscle fascia and provide a communication between the deep and superficial venous systems (Fig. 30.3A). Under normal circumstances, the valves in the perforating system prevent the high pressure from the deep venous system from being transmitted to the low-pressure superficial venous system. During relaxation of the calf muscles, blood may flow from the superficial to the deep venous system when the pressure in the deep system is temporarily lower than the superficial compartment. Vein valves maintain the direction of flow.

PATHOPHYSIOLOGY OF CHRONIC VENOUS INSUFFICIENCY AND DEVELOPMENT OF VARICOSE VEINS

The pathophysiology of superficial venous disease can be divided broadly into the following major categories:

1. **Reflux:** Valvular incompetency within superficial, deep, or perforating veins can occur as either a primary event due to an inherent issue with the valve structure or secondary

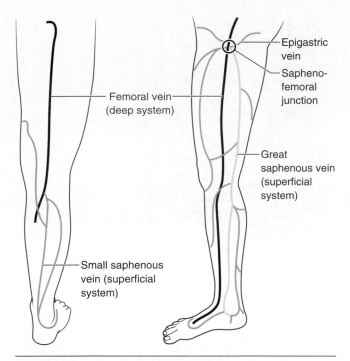

Figure 30.1 • Anatomy of superficial venous system of the lower extremity.

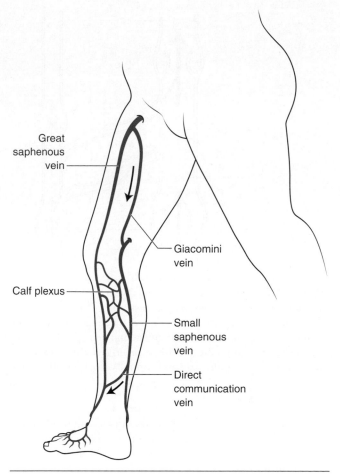

Figure 30.2 • Inter-saphenous communications between the great and small saphenous veins.

to dilatation of the vein wall. Reflux, as a primary cause, is more common in superficial veins rather than deep veins. Reflux results in monocyte-induced vein wall distension, retrograde flow, and distal venous hypertension within the involved veins.

2. **Obstruction:** Thrombosis in deep or superficial veins can result in subsequent fibrosis or obstruction of the venous outflow. This can result in venous reflux distal to the obstruction and result in further damage of the vein valves. Thrombosis can also result in scarring of the vein valves (without obstruction or fibrosis) and cause secondary venous reflux. This syndrome is referred to as "post-thrombotic syndrome (PTS)." Chronic venous insufficiency due to reflux and obstruction is more difficult to manage than chronic venous insufficiency from either reflux or obstruction alone.

At a cellular level, venous hypertension causes white cell sequestration and activation and red cell sludging. This also results in capillary dilation, increased permeability, and protein leakage leading to edema. Hemosiderin deposition results in hyperpigmentation. Fibrin cuff formation is also seen in the interstitium. Subcutaneous thickening also results from fat necrosis and liposclerosis. Venous ulcerations eventually result if venous hypertension continues. Venous ulcerations are typically seen in the medial or lateral malleolar area. Reflux within the GSV generally results in ulceration over the medial malleolus ulceration, while reflux within the SSV results in ulceration over the lateral malleolus.

SIGNS, SYMPTOMS, AND CLINICAL HISTORY

Symptoms of venous claudication include aching, tiredness, heaviness, pain, throbbing, burning or stabbing sensation, or cramping in the affected extremity. These symptoms are generally associated with peripheral edema and some patients may have associated itching, restless legs, or numbness. The symptoms typically occur with prolonged standing and improve with leg elevation or walking.

Objective scoring systems such as the Clinical, Etiologic, Anatomic, Pathophysiologic (CEAP) classification or the Venous Severity Scoring (VSS) have been used. The CEAP system developed by the American Venous Forum (5) is the most commonly used system (Table 30.1).

On examination, the earliest stages of venous disease may consist of reticular veins or telangiectasias. Telangiectasias are also called spider veins (Fig. 30.4A) and mostly these are asymptomatic but may represent underlying more extensive venous disease. Reticular veins (Fig. 30.4B), also known as feeder veins, are the dilated blue and green veins beneath the skin surface. Reticular veins are usually considered a cosmetic problem since these medium-sized veins generally do not lead to substantial medical symptoms or complications. Varicose veins are the larger ropelike veins that may be present in the great saphenous vein, small saphenous vein, AASV, and PASV (Fig. 30.4C). They may also be present as branch varicosities, particularly in patients several years after surgical stripping.

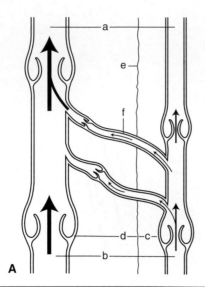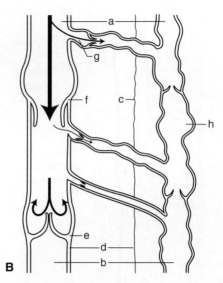

Figure 30.3 • **A:** Illustration of normal vein flow in the lower extremity (see text for details). *(a)* Proximal; *(b)* distal; *(c)* superficial compartment and vein; *(d)* deep compartment and vein; *(e)* muscle fascia; *(f)* flow from superficial to deep veins. **B:** Illustration of venous flow when chronic venous insufficiency occurs (i.e., abnormal flow from deep to superficial veins) (see text for details). *(a)* Proximal; *(b)* distal; *(c)* muscle fascia; *(d)* deep compartment and vein; *(e)* normal competent valve; *(f)* abnormal incompetent valve in deep venous system; *(g)* abnormal flow from the deep to the superficial vein; *(h)* abnormal dilated superficial vein. (Adapted from Beebe-Dimmer JL, Pfeifer JR, Engle JS, et al. The epidemiology of chronic venous insufficiency and varicose veins. *Ann Epidemiol.* 2005;15:175–184.)

An initial history should include documentation of the timing of the onset of varicosities to differentiate primary varicose veins versus secondary varicose veins. A history of deep venous thrombosis (DVT), superficial phlebitis, and trauma should be elicited. Any prior history of sclerotherapy, ablative therapy, and surgical therapy is important to note. Other systemic causes of leg edema and leg discomfort need to be ruled out. Appropriate assessment should be planned if other systemic causes of edema are noted. Realistic expectations must be discussed with the patient if other causes of edema are coexistent.

NON-INVASIVE VASCULAR TESTING

Non-invasive ultrasound plays a very important role in the assessment of superficial venous disease. Understanding and interpreting the duplex ultrasound findings prior to planning a procedure is crucial. In addition, duplex ultrasound is vital in guiding these procedures.

Table 30.2 summarizes the data elements that need to be captured during duplex ultrasound testing of superficial venous disease. This will help the interventionalist in determining the appropriate endoluminal procedure (s). A color duplex ultrasound machine should be used. A high-frequency linear array transducer of 7 to 13 MHz is the most appropriate probe for lower extremity superficial vein evaluation, but a curvilinear array transducer of 3.5 to 5 MHz may be needed for obese patients. B-mode machine images of the superficial (Fig. 30.5) and deep veins are obtained in both longitudinal and transverse views. Knowledge of variation in lower extremity vein anatomy and appearance on ultrasound is important (6).

Venous Incompetence or Venous Reflux Testing

Incompetence within the vein can be tested with the patient positioned in the reverse Trendelenburg position, applying distal calf compression (i.e., provides augmentation of venous flow), and assessing for the presence of distal reflux. Distal reflux on ultrasound lasting more than 2 seconds is considered to be diagnostic of reflux in most laboratories. The Valsalva maneuver is also used to detect reflux.

TABLE 30.1	The Clinical, Etiologic, Anatomic, Pathophysiologic (CEAP) Classification System for the Evaluation of the Severity of Venous Disease

"C": clinical

    C0: no visible venous disease
    C1: telangiectasias or reticular veins
    C2: varicose veins
    C3: edema
    C4: skin changes without ulceration
    C5: skin changes with healed ulceration
    C6: skin changes with active ulceration

"E": etiology (primary vs. secondary)

"A": anatomy (defines location of disease within superficial, deep, and perforating venous systems)

"P": pathophysiology (reflux, obstruction, or both)

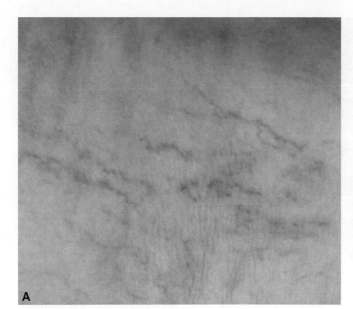

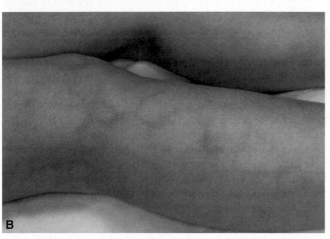

Figure 30.4 • **A:** Clinical appearance of spider veins or telangiectasias. **B:** Clinical appearance of reticular veins. **C:** Varicose vein in the distribution of the great saphenous vein.

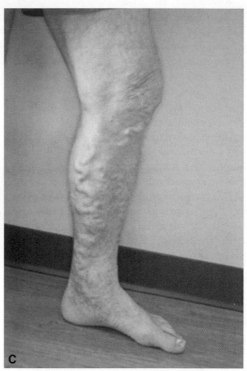

TABLE 30.2	Data Elements Captured during Duplex Ultrasonography for Evaluation of Superficial Venous Disease

1. Map saphenous vein segments that are incompetent

2. The extent of reflux in the saphenous veins and diameter of saphenous veins

3. The number, location, diameter, and function of incompetent perforating veins

4. Branch varicosities that show reflux

5. Veins that are hypoplastic, atretic, absent, or have been removed for bypass grafting or stripped

6. The state of the deep venous system including competence of valves and presence of thrombosis (acute, chronic, or subacute)

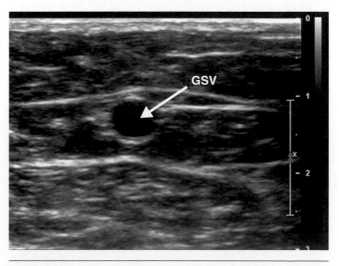

Figure 30.5 • Great saphenous vein (GSV) in transverse section within the saphenous fascia.

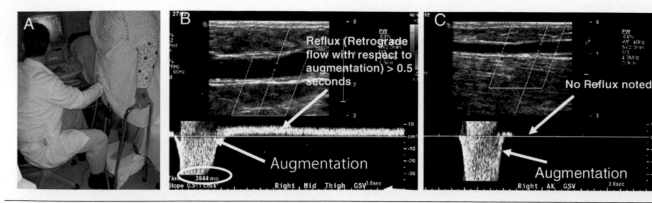

Figure 30.6 • **A:** Standing venous reflux test. **B:** Great saphenous vein with reflux of >0.5 second demonstrated following augmentation maneuver. **C:** Great saphenous vein without evidence of reflux following augmentation maneuver.

The diagnostic feature of reflux is the presence of distal flow in the vein during the Valsalva maneuver.

However, the Union Internationale de Phlébologie (UIP) consensus statement recommends testing reflux with the patient in the standing position and that the extremity in which the reflux testing is being performed should not be weight bearing (Fig. 30.6A) (7). Venous reflux is considered to be present if the retrograde flow (i.e., reverse direction to physiologic flow) lasts for more than 0.5 seconds (Fig. 30.6). Reflux can be elicited by calf squeeze for assessment of proximal veins or foot squeeze for assessment of calf veins. We use a pneumatic cuff inflation and deflation technique to squeeze and relax the calf in all patients who are able to tolerate these maneuvers.

CONSERVATIVE MANAGEMENT OF SUPERFICIAL VENOUS DISEASE

Conservative management for superficial venous disease includes exercise, leg elevation, and compression therapy. Exercises that activate the calf musculovenous pump such as ankle flexion, walking, or running for at least 30 minutes daily should be recommended to all patients (8).

Leg elevation, although impractical in most patients, is recommended for 15 to 20 minutes several times a day to reduce edema. Elevation of the foot end of the bed (by placing 2- to 3-in. blocks) may be recommended in patients who are able to tolerate this position. This provides a reverse Trendelenburg position at night and improves edema.

Other medical and cardiac conditions that result in edema should be appropriately treated. Considering other etiologies such as spinal stenosis and moderate to severe peripheral arterial disease in association with venous disease is very important. The therapy for venous disease should then be tailored for the individual patient.

Compression therapy is the most important component in the management of venous disease. Significant amounts of time must be spent counseling the patient (MD or nurse or other mid-level provider) regarding the advantages of compression therapy and the method of application. Compression therapy is in fact a lifestyle modification for these patients. Counseling increases the compliance of compression therapy significantly. Compression therapy results in reduction of the vein diameter (which increases the flow velocity), activation of fibrinolytic activity, and improvement in lymphatic outflow. This reduces venous reflux and prevents venous pooling in the ankles and decreases venous pressure resulting in reduction of edema.

It is extremely important to remember that thromboembolic device (TED) hoses and ACE wraps are not considered to be appropriate therapies for venous disease management in ambulatory patients. Inappropriately applied compression can also result in a tourniquet effect. Elastic graduated compression stockings are available in a variety of classes (Table 30.3).

TABLE 30.3 Types of Compression Stockings

Pressure of the Stockings (mm Hg)	Suggested Indications
15–20	Mild edema or ache, telangiectasias, older/frail patients who are unable to tolerate heavier compression
20–30	Ache or swelling of limb(s), telangiectasias, reticular veins, medium-sized varicose veins
30–40	Symptomatic varicose veins, venous ulceration, post-phlebetic syndrome
40–50	Venous ulceration, post-phlebetic syndrome, and lymphedema

TABLE 30.4	Available Systems for Delivery of Laser and Radiofrequency Ablation for the Treatment of Superficial Venous Disease

System
Laser
AngioDynamics—www.angiodynamics.com
Biolitec—www.biolitec.com
Diomed —www.diomedinc.com
Dornier MedTech—www.dornier.com
Vascular Solutions—www.vascularsolutions.com
Radiofrequency
VNUS Medical Technologies—www.vnus.com

Other forms of compression therapy including medium and short stretch bandages, inelastic wraps (e.g., CIRCAID wraps), and multilayer wraps are also available. A venous interventionalist should have a basic knowledge of the various types of compression therapies to facilitate appropriate patient management.

MINIMALLY INVASIVE PROCEDURES FOR SUPERFICIAL VENOUS DISEASE

Endoluminal Venous Ablation

Outpatient-based endoluminal ablative therapies have become quite popular in several medical specialties due to their relative simplicity. Laser and radiofrequency (RF) ablation has been widely embraced by patients with high satisfaction rates (Table 30.4).

Laser is an acronym for "light amplification by stimulated emission of radiation." Endovenous laser therapy (EVLT) uses thermal injury to induce non-thrombotic occlusion of the treated veins. One theory suggests that steam bubbles are formed at the laser tip causing diffuse thermal damage to the vein wall. Laser treatment has been found to produce carbonization of the vein wall (9). A variety of laser wavelengths are used, including 810, 940, 980, 1064, and 1320 nm (10).

VNUS® Medical Technologies Inc. (San Jose, CA) is the only company that manufactures RF generators and catheters in the United States. The VNUS Closure™ catheter that was initially used required a continuous pullback technique. ClosureFast™ was launched in 2006 with segmental ablation capability. This RF catheter uses thermal energy derived from a bipolar catheter. This generates heat up to 85 to 120°C. An in-built feedback mechanism monitors the vein wall impedance and the energy delivery is adjusted accordingly.

Generally these procedures are done in the outpatient setting. The patient is brought to the outpatient surgical suite. The leg on which the ablation is planned is prepped in the usual fashion with alcohol or betadine solution. Patients receive either pre-operative oral diazepam or peri-procedural conscious sedation at the discretion of performing physician. We use conscious sedation with intravenous midazolam and fentanyl. Institutional protocols for monitoring must be followed if conscious sedation is used.

COMMON PROCEDURAL STEPS FOR RADIOFREQUENCY ABLATION AND ENDOVENOUS LASER THERAPY

1. The saphenous vein should be mapped prior to the ablation from the groin to the calf. The vein is identified within the saphenous fascia (Fig. 30.5) and the surface of the skin is marked (Fig. 30.7A and B). The accessory saphenous veins and superior epigastric veins are identified and marked.
2. Access to the vein is obtained below the level of the knee with a 21-gauge micropuncture needle under ultrasound guidance. A 0.018″ wire is then passed into the vein and the needle removed (Fig. 30.7C).

SPECIFIC STEPS FOR ENDOVENOUS LASER THERAPY

1. A 5-Fr. introducer sheath is passed over the 0.018″ wire and the wire is removed (Fig. 30.8A).
2. A 0.035″ J wire is passed through the sheath (Fig. 30.8B).
3. A 4-Fr. sheath is then passed over the J wire (Fig. 30.8C).
4. The laser fiber is exchanged for the J guidewire (Fig. 30.8D).
5. The tip of the laser fiber is confirmed to be no closer than 2 cm from the saphenofemoral or saphenopopliteal junction using ultrasound guidance (Fig. 30.8E).

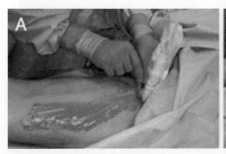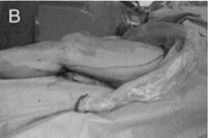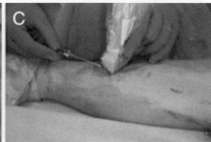

Figure 30.7 • A–C: Procedural steps common to radiofrequency ablation and endoluminal laser ablation of superficial veins (see text for details).

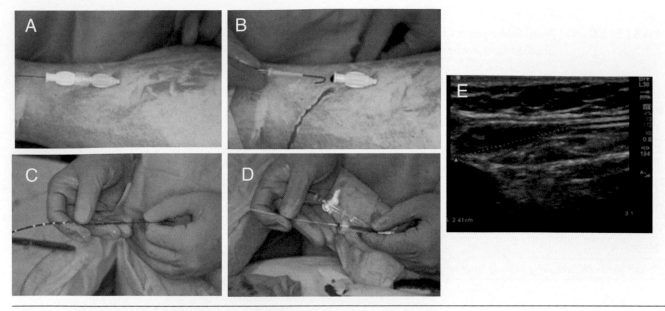

Figure 30.8 • A–E: Procedural steps specific to endovenous laser ablation of superficial veins (see text for details).

SPECIFIC STEPS FOR RADIOFREQUENCY ABLATION

1. A 7-Fr. introducer sheath is passed over the 0.035″ wire. The RF catheter is passed through the introducer (Fig. 30.9A).
2. The catheter tip is confirmed by ultrasound to be no closer than 2.5 cm from the saphenofemoral or saphenopopliteal junction (Fig. 30.9B).

Once the position of the catheter tip (for RF) or fiber tip (for EVLT) is confirmed, tumescent anesthesia composed of a solution of 0.1% lidocaine (100 to 300 ccs) and bicarbonate is infiltrated along the saphenous vein within the saphenous fascia. A 0.1% lidocaine solution with 1:1,000,000 epinephrine has also been used. A maximum lidocaine dose of 35 mg/kg is considered to be safe (11). Infiltration can be performed with prefilled syringes or with peristaltic pumps that help decrease the procedural time.

Tumescent anesthesia has three functions: (1) it provides local anesthesia, (2) it causes venospasm and collapse of the vein over the RF catheter or laser fiber, and (3) it acts as "heat sink" to absorb the heat generated by EVLT or RF, which prevents thermal injury of adjacent structures and the overlying skin.

Once tumescent anesthesia is performed, the patient is placed in the Trendelenburg position (this is particularly important for RF ablation as contact of the catheter with the vein wall is vital for detection of impedance and heat generation). The RF catheter is pulled back in 7-cm segments, whereas laser fibers are pulled back continuously. The vein occludes as the RF or laser energy is delivered during the pullback.

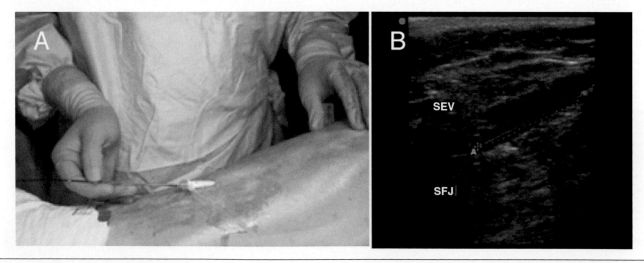

Figure 30.9 • A,B: Procedural steps specific to radiofrequency ablation of superficial veins (see text for details). SFV, saphenofemoral junction; SEV, superficial epigastric vein.

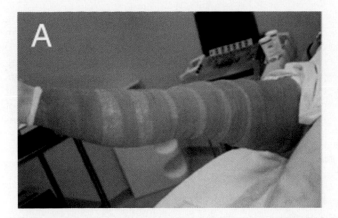
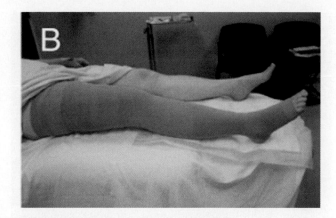

Figure 30.10 • Care of patient following radiofrequency or laser ablation of superficial veins. **A:** The leg is initially wrapped with a compression wrap. **B:** Compression stocking is applied over the compression wrap.

Adjunct procedures such as foam sclerotherapy or stab phlebectomy may be performed in the same setting or can be staged at a later time at the discretion of the performing physician. The leg is then wrapped with compression wraps (Fig. 30.10A and B) to absorb the moisture that is expected to drain over the next 3 to 4 days. The wraps are held in place by a compression stocking (15 to 20 mm Hg or 20 to 30 mm Hg compression).

Patients must be instructed to stay active post-operatively. The wraps are removed when the patients return for a venous duplex in 3 to 5 days.

Although the incidence of DVT and pulmonary embolism (PE) are quite low (12) following these procedures, several clinicians use subcutaneous injections of prophylactic dose anti-coagulant (i.e., unfractionated or low-molecular weight heparin) for 1 week following the procedure. However, there are no data to support this practice. Follow-up is suggested within 1 week to assess for complications (Table 30.5).

Success Rates

The primary success rate, typically defined as occlusion of the ablated vein lumen without flow, is achieved in more than 95% of patients at 3 years for EVLT, and 90% of patients at 4 years with RF ablation (using the older Closure™ catheter) (13). The new-generation RF catheter ablation (Closure-FAST) is believed to have a higher success rate of 94% at 2 years (14).

Sclerotherapy

Liquid sclerotherapy is used in the treatment of patients with telangiectasias and reticular veins. Available sclerosants are listed in Table 30.6. Visual sclerotherapy is performed using 30- to 33-gauge needles and 3-cc syringes. Having a physician extender such as a nurse or a physician assistant would be an effective strategy for a successful vein practice (15).

FOAM SCLEROTHERAPY

Detergents can be mixed with air or CO_2 to generate a foam that achieves the same desired end point using lower concentrations of sclerosant as compared with liquid sclerotherapy (Fig. 30.11). Ultrasound guidance can also be used to perform foam sclerotherapy. Detailed discussion of this technique is beyond the scope of this chapter. However, it is a helpful adjunct technique for the treatment of tortuous branches and larger reticular branches following thermal

TABLE 30.5 Complications from Endoluminal Ablative Therapy

Complications
• DVT and pulmonary embolus
• Phlebitis
• Bruising
• Cutaneous nerve injury—calf GSV or distal SSV ablation is more likely
• Hyperpigmentation
• Skin burns
• Ecchymosis
• Paresthesias
• Foot drop in small saphenous ablation

DVT, deep venous thrombosis; GSV, great saphenous vein; SSV, small saphenous vein.

TABLE 30.6 Sclerosants

Detergents	Hypertonic and Ionic Solutions
1. Sodium morrhuate	1. Hypertonic saline
2. Ethanolamine oleate	2. Sclerodex
3. Sotradecol	3. Polyiodinated iodine
4. Polidocanol	
5. Glycerin	

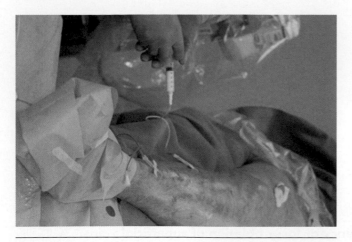

Figure 30.11 • Foam sclerotherapy of branch varicosities.

ablation treatment for truncal saphenous varicosities. An interventionalist should attend advance sclerotherapy courses to understand the technique and its potential adverse effects (16,17).

Foam sclerotherapy, at higher concentrations, has also been used in treatment of truncal saphenous varicosities and large varicose veins. Finally, it can be used in treating incompetent perforators.

Percutaneous Microphlebectomy

Ambulatory stab avulsion phlebectomy, ambulatory phlebectomy, mini-surgical phlebectomy, Muller's phlebectomy, or percutaneous microphlebectomy are office-based procedures by which varicose veins are exteriorized and avulsed through multiple stab incisions.

The veins are first marked in the standing position or identified on the procedure table with ultrasound assistance. The skin is anesthetized with tumescent anesthesia as described above (see p. 448). Parallel to the markings, millimeter stab incisions are made every 5 to 10 cm through which the varicose vein is grasped using phlebectomy hooks. The vein is then exteriorized (Fig. 30.12) using hemostats. The vein is extracted until it breaks. This procedure is completed until the

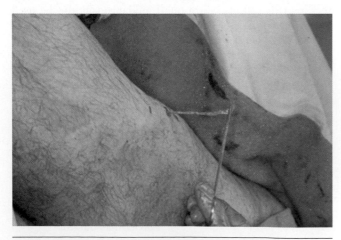

Figure 30.12 • Exteriorizing the vein during ambulatory phlebectomy.

vein is completely extracted. The incisions are closed using Steri-Strips. This procedure can be performed separately or in combination with ablation of the saphenous veins.

The most frequent complications encountered during phlebectomy include blister formation, hyperpigmentation, telangiectasia matting, and "hotspots" (18,19). Infrequent complications can also include inadvertent exteriorization of nerves instead of veins. Knowledge of the superficial venous anatomy is clearly of paramount importance.

At the completion of the procedure, the leg on which phlebectomy was performed is wrapped with compression bandages similar to that described following ablation therapies.

Perforator Incompetence Management

Although Subfascial Endoscopic Perforator Surgery (SEPS) was a significant advancement when compared to open ligation, this technique has faced complications such as surgical site infection and inability to ligate the distal perforators (20). RF ablation (using VNUS Closure radio-frequency stylet (RFS) catheter, San Jose, CA) is a minimally invasive technique to ablate incompetent perforator veins (IPVs). However, performing this technique requires advanced ultrasound skills. Most vascular technologists do not scan for IPVs. These need to be scanned while the patients are sitting on the edge of the table with feet dangling. Reflux may be elicited using calf or foot squeeze maneuvers.

Laser ablation and foam sclerotherapy is also performed to ablate IPVs. However, in this section, only the FDA-approved Closure RFS catheter (VNUS; Medical Technologies, Inc., San Jose, CA) technique for ablation of IPVs is described. This has advantages over other techniques as one can ablate the distal, lateral calf, or thigh perforators. With the RFS stylet, one can monitor impedance feedback and confirm intraluminal access. The ablation energy delivery with RF is focal and this is beneficial as the perforators run in close proximity with the accompanying arteries.

Technique

- The patient is positioned on the examination chair in a reversed Trendelenburg position.
- The below-knee area is prepped in the usual sterile fashion.
- The perforators are marked on the skin following location using ultrasound.
- IPVs are identified in the transverse and long axes. The presence of a registered vascular technologist with considerable experience in vascular ultrasound may be very helpful, particularly during the initial experience.
- The skin is infiltrated with 1 to 2 mL of 1% lidocaine.
- A micropuncture needle is used to access the IPV and is exchanged for a 0.018″ wire.
- A stylet is then passed over the guidewire (Fig. 30.13).
- A small incision is made with a scalpel to facilitate delivery of the rigid stylet.
- Intravascular position of the stylet is confirmed by venous blood flashback and/or impedance $< 400\ \Omega$.
- The stylet tip is placed just below the deep fascia and at least 5 mm from both the skin surface and the deep vein.
- The trocar is removed from the stylet.
- External compression with the ultrasound probe is applied to empty the vein segment and improve electrode contact with the vein wall.

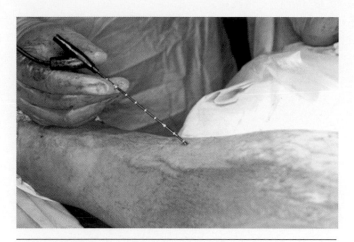

Figure 30.13 • Stylet passed into the incompetent perforator vein.

- Two to four milliliters of 1% lidocaine is injected around the target vein.
- The patient is placed in the Trendelenburg position.
- The RF generator temperature is set by default at 85°C.
- RF energy is delivered for 60 to 90 seconds at the 3, 6, 9, and 12 o'clock positions.
- Ablation is confirmed by lack of flow in the perforator.
- A 4 × 4 gauze is applied over treated perforators and compression wraps are applied around the leg from the ankle to the knee, as described previously.
- A follow-up duplex scan is performed within 1 week to rule out the presence of a DVT and confirm vessel occlusion.

Hingorani et al. (21) have published the first small study reporting outcomes following RF ablation of IPVs. In 32 patients with 82 IPVs, the immediate success rate at 1 month was 88%. No local or systemic complications were noted.

CONCLUSION

Almost all types of superficial or perforator vein reflux can be treated with a high degree of success using endovascular techniques in a single setting or in a staged manner. Knowledge of venous anatomy, physiology, and duplex ultrasound skills is an absolute requirement for a practicing interventionalist prior to performing these interventions. Surgical therapy should be reserved for large, tortuous or aneurysmal superficial veins or varicose veins in association with AV malformations.

References

1. Abenhaim L, Kurz X. The VEINES study (VEnous Insufficiency Epidemiologic and Economic Study): an international cohort study on chronic venous disorders of the leg. VEINES Group. *Angiology.* 1997;48:59–66.
2. Heit JA. Venous thromboembolism epidemiology: implications for prevention and management. *Semin Thromb Hemost.* 2002;28(suppl 2):3–13.
3. Kistner RL. D. Eugene Strandness Memorial Lecture: Foresight 2020: creating the venous vision. *J Vasc Surg.* 2007;46:163–168.
4. Caggiati A, Bergan JJ, Gloviczki P, et al. Nomenclature of the veins of the lower limbs: an international interdisciplinary consensus statement. *J Vasc Surg.* 2002;36:416–422.
5. Nicolaides AN. Investigation of chronic venous insufficiency: a consensus statement (France, March 5–9, 1997). *Circulation.* 2000;102:E126–E163.
6. Cavezzi A, Labropoulos N, Partsch H, et al. Duplex ultrasound investigation of the veins in chronic venous disease of the lower limbs—UIP consensus document. Part II. Anatomy. *Eur J Vasc Endovasc Surg.* 2006;31:288–299.
7. Coleridge-Smith P, Labropoulos N, Partsch H, et al. Duplex ultrasound investigation of the veins in chronic venous disease of the lower limbs—UIP consensus document. Part I. Basic principles. *Eur J Vasc Endovasc Surg.* 2006;31:83–92.
8. Fronek HS. Conservative management of venous disease. In: Fronek HS, ed. *Fundamentals of Phlebology: Venous Disease for Clinicians.* Oakland, CA: American College of Phlebology; 2004:33–40.
9. Schmedt CG, Sroka R, Steckmeier S, et al. Investigation on radiofrequency and laser (980 nm) effects after endoluminal treatment of saphenous vein insufficiency in an ex-vivo model. *Eur J Vasc Endovasc Surg.* 2006;32:318–325.
10. Darwood RJ, Gough MJ. Endovenous laser treatment for uncomplicated varicose veins. *Phlebology.* 2009;24(suppl 1):50–61.
11. Klein JA. Tumescent technique for regional anesthesia permits lidocaine doses of 35 mg/kg for liposuction. *J Dermatol Surg Oncol.* 1990;16:248–263.
12. Mozes G, Kalra M, Carmo M, et al. Extension of saphenous thrombus into the femoral vein: a potential complication of new endovenous ablation techniques. *J Vasc Surg.* 2005;41:130–135.
13. Nijsten T, van den Bos RR, Goldman MP, et al. Minimally invasive techniques in the treatment of saphenous varicose veins. *J Am Acad Dermatol.* 2009;60:110–119.
14. Dietzek A. Two-year follow-up data from a prospective, multicenter study of the efficacy of the ClosureFAST catheter. In: *35th Annual Veith Symposium*; November 19, 2008; New York.
15. Parsons ME. Sclerotherapy basics. *Dermatol Clin.* 2004;22:501–508, xi.
16. Breu FX, Guggenbichler S. European consensus meeting on foam sclerotherapy, April 4–6, 2003, Tegernsee, Germany. *Dermatol Surg.* 2004;30:709–717; discussion 17.
17. Breu FX, Guggenbichler S, Wollmann JC. Duplex ultrasound and efficacy criteria in foam sclerotherapy from the 2nd European consensus meeting on foam sclerotherapy 2006, Tegernsee, Germany. *Vasa.* 2008;37:90–95.
18. Olivencia JA. Minimally invasive vein surgery: ambulatory phlebectomy. *Tech Vasc Interv Radiol.* 2003;6:121–124.
19. Olivencia JA. Ambulatory phlebectomy turned 2400 years old. *Dermatol Surg.* 2004;30:704–708; discussion 8.
20. Sybrandy JE, van Gent WB, Pierik EG, et al. Endoscopic versus open subfascial division of incompetent perforating veins in the treatment of venous leg ulceration: long-term follow-up. *J Vasc Surg.* 2001;33:1028–1032.
21. Hingorani AP, Ascher E, Marks N, et al. Predictive factors of success following radio-frequency stylet (RFS) ablation of incompetent perforating veins (IPV). *J Vasc Surg.* 2009;50:844–848.

INDEX

Page numbers followed by f and t indicate figures and tables, respectively.